# Monoclonal Antibodies
# in Clinical Medicine

# Monoclonal Antibodies in Clinical Medicine

edited by

ANDREW J. MCMICHAEL   AND   JOHN W. FABRE

*Nuffield Department of Medicine, John Radcliffe Hospital, Headington, Oxford. OX3 9DU*

*Nuffield Department of Surgery, John Radcliffe Hospital, Headington, Oxford. OX3 9DU*

1982

ACADEMIC PRESS

*A Subsidiary of Harcourt Brace Jovanovich, Publishers*

LONDON  NEW YORK  PARIS  SAN DIEGO  SAN FRANCISCO  SAO PAULO  SYDNEY  TOKYO  TORONTO

ACADEMIC PRESS INC. (LONDON) LTD.
24/28 Oval Road
London NW1


United States Edition published by
ACADEMIC PRESS INC.
111 Fifth Avenue
New York, New York 10003

*British Library Cataloguing in Publication Data*
Monoclonal antibodies in clinical medicine.
   1. Immunoglobulins  2. Gammopathies, Monoclonal
   I. McMichael, A.    II. Fabre, J.
   616.079'3      QR186.7

*Library of Congress Catalog Card Number*: 81–71580

ISBN: 0-12-485580-6

Phototypeset by Oxford Verbatim Limited
Printed in Great Britain by St. Edmundsbury Press, Bury St. Edmunds.

# Contributors

Z. ABDULAZIZ
  *Nuffield Department of Pathology, John Radcliffe Hospital, Oxford. OX3 9DU*
D. ANSTEE
  *South Western Regional Transfusion Centre, Southmead Road, Bristol. BS10 5ND*
C. BARBATIS
  *Nuffield Department of Pathology, University of Oxford, John Radcliffe Hospital, Oxford. OX3 9DU*
J. M. BASTIN
  *Nuffield Department of Medicine, John Radcliffe Hospital, Oxford. OX3 9DU*
P. C. L. BEVERLEY
  *Imperial Cancer Research Fund, Human Tumour Immunology Group, University College Hospital Medical School, University Street, London. WC1E 6JJ*
J. F. BRADLEY
  *Nuffield Department of Pathology, University of Oxford, John Radcliffe Hospital, Oxford. OX3 9DU*
J. BURNS
  *Nuffield Department of Pathology, University of Oxford, John Radcliffe Hospital, Oxford. OX3 9DU*
J. P. CAEN
  *Unite 150 INSERM, Department of Haemostasis and Thrombosis, Hopital Saint Louis, 2 Place du Dr. A. Fournier, 75476 Paris Cedex 10, France.*
A. R. M. COATES
  *MRC Unit for Laboratory Studies of Tuberculosis, Royal Postgraduate Medical School, Ducane Road, London. W12 0HS*
S. COHEN
  *Department of Chemical Pathology, Guy's Hospital Medical School, London. SE1 9RT*
B. COSIMI
  *Transplantation Immunology Unit, Massachusetts General Hospital and Department of Surgery, Harvard Medical School, Boston, Mass. 02114 U.S.A.*
A. C. CUELLO
  *Departments of Pharmacology and Human Anatomy, · (Neuroanatomy/Neuropharmacology Group), Oxford University, Oxford.*
R. DALCHAU
  *Blond McIndoe Centre, Queen Victoria Hospital, East Grinstead, Sussex. RH19 3D2*

A. J. S. DAVIES
: *Divisions of Biology and Chemistry, Chester Beatty Research Institute, Institute of Cancer Research, Fulham Road, London. SW3 6JB*

D. DELIA
: *Membrane Immunology Laboratory, Imperial Cancer Research Fund, Lincoln's Inn Fields, London. WC2A 3PX*

D. C. EDWARDS
: *Divisions of Biology and Chemistry, Chester Beatty Research Institute, Institute of Cancer Research, Fulham Road, London. SW3 6JB*

M. A. EPSTEIN
: *Department of Pathology, University of Bristol Medical School, University Walk, Bristol. BS8 1TD*

J. W. FABRE
: *Blond McIndoe Centre, Queen Victoria Hospital, East Grinstead, Sussex. RH19 3DZ*

K. A. FLEMING
: *Nuffield Department of Pathology, University of Oxford, John Radcliffe Hospital, Oxford. OX3 9DU*

K. C. GATTER
: *Nuffield Department of Pathology, John Radcliffe Hospital, Oxford. OX3 9DU*

W. GERHARD
: *The Wistar Institute of Anatomy and Biology, 36th Street at Spruce, Philadelphia, PA 19104, U.S.A.*

A. M. GOATE
: *Nuffield Department of Pathology, University of Oxford, John Radcliffe Hospital, Oxford. OX3 9DU*

G. GOLDSTEIN
: *Ortho Pharmaceutical Corporation, Immunobiology Division, Raritan, New Jersey 08869, U.S.A.*

P. GOODFELLOW
: *Imperial Cancer Research Fund, Lincoln's Inn Fields, London. WC2A 3PX*

M. F. GREAVES
: *Membrane Immunology Laboratory, Imperial Cancer Research Fund, Lincoln's Inn Fields, London. WC2A 3PX*

E. HABER
: *Cardiac Unit, Department of Medicine, Massachusetts General Hospital, Boston, Mass. 02114, U.S.A.*

G. JANOSSY
: *Department of Immunology, Royal Free Hospital School of Medicine, Pond Street, London. NW3 2QG*

H. S. KAPLAN
: *Cancer Biology Research Laboratory, Stanford University School of Medicine, Stanford, CA 94305, U.S.A.*

A. P. KENDAL
: *Centre for Disease Control, Building 7, Room 112, Atlanta, Georgia 30333, U.S.A.*

N. KIEFFER
Unite 150 INSERM, Department of Haemostasis and Thrombosis, Hopital Saint Louis, 2 Place du Dr. A. Fournier, 75475 Paris Cedex 10, France.

J. KIRKLEY
Nuffield Department of Surgery, John Radcliffe Hospital, Oxford. OX3 9DU

E. S. LENNOX
MRC Laboratory of Molecular Biology, Hills Road, Cambridge. CB2 2QH

J. LIFTER
Ortho Pharmaceutical Corporation, Immunobiology Division, Raritan, New Jersey 08869, U.S.A.

D. Y. MASON
Nuffield Department of Pathology, John Radcliffe Hospital, Oxford. OX3 9DU

J. O'D MCGEE
Nuffield Department of Pathology, University of Oxford, John Radcliffe Hospital, Oxford. OX3 9DU

A. MCMICHAEL
Nuffield Department of Medicine, John Radcliffe Hospital, Headington, Oxford. OX3 9DU

C. MILSTEIN
MRC Laboratory of Molecular Biology, Hills Road, Cambridge. CB2 2QH

D. A. MITCHISON
MRC Unit for Laboratory Studies of Tuberculosis, Royal Postgraduate Medical School, Ducane Road, London. W12 0HS

R. MITTLER
Ortho Pharmaceutical Corporation, Immunobiology Division, Raritan, New Jersey 08869, U.S.A.

J. A. MORTON
Nuffield Department of Pathology, University of Oxford, John Radcliffe Hospital, Oxford. OX3 9DU

M. NAIEM
Nuffield Department of Pathology, John Radcliffe Hospital, Oxford. OX3 9DU

J. R. G. NASH
Nuffield Department of Pathology, John Radcliffe Hospital, Oxford. OX3 9DU

R. NEWMAN
Membrane Immunology Laboratory, Imperial Cancer Research Fund, Lincoln's Inn Fields, London. WC2A 3PX

J. R. NORTH
Department of Pathology, University of Bristol Medical School, University Walk, Bristol. BS8 1TD

L. OLSSON
Cancer Biology Research Laboratory, Stanford University Medical Centre, Stanford, CA 94305, U.S.A.

A. RAUBITSCHEK
Cancer Biology Research Laboratory, Stanford University Medical Centre, Stanford, CA 94305, U.S.A.

C. W. G. REDMAN
*Nuffield Department of Obstetrics and Gynaecology, John Radcliffe Hospital, Headington, Oxford. OX3 9DU*

W. C. J. ROSS
*Division of Biology and Chemistry, Chester Beatty Research Institute, Institute of Cancer Research, Fulham Road, London. SW3 6JB*

C. RUAN
*Unite 150 INSERM, Department of Haemostasis and Thrombosis, Hopital Saint Louis, 2 Place du Dr. A. Fournier, 75475 Paris Cedex 10, France.*

K. SIKORA
*Ludwig Institute for Cancer Research, MRC Centre, The Medical School, Hills Road, Cambridge. CB2 2QH*

E. SOLOMON
*Imperial Cancer Research Fund, Lincoln's Inn Fields, London. WC2A 3PX*

H. STEIN
*Institute for Pathology, Christian Albrechts University, Kiel, West Germany.*

G. M. STIRRAT
*Nuffield Department of Obstetrics and Gynaecology, Bristol Maternity Hospital, Bristol. BST AD6*

C. A. SUNDERLAND
*Nuffield Department of Obstetrics and Gynaecology, Bristol Maternity Hospital, Bristol. BST AD6*

P. E. THORPE
*Drug Targeting Laboratory, Imperial Cancer Research Fund, Lincoln's Inn Fields, London. WC2A 3PX*

G. TOBELEM
*Unite 150 INSERM, Department of Haemostasis and Thrombosis, Hopital Sain. Louis, 2 Place du Dr. A. Fournier, 75475 Paris Cedex 10, France.*

L. VODINELICH
*Membrane Immunology Laboratory, Imperial Cancer Research Fund, Lincoln's Inn Fields, London. WC2A 3PX*

# Preface

It is only 7 years since G. Kohler and Cesar Milstein published their work on the production of mouse monoclonal antibodies to sheep erythrocytes, but in that short time monoclonal antibodies have had an astonishing impact on almost every facet of biology. They are now beginning to be used in clinical practice and there can be little doubt that in the next few years they will have as profound and wide-ranging an influence on clinicians as they have had in the past few years on laboratory scientists. As is illustrated in innumerable examples in this volume, every aspect of clinical medicine – diagnosis, prognosis, understanding of pathophysiology, therapy and prophylaxis – will be enormously enhanced by the advent of monoclonal antibodies.

A wealth of benefits in clinical application lay before us. Quite clearly, however, the promise of monoclonal antibodies will be most fully and rapidly realised only if clinicians are aware of their potential benefits, and if laboratory scientists with clinical interests apply themselves to the relevant problems. At this early stage it is difficult for those not directly involved with monoclonal antibodies to assimilate disconnected papers, or to understand the background and look to the future. It is particularly with this in mind that this volume was produced, and we hope that it will serve as a milestone in the dissemination of awareness of the clinical benefits that lie ahead, and thereby hasten their becoming a reality.

The production of monoclonal antibodies represented the culmination of much basic biological research on cell fusion. Their clinical application will be an excellent example of how even the most basic research can have quite unexpected and profound clinical value and it is salutory to stress that point in a volume such as this. All of us who work with monoclonal antibodies owe a large debt of gratitude to Dr. Cesar Milstein, not only because it was largely due to his pioneering work with Dr. G. Kohler that monoclonal antibodies are a reality today, but also because of the generosity with which he distributed, from the earliest days, his myeloma lines to all of those interested in the field. We are therefore delighted and much honoured that he agreed to write the introductory chapter of this book, as it forms a most appropriate and informative background for the succeeding chapters.

We could not hope, even in a volume of this size, to be fully comprehensive, but we have tried to give an idea of the scope that exists for clinical application, and have chosen subjects where monoclonal antibodies are already or will very likely soon be of clinical benefit. Within each subject we have sought illustrative chapters; for example the chapters on influenza and Epstein-Barr viruses represent virology, although monoclonal antibodies have been made against a large number of different viruses. The last section of the book consists of 4 chapters giving detailed methodology on the production and use of monoclonal antibodies. We felt that a detailed exposition of the practical aspects of monoclonal antibodies would be invaluable to many readers, as this is rarely given in the literature and quite obviously, however valuable monoclonal antibodies might be, their value is diminished if one has difficulty producing them or cannot put them to optimal use.

It is our hope that the book will have a broad educative function and reach a diverse readership. With this in view, the authors were asked to make their chapters accessible to non-specialists, and they have done this admirably well. We are grateful to all the authors for their contributions, which were submitted within a 3 month period and include much unpublished data. The book should therefore be as current as any major journal issue at the time of publication. We are grateful to Peter Brown of Academic Press who initiated and encouraged the project, to Jean Broadis, Eunice Berry and Rosemary Bryan for expert secretarial assistance, and to Phyllis Hildreth for help with the index and appendices.

*June 1982*

*A. J. McMichael*
*J. W. Fabre*

# Contents

Contents xiii

# A   INTRODUCTION

# 1 Monoclonal Antibodies from Hybrid Myelomas: theoretical aspects and some general comments

C. MILSTEIN

*MRC Laboratory of Molecular Biology, Hills Road, Cambridge. CB2 2QH.*

## I INTRODUCTION

Antibody producing lymphoid cells from immunized animals have a very short life when cultured under *in vitro* conditions. Individual myeloma cell lines can be grown permanently in culture, but the antibody they produce does not express a pre-defined specificity. When both types of cells are fused, hybrids can be derived which retain the essential properties of (a) permanent growth, and (b) production and secretion of antibody with a pre-defined specificity. Since the hybrid cells can be cloned, it is possible to dissect the heterogeneous response of an animal (Fig. 1·1). The procedure therefore permits the derivation of

*C. Milstein*

clean reagents directed against very well defined antigenic determinants, regardless of the complexity of the immunogen: this allows a new
strategic approach to a wide variety of problems, and its impact in the
field of clinical medicine is the object of this book.

Although the experimental set up looks simple and straightforward,
the development of the technique was the result of many years of
fundamental development in unconnected areas of cell biology and
immunology. The discovery of cell hybrids formed by spontaneous
fusions of two different cells in culture was discovered in 1960, but this
was a very rare event with little practical importance. The exploitation

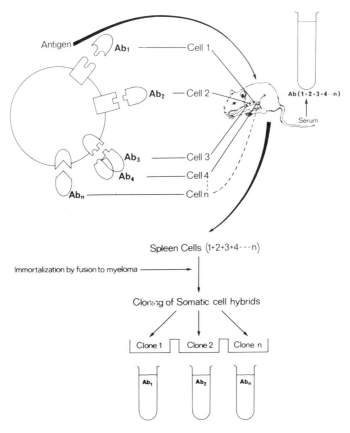

FIG. 1·1 Hybrid myelomas allow dissection of the immune response. The response of
an animal to an antigen is very complex. But each antibody is synthesized by individual
cells. These can be immortalized by cell fusion to provide an inexhaustible supply of
monoclonal antibody (from Milstein and Lennox, 1980).

of the phenomenon for research purposes was made practical by further developments permitting the increase of fusion efficiency and the selection of hybrid cells. (For a comprehensive review of the historical developments, see Ringertz and Savage, 1976). In the following 10 years, somatic cell hybrids were extensively used for two purposes; namely for gene mapping and for studies of gene expression and differentiation. The immortalization of a given differentiated function and the use of hybrid cells as a permanent source of specific products, in this case monoclonal antibodies, added a new application to somatic cell hybrids.

## II DERIVATION AND SELECTION OF HYBRID MYELOMAS SECRETING SPECIFIC ANTIBODY

The procedure first used for the derivation of anti sheep red cells (Kohler and Milstein, 1975) and schematically described in Fig. 1·2 requires myeloma cell lines, well adapted to permanent growth in cell culture conditions, but including genetic deficiencies which do not allow them to grow under certain conditions. The most commonly used are mutants lacking the enzymes hypoxanthine guanine ribosyl transferase or thymidine kinase. The mutants are usually selected among those able to grow in the presence of azaguanine or bromodeoxyuridine. Such mutants are resistant to these DNA analogues, because they lack enzymes of the salvage pathway. For the same reason, they are unable to incorporate externally supplied hypoxanthine or thymidine. When endogenous synthesis of DNA precursors is blocked with aminopterin, the cells die, even when hypoxanthine or thymidine are also included (HAT medium) (Szybalski *et al.*, 1962). Hybrids between them and spleen cells, which contain the wild type salvage pathway enzymes can then be selected from the parental components as the only cells that actively multiply in HAT medium.

The growing hybrids coexpress certain genotypic and phenotypic characteristics of both parental cells, but there are restrictions, which will be discussed later. When selected parental myelomas are used, the majority of the hybrid cells express antibody molecules derived from the lymphoid cells (e.g. spleen) of the immunized animal. Among those hybrids, some may express and secrete desired antibodies. Such hybrid cells can be individually isolated, and grown as clones secreting a specifically selected antibody (Fig. 1·3).

Practical problems and strategic approaches have been extensively reviewed (Galfre and Milstein, 1981; and see Chapter 21). The

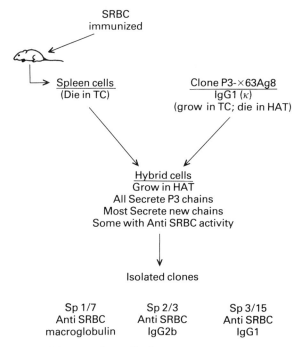

FIG. 1·2 Fixation of the specific antibody production of a transient spleen cell in a permanent tissue culture line (from Milstein and Kohler, 1977).

response of an animal to a given immunogen usually results in the stimulation of a highly heterogeneous population of cells, each secreting different antibody molecules. The hybrid myelomas represent a cross-section of the heterogeneous population (Fig. 1·1). Among those, some will secrete antibody molecules exhibiting desired properties. It follows that the successful derivation of desired lines will largely depend on the appropriate immunization of the animal, and on the ability of the experimenter to select the desired clones from among the large number of hybrid clones randomly produced.

Immunogens are often complex structures, or impure substances, but these factors are of little importance, provided that the desired responses can be induced, and not less importantly, that the relevant antibody can be specifically recognized in the presence of the contaminating components (Williams *et al.*, 1977). For instance, the antibodies induced to impurities of an interferon crude preparation are totally ignored by testing the ability of the antibody to neutralize or remove interferon activity (Secher and Burke, 1980). A monoclonal antibody specifically recognizing thymocytes can be recognized, be-

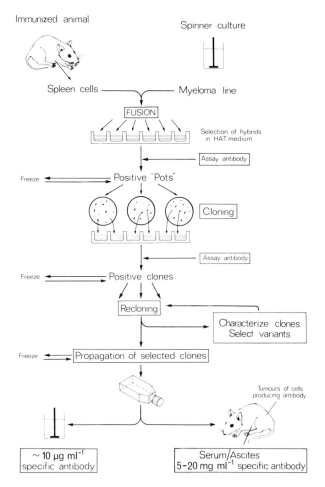

FIG. 1·3 Usual steps involved in the derivation and cloning of antibody producing hybrid myelomas (from Galfre and Milstein, 1981).

cause it will bind to thymocytes, but not to peripheral lymphocytes (McMichael *et al.*, 1979). Here, unlike the case of interferon, antibodies to thymocytes which also recognize peripheral lymphocytes are not ignored in a simple binding assay. This introduces certain complications in screening procedures.

On the other hand, complex antigenic mixtures may contain dominant immunogenic components. These may effectively decrease the response to a desired antigen, in which case partial purification of the antigen in question may become essential. One general way to achieve such partial purification is by using monoclonal antibodies as immunoadsorbants to remove such impurities (Milstein and Lennox, 1980, and see chapter 22). Other approaches involving special immunization schedules, *in vitro* stimulation, induction of tolerance to unwanted specificities etc, are being explored in several laboratories. With time, they may greatly facilitate the search for clones producing specific antibodies.

Desired antibody properties, however, are not only specific recognition of antigen: other no less critical considerations include cross reactivity, avidity and other thermodynamic or kinetic parameters, cytotoxicity or agglutination properties etc. All these considerations are of paramount importance for the selection of hybrid lines, and due consideration of them must be given at the experimental design stages. Indeed, it has been the experience of many laboratories that after deriving a hybrid line secreting the desired antibody specificity, on subsequent tests, the monoclonal antibody did not perform as it was expected to . For instance, it did not have sufficient avidity to perform well in radioimmunoassays, or it was not a good haemagglutinator.

To avoid such disappointments, one must use screening methods which will test the activity of prospective clones, not only for one property, namely recognition of antigen, but also for other desired ones. If high avidity is required, appropriate conditions should be used, so that low avidity antibodies will be scored negative. This may require more extensive screening, but will serve to recognize the importance of correct immunization schedules. In future, more serious considerations will have to be given to enhancement or preselection of cells expressing specific antibody, as a way of simplifying the screening procedures.

## III SUCCESSFUL HYBRIDS SELECTIVELY EXPRESS ANTIBODY SECRETION

The preparation of hybrid lines by the conventional procedure is by itself selective, and does not require, for instance, the removal of T cells (Milstein, *et al.*, 1977). Although spleen cells of a hyperimmune animal typically contain 1% of cells actively secreting antibody, the successful hybrids derived from them are likely to include 10% of hybrid myelomas actively secreting specific antibody. Even more revealing is the fact that while about 5% of spleen cells actively secrete immunoglobulin of any description, the successful hybrid clones are much enriched. At best, over 90% of the hybrids secrete immunoglobulin (Table 1·1). This highest figure was obtained when the rat myeloma

Y3/Ag 1.2.3 was used in fusions with rat spleen cells. Other combinations were less successful, and in this connection, the importance of the myeloma parental line should not be overlooked in normal practice.

TABLE 1·1
Preferential expression of immunoglobulin
secretion by hybrid myelomas
(data from Clark and Milstein, 1981)

|  |  | % Ig-secreting |
| --- | --- | --- |
| Spleen cells |  | 5 |
| Hybrid clones: |  |  |
| Myeloma | × Spleen |  |
| Mouse NSI | Mouse | 70 |
| Mouse NSO | Mouse | 45 |
| Mouse NSI | Rat | 25 |
| Rat Y3 | Rat | 95 |
| Rat YB2/0 | Rat | 85 |
| Rat Y3 | Mouse | 80 |
| Rat YB2/0 | Mouse | 50 |

Values are rounded averages. NSI refers to NSI/1 Ag 4·1;
NSO to the non-secretors NSO/u and X63/Ag 8·653; Y3
refers to Y3 Ag 1·2·3, and YB2/0 to the non-secretor YB2/3·0
Ag 20.

The enrichment for the antibody secretion phenotype seems to have several causes. One of them may be related to preferential recovery of hybrids involving actively dividing cells. Actively dividing cells, in a stimulated animal, are enriched with antibody-producing cells triggered by the antigenic challenge. Another factor which probably introduces an enrichment factor is brought about by phenotypic complementation. A B cell may express, but not secrete antibody. The actively screening myeloma cell confers to the hybrids the high secretion phenotype (Levy and Dilley, 1978) (Laskov *et al.*, 1978) (Raschke, 1980). In a hyperimmune spleen, there are many cells which do not actively secrete antibody, while the hybrid derivatives do. The final, and in some respects the most interesting, selectivity is that the recovered hybrids are derived from fusions with B cells, at least when the rat myeloma Y3 is used for parental fusions (Clark and Milstein, 1981). This means that removal of T cells before fusion may not be a useful preselection.

## IV ARE MONOCLONAL ANTIBODIES A RANDOM REPRESENTATION OF THE ANTIBODIES OF THE IMMUNIZED ANIMAL?

From what I have said above, it is clear that the hybrids are not from a random representation of the spleen cell population. Leaving aside the advantage of this enrichment, it is important to know if the selectivity introduces a bias in the antibodies which are expressed. In other words: are the antibodies produced by the permanently established hybrids a cross-section of the antibodies produced by the immunized animal?

In general, this is so, and it is for this reason that the immunization of the animal prior to fusion is of the utmost importance to the derivation of monoclonal antibodies. Clearly, if the animal does not contain the cells expressing the desired antibody, the hybrid myeloma method cannot immortalize it. This may seem a redundant statement, but it often explains unnecessary experimental failures.

However, there are specific cases when a given antibody-secreting cell may give rise to antibodies which are lethal to the hybrid. For instance, if the antibody is directed against a structure of the parental myeloma, in the presence of complement, lysis may occur.

The difference between the antibody produced by the animal and the cross-section of monoclonal antibodies derived from the same immunized animal, refers to the type of cell which is immortalized by fusion, and to the *in vivo* antibody turnover. Above, I have already mentioned that survival of hybrids was biased towards certain types of spleen cells. It is quite possible that the best hybrids are with cells which are not the best antibody-secreting plasma cells (Claflin and Williams, 1978). Indeed, such best secretors may be no longer dividing cells, and unable to give viable hybrids.

The antibody present in the serum of an animal at any single stage of immunization is the composite of the production of antibodies by certain types of cells over a period of days, depending on the half life of the antibody *in vivo*. The monoclonal antibodies originate from a cross-section of slightly different cell population which is taken at a particular moment.

All this, interesting as it is from a theoretical point of view, provides no justification for statements like "Monoclonal antibodies are not so good as conventional antibodies for . . . etc". Monoclonal antibodies, or appropriate mixtures of them, should theoretically be as good, in fact should be better, than any antiserum prepared in the same animal.

Why is it then, that the avidity achieved by the monoclonal anti-bodies isolated in one screening usually does not match the available antisera? The reason may be one of many, or a combination of them, and two need careful scrutiny in any particular case. Antisera are usually prepared following immunization routines developed over a number of trials and errors in different species and strains of animals. After finding that guinea pigs give the best antibodies in comparison with rats, mice, rabbits etc, it is not likely that mouse or rat monoclonal antibodies will match the best fraction of the guinea pig antiserum.

It is often the case that the antibody used for a radioimmunoassay represents only a small fraction of the antiserum prepared. If high avidity antibodies comprise only 5% of the total, it is not surprising that only one out of 20 monoclonal antibodies will have the desired high avidity, unless the screening is designed to ignore the low avidity ones.

## V UNUSUAL SEROLOGICAL PROPERTIES OF MONOCLONAL ANTIBODIES

Monoclonal antibodies have some serological properties which, at first sight, may appear odd. Serological methods were developed over many years, and they had to cope with antibody mixtures. There is nothing unexpected about a bivalent antibody molecule and a mono-valent antigen giving a non-precipitating antigen-antibody reaction. Yet, serologists are not used to that, since they usually deal with antigens which are not monovalent in terms of the polyclonal antisera.

A number of unexpected properties are easy to trace back to this essential difference. An antiserum may be stable for instance, to freeze-drying, to iodination, or to some other physical or chemical treatment. But that stability may be a composite of some antibody molecules being stable, and others being labile. If 50% are stable, the total loss of titre will be one dilution, which may pass unnoticed. The equivalent mono-clonal antibody has a 50% chance of being stable, in which case it will be more stable than the serum, but it also has a 50% chance of being labile. Standard treatments to antisera, which often leads to a tolerable loss of activity, are disastrous with certain monoclonal antibodies, and predictions about their behaviour and stability are more difficult to make.

It has been observed that labelled monoclonal antibodies can diffuse through precipitation lines in double diffusion Ouchterlony plate (Lachmann *et al.*, 1980). This appears to break the rule that precipitation lines act as diffusion barriers. The reason is probably a very simple one. Labelled monoclonal antibodies, in the presence of a polyvalent antiserum, can saturate an antigenic site without dissolving a precipitate. This is another example of an unusual property which, nevertheless, is easy to explain by the difference in behaviour of a complex mixture and the separated components.

Cytotoxicity reactions with monoclonal antibody, like precipitation, require multiple sites, but in addition, the distribution of the sites in the cell surface may be critical. Synergistic cytotoxicity with two different monoclonal antibodies recognizing rat histocompatibility antigens provides an excellent example of this phenomenon (Fig. 1·4). If one is searching for certain antibodies by cytotoxicity tests, the monoclonality of the reagents conspires against their identification, but the monoclonal reagents, once isolated, become powerful tools. One of the monoclonal anti-rat histocompatibility antigens could be used to sensitize rat red cells, which were only lysed in the presence of other antibodies. This permitted the development of a Jerne plaque assay of cells secreting "non-lytic" antibody, by means of red cells pre-treated with a previously isolated synergistic monoclonal antibody (Howard and Corvalan, 1979).

On the other hand, there are other unusual properties, much more difficult to explain. There have been examples of three monoclonal antibodies reacting against independent sites of a single molecule, which, nevertheless, failed to precipitate it (Lachmann *et al.*, 1980).

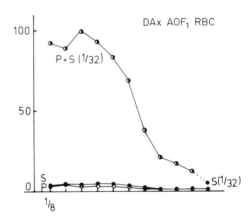

FIG. 1·4 The combined effect of two monoclonal antibodies is demonstrated by the lysis of rat red blood cells. The two monoclonal antibodies recognize two independent sites (labelled P and S) of the same histo-compatibility antigen. The red cells have been made radioactive with $^{51}Cr$ and the cell lysis is measured by the release of the radioactivity to the extracellular medium following addition of antibody and complement. Each antibody separately does not affect the cells but the two together completely disrupt them. The antibodies were diluted twofold from 1/8. When P and S were mixed S was used at a dilution of 1/32 throughout. (from Howard *et al.*, 1979).

Indirect haemagglutination with a given monoclonal anti SRBC was found to be negative, with no obvious explanation (Galfre *et al.*, 1979). The precise reasons may involve structural features or steric constraints, but the result emphasizes the individuality of reactivities to be expected. Complex mixtures (which the usual antisera are) are to a certain extent self-correcting and blur the individuality of each antibody species.

The specificity of a monoclonal antibody derives from its purity, but does not preclude cross-reactivity, due to recognition of similar antigens, or identical determinants located on different antigens. This is particularly relevant in complex situations, like expression of cell surface antigens, where a common antigenic determinant could be expressed in different molecules: for instance, a common segment of evolutionarily related proteins, a carbohydrate moiety etc. On the other hand, lack of reactivity with a monoclonal antibody does not prove absence of the antigen, since such a reaction could be affected by changes in the environment of the antigenic determinant.


## VI CONCLUDING REMARKS

Because monoclonal antibodies are defined chemical entities as opposed to undefined mixtures, they are slowly replacing conventional antisera in standard kits for clinical and other serological tests. Their impact over a wide spectrum of medical problems is well exemplified in the different chapters of this book. Many areas of basic biology, including cellular, subcellular and molecular structure and assembly, the nervous system and differentiation, are beginning to use the strategic advantages that cloning of antibody producing cells affords. Industry is turning its attention to the possible advantages that monoclonal antibodies may offer for the purification of biological extracts.

Thus the monoclonal antibody strategy is providing important new approaches to innumerable medical and other problems. Other developments are ripe for serious exploration. Preparation of antibodies in species other than mice or rats is an obvious next step. Considerable efforts towards developing reliable methods for the *in vitro* production of human antibodies are being made. This is the subject of the following chapter, and I do not need to discuss it further. However, the problem has much wider implications, since the importance of other species like farm animals and pets is at present overshadowed by medical priorities.

It is clear that chemical modifications of the monoclonal antibodies are likely to be of overwhelming importance. Such modifications are necessary as a way of visualizing the target recognized by the antibody when the purpose is diagnostic. Those most commonly in use involve the introduction of a fluorescent, radioactive or enzymatic tag, aimed at immunocyto-chemistry or radioimmuno and other binding assays. Other uses will also need chemical modifications, and the most exciting at present involve the attachment of toxic substances as a way of targeting of cytotoxic drugs (see chapter 7). The preparation of immunoadsorbant columns also involves a chemical modification, and the use of monoclonal antibodies may have a great impact in the strategy for the purification of either natural products or proteins manufactured by genetically engineered bacteria. The manufacture of a human hormone or interferon using recombinant bacteria requires a very exacting purification of the final product, and immunoadsorbants with monoclonal antibodies may provide the answer (Secher and Burke, 1980, and see chapter 22).

The industrial production of monoclonal antibodies using animals may be an unwise proposition in commercial terms, as well as ethically objectionable. The development of alternatives involving mass culture methods is likely to be more valuable in the long run. Technical developments in media, culture conditions and automation to the point where production in culture is cheaper than in animals may be much nearer than many people suspect.

It is possible that further ahead, antibodies will themselves be produced in bacteria (Milstein and Kohler, 1977). However, the strictly commercial advantages of this, over the myeloma cell culture method, are not as obvious as they may seem at first sight. In any case, the bacterial approach is, in my view, unlikely to be advantageous until the system is developed to secrete the antibody into the culture medium as myeloma cells do.

As mentioned before, the individuality of monoclonal antibodies is likely to introduce complications, as well as great advantages. It should surprise no one if monoclonal antibodies selected for their excellent performance for the preparation of iodinated derivatives are very poor for the preparation of fluoresceinated derivatives. The expertise commercial companies will require for the correct selection and individual assessment of each monoclonal antibody is well above the less demanding expertise required for the preparation of equivalent antisera. On the other hand, the consistency of monoclonal antibodies will facilitate standardization of commercial production, and the gentle expert touch of the researcher will be less likely to match the advantages derived from the large scale screening and the standardization available to industry.

The *in vitro* production of antibodies offers other exciting possibilities.

The use of aminoacids containing $^3$H, $^{14}$C, $^{35}$S etc. for the preparation of suitably internally labelled monoclonal antibody is an alternative approach to chemical modification. The advantages of such internally labelled proteins in immunocytochemistry has been stressed elsewhere (Cuello *et al.*, 1980 and see chapter 17). Other internal modifications could involve the use of amino acids analogues, and these could introduce changes in the physio-chemical properties of the antibodies.

Much more drastic modifications to antibodies which have been made possible by the cloning of antibody-producing cells, are likely to be primary sequence changes introduced by somatic cell genetics, and recombinant techniques. Although the frequency of structural mutants of immunoglobulin-producing cells in culture is low, they have been detected (Milstein *et al.*, 1976). Selection of appropriate mutants is being actively investigated, and the possibility of selection of "class switch" mutants, i.e. mutants expressing the same heavy chain V region associated with a different C region, has been suggested by the studies of Preud'homme *et al.*, 1975; Liesegang *et al.*, 1978; and Kohler and Shulman, 1980.

Even more ambitious is to introduce structural changes by isolating the corresponding genes or DNA fragments of a given antibody, and to separately modify the sequences coding for light and heavy chains (Milstein, 1980). In this way, the V region of a mouse antibody could be "stitched" to a human C region. This is more than of academic interest, since it may be quite difficult to prepare certain human monoclonal antibodies which may require as parental cells those from a lymphoid organ of a suitably hyperimmunized person.

Direct modifications of the complementarity determinant residues with a view to changing the fine specificity of the antibody will require a better understanding of the protein folding problem, of the effect of amino acid modifications on tertiary structure, and of protein-ligand interactions.

All these possibilities, exciting as they are, are contingent on considerable developments in our understanding of gene expression and transfection, particularly in connection with the expression of secreted multichain molecules of the type of immunoglobulins. We do not even know yet whether such experiments are to be done in bacteria, or in animal cells. Once again, basic developments in molecular biology must take priority.

REFERENCES

Claflin, L. and Williams, K. (1978). *Curr. Top. Microbiol. Immunol.* **81**, 107–199.

Clark, M. R. and Milstein, C. (1981). *Somatic Cell Genetics* (in press). Cuello, A. C., Milstein, A. and Priestley, J. V. (1980). *Brain Res. Bull.* **5**(5) (in press).

Galfre, G. and Milstein, C. (1981). *Meth. Enzymol.* **7B**, 3–46.

Galfre, G., Milstein, C. and Wright, B. (1979). *Nature* **277**, 131–133.

Howard, J. C. and Corvalan, J. R. F. (1979). *Nature* **278**, 449.

Howard, J. C., Butcher, G. W., Galfre, G., Milstein, C. and Milstein, C. P. (1979). *Immunol. Rev.* **47**, 139–173.

Kohler, G. and Milstein, C. (1975). *Nature* **256**, 495–497.

Kohler, G. and Shulman, M. J. (1980). *Eur J. Immunol.* **10**, 467–476.

Lachmann, P. J., Oldroyd, R. G., Milstein, C. and Wright, B. W. (1980). *Immunology* **41**, 503–515.

Laskov, R., Kimm, K. J. and Asofsky, R. (1978). *Curr. Top. Microbiol. Immunol.* **81**, 173–175.

Levy, R. and Dilley, J. (1978). *Proc. natn. Acad. Sci. U.S.A.* **75**, 2411–2415.

Liesegang, B., Radbruch, A. and Rajewsky, K. (1978). *Proc. natn. Acad. Sci. U.S.A.* **75**, 3901–3905.

McMichael, A. J., Pilch, J. R., Galfre, G., Mason, D. Y., Fabre, J. W. and Milstein, C. (1979). *Eur. J. Immunol* **9**, 205–210.

Milstein, C. (1981). *Proc. R. Soc. Lond.* **B211**, 393–412.

Milstein, C. and Kohler, G. (1977). *In* "Antibodies in Human Diagnosis and Therapy" (E. Haber and R. M. Krause, Eds), pp. 271–284. Raven Press, New York.

Milstein, C. and Lennox, E. (1980). *In* "Current Topics in Developmental Biology: Developmental Immunology" (M. Friedlander, Ed.), Vol. 14, pp. 1–32. Academic Press, London and New York.

Milstein, C., Adetugbo, K., Cowan, N. J., Kohler, G., Secher, D. S. and Wilde, C. D. (1977). *Cold Spring Harb. Symp.* **XLI**, 793–802.

Preud'homme, J. L., Birshtein, B. K. and Scharff, M. D. (1975). *Proc. natn. Acad. Sci. U.S.A.* **72**, 1427–1430.

Raschke, W. C. (1980). *Biochim, biophys. Acta* **605**, 113–145.

Ringertz, N. R. and Savage, R. E. (1976). *In* "Cell Hybrids". Academic Press, London and New York.

Secher, D. S. and Burke, D. C. (1980). *Nature* **285**, 446–450.

Szybalski, W., Szybalska, E. H. and Ragin, G. (1962). *Natn. Cancer Inst. Monogr.* **7**, 75–89.

Williams, A. F., Galfre, G. and Milstein, C. (1977). *Cell* **12**, 663–673.

# 2 Monoclonal Human Antibodies: a recent development with wide-ranging clinical potential

Henry S. Kaplan, Lennart Olsson and
Andrew Raubitschek

*Cancer Biology Research Laboratory, Stanford University School
of Medicine, Stanford, CA 94305, U.S.A.*

## I INTRODUCTION

The development by Kohler and Milstein (1975, 1976) of the mouse hybridoma procedure for monoclonal antibody production opened a new era in immunology. The clonal selection and immortality of hybridoma cell lines assure the monoclonality, monospecificity and permanent availability of their antibody products, thus liberating immunologists from the constraints and difficulties previously associated with the preparation and use of heteroantisera. The monoclonality of hybridoma antibodies can readily be verified by simple procedures (Oi and Herzenberg, 1979), and titer is limited only by cell culture volume. Antibody titer can be greatly augmented by intra-peritoneal mouse ascites fluid passage.

For diagnostic and therapeutic applications in man, it would obviously be desirable to produce human rather than mouse or other rodent antibodies. The clinical use of xenoantibodies is likely to be severely limited by the fact that they are foreign proteins. Although human immunoglobulin-producing cells have been fused to mouse myeloma cells to create chimeric hybridomas (Schwaber, 1975; Levy and Dilley, 1978), most such hybrids have, with rare exceptions (Schlom *et al.*, 1980), tended to be highly unstable due to the selective loss of human chromosomes. The alternative approach of transforming human B-lymphocytes with the Epstein-Barr virus (EBV) also appears to have limited practical usefulness because such cultures have tended to cease antibody production after a variable period (Steinitz *et al.*, 1977; Zurawski *et al.*, 1978; Koskimies, 1979). We have succeeded in producing human-human hybridomas secreting monoclonal antibodies of predefined antigenic specificity by fusing primed human lymphoid cells with HAT-sensitive human myeloma cells (Olsson and Kaplan, 1980). In this contribution, we briefly review the present "state of the art" with respect to the production of human monoclonal antibodies, and consider the potential applications of such antibodies in clinical medicine.


## II  TECHNICAL CONSIDERATIONS

Murine myeloma cell lines have usually been selected for 8-azaguanine resistance in a single step procedure by cloning the parental myeloma cells in soft agar in the presence of 8-azaguanine (8-AG). The human myeloma cell line U-266, established and characterized by Nilsson *et al.* (1970), was selected for use in our experiments. We initially tried to select 8-AG resistant mutants in semi-solid agar culture medium; our early attempts were unsuccessful, though we have subsequently succeeded by using macrophage feeder layers. We therefore turned to the use of liquid cultures for the selection of 8-AG resistant mutants of the U-266 cell line. A large inoculum of U-266 cells was grown in RPMI-1640 medium supplemented with 15% fetal calf serum (FCS) and 20 $\mu$g/ml of 8-AG. After five days, at least 99% of the cells were dead. The viable cells were isolated and reincubated with 20 $\mu$g/ml 8-AG for another three days. Viable myeloma cells were again isolated and reseeded in RPMI-1640 with 15% FCS and 5 $\mu$g/ml 8-AG. Visible cell growth could be observed in this culture within one week. The 8-AG concentration was then increased to 10 μg/ml, and after approximately one additional week, as growth resumed, the analog concentration was further increased to 15 μg/ml, and about one week later to 20 μg/ml, without any further inhibition of cell growth. The cell culture was then expanded in RPMI-1640 with 15% FCS and 20 μg/ml 8-AG, and cloned in microtiter plates by the limiting dilution procedure. The fastest growing clone, which had a cell population doubling time of about 18–20 hours in exponential growth phase, was selected for use in human hybridoma production.

This clone was identified as SKO-007 in the Stanford University Biological Organism Registry. These cells died, as expected, when incubated in modified ("human") HAT medium (containing hypoxanthine $10^{-4}$M, aminopterin $4 \times 10^{-8}$M, and thymidine $1 \cdot 5 \times 10^{-6}$M). A relatively low aminopterin concentration was used in order to obtain a maximum yield of hybridomas. The SKO-007 cell line was found to fuse readily with human lymphoid cells in the presence of polyethylene glycol (PEG). The HLA phenotype of this line (determined by Dr. Rose Payne, Department of Medicine, Stanford University Medical Center) is HLA-A2, A3, B7, BW60, BW6, CW3, and its karyotype (determined by Drs. Barbara Kaiser-McCaw and Frederick Hecht, Southwest Biomedical Research Institute, Tempe, Arizona) is 44, X, −8, −17, −18, +2mar., +2min, t(1;1), t(2,?). t(3;?), t(11;?).

The parental lymphocytes used as fusion partners must be in certain stages of differentiation in order to be readily fusable with the parental myeloma cells. This requirement is rather easily met in the murine hybridoma system, since antigen can be presented repetitively *in vivo* and the primed spleen cells can be harvested at the optimal time for fusion. For obvious reasons, this is possible only under exceptional cirumstances (cf. Olsson and Kaplan, 1980) in the human-human system. We have therefore used mitogen stimulation *in vitro* in order to enhance the fusability of human peripheral blood lymphocytes (PBL) (Table 2·1). Pokeweed mitogen (PWM) significantly increased the yield of antibody-producing hybrids, whereas lipopolysaccharide was without effect. The more complex system described by Hoffmann (1980) also gave excellent polyclonal stimulation responses.

The development of optimal methods for priming human lymphocytes with specific antigen will be crucial to the success of the human-human monoclonal hybridoma antibody technique. Most investigators concerned with this problem have attempted to prime human lymphocytes *in vitro* (Hoffman *et al.*, 1973; Dosch and Gelfand, 1977; Delfraissy *et al.*, 1977). Such systems allow the induction of primary immune responses against a given antigen, but the important secondary immune response

TABLE 2·1

Hybridoma Ig production by human lymphocytes fused with SKO-007 human myeloma cells

| Source of lymphocytes | Wells seeded Total number | Wells with viable hybrids Number | Per cent | Wells with IgG production[a] Number positive | Per cent positive | Wells with IgM production[a] Number positive | Per cent positive |
|---|---|---|---|---|---|---|---|
| Spleen | 288 | 176 | 61 | 107 | 37 | 64 | 22 |
| PBL[b], unstimulated | 288 | 94 | 33 | 45 | 16 | 37 | 13 |
| PBL[b] stimulated 7 days with LPS 50 $\mu$g ml$^{-1}$ prior to fusion | 288 | 88 | 31 | 51 | 18 | 46 | 16 |
| PBL[b] stimulated 5 days with PWM 25 $\mu$g ml$^{-1}$ prior to fusion | 288 | 242 | 84 | 146 | 51 | 134 | 47 |

[a]  IgG and/or IgM production detected by radioimmunoassay 21 days after fusion.
[b]  Peripheral blood mononuclear cells isolated from buffy coats on Ficoll-Hypaque gradients.

has hitherto not been reported to occur following *in vitro* priming. Alternatively, we have recently attempted to prime human PBL with antigen *in vivo* after inoculating them intrasplenically into immuno-suppressed mice, and then to fuse such antigen-primed human PBL with human myeloma cells in order to generate human-human hybridomas. Details of these experiments will be reported elsewhere (Olsson *et al.*, in preparation).

The SKO-007 myeloma cell line produces IgE($\lambda$). Each hybridoma derived from SKO-007 is therefore likely to produce several different immunoglobulin molecules as a result of the permuted assembly of the heavy and light chains encoded by the genes of the lymphoid and myeloma cell precursors. This tends to reduce the yield of the desired monoclonal antibody product of the hybridoma. It would be advanta-geous if human-human hybridomas could be established from a non-producer myeloma cell line, since the cloned progeny of such hybrids should produce only a single type of immunoglobulin molecule. We have attempted to select a non-producer variant of the SKO-007 line by labeling producer cells with fluoresceinated anti-$\lambda$ antibody to dis-tinguish between myeloma cells with and without $\lambda$-light chain secretion, followed by separation of the fluorescent and non-fluorescent cells with the aid of a fluorescence-activated cell sorter (FACS-III, Becton-Dickinson Co.). Although some cultures appeared to be negative for Ig-production soon after sorting and cloning, they have all eventually become positive for at least light chain secretion. Thus, we have been unsuccessful to date in our efforts to select a non-producer variant of the SKO-007 human myeloma cell line. Another approach is to use malig-nant cell lines of B- or pre-B lymphocytic origin, rather than myelomas. It is possible that some malignant human lymphoma cell lines may support Ig secretion after fusion with human lymphocytes; our current experiments have provided preliminary results which encourage further work along these lines.

Various factors may influence the success or failure of a given cell fusion. The technique itself involves a number of steps, each with a certain variability; these will have to be individually analyzed and opti-mized to improve reproducibility. Among the factors which may be highly detrimental to the outcome of a cell fusion is contamination of the parental myeloma cell line with mycoplasma. We have recently been faced with this problem in relation to our SKO-007 myeloma cell line. The cells started to fuse less reproducibly, and no hybrid cell growth was obtained. It was demonstrated by various techniques that the cells were mycoplasma contaminated, as was the parental U-266 line, despite an initially negative broth culture test. Most types of mycoplasma do not interfere with the fusion process itself; instead, they impair the viability of the resultant hybrids by depleting the HAT medium of thymidine and, to a lesser extent, hypoxanthine (Boyle *et al.*, 1981). Antibodies added to the culture medium may suppress (but not eliminate) the growth of mycoplasma. We have now successfully eliminated mycoplasma from several of our SKO-007 cultures by treatment with heat (41°C; Hayflick, 1960), with combinations of antibiotics, or both, followed by re-cloning. However, this episode underlines the necessity for careful routine examination of the parental myeloma cells for mycoplasma; it is particularly important to be aware of this possibility when hybrids are observed to grow poorly.

The presence of antibody in the spent culture fluids of hybridomas is most conveniently detected either by solid-phase radioimmunoassay (RIA) or by enzyme-linked immunosorbent assay (ELISA). The sensitivity of both assays is in the range of $10-50$ ng ml$^{-1}$. We now prefer the ELISA test, because it is extremely rapid and obviates the need to label secondary antibody with $^{125}$I. However, in some cases it may be preferable to use a microcytotoxicity assay to screen for hydridomas that are producing cytotoxic antibodies. For example, in our attempts to generate human-human hybridoma anti-HLA antibodies, we have used microcytotoxicity assays. In some cases, it may be necessary to concentrate antibody from the supernatants before reliable microcytotoxicity or agglutination assays can be performed. Unfortunately, none of these assays gives reliable information concerning the affinity of the detected antibodies. It may be presumed that monoclonal antibodies will have the same variability in avidity as antibodies generated in the intact organism. A few calculations have been made of the affinity of murine monoclonal antibodies (Frankel and Gerhard, 1979). However, since the majority of murine monoclonal antibodies produced to date have been directed against cell surface antigens, it has been difficult to study their affinities carefully. As the numbers of different monoclonal antibodies against a given antigen increase with the expansion of monoclonal hybridoma antibody technology, it will not suffice merely to demonstrate that they have the expected specificity. It will be necessary in addition to evaluate their avidity in order to select those antibodies with the highest avidity for a given antigen. Methods must therefore be developed to detect antibody-producing clones of high avidity early in the course of their growth.

## III POTENTIAL CLINICAL APPLICATIONS

The clinical domains in which human monoclonal antibodies may prove to be useful may conveniently be considered under the broad headings of diagnosis, treatment, and prophylaxis. It is also possible to consider the potential clinical applications of human monoclonal antibodies in relation to specific categories of disease. Both of these approaches have been helpful in our consideration of the subject.

## A.    General Considerations

### 1. DIAGNOSTIC APPLICATIONS

Mouse monoclonal antibodies have already proved to be extraordinarily powerful new reagents in laboratory investigations and in *in vitro* diagnostic procedures such as radioimmunoassays. The relative ease and low cost with which mouse monoclonal antibodies of high titer and high affinity can be produced in response to a broad range of specific antigens is likely to make them the reagents of choice for most *in vitro* diagnostic applications. However, there are indications that mouse antibodies may prove to be suboptimal with respect to human HLA histocompatibility testing. Human lymphocytes may also be able to discriminate subtypes or strains of infectious agents differing significantly in their pathogenicity for man. In these specific situations, and perhaps in others yet to be ascertained, human monoclonal antibodies may prove to have greater specificity and selectivity; if so, they are likely to have an assured role in *in vitro* diagnostic tests. It is also possible that serologic tests applied to the screening of human populations for cancer will prove to be more sensitive and/or reproducible when human rather than mouse or other rodent monoclonal antibodies are used as reagents. Finally, pathologists are likely to find important applications for the use of human monoclonal antibodies, followed by secondary enzyme-conjugated heteroantibodies, in immunohistological and immunohistochemical diagnostic procedures.

However, diagnostic applictions within the human body are likely to constitute a much more important segment of the diagnostic use of human monoclonal antibodies. Perhaps the single most important application will occur in the imaging of radionuclide conjugated human monoclonal antibodies in patients with biopsy evidence of a malignant neoplasm. As indicated below, there is reason to anticipate that labelled human monoclonal antibodies will have important advantages over presently available radionuclide imaging techniques, not only in delineating the extent of primary neoplasms but also in the detection of macro- and perhaps even of micro-metastases. Another potentially very

important radionuclide imaging application is the detection and delineation of vascular and degenerative lesions. Of these, undoubtedly the
single most important group are acute myocardial infarcts. Monoclonal
antibodies have already been successfully developed which can detect
antigens specific to canine cardiac muscle myosin and have thus been
applied successfully to the imaging of experimental myocardial infarcts
(Khaw *et al.*, 1980). It is likely that human monoclonal antibodies
specific for human cardiac myosin can also be generated. Such antibodies would be useful not only in the initial diagnosis of acute myocardial infarction, but, since the radiation exposure entailed in their
administration would be negligible, they could be used at serial
intervals to follow the course of the healing process, thus providing
important additional guidance to cardiologists in the management of
such patients. Finally, radionuclide-labeled monoclonal antibodies
specific for the antigens of various pathogenic viruses, bacteria, fungi,
and parasites may some day facilitate the differential diagnosis of
lesions in internal organs such as the lung, brain, or liver, thus decreasing the need for invasive diagnostic procedures such as thoracotomy,
craniotomy or laparotomy and biopsy.

2. THERAPEUTIC APPLICATIONS

Human monoclonal antibodies will almost certainly prove effective in
the treatment of selected types of infectious disease. They are likely to
have their greatest role in the treatment of acute viral illnesses, for
which presently available antibiotics are known to be ineffective. Their
use will be particularly important in immunologically compromised
patients, such as chemically immunosuppressed organ and tissue
transplant recipients, who are known to be at risk of infection with
cytomegalovirus and various opportunistic organisms. Monoclonal
antibodies may also be therapeutically useful in the management of
infectious diseases caused by bacterial, fungal, and parasitic agents for
which no effective antibiotic or other specific chemotherapy is presently
available. In addition to their direct neutralizing or inactivating effects
on such agents, monoclonal antibodies of appropriate specificity can be
conjugated to antibiotics and then targeted to achieve significantly
higher local antibiotic concentrations in foci of infection, while reducing
antibiotic levels in unaffected tissues. This approach may be particularly
advantageous for certain fungal infections which must be treated with
potentially hazardous antibiotics such as Amphotericin B, the nephrotoxicity of which might thus be obviated. Finally, as indicated in the
section on neoplastic disease below, the adjuvant treatment of micro-

metastasis with human monoclonal antibodies may well prove to be their most significant clinical application.

## 3. PROPHYLACTIC APPLICATIONS

Technologies are already available for the administration of many classes of pharmaceutical agents in depot form: such preparations are slowly released within the body over a period of many months, and the time course of their release may be predicted or monitored to ascertain when a replacement injection becomes necessary. If these timed-release technologies can be successfully applied to the delivery of human monoclonal antibodies, effective prophylaxis against a spectrum of viral and perhaps other infectious diseases might become feasible. Effective human monoclonal antibody prevention of the common cold would undoubtedly be a widely acclaimed boon to all mankind. Another important example is hepatitis B virus, which is endemic to large populations in parts of Africa and South-East Asia. Although effective vaccines for hepatitis B virus now exist, their usefulness in endemically infected populations is severely limited by the fact that most initial infections occur in newborn infants whose immune systems are not sufficiently developed to respond to vaccination. If such newborn infants could be protected for the first six to twelve months of life by the administration of passive human monoclonal antibody to the hepatitis B virus surface antigen, they could then be vaccinated, and the vicious circle of virus transmission from parent to offspring thus effectively interrupted. Human monoclonal antibodies should also prove useful in preventing cytomegalovirus and other opportunistic infections in organ transplant recipients before and during the administration of chronic immunosuppressive chemotherapy. They may even be effective in the prevention of diseases due to certain parasites and to so-called slow viruses.

## B. Specific Applications

### 1. TRANSPLANTATION IMMUNITY

Patients receiving homografts of various types are generally pretreated with immunosuppressive drugs and/or irradiation in order to reduce the risk of graft rejection. Such rejection is mainly due to recipient T-lymphocyte-mediated cytotoxic activity. However, many immuno-suppressive drugs also impair B-lymphocyte responses and thus increase susceptibility to infection. It would be highly desirable if T-cell-mediated immunologic function could be selectively suppressed in the graft recipient, leaving B-cell immunity and resistance to infection intact. Human monoclonal hybridoma antibodies with specificity against human cytotoxic T-lymphocyte subsets would therefore be highly useful reagents in the pretreatment of homograft recipients. Moreover, in the particular case of patients who must undergo bone marrow transplantation for the treatment of leukemia or marrow aplasia, an additional life-threatening complication caused by the T-lymphocytes of the donor marrow is that of graft-versus-host disease (GVHD). Pretreatment of the donor marrow with a monoclonal antibody which selectively kills human cytotoxic T-lymphocytes may significantly decrease or even eliminate the problem of GVHD in bone marrow transplant recipients. Experiments in animals, particularly mice, have already yielded encouraging evidence of the efficacy of anti-T-lymphocyte antibodies in preventing GVHD following bone marrow transplantation.

In addition, it is apparent that human monoclonal hybridoma antibodies will also be useful in controlling the often rather complicated infectious diseases that occur in recipients of homografts. Some of these infectious diseases are due to the current methods for induction of immunosuppression (and should thus be minimized by the use of specific T-lymphocyte antibodies), but others are related to the underlying disease of the graft recipient. it can thus be expected that the administration of human monoclonal hybridoma antibodies will be an important new form of supportive treatment for such patients.

## 2. FERTILITY CONTROL

Several steps in the human reproductive process appear to be susceptible to immunological intervention (Diczfalusy, 1975). Sperm-immobilizing antibodies have been found in the sera of women with otherwise unexplained sterility (Isojima *et al.*, 1972). These antibodies, of both IgG and IgM classes, appear to be directed against antigens in seminal plasma. It is thus quite conceivable that human monoclonal antibodies could be generated against the same seminal plasma antigens, and administered passively in long-acting depot form to women of reproductive age. Another promising approach stems from the essential role of human chorionic gonadotrophin (HCG) in the maintenance of pregnancy. The amino acid sequences of the $\alpha$ and $\beta$ subunits of HCG have been known for several years (Carlsen *et al.*, 1973; Morgan *et al.*, 1975). It has been established that a fragment of approximately 28 amino acids at the carboxy-terminus of the $\beta$ subunit of hCG is not present in the $\beta$ subunit of other glycoprotein hormones such as human luteinizing hormone (hLH), and heterologous antibodies to the $\beta$ subunit of hCG have been shown to have the ability to discriminate between hCG and hLH (Ross *et al.*, 1972). Subhuman primates actively immunized with the $\beta$ subunit of hCG coupled to sulphanilic acid or to tetanus toxoid developed antibodies which reacted not only with the $\beta$ subunit but with native hCG, and not with other glycoprotein hormones (Stevens, 1975; Talwar *et al.*, 1976). Such animals manifested disruption of ovulation for a period of two to three months after immunization, and were apparently infertile during this interval. Women to whom the hapten-coupled hCG was administered also developed antibodies to hCG and to pituitary luteinizing hormone(LH) (Stevens, 1975). Mitchison (1975) has cautioned that active immunization against hCG or its $\beta$ subunit might (at least in some individuals) prove to be irreversible, and suggested that the administration of passive antibody to the $\beta$ subunit of hCG would be a preferable approach. The generation of high titer human monoclonal antibodies to the $\beta$ subunit of hCG now appears to be quite feasible. Repeated administration of such antibody in depot form should, in principle, be entirely safe and well tolerated. However, whether this approach would prove realistic with respect to cost and to the logistics of the repeated injection of large populations of women remains problematical.

3. NEOPLASTIC DISEASE

The availability of human monoclonal antibodies directed against cell membrane antigens phenotypically distinctive for various specific types of human neoplasms would open the way to new immunodiagnostic and immunotherapeutic applications which might well have major prognostic signficance. Although many diagnostic techniques now exist for the detection of macrometastases, no practical procedures are currently available for the detection of micrometastases. Adjuvant chemotherapy is now widely used for the attempted eradication of micrometastases in patients with leukemias, lymphomas, breast cancers, and certain other types of neoplasms; although the efficacy of selected drug combinations has been demonstrated in some of these clinical situations, it is far from optimal even in the most favourable circumstances. Neoplasms such as small cell carcinoma of the lung, carcinoma of the breast and ovary, melanomas, non-Hodgkin's lymphomas, and leukemias are usually highly responsive to chemotherapy or combined modality therapy. Yet, despite the fact that patients with these types of tumors often enter complete remission, with the apparent disappearance of all signs of tumor, many of them later relapse and die with progressively growing neoplasms. Human monoclonal antibodies capable of eradicating such micrometastases might prevent many of these relapses and thus convert complete remissions into true cures.

The fact that mouse monoclonal antibodies to the cell membrane antigens of some types of human neoplasms have been successfully produced (Brown *et al.*, 1980; Mitchell *et al.*, 1980; Dippold *et al.*, 1980) makes it very likely that similar monoclonal antibodies of human origin can also now be obtained. However, whether such human monoclonal antitumor antibodies would be of sufficiently high titer and affinity to be clinically useful remains to be ascertained. Various techniques of presentation of human tumor cell membrane antigens will have to be explored to determine which technique of priming elicits human monoclonal antibody of highest titer and affinity. Procedures to be investigated include the use of intact human tumor cells *in vitro*, the use of cell membrane fractions isolated from tumor cell lysates, and the use of affinity chromatography-purified tumor cell membrane antigens. Convenient assay methods are already available to screen candidate hybridomas for the production of antibodies capable of binding to specific populations of human tumor cells. Purification of the relevant cell membrane antigen will be required before quantitative tests of antibody affinity can be carried out for human monoclonal antibodies with promising characteristics. After human monoclonal antibodies to one or more specific types of human neoplasms have been generated and cultures amplified sufficiently to harvest and purify large amounts of antibody, clinical studies will proceed through the usual sequence of Phase I, II, and III trials.

### (a) *Phase I Studies*

The major objective of Phase I studies with candidate human monoclonal antibodies will be to rule out the occurrence of life-threatening toxic reactions, to assess the frequency and severity of morbid reactions, and to establish acceptable dose levels for diagnostic and therapeutic use. Subjects for these studies will be patients with advanced neoplastic disease, of the type used to generate the corresponding hybridoma antibody, who have relapsed after maximally tolerated conventional therapy or who for other reasons are not deemed to be suitable candidates for conventional therapy. In patients with large tumor masses, mixtures of cold and radiolabelled monoclonal antibodies may be administered to verify antibody localization by imaging studies. Renal scans should also be performed to determine whether immune complex deposition has occurred. Although objective evidence of tumor regression is unlikely to occur in patients with large body burdens of tumor following administration of test doses of hybridoma antibodies, any such responses would of course be of interest to note. Tumor-bearing patients with advanced disease may be complement-depleted due to cachexia, making it even less likely that significant cytotoxic responses will occur due to the binding of autologous complement to tumor-bound antibody. The sera of Phase I patients will need to be monitored at serial intervals during the repeated administration of human monoclonal antibodies to determine whether they are making anti-idiotype antibodies, which might conceivably lead to undesirable secondary reactions. Such Phase I trials will gradually be extended to include a broad spectrum of neoplasms as additional specific human monoclonal antibodies are generated and pass rigorous testing *in vitro*.

## (b) *Phase II diagnostic studies*

Despite such diagnostic advances as lymphangiography, computed tomography, radioisotopic scans with selective radionuclides such as $^{67}Ga$, $^{99m}Tc$ and $^{111}In$, and ultrasonography, the detection of micro- and very small macrometastases is still not feasible. New techniques of markedly greater sensitivity and specificity are urgently needed, and, if available, would have a major impact on cancer management. For example, decisions concerning the need for adjuvant chemotherapy in patients with cancer of the breast, melanoma, or osteogenic sarcoma could be made on a much more selective basis; patients who present evidence of micrometastases could be spared surgical procedures such as mastectomy or limb amputation. Moreover, the differential diagnosis of tumor from chronic infection in patients who may be relapsing after prior chemotherapy and/or radiotherapy is frequently extremely difficult. Immunologic reagents labeled with radionuclides have long seemed the only approach which could offer the requisite specificity (Order, 1976; Pressman, 1980). However, the many problems associated with the use of classical heteroantisera for this purpose have hampered progress. The possibility of generating monoclonal antibodies to the cell surface antigens which define the phenotypes of a spectrum of human malignancies thus opens the way to systematic and critical studies of the radioimmunodiagnostic detection of metastatic disease and the differential diagnosis of neoplastic manifestations versus other types of disease processes.

For immunodiagnostic imaging, recent theoretical studies (Rockoff *et al.*, 1980) suggest that an uptake ratio of 5 or higher will be needed to detect small (1 cm² cross-sectional area) tumors 5 cm beneath the surface. Successful imaging of human tumors has now been achieved with heterologous [131]I labeled goat antisera raised against CEA, αFP, and hCG (Mach *et al.*, 1980; Goldenberg *et al.*, 1980; Kim *et al.*, 1980). Anti-CEA has also been used for lymphoscintigraphy (DeLand *et al.*, 1980). Goat [131]I anti-CEA and anti-ferritin have also had initial clinical trials in the treatment of intrahepatic neoplasms (Ettinger *et al.*, 1979; Order *et al.*, 1980). These exploratory studies with heterogeneous heterologous antisera have demonstrated problem areas which may well be resolved by the use of human monoclonal antibodies. It has now been demonstrated in human melanoma that most heterologous monoclonal antibodies do not recognize antigens specific for melanoma cells alone (Old, 1981). However, the autologous sera of 4 of 75 patients recognized their own melanomas; another 5 recognized their own tumors plus those of other melanoma patients. These observations are encouraging with respect to the likelihood that human monoclonal antibodies will yield more specific labeling ratios.

Another aspect of specificity lies in the distribution of the injected antibody. The problem is illustrated by a study (Khaw *et al.*, 1980) involving imaging of experimental canine myocardial infarcts with antibodies to cardiac muscle myosin. Gamma scintigrams showed a large hepatic uptake, a difficulty brought about either by specific binding of foreign immunoglobulin or nonspecific uptake of partially denatured proteins. Preliminary studies with mice in this laboratory indicate that different methods of radiolabeling antibody may cause varying amounts of denaturation, thus altering the distribution of the injected radiolabeled antibody. Nelson and Manning (1980) have shown that different heterologous antibodies and their fragments have varying half lives when transfused into rodents. In principle, human antibody and its fragments should be less subject to nonspecific uptake in the liver and thus remain in circulation significantly longer, being depleted only by specific antigen-antibody reactions. Human antibody also should not be immunogenic, thus permitting its repeated administration without inducing sensitivity. For the purpose of imaging, [123]I, [111]In, and [99m]Tc should be superior to [131]I.

It is clear from studies with animal and human tumors that blocking or enhancing antibody can play an important role in the tumor-host relationship. With the advent of monoclonal antibodies this relationship can be probed in more detail in animal model systems. Such studies should reveal the type of antibody preparation and labeling methods which will minimize the chance of enhancing tumor growth and maximize specific labeling. Systematic Phase II clinical investigations can then be undertaken to critically assess the sensitivity, specificity, and limits of resolution of primary and metastatic tumor imaging with radiolabeled human monoclonal antibodies, and to establish, for a spectrum of human types, whether this new diagnostic approach is indeed superior to presently available procedures.

(c)  *Phase III therapeutic studies*

There is little reason to anticipate that specific immunotherapy with human monoclonal hybridoma antibodies could succeed in eradicating bulky tumor masses. Unless remarkable regressions are observed during Phase I trials, it would seem unrealistic to plan on the use of hybridoma antibodies as a primary form of cytoreductive treatment, either alone or in combination with other treatment modalities. Instead, it seems more realistic to ask whether cytotoxic hybridoma antibodies can eradicate residual micrometastases in patients with various types of neoplastic disease who have achieved complete remissions with conventional therapy. If so, permanent cure can be offered to a high proportion of patients with non-Hodgkin's lymphomas, leukemias, small cell carcinoma of the lung, carcinoma of the breast, carcinoma of the ovary, and perhaps carcinoma of the colon and rectum who would otherwise be destined to develop relapses leading to their demise.

Phase III studies will require carefully designed prospective randomized clinical trials, in which patients who have entered complete remission on conventional treatment are randomly allocated either to no further treatment or to treatment with human monoclonal antibodies of the desired antitumor specificity. Since the natural cytotoxicity of such antibodies alone is likely to be insufficient to assure the eradication of all residual tumor cells, some form of amplification of the cytotoxic activity of these reagents will probably have to be employed. At present, the most promising approaches appear to be the conjugation of human monoclonal antitumor antibodies to an $\alpha$-particle-emitting radionuclide such as radium ($^{224}$Ra) or astatine ($^{211}$At; Neirinckx *et al.*, 1973), to chemotherapeutic agents such as the alkylating agent cyclophosphamide or the anthracycline adriamycin, or to the A chains of toxins such as ricin and diphtheria toxin (Thorpe *et al.*, 1978 and see chapter 7).

There are of course many potential pitfalls in the use of human monoclonal antibodies in specific adjuvant immunotherapy of human neoplastic disease. There is already evidence (Ritz *et al.*, 1980) that some tumor cell membrane antigens are readily shed from the cell surface and that these antigens may exist in soluble form in the blood stream in sufficient concentration to bind much or all of the administered antibody, thus preventing its binding to the tumor cell population. Antigenic modulation may also occur following the administration of monoclonal antibody, thus temporarily denuding the membranes of surviving tumor cells of antigen to which the next administered dose of antibody could bind (Rosenthal *et al.*, 1980). This possibility would have to be taken into account in determining optimal schedules of administration of antibodies to such patients.

It is now increasingly doubtful that true tumor-specific antigens exist (Old, 1981). Instead, most tumor-associated cell membrane antigens appear to be embryonic or differentiation antigens which are also expressed on certain subpopulations of normal cells, either during embryonic development or at a specific stage in the differentiation pathway of the cells of origin of the tumor. If human monoclonal antibodies could be rendered sufficiently cytotoxic to eradicate residual tumor cell populations, it is likely that they would also kill many of the antigenically related normal embryonic or differentiating cells. However, except for the special instance of true stem cells, the normal subpopulation thus eliminated could readily be replenished by regeneration from more undifferentiated precursors.

A more serious concern is that of antigenic heterogeneity, a phenomenon well documented for AKR mouse lymphomas (Olsson and Ebbesen, 1979) and human tumors (Taupier *et al.*, 1981). This process is due to evolution of subclones of tumor cells on the surface membranes of which antigen expression is either altered or deficient. Such subpopulations would bind little or no monoclonal antibody of any one idiotype, and would thus fail to be killed and could grow out selectively to render the recurrent tumor resistant to retreatment. It may be possible to circumvent this problem by using combinations of human monoclonal antibodies, each with preferential activity against a different cell membrane antigen shared by the cells of a given type of neoplasm. Such a "cocktail" of human monoclonal antibodies would be more likely to bind to essentially all of the residual tumor cell population, and thus to increase the probability of complete tumor cell eradication.

## C. SIDE EFFECTS

Monoclonal hybridoma antibody products are derived from cells that have the phenotypic characteristics of malignant cells. This raises the question of the potential biohazard of products derived from such cells, especially with respect to the possible release of oncogenic viruses. The human myeloma cell line SKO-007 has been carefully investigated for the possible presence of such transforming agents. The culture fluids are negative for reverse transcriptase-bearing particles of retroviral density, and there has been no instance to date in which non-malignant human cells co-cultivated with SKO-007 or U-266 cells have become transformed. Moreover, Ig products obtained from human hybridomas can be highly purified and treated with non-ionic detergents, which rapidly inactivate retroviruses without impairing the biological activity of the antibody. However, it is obvious that each hybridoma antibody product will have to be tested very carefully to rule out contamination with viral, bacterial, parasitic, or oncogenic agents, before such products are introduced clinically.

Monoclonal antibodies, like any other Ig, may elicit an anti-idiotype reaction that may result in inactivation of the monoclonal antibody in respect to its reactivity against its target antigen. It is therefore a theoretical possibility that the repeated injection of monoclonal antibodies may result in immunization against the idiotype of the monoclonal antibody, resulting in the abrogation of its biological activity. It is also conceivable that anti-idiotype reactions could, in rare instances, lead to secondary complications in the host. Experiments in mice have not been hampered by anti-idiotype reactions, suggesting that the risk of their occurrence is low. However, experience with the administration of monoclonal antibodies is still too limited to provide reliable risk estimates for this problem or for other complications monoclonal antibody treatments may generate. It will therefore be important to document all such reactions and complications, or their non-occurrence, very carefully during the conduct of Phase I clinical trials with human monoclonal antibodies.

REFERENCES

Boyle, J. M., Hopkins, J., Fox, M., Allen, T. D. and Leach, R. H. (1981). *Expl. Cell Res.* **132**, 67–72.
Carlsen, R. B., Bahl, O. P. and Swaminathan, N. (1973). *J. biol. Chem.* **248**, 6810–6827.
DeLand, F. H., Kim, E. E. and Goldenberg, D. M. (1980). *Cancer Res.* **40**, 2997–3000.
Delfraissy, J.-F., Galanaud, P., Dormont, J. and Wallon, C. (1977). *J. Immunol.* **118**, 630–635.
Diczfalusy, E. (1975). *Acta Endocrinol.* [Suppl.] **194**, 13–29.
Dosch, H. M. and Gelfand, E. W. (1977). *J. Immunol.* **118**, 302–308.

Ettinger, D. S., Dragon, L. H., Klein, J., Sgagias, M. and Order, S. E. (1979). *Cancer Treat. Rep.* **63**, 131–134.

Frankel, M. E. and Gerhard, W. (1979). *Molec. Immunol.* **16**, 101–106.

Goldenberg, D. M., Kim, E. E., DeLand, F. H., Bennett, S. and Primus, F. J. (1980a). *Cancer Res.* **40**, 2984–2992.

Goldenberg, D. M., Kim, E. E., DeLand, F. H., Van Nagell, J. R., Jr. and Javadpour, N. (1980b). *Science* **208**, 1284–1286.

Hayflick, L. (1960). *Nature* **185**, 738–784.

Hoffmann, M. K. (1980). *Proc. natn. Acad. Sci. U.S.A.* **77**, 1139–1143.

Hoffmann, M. K., Schmidt, D. and Oettgen, H. F. (1973). *Nature* **243**, 408–410.

Isojima, S., Tsuchiya, K., Koyama, K., Tanaka, C., Naka, O. and Adachi, H. (1972). *Am. J. Obstet. Gynec.* **112**, 199–207.

Khaw, B. A., Fallon, J. T., Strauss, H. W. and Haber, E. (1980). *Science* **209**, 295–297.

Kim, E. E., DeLand, F. H., Nelson, M. O., Bennett, S., Simmons, G., Alpert, E. and Goldenberg, D. M. (1980). *Cancer Res.* **40**, 3008–3012.

Kohler, G. and Milstein, C. (1975). *Nature* **256**, 495–497.

Kohler, G. and Milstein, C. (1976). *Eur. J. Immunol.* **6**, 511–519.

Koskimies, S. (1979). *Scand. J. Immunol.* **10**, 371 (abstract).

Levy, R. and Dilley, J. (1978). *Proc. natn. Acad. Sci. U.S.A.* **75**, 2411–2415.

Mach, J.-P., Carrel, S., Forni, M., Ritschard, J., Donath, A. and Alberto, P. (1980). *New Engl. J. Med.* **303**, 5–10.

Mitchison, N. A. (1975). *Acta Endocrinol. [Suppl.]* **194**, 405–413.

Morgan, F. J., Birken, S. and Canfield, R. E. (1975). *J. biol. Chem.* **250**, 5247–5258.

Neirinckx, R. D., Myburgh, J. A. and Smit, J. A. (1973). *In* Symposium on "New Developments in Radiopharmaceuticals and Labelled Compounds" pp. 171–175. International Atomic Energy Agency, Vienna.

Nelson, S. J. and Manning, D. M. (1980). *J. Immunol.* **75**, 2339–2343.

Nilsson, K., Bennich, H., Johansson, S. G. O. and Pontén, J. (1970). *Clin. Exp. Immunol.* **7**, 477–489.

Oi, V. T. and Herzenberg, L. A. (1979). *In* "Selected Methods in Cellular Immunology" (B. B. Mishell and S. M. Shiigi, Eds), pp. 351–372. W. H. Freeman, Pub., San Francisco.

Old, L. J. (1981). *Cancer Res.* **41**, 361–375.

Olsson, L. and Ebbesen, P. (1979). *J. natn. Cancer Inst.* **62**, 623–627.

Olsson, L. and Kaplan, H. S. (1980). *Proc. natn. Acad. Sci. U.S.A.* **77**, 5429–5431.

Order, S. E. (1976). *Radiology* **118**, 219–223.

Order, S. E., Klein, J. L., Ettinger, D., Alderson, P., Siegelman, S. and Leichner, P. (1980). *Int. J. Radiation Oncology Biol. Phys.* **6**, 703–710.

Pressman, D. (1980). *Cancer Res.* **40**, 2960–2964.

Ritz, J., Pesando, J. M., Notis-McConarty, J. and Schlossman, S. F. (1980). *J. Immunol.* **125**, 1506–1514.

Rockoff, S. D., Goodenough, D. J. and McIntire, K. R. (1980). *Cancer Res.* **40**, 3054–3058.

Rosenthal, K. L., Tompkins, W. A. F. and Rawls, W. E. (1980). *Cancer Res.* **40**, 4744–4750.

Ross, G. T., Vaitukaitis, J. L. and Robbins, J. B. (1972). *In* "Structure Activity Relationships of Protein and Polypeptide Hormones" (M. Margoulies and F. C. Greenwood, Eds), Vol. 241, pp. 153–157. Excerpta Med., Amsterdam.

Schlom, J., Wunderlich, D. and Teramoto, Y. A. (1980). *Proc. natn. Acad. Sci. U.S.A.* **77**, 6841–6845.

Schwaber, J. (1975). *Expl. Cell Res.* **93**, 343–354.

Steinitz, M., Klein, G., Koskimies, S. and Mäkelä, O. (1977). *Nature* **269**, 420–422.

Stevens, V. C. (1975). *Acta Endocrinol. (Suppl,)* **194**, 357–369.

Talwar, G. P., Sharura, N. C., Dubey, S. K., Salahuddin, M., Das, C., Ramakrishnan, S., Kumar, S. and Hingorani, V. (1976). *Proc. natn. Acad. Sci. U.S.A.* **73**, 218–222.

Taupier, M. A., Loken, M. R., Kearney, J. F., Leibson, P. J. and Schreiber, H. (1981). *Proc. Am. Ass. Cancer Res.* **22**, 294 (abstract).

Thorpe, P. E., Ross, W. C. J., Cumber, A. J., Hinson, C. A., Edwards, D. C. and Davies, A. J. S. (1978). *Nature* **271**, 752–755.

Zurawski, V. R., Jr., Haber, E. and Black, P. H. (1978). *Science* **199**, 1439–1441.

# B  IMMUNOLOGICAL ASPECTS

# 3 Immunoregulatory Changes in Human Disease Detected by Monoclonal Antibodies to T Lymphocytes

GIDEON GOLDSTEIN, JOHN LIFTER AND
ROBERT MITTLER

*Ortho Pharmaceutical Corporation, Immunobiology
Division, Raritan, New Jersey 08869, U.S.A.*

# 1 INTRODUCTION

## A. Immune Alterations Associated with Human Disease

During the past ten years enormous strides have been made in understanding how the immune system participates in maintaining bodily homeostasis. It is now well established that alterations of immune function occur in a large number of human diseases and these alterations include inappropriate hyperimmune responsiveness and immune depression. In disorders such as immune deficiency, infection and cancer, reduced responses are permissive or perpetuating factors; by contrast in allergic or autoimmune disease, aberrant and intensified immune responses appear to be involved in the pathogenetic mechanisms. Lastly, aging can be thought of as a predisposing condition permitting aberrant or depressed immune responses, and autoimmunity and predisposition to cancer and infection may be a consequence of these changes. Both the complexity of the immune system itself plus the myriad of chemical and hormonal interactions that can modulate the immune response have contributed to the difficulty of measuring the immune status of a given individual.

## B. Early Methods of Evaluating the State of the Immune System

Previously immunological defects, particularly T cell defects, have been detected by measuring the functional status of the immune system. Tests designed to evaluate the immune response, such as the antibody response to or cutaneous reactivity with a given antigen, have proven unsatisfactory for routine use because of the high variability of these responses, even in normal individuals. Similarly, the evaluation of lymphocyte responsiveness to mitogens and in mixed lymphocyte culture have not proven generally useful because these parameters only decline with extremely severe abnormalities. Lastly, enumeration of T cells with the well known E-rosette assay has been shown to possess a high degree of variability due to a lack of standardization of specific test procedures. As a consequence of these shortcomings, it has become increasingly evident that more reliable and quantitative techniques are needed to evaluate immune status in man.

## C. Immune System Consists of Discrete Subsets of Cells

Out of the need to measure the immune status, a new approach was developed based upon the precise recognition of the immune system's functional components. From work with mice, it is now recognized that the immune system consists of functionally discrete subsets of T cells which can be identified by their cell surface differentiation antigens (Cantor and Boyse, 1975; McKenzie and Potter, 1979; Jandinski *et al.*, 1976). In mice these surface markers were originally recognized by alloantisera generated by reciprocal immunizations of inbred mice strains with lymphocytes (Shen *et al.*, 1978). Direct application of this work to man was attempted with adsorbed heteroantisera generated by immunizations of rabbits or goats with human lymphocytes. These techniques did not prove to be of practical value for widespread use because of considerable batch variations, frequent low titers and the extensive tissue absorptions required to obtain specificity (Strelkauskas *et al.*, 1978; Moretta *et al.*, 1976; Wybran and Fudenberg, 1971). However these reagents did provide provocative indications that alterations of functional subsets of T cells, identified by these antisera to cell surface antigens, were a feature of several diseases.

The advent of hybridoma technology, whereby tumor clones can be generated to secrete desired monoclonal antibodies, has ushered in a new era (Kohler and Milstein, 1975; Barnstable *et al.*, 1978; Trucco *et al.*, 1978; Koprowski *et al.*, 1978). Utilizing this methodology, highly specific and reproducible reagents have been produced to identify and enumerate functional subsets of lymphocytes and these reagents have already provided entirely new information as to immune abnormalities in human disease, as will be described below.

## II GENERATION OF MONOCLONAL ANTIBODIES

The production and characterization of hybridomas producing antibodies to human T lymphocytes have been described in detail (Kung *et al.*, 1979, 1980; Reinherz *et al.*, 1979a–d, 1980a,b; Greaves *et al.*, 1981). Briefly, the antibodies are generated in a mouse hybridoma system, as described by Kohler and Milstein (1975), by immunizing mice with human E-rosette purified peripheral lymphocytes, thymocytes, T cell lines or leukemic T cells. The resulting antibodies are selected by screening the hybridoma supernatants by indirect immunofluorescent

staining and flow cytometric analysis on various lymphocyte populations. Hybridomas of interest are cloned and recloned and selected
hybridomas are passed by peritoneal passage to produce ascitic fluid in
mice. The reactivities of the OKT reagents are illustrated in Table 3·1.

To our knowledge only OKT3, OKT4 and OKT5/OKT8 antibodies
are solely represented on T lineage cells. OKT1 is present only on T
cells in normal individuals yet is also detected on B cell lines (Fox *et al.*,
1981). OKT6 is restricted to thymocytes if lymphoid cells alone are
analyzed but is also found on Langerhans cells in the skin (Fithian *et al.*,
1981) and in certain neuroblastomas (Greaves *et al.*, 1981). OKT9
recognizes the transferrin receptor (Sutherland *et al.*, 1981) and is found
on dividing cells of all cell lineages. OKT10 (Janossy *et al.*, 1981a) is
found on cells at various stages of differentiation of both T and B cell
and myelomonocytic lineages. OKT11 recognizes the sheep red blood
cell receptor (Verbi *et al.*, 1981) and reacts with all peripheral T cells in
addition to a population whose phenotype is $OKT11^+,1^-,3^-,4^-,5^-$,
$8^-,OKM1^+$. These cells mediate natural killer activity (Zarling and
Kung, 1980) and antibody-dependent cellular cytotoxicity (Kay and
Horwitz, 1980); however, their lineage assignment remains controversial. OKIa1 is found on B cells, monocytes and certain tissue reticular cells in addition to activated T cells (Reinherz *et al.*, 1979d).
OKM1 is found on monocytes and granulocytes plus certain circulating
null cells and $OKT11^+$ cells (Breard *et al.*, 1980). While only a small
number of the OKT antibodies appear to be fully T cell specific it must
be emphasized that even the nonlineage-specific reagents can still
provide valuable information as to the state of T cell maturation and
function.

Many monoclonal antibodies are now being generated in other
laboratories and a number have demonstrated similar reactivities to the
OKT reagents. For example, a spectrum of pan-T antibodies, reactive
with the majority of circulating T cells include: 17F12 (Engleman *et al.*,
1980); T101 (Royston *et al.*, 1980); SK5 (Wang, *et al.*, 1980); 9·6
(Kamoun *et al.*, 1981); UCHT1 (Callard *et al.*, 1981) and 10·2 (Hansen
*et al.*, 1980a). In addition to the pan-T antibodies, a variety of monoclonal antibodies to T cell subsets and thymocytes have been produced
by other investigators: 3A1 (Haynes *et al.*, 1980); SK1,2,3,4 (Evans *et
al.*, 1981; Ledbetter *et al.*, 1981); 9·3 (Martin *et al.*, 1980; Hansen *et al.*,
1980b); NA1/34 (McMichael *et al.*, 1979) and 12E7 (Levy *et al.*, 1979).
In this review, we have largely confined ourselves to OKT reagents
because they have been used most extensively in clinical studies.

TABLE 3·1

Reactivity of monoclonal antibodies with human cells from various sources

| Monoclonal Antibody (OKT Series) | Bone marrow | | | Spleen | Thymus | | | Peripheral blood | | | | Cell lines | |
|---|---|---|---|---|---|---|---|---|---|---|---|---|---|
| | Stem Cells | Myeloid Series | Erythroid Series | | Early | Common | Late | E+ T Cells | E− B Cells | Null Cells | Monocytes | T | B |
| OKT1 | − | − | − | + | W[b] | W | + | + | − | − | − | + | + |
| OKT3 | − | − | − | + | W | W | + | + | − | − | − | + | − |
| OKT4 | − | − | − | + | − | + | +[c] | +[f] | − | − | − | + | − |
| OKT5 | − | − | − | + | − | + | +[d] | +[g] | − | − | − | + | − |
| OKT6 | − | − | − | − | − | + | − | − | − | − | − | + | − |
| OKT8 | − | − | − | + | − | + | +[e] | +[h] | − | − | − | + | − |
| OKT9 | − | NE[a] | NE | − | ± | ± | ± | − | − | NE | NE | + | + |
| OKT10 | + | + | NE | + | + | + | + | + | − | + | NE | + | + |
| OKT11A | ± | − | − | + | + | + | + | + | − | − | − | + | − |
| OKM1 | − | − | − | NE | − | − | − | − | − | + | + | − | NE |
| OKIa1 | + | − | − | + | − | − | − | −[i] | + | + | + | + | + |

a Not Evaluated
b Weak reactivity
c Upon removal of OKT6+ cells, approximately 72% of the cells are OKT4+
d Upon removal of OKT6+ cells, approximately 30% of the cells are OKT5+
e Upon removal of OKT6+ cells, approximately 31% of the cells are OKT8+
f Approximately 67% positive cells
g Approximately 31% positive cells
h Approximately 31% positive cells
i OKIa1 is expressed on activated T cells

## III FUNCTIONAL CHARACTERIZATION OF PERIPHERAL BLOOD LYMPHOCYTE POPULATIONS

OKT1* and OKT3 monoclonal antibodies have been shown to identify greater than 95% of circulating peripheral human T cells. Treatment of purified peripheral T cells with antibody and complement abolishes all known T cell functions such as T cell proliferation with mitogens or allogeneic stimulation, T cell mediated help during pokeweed mitogen driven antibody responses *in vitro*, T cell mediated suppression and the generation of cytotoxic T cells (CTL) in response to allogeneic targets in mixed lymphocyte culture. Within the OKT1/OKT3 population reside two phenotypically and functionally distinct subpopulations. These subpopulations are detected by monoclonal antibodies OKT4 and OKT8. OKT4 identifies 50–60% of normal human peripheral T cells and OKT8 identifies 30–40% of the T cell population. These two mutually exclusive subsets together represent greater than 95% of the human T cell pool and it remains uncertain whether peripheral cells lacking both OKT4 and OKT8 are truly T cells. Previous studies have shown that the OKT4$^+$ population contains cells capable of inducing both B cell differentiation and helping the development of alloreactive CTL precursors although it does not contain these precursors (Reinherz *et al.*, 1979b, c). The OKT8$^+$ population on the other hand contains alloreactive precursor and effector CTL as well as suppressor cells (Thomas *et al.*, 1981b). Thus, the two subsets are functionally identified as inducer/helper and suppressor/cytotoxic subsets, respectively.

Considerable interaction occurs between these two subsets, as is demonstrated by the following observations. The OKT4$^+$ subset has been shown to contain both radiosensitive and radioresistant populations (Thomas *et al.*, 1980, 1981a). Irradiation of the OKT4$^+$ population and subsequent co-culture of these cells with unirradiated OKT8$^+$ cells and B cells failed to suppress plaque forming cells (PFC) in a pokeweed mitogen (PWM) driven system. Addition of unirradiated OKT4$^+$ cells to this system resulted in marked suppression of PFC. Furthermore, when graded numbers of unirradiated OKT4$^+$ cells were added to PWM driven B cell cultures, the number of PFC generated did not follow a linear relationship with respect to added cells. The addition of relatively low numbers of those cells resulted in a plateau effect and

---

* OKT1 is an IgG₁ which does not fix complement. Cytotoxicity assays with OKT1 require use of a complement fixing α-mouse immunoglobulin as a second antibody.

subsequently, a diminution of the PFC response as the number of added cells increased. In contrast to this observation, when irradiated OKT4$^+$ cells were added in graded numbers to the B cell cultures, a linear dose response curve was generated with respect to PFC.

Taken together, the above observations suggest that radiosensitive cells within the OKT4$^+$ subset are required for the generation of suppressor function by interacting with the OKT8$^+$ population. In addition, this data suggests that within the radiosensitive OKT4$^+$ population may reside a novel suppressor cell bearing the OKT3$^+$,4$^+$, 8$^-$ phenotype. This hypothesis is further supported by the observations of Thomas *et al.* (1981c) that small numbers of activated OKT4$^+$ cells (which retain the OKT4$^+$ phenotype following PWM activation) were able to suppress B cell differentiation by fresh OKT4$^+$ cells. In a recent report, Uchiyama *et al.* (1981a, b) described somewhat similar findings. These investigators described a monoclonal antibody (antiTac) which reacts only with a subpopulation of mature PWM activated T cells. When both the Tac$^+$ and Tac$^-$ populations were functionally analyzed for inducer/helper and suppressor/cytotoxic functions it was found that the Tac$^+$ population contained radioresistant help and radiosensitive suppression as well as CTL activity against allogeneic targets. In contrast, the Tac$^-$ population contained only radiosensitive helper cells.

In addition to the OKT8$^+$ subset functioning as suppressors of B cell differentiation and immunoglobulin production, they also serve as CTL in the *in vitro* generation of hapten altered (trinitrophenyl-TNP) self-reactive human cytotoxic T lymphocytes. Studies directed toward a better comprehension of the role of T-T interaction in the generation of these killer cells (Friedman *et al.*, 1981) have concluded that while the cytotoxic effector function is contained within the OKT8$^+$ subset, optimal cytotoxic responses to altered self-antigens required the presence of both OKT4$^+$ and OKT8$^+$ cells. These observations suggest that cooperation between these subsets is essential for maximal amplification of killing. The following observations support this concept: (1) OKT4$^+$ cells and not OKT8$^+$ cells generate helper factors during a mixed lymphocyte reaction and these amplify TNP altered self-reactive CTL responses and (2) helper factors by-pass the need for OKT4$^+$ OKT8$^+$ interaction in the CTL response. Taken together, these observations demonstrate the importance of functional T-T interactions in the immunoregulation of both T and B cell differentiation.

## IV ANALYSIS OF LYMPHOCYTE DIFFERENTIATION AND MATURATION IN LYMPHOID TISSUES USING MONOCLONAL ANTIBODIES

Monoclonal antibodies have been generated that recognize differentiation antigens which appear (or disappear) at precise stages of cell maturation. With the availability of such reagents, a number of laboratories have begun to study the ontogeny of T and B lymphocytes and their microanatomical locations within the lymphoid tissues. The following is a brief summary of some of these studies.

### A. THYMUS

In the thymus, cell maturation associated with the appearance or disappearance of cell surface antigens appears to follow the direction of cortex to medulla. $TdT^+$ (terminal deoxynucleotidyl transferase) blasts beneath the thymic capsule are $OKT10^+$ and lack other T cell markers. These cells are especially prominent in the fetal thymus (Bradstock *et al.*, 1980). The majority of cortical lymphocytes (common thymocytes) bear thymocyte specific antigens, while the medullary cell pattern approximates the staining of peripheral T cells. More specifically, the phenotype of typical cortical (common) thymocytes was $TdT^+$, $OKT6^+,10^+,4^+,5^+,8^+,11^+$, while the phenotype of typical medullary (mature) thymocytes was $OKT11^+,1^+,3^+$ and either $OKT4^+$ or $OKT5/OKT8^+$ (Reinherz *et al.*, 1980b). Noteworthy were 10–15% of thymocytes showing intermediate phenotypes between cortical and medullary thymocytes (Tidman *et al.*, 1981). It appears that TdT, then OKT6, and finally OKT10 are lost during maturation. Simultaneously, the expression of OKT3,4,8 and HLA-A,B,C is generated. These findings, along with the occasional presence of $TdT^+$ cells (cortical phenotype) in the medulla, suggested that differentiation proceeded in a continuous pattern from the cortex to the medulla (Janossy *et al.*, 1981a) (Fig. 3·1).

### B. BONE MARROW

Analysis of T lymphocyte populations in the bone marrow (BM) revealed two groups of cells: (1) lymphocytes of peripheral T cell phenotype and (2) putative T lymphoid precursors. The differentiation antigens ex-

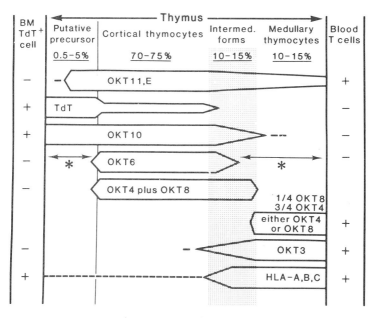

FIG. 3·1 Scheme of human thymocyte differentiation based on reactivity with mono-clonal antibodies with membrane antigens and terminal deoxynucleotidyl transferase. Positivity of cell populations is shown by horizontal bars; dotted lines indicate barely detectable or very weak positivity on a few cells. OKT6$^+$ cells simultaneously express both OKT4 and OKT8, whereas OKT6$^-$ cells (asterisks) are heterogeneous: putative precursors which are large TdT$^+$ blasts (OKT11$^+$,10$^+$) resembling bone marrow TdT$^+$ cells (which are also OKT10$^+$); medullary thymocytes which have already been segregated into inducer/helper (OKT4$^+$, OKT8$^-$ majority) and suppressor/cytotoxic cell types (OKT8$^+$, OKT4$^-$; minority). There are a number of identifiable inter-mediary forms (stipled area) between cortical and medullary thymocytes. (data from Tidman *et al.*, 1981)

pressed in the former population were exclusively of T lymphoid lineage (OKT3, OKT11 and OKT4 or OKT8) and were absent on bone marrow precursors. These antigens are generated on T cells within the thymus and cells bearing these antigens apparently enter the bone marrow from the blood after maturing in the thymus. In contrast, the differentiation antigens expressed in the precursor population (OKT10, TdT) were not lineage specific since OKT10 reacts with both early hematopoietic stem cells (BM TdT$^+$ cells, myeloblasts, pro-myelocytes and some myelocytes) and various derivatives of these precursors (thymocytes and B lymphocytes). There were no transi-tional forms demonstrated between these distinct populations of T cell precursors and mature T cells. (Janossy *et al.*, 1981b; Crawford *et al.*, 1981a).

## C. Lymph Nodes

T cells and B cells are well known to occupy separate compartments in human lymph nodes with the former being restricted to paracortical areas and the latter to the follicular regions and medullary cords. Recently, analysis of T lymphocyte populations in human lymph nodes has revealed that the majority of cells in paracortical areas are $OKT1^+, 3^+, 4^+$ cells (inducer/helper subset); whereas, the majority of cells in the primary follicles are B cells by virtue of their reactivity with anti-IgM antibodies and OKIa1. However, some $OKT1^+, 3^+, 4^+$ cells were located in the germinal centers of the follicles and the presence of these cells in this area could indicate their inducer role in relation to the formation of antibody forming cells in germinal centers. $OKIa1^+$ interdigitating reticular cells were closely associated with the $OKT4^+$ cells. It is possible that this association reflects their role in the presentation of antigen to T lymphocytes (Poppema *et al.*, 1979, 1981; Bhan *et al.*, 1980). $OKT8^+$ cells were present in the paracortical areas but did not show a particular association with $OKIa1^+$ interdigitating reticular cells.

## D. Tonsils

Tonsillar architecture typically contains paracortical T cell areas and germinal centers consisting of B lymphocytes in a well defined follicular area. Analysis of lymphocyte populations in human tonsils demonstrated that the majority of T cells in the paracortical region were $OKT4^+$. These cells were closely associated with $OKIa1^+$ interdigitating cells (Janossy *et al.*, 1980; Heusermann *et al.*, 1974; Kaiserling and Lennert, 1974; Lampert *et al.*, 1982). As seen in the lymph nodes, this association between $OKIa1^+$ cells with $OKT4^+$ cells could indicate their role in the presentation of antigen to T cells. Also, the lymphocyte corona of the tonsils contained a small number of $OKT4^+$ cells and $OKT8^+$ cells (Tidman *et al.*, 1981).

# V METHODOLOGIES OF T CELL ENUMERATION FOR CLINICAL EVALUATION

Microscopic or flow cytometric techniques may be used to enumerate the T lymphocyte subpopulations in peripheral blood. Depending on the instrumentation or methodology these analyses can be performed on whole blood, buffy coat preparations, or mononuclear cells isolated by Ficoll-Hypaque density gradient centrifugation (Hoffman *et al.*, 1980; Kung and Goldstein, 1980; Reinherz *et al.*, 1979c,d, 1980b). Flow cytometric techniques may employ direct immunofluorescence, in which the monoclonal antibody is conjugated with a fluorescent dye, or indirect immunofluorescence, in which the monoclonal antibody bound to the cell surface is visualized with a second fluorescent antibody directed against the monoclonal immunoglobulin. Microscopic techniques include direct and indirect immunofluorescence, direct or indirect visualization utilizing monoclonal antibodies or second antibodies conjugated with colloidal gold (De Waele *et al.*, 1981a), and direct or indirect visualization utilizing antibodies conjugated to enzymes (Druguet and Pepys, 1977; Pepys and Pepys, 1980; Pepys *et al.*, 1981). Good correlations between these methodologies may be obtained if adequate attention is given to counting statistics.

## VI MONOCLONAL ANTIBODIES IN CLINICAL MEDICINE

### A. MEASUREMENTS OF CIRCULATING CELLS

Monoclonal antibodies are providing new dimensions to the diagnosis of human disease and may well provide new clinical parameters to monitor and diagnose disease. Using the techniques enumerated above, they can be used to describe T lymphocytes, their subpopulations and state of activation in tissue sections, exudates and blood. To date most work with these reagents has concentrated on describing circulating blood lymphocytes and this review will concentrate on these changes. Monoclonal antibodies can determine the proportions and absolute numbers of T cells and T cell subsets. The ratio of inducer/suppressor cells (OKT4/OKT8) in peripheral blood appears to be a particularly significant parameter. The physiological state of T cells (resting or activated) can also be evaluated using, for example, the reactivity of OKT9, OKT10 and OKIal monoclonal antibodies since they react with antigens that are expressed during replication or activation of T cells. In the following section, clinical disorders in which distinct abnormalities in some of these parameters are observed will be discussed.

## B. DIAGNOSTIC APPLICATIONS OF MONOCLONAL ANTIBODIES

### 1. CANCER

#### (a) *Lymphoid Malignancies*

Monoclonal antibodies are of great utility for classifying leukemias and lymphomas. These reagents clearly distinguish between T and B cell leukemias and provide information on the differentiation of T cell malignancies. Thus the T cell leukemias of infancy represent early thymic stages of differentiation (the majority of acute lymphoblastic leukemias are reactive with either OKT10 alone or OKT9 and OKT10), whereas cutaneous T cell lymphomas, such as Sezary syndrome, represent maligancies of a more mature T cell phenotype (OKT4) (Reinherz *et al.*, 1980b; Kung *et al.*, 1981; Berger *et al.*, 1979). Acute lymphoblastic leukemias (ALL) are usually classified with monoclonal antibodies into T cell leukemias (OKT11$^+$, OKIal$^-$, CALLA$^-$, BA-1$^-$) versus common ALL (OKT11$^-$, OKIal$^+$, CALLA$^+$, BA-1$^+$) (Kersey *et al.*, 1981; Ritz *et al.*, 1980; Abramson *et al.*, 1981). (CALLA is a leukemia-associated antigen found in patients with ALL and some patients with chronic myelocytic leukemia (CML) and BA-1 is a monoclonal antibody that identifies a determinant primarily expressed on cells of human B lymphocyte lineage that is lost when these cells terminally differentiate into plasma cells).

Recently, preliminary work in typing non-Hogdkin lymphomas demonstrated the presence of large cell histiocytic lymphomas bearing the phenotype OKT9$^+$,10$^+$, OKIal$^-$ in addition to surface immuno globulins (SIgG$^+$) (Aisenberg and Wilkes, 1981). Based on the facts that OKT9 and OKT10 antigens are not lineage specific and that plasma cells lack the DR antigen, the data suggested that these neo-plasms represented the expansion of a clone of B lymphocytes which have lost the DR antigen and are on the pathway to plasma cell differentiation. Further investigation is needed in order to understand both the significance and the frequency of this unusual phenotype in lymphocyte differentiation. Leukemia classification with monoclonal antibodies is addressed more fully by Greaves *et al.* in this volume (see chapter 6).

#### (b) *Non-Lymphoid Malignancies*

The immunoregulatory status in patients with cancer is a field requir-ing extensive exploration since both animal and human data suggest that maligancy may be associated with a state of immunosuppression. Furthermore, many treatment modalities used in cancer, including X-irradiation and cytotoxic drugs, may themselves be immuno-suppressive. Preliminary data have been obtained in lung cancer, breast cancer and squamous cell carcinoma associated with psoralen/ ultraviolet-A radiation therapy (PUVA) for psoriasis.

Any analysis of lung cancer patients must be appropriately analyzed to allow for the effects of smoking because smoking itself causes a leukocytosis including a lymphocytosis and, in subjects with a very heavy smoking history, is associated with a lowered OKT4/OKT8 ratio (Ginns *et al.*, 1981). Patients with primary squamous cell carcinoma had changes, but these could be attributed to their heavy smoking history. Patients with primary adenocarcinoma revealed a decrease in OKT8$^+$ cells. The most striking change, unrelated to smoking history, was recorded in patients with secondary metastases in lung (various primaries). These patients showed a reduced OKT4/OKT8 ratio due to an increase in the proportion of OKT8$^+$ cells. Thus each type of lung cancer was associated with a distinctive pattern of T lymphocytes as enumerated by monoclonal antibodies. Metastatic carcinoma in particular appeared to be associated with immunosuppression as judged by a low OKT4/OKT8 ratio. This of itself is an important finding but it leaves unanswered the question of whether immunosuppression preceded tumor metastases and in fact permitted it or whether metastatic tumors themselves induce a state of immunosuppression, as is suggested from experimental studies in animals (Lau *et al.*, 1982).

Preliminary findings in breast cancer (W. De Cock, personal communication) in newly diagnosed untreated patients have also revealed that patients staged as having localized disease appear to have normal proportions of T cells and OKT4 and OKT8 cells, whereas, patients in which neoplastic spread is detectable at presentation have a lowered OKT4/OKT8 ratio suggestive of an immunosuppressed state.

Untreated patients with psoriasis have a normal OKT4/OKT8 ratio (R. Edelson, personal communication; Moscicki *et al.*, 1981) while a low ratio was found in patients on long-term PUVA therapy. Ultraviolet irradiation appears to reduce the level of OKT4 cells transiently and this reduction may play a role in the altered immune state (immuno-suppressive effect) observed after treatment (Morison *et al.*, 1981). Two psoriatic patients undergoing chronic PUVA therapy developed squamous cell carcinoma of the skin, and these patients had the lowest OKT4/OKT8 ratios, suggesting that in this instance that the immuno-suppressed state permitted the emergence of clinical cancer.

These preliminary studies indicate that immunosuppression may be a feature of certain malignancies, particularly the metastatic state, and that these analyses need to be expanded and extended.

## 2. INFECTIOUS DISEASE

The immunoregulatory status of T cell subsets has been studied in relatively few infectious diseases to date. Nevertheless, preliminary findings indicate that distinct immunoregulatory changes occur for different classes of microorganisms and that these alterations may be closely related to the course of the disease.

### (a) *Viral*

(i). *Infectious mononucleosis*   Immune alterations in infectious disease play a major role in disease outcome. In acute and convalescent phases of infectious mononucleosis (IM) the following changes were found in the peripheral blood lymphoid population (Fig. 3·2). First, a massive increase in OKT8$^+$ T cells during acute IM; many of these cells expressed the DR antigen (OKIa1$^+$) as a sign of activation and had the morphology of the large atypical cells characteristic of IM (Crawford *et al.*, 1981b; Tosato *et al.*, 1979; Johnson *et al.*, 1978). Second additional antigens displayed were OKT9 and OKT10, again probably indicative of activation and proliferation. The expansion of the OKT8$^+$ subset resulted in a reversal of the OKT4/OKT8 ratio ($<$1) (De Waele *et al.*, 1981b). It is thought that the Epstein-Barr virus infection in IM, which primarily involves B cells, may trigger proliferation and activation of T suppressor/cytotoxic cells and that these may play a role in suppressing the virally induced B cell activation and proliferation. In contrast to the acute course, convalescence was associated with a return to normal of T cell subset distribution, a decrease in activated T cells and restoration of immune function (Reinherz *et al.*, 1980c).

(ii). *Cytomegalovirus*   Patients with acute cytomegalovirus (CMV) mononucleosis and renal transplant patients with symptomatic primary CMV disease revealed an absolute decrease in OKT4$^+$ T cells and an increase in OKT8$^+$ T cells resulting in a decrease in the OKT4/OKT8 ratio in acute CMV infection. This reversal in the OKT4/OKT8 ratio accompanied an observed lymphocyte hyporesponsiveness (Carney *et al.*, 1981) which may contribute to the prolonged illness characteristic of the virus, and to the increased risk of bacterial and fungal superinfections that have been described (Rubin *et al.*, 1977). In parallel with clinical recovery, both subset distributions and mitogen responses returned to normal levels (Rubin *et al.*, 1981). One patient clearly displayed this pattern on four separate occasions— at the time of acute illness, and then 22, 64 and 105 days after the onset of symptoms. At these times, OKT4/OKT8 ratios of 0·48, 0·60, 0·86 and 1·2 resulted respectively. These parameters therefore, may thus serve as useful indicators in following both the course of infection and the response of the patient to therapy.

(iii). *Hepatitis B virus*   Patients with acute hepatitis B virus infection (HBV) revealed a decrease in the OKT4/OKT8 ratio due to an

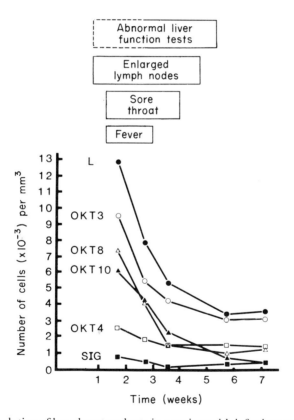

FIG. 3·2 Evolution of lymphocyte subsets in a patient with infectious mononucleosis. Absolute numbers of peripheral lymphocytes (L) and of OKT3+, OKT8+, OKT10+, OKT4+ and surface-immunoglobulin (SIG) positive lymphocytes are plotted as a function of time after the onset of symptoms. The presence of the main clinical signs and symptoms is indicated at the top. (data from De Waele *et al.*, 1981b)

increase in OKT8$^+$ T cells. (H. Thomas *et al.*, 1981; Bach and Bach, 1981). Restoration of this imbalance occurred upon clearance of the hepatitis B antigen and appearance of hepatitis B antibody. In patients with chronic active hepatitis due to hepatitis B virus the OKT4/OKT8 ratio was also decreased. In subjects with normal hepatic histology (positive carrier) normal subset distributions were found, whereas in patients with chronic hepatitis due to hepatitis B virus the low OKT4/OKT8 ratio was due to a decrease in the absolute numbers of OKT4$^+$ T cells rather than an increase in OKT8$^+$ T cells as observed in acute type B hepatitis.

(iv). *Hepatitis A virus* In hepatitis A the OKT4/OKT8 ratio was increased (H. Thomas, personal communication). This provides an interesting contrast to hepatitis B infection. For hepatitis B, the low OKT4/OKT8 ratio was associated with a prolonged clinical course and the ratio did not normalize until the virus was eliminated, as evidenced by the disappearance of circulating core antigen E and the appearance of antibodies. By contrast hepatitis A provoked a high OKT4/OKT8 ratio and was invariably associated with rapid clinical recovery. These findings suggest that some microorganisms may generate spurious suppressive signals which impair the vigor of the immune response, thereby permitting the organisms to proliferate unchecked and cause a more prolonged clinical infection. It may be that immunosuppressive peptides isolated from microorganisms, e.g. cyclosporin A, have evolved to fulfill this particular function in the host-parasite relationship.

(b) *Bacterial*

(i). *Leprosy* Patients with lepromatous leprosy, whose disease was associated with erythema nodosum leprosum (ENL), demonstrated an increased percentage of OKT4$^+$ T cells and a decreased percentage of OKT8$^+$ T cells. This resulted in an increased OKT4$^+$/OKT8$^+$ ratio (Bach *et al.*, 1981). These alterations in T cell surface markers are in good agreement with *in vitro* functional studies which demonstrated both elevated proliferative responses to mitogens (PHA) and depressed Con-A induced suppressor T cell activity (Lim *et al.*, 1975). It is suggested that this imbalance between T cell subsets might contribute to the occurrence of ENL reactions in these patients. In contrast, patients with lepromatous leprosy without ENL or tuberculoid forms of leprosy exhibited a normal immunological profile with monoclonal antibodies. Despite this there was a moderate decrease of proliferative responses to mitogens and impaired delayed-type hypersensitivity reactions (Bach and Bach, 1981). Further analysis of this heterogeneous group of disorders is needed in order to understand the complexity of these immune abnormalities.

(c) *Fungal*

(i). *Histoplasmosis* T cell subsets were studied during an epidemic of histoplasmosis. Acute histoplasmosis was associated with a low OKT4/ OKT8 ratio which reverted to normal if clinical recovery occurred within 6–10 weeks. Prolonged clinical disease was associated with prolongation of the OKT4/OKT8 ratio abnormality. Some patients who developed pulmonary cavitary forms of the disease with hypersensitivity and/or erythema nodosum exhibited elevated OKT4/ OKT8 ratios (R. Rubin, personal communication; Payan *et al.*, 1982).

Again these findings suggest that the microorganisms utilize immunosuppressive signals as part of their attack armamentarium and that the hypersensitivity phase of the disease may be due to other immunopathological mechanisms, perhaps autoimmune or allergic.

While these studies in infectious disease represent only an early beginning, analysis of these immunological changes should reveal new insights into the various factors determining the balance in host-parasite relations. If chronicity is widely due to spurious immunosuppressive signals generated by the invading microorganism, it raises the exciting possibility that immunoregulatory therapy could override this effect and provide a new treatment modality for some infectious diseases.

3. IMMUNE DEFICIENCY

The most common form of immune deficiency is common variable immune deficiency with acquired hypogammaglobulinemia. The majority of these cases have low OKT4/OKT8 ratios and in preliminary studies *in vitro* depletion of $OKT8^+$ T cells permits the development of pokeweed mitogen stimulated production of immunoglobulin by B cells (L. Chess, personal communication).

Other patients with acquired hypogammaglobulinemia revealed immunological abnormalities in T cell subsets ranging from a reduction of $OKT4^+$ T cell number and/or function to an increase of activated $OKT8^+$ T cells, as detected by the presence of the DR antigen. Some patients exhibited anti-helper T cell autoantibodies, but it is uncertain whether these antibodies were responsible for these changes (Thomas *et* al., 1981b; Reinherz et al., 1981 a, b; Rubinstein et al., 1981). It appears that hypogammaglobulinemia is generally associated with a lowered OKT4/OKT8 ratio, representative of either reduced helper activity or increased suppressor activity; however, at this time it is not possible to determine if the altered subset distribution is the cause or an effect of the disease.

Patients with primary immunodeficiencies exhibited a wide diversity of changes in T cell subset populations. Many patients demonstrated both decreased proportions of $OKT4^+$ T cells and increased proportions of $OKT8^+$ T cells resulting in a reversal of the normal OKT4/OKT8 ratio (Pandolfi et al., 1981; Bach and Bach, 1981; Phan-Dinh-Tuy et al., 1981). A variety of patterns have been detected and it is clearly necessary to extend these observations which may well result in a more definitive classification of primary immune deficiencies in terms of precise stages of maturational arrests.

4.  AUTOIMMUNE DISEASE

(a)  Rheumatic

(i). Rheumatoid arthritis   Patients with inactive rheumatoid arthritis (RA) were indistinguishable from controls with respect to their T cell levels and OKT4/OKT8 ratios. In contrast, patients with active RA had an elevated percentage of $OKT4^+$ cells, a reduced percentage of $OKT8^+$ cells and a decreased absolute number of $OKT8^+$ cells, resulting in an elevated OKT4/OKT8 ratio (Veys et al., 1981, 1982). This suggests that increased helper activity or decreased suppressor activity is associated with rheumatoid arthritis, a finding consonant with previous functional studies (Keystone et al., 1980).

Clinical studies in patients with active RA are currently underway using the antihelminthic drug levamisole (Janssen, 1976) and the immunoregulatory synthetic pentapeptide TP-5, which represents the active fragment of thymopoietin (Goldstein et al., 1979). Very preliminary monitoring of these regimens suggests that patients responding to treatment exhibit a fall of the previously elevated OKT4/OKT8 ratio levels (Fig. 3·3), and this may in turn explain the therapeutic mechanism of these immunoregulatory compounds.

(ii). Systemic lupus erythematosus   There are conflicting data concerning concerning the T cell subset alterations in patients with systemic lupus erythematosus (SLE). Morimoto et al., (1980a) showed a reduction in $OKT8^+$ ($OKT5^+$) T cells in active SLE patients, and concluded that a

significant correlation existed between the level of the OKT8⁺
(OKT5⁺) cells and clinical disease activity. The finding of autoantibodies to OKT8 (OKT5) T cells during active stages was postulated as
a possible mechanism to account for the decrease in the OKT8 T cell
population (Morimoto *et al.*, 1980b). It is important to note that
Morimoto *et al.*, may have specifically chosen a population of SLE
patients with autoantibodies and, therefore, may have evaluated a
selective group of SLE patients. In contrast to these findings,
Chatenoud and Bach (1981) and Chess *et al.*, (personal communication) observed a normal to increased level of OKT8⁺ T cells in the
majority of patients with active SLE. It should be noted, however, that
most patients studied by Chatenoud and Bach received maintenance
steroid therapy at the time of T cell analysis and that this may have
perturbed the underlying changes. Chess *et al.*, however, studied
untreated patients with active SLE. While additional studies are re-

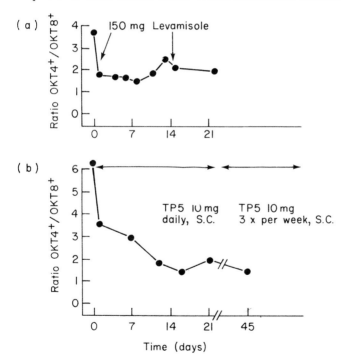

FIG. 3·3 Rheumatoid Arthritis. Change in immunoregulatory ratio (OKT4/OKT8)
with two immunomodulating agents, TP5 and Levamisole. (a) Arrows indicate the
time (days) levamisole was administered. (b) Arrows indicate the time (days) two
dosage schedules in which TP5 was administered by sub-cutaneons (S.C.) injection.
(data from Veys *et al.*, 1981a).

quired to evaluate T cell alterations in this disorder, preliminary findings suggest that the impaired suppression, which is a hallmark of SLE, may be due to defects in the immunoregulatory circuitry rather than a simple decrease of OKT8$^+$ T cells.

(iii). *Sjogren's syndrome*   Patients with Sjogren's syndrome, a disease characterized by lymphoid infiltration of exocrine glands and circulating autoantibodies (Tannenbaum *et al.*, 1975; Alspaugh and Tan, 1975) exhibited a marked increase in the proportion of OKT4$^+$ T cells and a decrease in OKT8$^+$ T cells in the peripheral blood. The increased OKT4/OKT8 ratio correlated well with the degree of lymphoid infiltration in lip biopsies, but not to specific autoantibodies or rheumatoid factor (Fox *et al.*, 1982). This suggests that the increased ratio is associated with but not necessarily the cause of the presence of autoantibodies.

(b) *Gastrointestinal*

(i). *Primary biliary cirrhosis*   Patients with primary biliary cirrhosis (PBC) demonstrated a significant reduction in the OKT4/OKT8 ratio due to a decrease in the OKT4$^+$ T cells in early PBC and a reduction of both OKT4$^+$ and OKT8$^+$ T cells in late PBC compared to normal controls and patients with extrahepatic cholestasis (Routhier *et al.*, 1980). A better prognosis resulted when patients exhibited a low OKT4/OKT8 ratio, shown to be associated with granulomatous changes, as compared to patients with a high OKT4/OKT8 ratio, without granulomatous changes, who manifested rapidly progressive disease (H. Thomas, personal communication). Treatment with cyclosporin A, a cyclic polypeptide, increased the proportion of OKT8$^+$ T cells and this was associated with clinical improvement. Although cyclosporin A appeared to act on the regulatory balance of the immune system, its role may be limited by renal toxicity and the possibility of an increased incidence of tumors, as shown with other immunosuppressants.

(ii). *Chronic active hepatitis*   Patients with autoimmune chronic active hepatitis exhibited an elevated OKT4/OKT8 ratio (Thomas, *et al.*, 1981). Concanavalin A proved ineffective in activating the OKT8$^+$ T cells in these patients which suggested that either a deficiency in suppressor activity or a defect in the suppressor cells themselves, rather than hyperactivity of the OKT4$^+$ T cells, may be responsible for the disease etiology (Hodgson *et al.*, 1978).

(c) *Neurologic*

(i). *Multiple sclerosis* There are some mild conflicts in the data concerning the T cell subset alterations in patients with multiple sclerosis (MS). Bach *et al.*, (1980) found that in patients with acute phase MS, the proportion of OKT4$^+$ cells increased and the proportion of OKT8$^+$ T cells decreased when compared to patients in remission or normal controls. This resulted in an elevated OKT4/OKT8 ratio. Interestingly, the absolute number of T cells (OKT3$^+$) was not significantly different in all forms of MS compared to controls. In contrast, Reinherz *et al.*, (1980d) reported a reduced percentage of OKT3$^+$ T cells in all patients with MS due to a selective decrease of OKT8$^+$ cells during periods of acute exacerbation, and a reappearance of OKT8$^+$ cells during periods of disease inactivity. This resulted in an increased OKT4/OKT8 ratio in patients with acute MS and a normalization of this ratio during periods of disease inactivity. The presence of a high OKT4/OKT8 ratio (lack of suppression) with active disease, recognized by both groups, is a provocative finding in relation to the pathogenesis of this disease.

(ii). *Myasthenia gravis* Patients with myasthenia gravis demonstrated an increased OKT4/OKT8 ratio due to a decrease of suppressor cells as determined by OKT8 reactivity and an *in vitro* mixed lymphocyte reaction. Patients also showed an increase in immature T cells, as defined by their simultaneous reaction with OKT4 and OKT8. Thymectomy resulted in the rapid removal of these immature cells, and a greater increase in the OKT4/OKT8 ratio (Berrih *et al.*, 1981). This suggests that clinical myasthenia gravis is associated with an increased OKT4/OKT8 ratio with thymectomy exacerbating this abnormality. These findings are consistent with an autoimmune etiology for myasthenia gravis, and the findings following thymectomy are consistent with the known effect of thymectomy in causing a loss of suppressor cells in animals.

(d) *Other*

Other autoimmune diseases for example, pemphigus vulgaris (Safai *et al.*, 1978; Berger *et al.*, 1981), hemolytic anemia (Bach and Bach, 1981), red cell aplasia and neutropenia (Callard *et al.*, 1981) and membranous glomerulonephritis (Chatenoud *et al.*, 1982; Chatenoud and Bach, 1981), revealed an increased OKT4/OKT8 ratio. Further work is needed in order to firmly establish whether these aberrations are truly associated with these diseases.

The general picture that emerges from most of these putative auto-immune diseases is that there does indeed seem to be a lack of suppressor cells as detected by the clinical state, functional assays and the OKT4/OKT8 ratio. One striking exception is SLE and in this case the present evidence is that the lack of suppression is due to defects in immunoregulatory circuits other than the lack of OKT8$^+$ T cells (L. Chess, personal communication).

## 5. ALLERGY

Patients with active atopic dermatitis (AD) revealed a selective reduction in the OKT8$^+$ T cells (17 out of 22 patients), a reduced percentage of OKT3$^+$ cells and normal levels of OKT4$^+$ T cells, resulting in an increase in the OKT4/OKT8 ratio (Leung et al., 1981). In contrast, healthy controls, patients with other skin diseases or respiratory allergic disease and 5 patients with a past history of AD with no active skin disease at the time of study revealed normal levels of OKT8$^+$ T cells. These findings suggested an association between active AD and reduced OKT8$^+$ cells, but further studies are required to substantiate this hypothesis.

In addition, a proportion of patients with hayfever due to ragweed pollen also revealed an increase in the OKT4/OKT8 ratio (Alexander and Norman, unpublished observations) but these very preliminary findings require extension.

## 6. AGING

Aging mice show clear abnormalities of their immune system and it has been suggested that this is related to thymic involution (Weksler et al., 1978; Goldberg et al., 1982). Similarly, older humans have detectable functional changes in their immune system (Inkeles et al., 1977; Weksler and Hutteroth, 1974). Moody et al., (1981) have shown that the T cell subsets in aging humans show a corresponding abnormality. They found an increase in the OKT4 subset and a decrease in the OKT8 subset, resulting in an elevated OKT4/OKT8 ratio. W. De Cock, et al. (personal communication) found that whereas half their aged population had this abnormality, one quarter showed normal OKT4/OKT8 ratios and the remaining quarter actually had low OKT4/OKT8 ratios. These findings suggest that the equilibrium of immuno-regulation is disturbed with aging, and that the majority of the elderly have moved towards a state of reduced suppression while another sizeable population has a relative increase in suppression. These findings are provocative with respect to susceptibility to disease with aging.

7. TRANSPLANTATION

(a) *Renal*

The monitoring of T cell subset levels and interrelationships has focused predominantly on immunosuppressed renal allograft recipients (Colvin *et al.*, 1981a). In the first few months following transplantation significant shifts of T cell subset ratios occurred. A normal to high OKT4/OKT8 ratio was permissive for renal allograft rejection, whereas rejection was rare in the presence of a low OKT4/OKT8 ratio. Studies showed this latter pattern to be associated with a higher risk of infection or even possibly due to activation of cytomegalovirus infection. Heavy immunosuppression in transplantation appeared to activate latent viruses, especially herpes simplex and cytomegalovirus (Cosimi *et al.*, 1981a, b). Therefore, the challenge now is not only to suppress allograft rejection but to individualize dosage regimens to prevent organ rejection without heightening the risk of infection. While it is not possible at this time to predict the precise time of rejection using this methodology, monitoring of immunosuppressive therapy enables the identification of patients at risk for rejection or infection, the institution of proper therapy and the successul monitoring of the patients' responses to therapy. This topic is more completely discussed in chapter 4 of this volume.

(b) *Bone Marrow*

Patients receiving bone marrow transplants for the treatment of acute leukemia or aplastic anemia demonstrated reduced levels of OKT4 and OKT8 cells post-transplant, resulting in a decrease in the OKT4/OKT8 ratio. $OKT8^+$ T cells began to recover within 3 months after transplant and subsequently remained at abnormally high levels for periods of several years (Atkinson *et al.*, 1982; de Bruin *et al.*, 1981). This reversal of the normal OKT4/OKT8 ratio occurred regardless of whether the recipient received an allogeneic, syngeneic or autologous transplant, and regardless of whether or not acute or chronic graft-versus-host disease (GVHD) developed. Recovery of the $OKT8^+$ subpopulation correlated with increasing time post-transplant and not with resolution of acute or chronic GVHD. These results do not support the findings of Reinherz *et al.* (1979e) who reported a total absence of the suppressor/cytotoxic subset in acute GVHD and that the reappearance of this subpopulation preceded the cessation of disease activity.

# VII THE FUTURE OF MONOCLONAL ANTIBODIES TO HUMAN T-LYMPHOCYTES

## A. Increased Understanding of Immunoregulation

It is well established that the immune system consists of a multitude of cellular components that interact in a balanced fashion. The overall responsiveness of the system is affected by both chemical and endocrine signals and modifications of its cellular constituents. Imbalance of any one of these parameters, singly or in combination, could each contribute to immune abnormalities. Previously, the analysis of immunologic alterations that occur in human disease has relied upon measuring the functional status of the immune system. The recent application of hybridoma technology using monoclonal antibodies based upon the precise recognition of the functional components of the immune system offers the potential for expanding our understanding of immunoregulation in man and for detecting immunoregulatory abnormalities that occur in disease.

## B. Enhanced Detection of Immunoregulatory Disorders

Although studies with monoclonal antibodies are still in their infancy it is clear already that distinct patterns are emerging. In advanced cancer, chronic infections and certain immunodeficiencies an imbalance favoring excess suppression can be detected. By contrast in a number of putative autoimmune diseases and certain allergic diseases an imbalance with deficient suppression can be detected. In aging the immune system appears to become imbalanced, usually in the direction of defective suppression but also in some cases in the direction of enhanced suppression.

It is clear that these early studies will need to be expanded over the next few years with the development of a full description of these diseases in terms of the immunoregulatory abnormalities detected by monoclonal antibodies to differentiation antigens defining functional subsets of lymphocytes. Also of great interest will be the study of diseases such as diabetes, atherosclerosis and hypertension where immune mechanisms are implicated in the pathogenesis but not yet clearly established.

Several examples can be cited to highlight the immediate clinical utility of monoclonal antibodies. For example, one patient with multiple sclerosis exhibited a defect in suppressor T cells one week before the clinical onset of an exacerbation (Bach *et al.*, 1980). Four out of five patients at risk for primary CMV infection developed a reversal of their OKT4/OKT8 ratio in conjunction with the onset of acute CMV infection (Rubin *et al.*, 1981). One renal transplant patient without CMV infection, but with four separate opportunistic infections postoperatively, was shown to have a markedly decreased OKT4/OKT8 ratio, a ratio indicative of an increased susceptibility to infection. Finally, the OKT4/OKT8 ratio provided important clues for the differential diagnosis of patients with a fever of unknown origin (FUO) and other manifestations of inflammatory disease, e.g. influenza, S. viridans, S. aureus (R. Rubin, personal communication). Thus, although the utility of lymphocyte subpopulation measurement in clinical disease is only at an early stage, it is possible that such information will be useful not only in predicting the risk of infection and categorizing the type of infection, but also in helping the clinician to understand the host's immune response to the infection.


C. MONITORING THERAPEUTIC PROGRESS

The monitoring of a patient's response to therapy utilizing monoclonal antibodies to T cell subsets has revealed information concerning the type of disease, the course of the disease and the dosage regimen needed to control the disease process. For example, the immunosuppressive therapy used in transplantation and the rejection processes that follow placement of the graft appear to activate latent virus e.g. cytomegalovirus. CMV has been shown to be an important pathogen in renal transplant patients, causing a variety of infectious disease syndromes, predisposing to potentially lethal superinfection and, perhaps, producing allograft dysfunction. The monitoring of T cell subsets with monoclonal antibodies has enabled a reduction in the dose of immunosuppressive drugs administered, without jeopardizing organ rejection, and has led to positive effects on the course of the CMV infection. This lymphocyte population data has also allowed the clinician to distinguish between two types of kidney damage, that caused by CMV infection (diffuse glomerulopathy) or that caused by the rejection process (tubulointerstitial changes), thus permitting proper therapy to be instituted (Richardson *et al.*, 1981). Finally, the risk of organ rejection can be predicted by monitoring the OKT4/OKT8 ratio and proper therapy can be instituted accordingly.

Patients with rheumatoid arthritis (RA) revealed an increased OKT4/OKT8 ratio due to a decrease on OKT8$^+$ T cells. Administration of the immunoregulatory synthetic peptide TP-5 or the anti-helminthic drug levamisole to patients with active RA demonstrated both a normalization of this ratio and the induction of clinical remission. It is apparent that while the monitoring of therapeutic regimens with monoclonal antibodies is still in an early stage this technology has already proven invaluable in the successful evaluation of various immunoregulatory and immunosuppressive therapies.

### D. Novel Therapeutic Applications

Monoclonal antibodies offer the potential for the production of a highly specific therapeutic agent which can be reproducibly manufactured to clinical standards of purity and consistency. Pan-T reagents (OKT1, OKT3, OKT11), which react selectively with peripheral human T cells, are being developed for these purposes. For example, OKT3 (which appears to exert direct immunosuppressive activities as well as initiating the removal of T cells from the circulation) (Chang *et al.*, 1981) is currently being utilized *in vivo* as an immunosuppressive drug for patients undergoing acute rejection of histocompatible renal grafts and *in vitro* for the prevention of graft versus host disease in recipients of bone marrow transplants (see Chapter 4).

Monoclonal antibodies are also being developed for the treatment of leukemia (Miller *et al.*, 1981; Hatzubai *et al.*, 1981; Ritz *et al.*, 1980). In this procedure, leukemic reactive monoclonal antibodies could be used to treat patients directly or to ablate leukemic cells in a patient's bone marrow sample *in vitro*, followed by the transplantation of the remaining bone marrow stem cells into the patient after whole body irradiation. A variation of this procedure might be the conjugation of monoclonal antibodies to specific toxins to selectively eliminate leukemic cells *in vitro* prior to transplantation. Experimental models demonstrating this technique have been successfully carried out.

The production of monoclonal antibodies by the hybridoma technique is clearly an innovative force in clinical immunology. In the area of human T cell differentiation, it is already clear that monoclonal antibodies to human T cell differentiation antigens offer the potential for expanding our understanding of immunoregulation in man and for detecting immunoregulatory abnormalities that occur in disease.

Furthermore, these reagents should have practical utility in evaluating immunoregulatory therapies and are currently being used as therapeutic agents themselves.

REFERENCES

Abramson, C. S., Kersey, J. H. and LeBien, T. W. (1981). *J. Immunol.* **126**, 83–88.
Aisenberg, A. C. and Wilkes, B. M. (1981). *J. exp. Med.* **152**, 1126–1131.
Alspaugh, M. and Tan, E. (1975). *J. clin. Invest.* **55**, 1067–1073.
Atkinson K., Hansen J. A., Storb, R., Goehle, S., Goldstein, G. and Thomas, E. D. (1982). *Blood* (in press).
Bach, M-A. and Bach, J-F. (1981). *Int. J. Immunopharmacol.* **3**, 269–273.
Bach, M-A., Phan-Dinh-Tuy, F., Tournier, E., Chatenoud, L., Bach, J-F., Martin, C. and Degos, J. D. (1980). *Lancet* ii, 1221–1223.
Bach, M-A., Chatenoud, L., Wallach, D., Phan-Dinh-Tuy, F. and Cottenot, S. (1981). *Clin. exp. Immunol.* **44**, 491–500.
Barnstable, C. J., Bodmer, W. F., Brown, G., Galfa, G., Milstein, C. and Williams, A. F. (1978). *Cell* **14**, 9–21.
Berger, C. L., Warburton, D., Raafat, J., LoGerfo, P., and Edelson, R. L. (1979). *Blood* **53**, 642–651.
Berger, C. L., Kung, P. C., Goldstein, G., DePietro, W. Takezaki, S., Chu, A., Fithian, E. and Edelson, R. L. (1981). *Int. J. Immunopharmacol.* **3**, 275–282.
Berrih, S., Gaud, C., Bach, M-A., LeBrigand, H., Binet, J. P. and Bach, J-F. (1981). *Clin. exp. Immunol.* **45**, 1–8.
Bhan, A. I., Reinherz, E. L., Poppema, S., McCluskey, R. T. and Schlossman, S. F. (1980). *J. exp. Med.* **152**, 771–782.
Bradstock, K. F., Janossy, G., Pizzolo, G., Hoffbrand, A. V., McMichael, A., Pilch, J. R., Milstein, C., Beverley, P. and Bollum, F. J. (1980). *J. natn. Cancer Inst.* **65**, 33–42.
Breard, J., Reinherz, E. L., Kung, P. C., Goldstein, G. and Schlossman, S. F. (1980). *J. Immunol.* **124**, 1943–1948.
Callard, R. E., Smith, C. M., Worman, C., Linch, D., Cawley, J. C. and Beverly, P. C. L. (1981). *Clin. exp. Immunol.* **43**, 497–505.
Cantor, H. and Boyse, E. A. (1975). *J. exp. Med.* 141, 1376–1389.
Carney, W. P., Rubin, R. H., Hoffman, R. A., Hansen, W. P., Healey, K. and Hirsch, M. S. (1981). *J. Immunol.* **126**, 2114–2116.
Chang, T. W., Kung, P. C., Gingras, S. P. and Goldstein, G. (1981). *Proc. natn. Acad. Sci. U.S.A.* **78**, 1805–1808.
Chatenoud, L. and Bach, M-A. (1981). *Kidney Int.* **20**, 267–274.
Chatenoud, L., Bach, M-A., Jungers, P. and Bach, J-F. (1982). *Immunol. Lett.* (in press).
Colvin, R., Cosimi, S. B., Burton, R., Goldstein, G., Kung, P. C., Rubin, R., Herrin, J. T., Fuller, T. C., Delmonico, F. L. and Russell, P. S. (1981). *In*, "Proc. of 8th Int. Congress of Nephrology" 990–996.

Cosimi, A. B., Colvin, R. B., Burton, R. C., Rubin, R. H., Goldstein, G., Kung P. C., Hansen, W. P., Delmonico, F. L. and Russell, P. S. (1981a). *N. Engl. J. Med.* **305**, 308–314.

Cosimi, A. B., Colvin, R., Burton, R. C., Winn, H. J., Rubin, R., Goldstein, G., Kung, P. C., Hoffman, R. A., Hansen, W. P. and Russell, P. S. (1981b). *Transpl. proc.* **XIII**, 1589–1593.

Crawford, D. H., Francis, G. E., Wing, M. A., Edwards, A. J., Janossy, G., Hoffbrand, A. V., Prentice, H. G., Secher, D., McConnell, I., Kung, P. C. and Goldstein, G. (1981a). *Br. J. Haemotol.* **49**, 209–217.

Crawford, D. H., Brickell, P., Tidman, N., McConnell, I., Hoffbrand, A. V. and Janossy, G. (1981b). *Clin. exp. Immunol.* **43**, 291–297.

de Bruin, H. G., Astaldi, A., Leupers, T., van de Griend R. J., Dooren, L. J., Schellekens, P. T. A., Tanke, H. J., Roos, M. and Vossen J. M. (1981). *J. Immunol.* **127**, 244–251.

De Waele, M., De Mey, J., Moeremans, M. and Van Camp. B. K. G. (1981a). *In* "Leukemia Markers" (W. Knapp, ed.). Academic Press; London and New York (in press).

De Waele, M., Thielmans, C. and Van Camp, B. K. G. (1981b). *N. Engl. J. Med.* **304**, 460–462.

Druguet, M. and Pepys, M. B. (1977). *Clin. exp. Immunol.* **29**, 162–167.

Engleman, E. G., Warnke, R., Fox, R. I., Dilley, J., Benike, C. J. and Levy, R. (1981). *Proc. natn. Acad. Sci. U.S.A.* **78**, 1791–1795.

Evans, R. L., Wall, D. W., Platsoucas, C. D., Siegal, F. P., Fikrig, S. M., Testa, C. M. and Good, R. A. (1981) *Proc. natn. Acad. Sci. U.S.A.* **78**, 544–548.

Fithian, E., Kung, P., Goldstein, G., Rubenfeld, M., Fenoglio, C. and Edelson, R. (1981). *Proc. natn. Acad. Sci. U.S.A.* **78**, 2541–2544.

Fox, R., Kung, P. and Levy, R. (1981). *In*, "Lymphocyte Differentiation" (N. Warner, Ed.) Academic Press, London and New York.

Fox, R. I., Carstens, S. A., Fong, S., Robinson, C.A., Howell, F. and Vaughan, J. H. (1982). *Arthritis Rheum.* (in press).

Friedman, S. M., Hunter, S. B., Irigoyen, O. H., Kung, P. C., Goldstein, G. and Chess, L. (1981). *J. Immunol.* **126**, 1702–1705.

Ginns, L. C., Goldenheim, P. D., Miller, L. G., Burton, R. C., Gillick, L., Colvin, R. B., Goldstein, G., Kung, P. C., Hurwitz, C. and Kazemi, H. (1981) *N. Engl. J. Med.* (submitted).

Goldberg, E. H., Goldstein, G., Boyse, E. A., Scheid, M. P. (1982). *Immunogenetics* (in press).

Goldstein, G. Scheid, M. P., Boyse, E. A., Schlesinger, D. H. and Van Wauwe, J. (1979). *Science* **204**, 1309–1310.

Greaves, M.F., Delia, D., Sutherland, R., Rao, J., Verbi, W., Kemshead, J., Hariri, G., Goldstein, G. and Kung, P. (1981). *Int. J. Immunopharmacol.* **3**, 283–299.

Hansen, J., Martin, P., Kamoun, M., Torok-Storb, B., Newman, M., Nowinski, R. and Thomas, E. (1980a). *Transpl. Proc.* **XIII**, 1133–1137.

Hansen, J., Martin, P. and Nowinski, R. (1980b). *Immunogenetics* **10**, 247–260.

Hatzubai, A., Maloney, D. G. and Levy, R. (1981). *J. Immunol.* **126**, 2397–2402.

Haynes, B. F., Mann, D. L., Hemler, M. E., Schroer, J. A., Shelhamer, J. H., Eisenbarth, G. S., Strominger, J. L., Thomas, C. A., Mostowski, H. S. and Fauci, A. S. (1980). *Proc. natn. Acad. Sci. U.S.A.* **77**, 2914–2918.

Heusermann, U., Stutte, H. J. and Muller-Hermelink, H. K. (1974). *Cell Tiss. Res.* **153**, 415–417.

Hodgson, H. J. F., Wands, J. R. and Isselbacher, K. J. (1978). *Proc. natn. Acad. Sci. U.S.A.* **75**, 1549–1553.

Hoffman, R. A., Kung, P. C., Hansen, W. P. and Goldstein, G. (1980). *Proc. natn. Acad. Sci. U.S.A.* **77**, 4914–4917.

Inkeles, B., Innes, J. B., Kuntz, M. M., Kadish, A. S. and Weksler, M. E. (1977). *J. exp. Med.* **145**, 1176–1187.

Jandinski, J., Cantor, H., Tadakuma, T., Peavy, D. L. and Pierce, C. (1976). *J. exp. Med.* **143**, 1382–1390.

Janossy, G., Tidman, N., Selby, W. S., Thomas, J. A., Granger, S., Kung, P. C., Goldstein, G. (1980). *Nature* **288**, 81–84.

Janossy, G., Thomas, J. A., Goldstein, G. and Bollum, F. J. (1981a). *In*, "Ciba Foundation Symposium 84" (J. H. Humphrey, Ed.), pp. 193–213. Pitman Medical, London.

Janossy, G., Tidman, N., Papageorgiou, E. S., Kung, P. C. and Goldstein, G. (1981b). *J. Immunol.* **126**, 1608–1613.

Janssen, P. A. J. (1976). *Prog. Res.* **20**, 347–83.

Johnsen, H. E., Madsen, M., Kristensen, T. and Kissmeyer-Nielson, F. (1978). *Acta. pathol. microbiol. scand.* **86**, 307–314.

Kaiserling, E., Stein, H. and Muller-Hermelink, H. K. (1974). *Cell Tiss. Res.* **155**, 47–55.

Kamoun, M., Martin, P. J., Hansen, J. A., Brown, M. A., Siadek, A. W. and Nowinski, R. C. (1981). *J. exp. Med.* **153**, 207–212.

Kay, H. D. and Horwitz, D. A. (1980) *J. clin. Invest.* **66**, 847–851.

Kersey, J. H., LeBien, T. W., Gajl-Peczalska, K., Nesbit, M., Jansen, J., Kung, P., Goldstein, G., Sather, H., Coccia, P., Siegel, S., Bleyer, A. and Hammond, D. (1981). *In*, "Leukemia Marker" (W. Knapp, Ed.) Academic Press, London and New York.

Keystone, E. C., Gladman, D. D., Buchanan, R., Cane, D. and Poplonski, L. (1981). *Arthritis Rheum.* **23**, 1246–1250.

Kohler, G. and Milstein, C. (1975). *Nature* (London) 256, 495–497.

Koprowski, H., Steplewski, Z., Herlyn, D. and Herlyn, M. (1978). *Proc. natn. Acad. Sci.* U.S.A. **71**, 3405–3409.

Kung, P. C. and Goldstein, G. (1980). *Vox Sanguinis* **39**, 121–127.

Kung, P. C., Goldstein, G., Reinherz, E. L. and Schlossman, S. F. (1979). *Science* **206**, 347–349.

Kung, P. C., Talle, M. A., DeMaria, M. E., Butler, M. S., Lifter, J. and Goldstein, G. (1980). *Transpl. Proc.* **XII** (Suppl. 1), 141–146.

Kung, P. C., Berger, C. L., Goldstein, G., LoGerfo, P. and Edelson, R. L. (1981). *Blood* **57**, 261–266.

Lampert, I. A., Pizzolo, G., Thomas, J. A. and Janossy, G. (1981). *J. Path.* (in press).

Lau, C. Y., Wang, E. Y. and Goldstein, G. (Unpublished observations).

Ledbetter, J. A., Evans, R. L., Lipinski, M., Cunningham-Rundles, C., Good, R. A. and Herzenberg, L. A. (1981). *J. exp. Med.* **153**, 310–323.

Leung, D. Y. M., Rhodes, A. R. and Geha, R. S. (1981). *J. Allergy Clin. Immunol.* (in press).

Levy, R., Dilley, J., Fox, R. I. and Warnke, R. (1979). Proc. *natn. Acad. Sci. U.S.A.* **76**, 6552–6556.

Lim, S. D., Jacobsen, R. R., Park, B. M. and Good, R. A. (1975). *Int. J. Lepr.* **43**, 95–100.

Martin, P. J., Hansen, J. A., Nowinski, R. C. and Brown, M. A. (1980). *Immunogenetics* **11**, 429–439.

McKenzie, I. F. C. and Potter, T. (1979). *Adv. Immunol.* **27**, 181–371.

McMichael, A. J., Pilch, J. R., Galfre, G., Mason, D. Y., Fabre, J. W. and Milstein, C. (1979). *Eur. J. Immunol.* **9**, 205–210.

Miller, R. A., Maloney, D. G., McKillop, J. and Levy, R. (1981). *Blood* **58**, 78–86.

Moody, C. E., Innes, J. B., Staiano-Coico, L., Incefy, G. S., Thaler, H. T., and Weksler, M. E. (1981). *Immunology* (in press).

Moretta, L., Ferrarin, M., Mingari, A., Moretta, A. and Webb, S. R. (1976). *J. Immunol.* **117**, 2171–2174.

Morimoto, C., Reinherz, E. L., Scholssman, S. F., Schur, P. H., Mills, J. A. and Steinberg, A. D. (1980a). *J. clin. Invest.* **66**, 1171–1174.

Morimoto, C., Reinherz, E. L., Abe, T., Homma, M. and Schlossman, S. F. (1980b). *Clin. Immunol. Immunopathol.* **16**, 474–484.

Morison, W. L., Parrish, J. A., Moscicki, R. and Bloch, K. J. (1981). *Clin. Res.* **29**, 608A.

Moscicki, R., Morison, W., Bloch, K. J., Parrish, J. and Colvin, R. B. (1981). *Clin. Res.* **29**, 373A.

Owen, J. J. T. and Ritter, M. A. (1969). *J. exp. med.* **129**, 431–437.

Pandolfi, F., Quinti, I., Frielingsdorf, F., Goldstein, G., Businco, L. and Aiuti, F. (1982). *clin. Immunol. Immunopathol.* **22**, 323–330.

Payan, D. G., Wheat, L. J., Ip, S., Hansen, W. P., Hoffman, R. A. Healey, C., Brahmi, Z. and Rubin, R. H. (1982). In "Proc. Interscience Conf. Antimicrobial Agents and Chemotherapy (in press).

Pepys, E. O. and Pepys, M. B. (1980). *J. Immunol. Methods* **32**, 305–314.

Pepys, E. O., Tennent, G. A. and Pepys, M. B. (1981). *Clin. exp. Immunol.* **46**, 229–234.

Phan-Dinh-Tuy, F., Durandy, A., Griscelli, C and Bach, M-A. (1981). *Scand. J. Immunol.* **14**, 193–200.

Poppema, S., Elema, J. D. and Halie, M. R. (1979). *Int. J. Cancer* **24**, 532–540.

Poppema, S., Bhan, A. K., Reinherz, E. L., McCluskey, R. T. and Schlossman, S. F. (1981). *J. exp. Med.* **152**, 30–41.

Reinherz, E. L., Kung, P. C., Goldstein, G. and Scholssman, S. F. (1979a). *J. Immunol.* **124**, 1312–1317.

Reinherz, E. L., Kung, P. C., Goldstein, G. and Schlossman, S. F. (1979b). *Proc. natn. Acad. Sci. U.S.A.* **76**, 4061–4066.

Reinherz, E. L., Kung, P. C., Goldstein, G. and Schlossman, S. F. (1979c). *J. Immunol.* **123** 2894–2896.

Reinherz, E. L., Kung, P. C., Pesando, J. M., Ritz, J., Goldstein, G. and Schlossman, S. F. (1979d). *J. exp. Med.* **150**, 1472–1482.

Reinherz, E. L., Parkman, R., Rappeport, J., Rosen, F. S. and Schlossman, S. F. (1979e). *New. Engl. J. Med.* **300**, 1061–1068.

Reinherz, E. L., Kung, P. C., Goldstein, G. and Schlossman, S. F. (1980a). *J. Immunol.* **124**, 1301–1307.

Reinherz, E. L., Kung, P. C., Goldstein, G., Levey, R. H. and Schlossman, S. F. (1980b). *Proc. natn. Acad. Sci. U.S.A.* **77**, 1588–1592.

Reinherz, E. L., O'Brien, C., Rosenthal, P. and Schlossman, S. F. (1980c). *J. Immunol.* **125**, 1269–1274.

Reinherz, E. L. Weiner, H. L., Hauser, S. L., Cohen, J. A., Distaso, J. A. and Schlossman, S. F. (1980d). *New Engl. J. Med.* **303**, 125–129.

Reinherz, E. L., Cooper, M. D., Schlossman, S. F. and Rosen, F. S. (1981). *J. clin. Invest.* **68**, 699–705.

Reinherz, E. L., Geha, R., Wohl, M. E., Morimoto, C., Rosen, F. S. and Schlossman, S. F. (1981b). *New Engl. J. Med.* **304**, 811–816.

Ritz, J., Pesando, J. M., Notis-McConarty, J., Lazarus, H. and Schlossman, S. F. (1980). *Nature* **283**, 583–585.

Routhier, G., Janossy, G., Epstein, O., Thomas, H. C. and Sherlock,S. (1980). *Lancet* ii, 1223–1226.

Royston, I., Majda, J., Baird, S., Meserve, B., Ivor, C. and Griffiths, J. (1980). *Blood* **54** (suppl 1) 106a.

Richardson, W. P., Colvin, R. B., Cheeseman, S. H., Tolkoff-Rubin, N. E., Herrin, J. T., Cosimi, A. B., Collins, A. B., Hirsch, M. S., McCluskey, R. T., Russell, P. S. and Rubin, R. H. (1981). *New. Engl. J. Med.* **305**, 57–63.

Rubin, R. H., Cosimi, A. B., Tolkoff-Rubin, N. B., Russell, P. S. and Hirsch, M. S. (1977). *Transplant.* **24**, 458–1164.

Rubin, R. H., Carney, W. P., Schooley, R. T., Colvin, R. B., Burton, R. C., Hoffman, R. A., Hansen, W. P., Cosimi, A. B., Russell, P. S. and Hirsch, M. S. (1981). *Int. J. Immunopharmacol.* **3**, 307–312.

Rubinstein, A., Sicklick, M., Mehra, V., Rosen, F. S. and Levey, R. H. (1981). *J. Clin. Invest.* **67**, 42–50.

Safai, B., Gupta, S. and Good, R. A. (1978). *Clin. exp. Dermat.* **3**, 129–134.

Shen, F. W., Hwang, S. M. and Boyse, E. A. (1978). *Immunogenetics* **6**, 389–396.

Strelkauskas, A. J., Schauf, V., Wilson, B. S., Chess, L. and Schlossman, S. F. (1978). *J. Immunol.* **120**, 1278–1282.

Sutherland, R., Delia, D., Schneider, C., Newman, R., Kemshead, J. and Greaves, M. (1981). *Proc. natn. Acad. Sci. U.S.A.* **78**, 4515–4519.

Tannenbaum, H., Pinkus, G., Anderson, L. and Schur, P. (1975). *Arthritis Rheum.* **18**, 305–314.

Thomas, H. C., Brown, D., Routhier, G., Janossy, G., Kung, P. C., Goldstein, G. and Sherlock, S. (1981). *Int. J. Immunopharmacol* **3**, 301–305.

Thomas, Y., Sosman, J., Irigoyen, O., Friedman, S. M., Kung, P. C., Goldstein, G. and Chess, L. (1980). *J. Immunol.* **125**, 2401–2408.

Thomas, Y., Sosman, J., Rogozinski, L., Irigoyen, O., Kung, P. C., Goldstein, G. and Chess, L. (1981a). *J. Immunol.* **126**, 1948–1951.

Thomas, Y., Sosman, J., Irigoyen, O., Rogozinski, L., Friedman, S. M. and Chess, L. (1981b). *Int. J. Immunopharmacol.* **3**, 193–201.

Thomas, Y., Rogozinski, L., Irigoyen, O., Friedman, S. M., Kung, P. C., Goldstein, G. and Chess, L. (1981c) *J. exp. Med.* **154**, 459–467.

Tidman, N., Janossy, G., Bodger, M., Granger, S., Kung, P. C. and Goldstein, G. (1981). *Clin. exp. Immunol.* **45**, 437–467.

Tosato, G., Magrath, I., Koski, I., Dooley, N. and Blaese, M. (1979). *New. Engl. J. Med.* **301**, 1133–1137.

Trucco, M. M., Stocker, J. W. and Cepellini, R. (1978). *Nature* (London) **273**, 666–668.

Uchiyama, T., Broder, S. and Waldmann, T. (1981a). *J. Immunol.* **126**, 1393–1398.

Uchiyama, T., Nelson, D. L., Fleisher, T. A. and Waldmann, T. A. (1981b). *J. Immunol.* **126**, 1398–1403.

Verbi, W., Greaves, M. F., Schneider, C., Konbet, K., Janossy, G., Stein, H., Kung, P. and Goldstein, G. (1982). *Eur. J. Immunol.* (in press).

Veys, E. M., Hermanns, P., Goldstein, G., Kung, P., Schindler, J. and Van Wauwe, J. (1981a). *Int. J. Immunopharmacol.* **3**, 313–319.

Veys, E. M., Hermanns, P., Schindler, J., Kung, P. C., Goldstein, G., Symoens, J. and Van Wauwe, J. (1982) *J. Rheumatol.* (in press).

Wang, C., Good, R. A., Ammeratti, P., Dymbort, G. and Evans, R. (1980). *J. exp. Med.* **151**, 1539–1544.

Weksler, M. E. and Hutteroth, T. H. (1974). *J. clin. Invest.* **53**, 99–104.

Weksler, M. E., Innes, J. B. and Goldstein, G. (1978). *J. exp. med.* **148**, 996–1006.

Wybran, J. H. and Fudenberg, H. H. (1971). *Trans. Ass. Am. Physns.* **84**, 239–244.

Zarling, J. M. and Kung, P. C. (1980). *Nature* **288**, 394–396.

# 4 Monoclonal Anti Human Lymphocyte Antibodies: their potential value in immunosuppression and bone marrow transplantation

GEORGE JANOSSY,[a] GIDEON GOLDSTEIN[b] AND
A. BENEDICT COSIMI[c]

[a] *Department of Immunology, Royal Free Hospital School of Medicine, Pond Street, London NW3 2QG.*
[b] *Ortho Pharmaceutical Corporation, Immunobiology Division, Raritan, New Jersey 08869. U.S.A.*
[c] *Transplantation Immunology Unit, Massachusets General Hospital and Department of Surgery, Harvard Medical School, Boston, Mass. 02114. U.S.A.*

## I INTRODUCTION

Immunosuppression and passive immunotherapy with heterologous antisera has been one of the major aims of experimental and clinical immunologists in the last two decades. Extensive studies in rodents, dogs and men have already defined the potential applications and, to some extent, the limitations of this approach. It is, therefore, obligatory to discuss the uses of monoclonal antibodies in the light of this previous experience. In this review we summarize the main similarities and differences in using conventional heterologous antisera as compared to monoclonal antibodies, and concentrate mainly on the potential uses of anti-lymphocyte reagents (anti-lymphocyte globulin, ALG). The most extensively characterized heterologous antisera of this kind have been made against human thymocytes and referred to as anti-thymocyte globulin (ATG).

The first well documented strong reduction in tuberculin and delayed type hypersensitivity reaction following the treatment of guinea pigs with rabbit anti-guinea pig ALG was demonstrated by Waksman and his colleagues in 1961. An upsurge of activities followed which coincided with the delineation of the main basic concepts of modern cellular immunology. After the administration of ALG and ATG longer skin allograft survivals as well as suppression of antibody responses to various antigens were demonstrated in rats and mice, and the survival of allogeneic kidney transplants in dogs has also been prolonged (Woodruff and Anderson, 1963; Gray *et al.*, 1964; Levey and Medawar, 1966; Monaco *et al.*, 1966). When the first successful results of clinical immunosuppression were also obtained with ATG (Starzl *et al.*, 1967) and these results were discussed at the Conference on Transplantation held at Santa Barbara (1967) it appeared that the age of ATG in clinical medicine had arrived. Nevertheless, the progress during the next 14 years has been frustratingly slow, and in retrospect it is easy to see the reasons why this was so (see below). The important point, however, is that during these years the role of ATG in clinical medicine has indeed been established (Table 4·1) and the most salient observations have been summarized at the two latest meetings of the Transplantation Society in New York and Boston (1976, 1980).

## II STANDARDIZATION OF ANTI THYMOCYTE GLOBULIN (ATG)

### A. PREPARATION OF ATG FOR USE *IN VIVO*

#### 1. PRODUCTION OF ANTISERA

Various experimental and commercial ATG and ALG preparations (made in rabbits and horses) were used as immunosuppressive agents in human kidney transplantation with variable success (reviewed by Groth, 1981). Since 1968 large quantities of well characterized horse-ATG (ATGAM; more than 30 separate large batches each comprising >20,000 vials of 250 mg IgG) were produced by the Upjohn Company. Many of these were distributed for multicentre prospective controlled trials bringing a new element of relative comparability into these studies. The brief principles of ATG production are described here in order to show some of the problems of standardization of conventional ATG. These are based on the methods used for the preparation of ATGAM by Wechter *et al.*, (1979).

Human thymocyte suspensions are freed of connective tissue. This tissue has to be removed because emulsions of whole organs used as immunogen would produce damaging antibodies to kidney glomerular basement membrane. Cell suspensions, pooled from 6 thymuses, are suspended in pertussis vaccine and emulsified in adjuvant. Repeated

TABLE 4·1

The major potential clinical uses of antisera and monoclonal antibodies to cells of the T lymphocyte lineage[a]

Treatment of patients *in vivo*[b]
  1. immunosuppression in
      a. renal transplants[1, 2, 7]
      b. skin allografts[1, 8]
      c. aplastic anaemia[1, 3]
      d. treatment of graft versus host disease[4]
  2. anti-leukaemia agents in
      a. T cell leukaemia/lymphoma (T-CLL, Sezary syndrome)[5]
      b. thymic acute lymphoblastic leukaemia (Thy-ALL)[9]

Treatment of bone marrow cell suspension *in vitro*[b]
  1. immunosuppression in allogeneic BM transplant; to prevent graft versus host disease[6, 10]
  2. anti-leukaemia antibody in autologous BM transplant; to eliminate residual Thy-ALL or T lymphoma prior to re-transplantation[11]

[a] Some of the key references about the uses of ATG in patients are as follows: 1. Cosimi (1981); 2. Monaco *et al.*, (1967); 3. Speck *et al.*, (1977); Grathwohl *et al.*, (1981); Marmont *et al.*, (1975); 4. Successful in Minnesota (Kersey *et al.*, 1981) but less effective in Seattle (Doney *et al.*, 1981); 5. Barrett *et al.*, (1976); Edelson *et al.*, (1979); 6. Rodt *et al.*, (1981). The following representative animal experiments are relevant: 7. Abaza *et al.*, 1966; 8. Monaco *et al.*, (1966b); Levey and Medawar. (1966); 9. Old *et al.*, (1967); 10. Kolb *et al.*, (1979). Rodt *et al.*, (1974); 11. Thierfelder *et al.*, (1977).

[b] The standardization procedures for the various administrations of ATG *in vivo* and *in vitro* are different. This is because the treatment of cells *in vitro* require more specific reagents than the ATG used *in vivo* (see text).

multiple injections (equivalent to 1-5 × $10^9$ thymocytes) are given fortnightly to horses at variable sites over a 3 month period. Plasma is pooled from several horses and IgG fractions are made using Rivanol. These batches are absorbed with erythocyte stroma (to reduce haemagglutin titer) and with insolubilized human plasma proteins. After the removal of Rivanol and the residual $\beta$-globulins, the sterile hepatitis B antigen free non-pyrogenic solution (pH 6.3) can be stored for longer than 2 years in sealed vials. Other preparations are sometimes also absorbed with human placenta but only exceptionally with other tissues. These technical points demonstrate that with relatively simple steps, such as the elimination of connective tissue from the immunizing material and some minimal absorption with erythocyte stroma, an effective production protocol can be designed. Further sophistication of the method (e.g. directed absorptions) with a material prepared in such a large scale cannot be achieved without uneconomically strenuous efforts.

2. STANDARDIZATION OF ANTI LYMPHOCYTE
GLOBULIN (ALG) AND (ATG)

The two major areas of investigations in respect of heterologous ATG preparations are the study of efficacy (assays of potency) and assays of cellular specificity. The first question is whether the ATG is an effective immunosuppressive drug when used *in vivo*, a different consideration from whether it is fully T lymphocyte specific. It is interesting to observe that during the first years of studies with ATG (until its possible use in bone marrow transplantation was brought forward; Rodt *et al.*, 1974, Thierfelder *et al.*, 1977) the second question was almost totally neglected or focussed exclusively on selected aspects of immediate concern such as the presence of antibodies to glomerular basement membrane, erythrocytes and platelets (see review by Lance *et al.*, 1973). In contrast, during the last three years monoclonal antibodies have been primarily analyzed for their cellular specificity, and until very recently little was known about their efficacy *in vivo* (see below).

(a) *Potential tests for efficacy*
These are "influenced" by our knowledge of how ATG might work (Fig. 4·1) and, irrespective of this theoretical knowledge, ultimately include controlled clinical trials. The preliminary role of assays of potency is to increase the chances of success *in vivo* and to restrict the clinical trials to the absolute minimum.
    Four major mechanisms may contribute to the immunosuppressive

effects of ATG (Fig. 4·1). First, lymphocytes are lysed by ATG in the presence of complement, and this process may contribute to the lymphocytopenia (Fig. 4·1(a); Monaco *et al.*, 1966). Nevertheless ATG preparations with similar suppressive capacity have often shown variable cytotoxic titers (Greaves *et al.*, 1969) and inhibit the immune system of mice which have low levels of lytic complement. Second, according to the "coating" or "blind-folding" theory (shown in Fig. 4·1(b) ) active ATG molecules bound to the surface of immune competent cells cover antigen specific receptors and/or interfere with other immune associated receptors (Brent *et al.*, 1967). This theory does not explain why the progeny of blind-folded lymphocytes are still devoid of immune activity. Nevertheless, the selective binding of ATG to certain

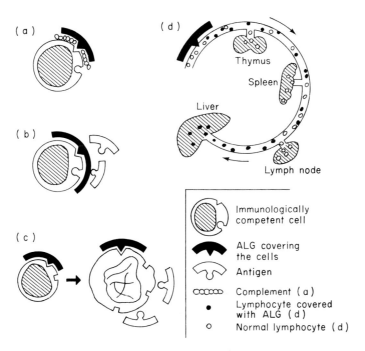

FIG. 4·1 Different hypotheses relating to the immunosuppressive actions of anti-lymphocyte antibodies. (a) Lymphoid cells are lysed by antibodies in the presence of complement. (b) The antigen specific receptors on the surface of lymphocytes are covered by the antibodies (blind-folding effect). (c) In the course of antibody induced blast transformation irrelevant clones are activated which are unresponsive to relevant antigens (and may secondarily diminish antigen specific responses; sterile activation). (d) Antibodies are bound to circulating lymphocytes; the covered cells are eliminated by phagocytosis in the liver and spleen ("opsonization").

receptors, such as binding sites for sheep erthyocyte (E), can be conveniently measured in the E-rosette inhibition test (Bach and Dormont, 1971). This proves to be a simple and valuable test for determining the titer of antibodies to these particular T cell specific sites. The ATG samples show a somewhat variable but reassuringly high (8,500–153,500) rosette inhibition titer (Wechter *et al.*, 1979). Third, some ATG preparations have mitogenic effects, which are frequently as powerful as the mitogenecity of phytohaemagglutinin, a strong T cell specific mitogen (Janossy and Greaves, 1972; Woodruff 1968). This could lead to the "sterile activation" of irrelevant clones of cells with no apparent immunological activity (Fig. 4·1(c) ). The importance of this finding is made doubtful by the observation that F(ab)₂ fragments of ATG are mitogenic but have no immunosuppressive effects (James, 1967). Finally, this observation already points to the importance of the Fc part of the IgG molecule in the immunosuppressive effects of ATG. Extensive studies by Martin (1969) and Greaves *et al.*, (1969) have indeed shown that the binding of ATG coated lymphocytes to macrophages ("opsonization" probably through Fc receptor attachment) shows the best correlation with the immunosuppressive effects seen *in vivo*. Cells covered by ATG are immediately cleared from the circulation causing lymphopenia (Gray *et al.*, 1964). These cells are eliminated by the liver and reticulo-endothelial system instead of reaching the lymphoid organs (Fig. 4·1(d); Martin 1969; Taub and Lance, 1968). This mechanism of action is in line with the clear demonstration that ATG exerts its effects of the recirculating lymphocyte populations which, in the mice and probably in man, includes a large subpopulation of T lymphocytes (Leuchars *et al.*, 1968; Nehlsen, 1971; Cantor, 1972). The fact that the recirculating T lymphocytes are more accessible to ATG actions than other "sessile" B lymphocytes and macrophages explains the T cell immunosuppressive properties of ATG even in the absence of true specificity for T cells (see below).

The opsonization test has so far been standardized only for murine cells and it is not yet available for human studies. Fortunately, the immunosuppressive potency of anti-human ATG preparations can be predicted with some certainty by studying the prolongation of skin allograft survival in Rhesus monkeys (Balner, 1971; Wechter *et al.*, 1979). Monkeys have numerous lymphocyte differentiation and transplantation antigens that are common with man (Balch *et al.*, 1977). Thus the ATG effects *in vivo* are likely to be similar in the two species. Most frequently a five dose course of 100 mg kg$^{-1}$ ATG is given on alternative days starting 2 days before skin grafting. This test also helps to exclude side effects related to ATG administration. The monkey skin allograft tests were used to confirm the absence of potentially lethal anti-glomerular membrane antibodies in the ATGAM preparations. The various batches analysed prolonged monkey skin allograft survival from the 7–10 days normal rejection time to 11½–40 days (Wechter *et al.*, 1979).

It is interesting to note that all four possible mechanisms of ATG action (Fig. 4·1) had relevance for the analysis of monoclonal antibodies. Ironically the monoclonal antibodies may help decisively in establishing the relative importance of these mechanisms (see below).

(b) *Specificity Tests*

These are most frequently restricted to the analysis of haemagglutinin and antiplatelet titers, which are clinically most relevant. As was indicated above ATG samples are absorbed with red cell stroma to decrease haemagglutinin titers (Wechter *et al.*, 1979) or with human placenta. Reactivity with other cells is frequently not given in the specifications of ATG preparations, but summarized in special studies which standardize heterologous antisera for diagnostic tests (reviewed in Greaves and Janossy, 1976; Janossy, 1981). These studies show that ATG strongly reacts with T and non-T cells including B lymphocytes (Fig. 4·2(e) ) as well as haemopoietic myeloid cells, their precursors and other tissues including kidney (Fig. 4·2(b) ).

It is important to emphasize that in spite of these impurities ATG is a far better choice than ALG, particuarly when this is made against B lymphoblastoid lines. These B cells share with bone marrow precursor cells some particularly richly expressed very immunogenic membrane moieties (HLA-DR Ia-like antigens) (Winchester *et al.*, 1977; Janossy *et al.*, 1977).

3. ATG IS IMMUNOSUPPRESSIVE IN MAN

In view of the reasonable results that can be achieved with azathioprine and prednisolone alone it is not unexpected that large numbers of patients have to be studied to document an improvement in long-term allograft survival following the addition of a third agent, ATG. These studies have progressed in successive stages since 1973 (Wechter *et al.*, 1979b). In the latest trials of cadaver kidney allografts obtained from unrelated donors the study group received a 4-week course of ATG following transplantation (10–20 mg kg$^{-1}$ daily). This was in addition to azathioprine and steroids which were also given to the control group. The comparisons of the two groups showed significantly fewer early rejection periods in the ATG-treated patients. The inclusion of a highly

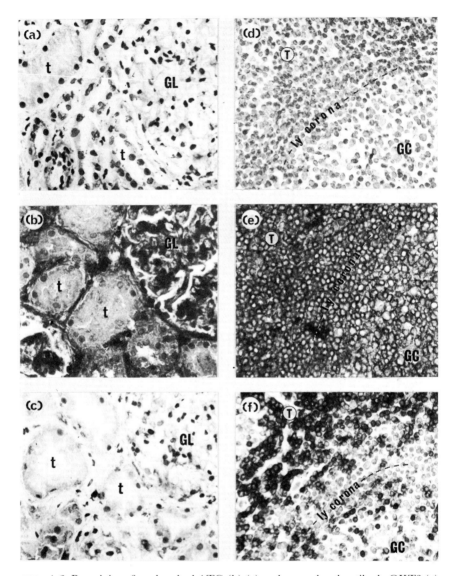

FIG. 4·2 Reactivity of unabsorbed ATG (b) (e) and monoclonal antibody OKT3 (c) (f) in kidney and lymph node. The sections of frozen kidney (a, b, c) and lymph node biopsies (d) (e) (f) were stained with immunoperoxidase. ATG stains cells diffusely in the lymph node with no apparent specificity for T cells in the paracortical area (T) or B cells in the lymphocyte corona and in the germinal centre (GC). ATG also stains the connective tissue and glomeruli (GL) in the kidney; (t): tubules. In contrast, OKT3 specifically stains T cells (T) but no B cells, and is also negative on kidney; (a) and (d) are controls with second layers only. Haemalum counterstain.

immunosuppressive agent such as ATG to an already intensive protocol could cause toxicity and more infections (e.g. cytomegalovirus). For this reason during ATG therapy the dose of steroids is decreased with clinical benefits (e.g. a decrease in avascular necrosis). As a result the occurrence of infections in the ATG group remains low while the functional allograft survival continues to be 10–13% higher (58% actuarial kidney survival at 2 years) than in the control group (47% at 2 years). Although these values have still not achieved statistical significance in individual hospitals (Cosimi, 1981), the kidney transplant registry (using observations on >1,500 cadaver allografts) shows that the inclusion of ATG in the protocol leads to a 10–11% improvement, which is statistically significant (p < 0·001, Jonasson *et al.*, 1982). At the same time the mortality rate is further reduced in the ATG group (<10% over 2 years) and compares favourably to any results reported for patients treated with azathioprine-prednisolone alone (Cosimi, 1981).

More definitive evidence for the immunosuppressive potency of ATG can be obtained more quickly during the treatment of acute rejection episodes in recipients of living-related-donor kidneys. In a group of 12 patients receiving only ATG rejection was reversed in every instance and 10 of the 12 allografts continue to function 6–36 months after transplantation. In contrast, of 12 patients treated with high dose steroids, rejection was reversed in only 10, and only 6 of 12 allografts were functioning 6–36 months later (Cosimi, 1981). In other similar series 1-year allograft survival invariably favoured the ATG-treatment group (70–80% versus 45–50%; Filo *et al.*, 1981, Light *et al.*, 1981; Nowygrod *et al.*, 1981).

Side effects of ATG included chills and fever (immediately after the dramatic drop of while blood cell count) as well as skin erythema, pruritis (18% of cases) and thrombocytopenia (10% of cases). In order to avoid phlebitis at the site of intravenous injection the ATG needs to be diluted with 250-1000 ml sterile saline and infused via a central venous catheter or an arterio-venous fistula. These latter effects may be due to the contaminating "irrelevant" antibodies in the ATG.

It is a paradox that in spite of the presence of cross-reactive antibodies certain ATG preparations induce bone marrow recovery in a proportion of patients with steroid resistant aplastic anaemia, although admittedly after some delay (Cosimi, 1981; Speck *et al.*, 1977). It has been shown that ATGAM contains antibodies to T cells of suppressor/cytotoxic function (anti-$TH_2$; Reinherz *et al.*, 1979; Janossy *et al.*, 1980) and these $TH_2$ positive cells are abnormally increased in a proportion of cases with selective neutropenia (Callard *et al.*, 1981) and aplastic anaemia (Lopez *et al.*, 1981). It is, therefore, reasonable to assume that the beneficial effects of ATGAM in aplastic anaemia and related disorders (which occur in a proportion of patients) may be due to these anti-suppressor/cytotoxic T cell antibodies and might be further improved by the elimination of antibodies to bone marrow precursor cells from the ATG preparation (see below). In the same disease the use of ALG (particularly if made against B lymphoid cell lines containing predominantly anti-HLA-DR but hardly any T cell specific antibody activity) could be disadvantageous because some myeloid precursor cells (CFUc) carry HLA-DR (Ia-like) antigens (Janossy *et al.*, 1978).

## B. Preparation of ATG for use *In Vitro*

### 1. ABSORPTIONS

In experiments with rodents, dogs and chicken the graft versus host reactive cell population can be eliminated by incubating the graft *in vitro* with antisera specific for T cells (Rodt *et al.*, 1974; Müller-Ruchholtz *et al.*, 1975; Kolb *et al.*, 1979; Ivanyi, 1980). For these purposes the human ATG preparations require extensive absorptions (reviewed in Greaves and Janossy, 1976 and Janossy, 1981).

Carefully monitored absorptions were used to prepare rabbit and horse antisera reacting with human thymocytes/T lymphocytes by Janossy *et al.*, 1977b; 1980) in order to prepare diagnostically useful reagents applied in sensitive immunofluorescence assays. Each absorption was carried out with $2\text{-}3 \times 10^8$ cells ml$^{-1}$ antiserum. Specific rabbit anti-human thymocyte/T lymphocyte serum (HuTLA) with no remaining cross-reactive antibodies to other cell types was obtained after absorptions with erythrocytes (2–4x), liver powder (2–4x), B-chronic lymphocytic leukaemia (CLL: 3–5x), B-lymphoid cell line (B-LCL; 1–2x) and acute myeloid leukaemia (AML: 2x) or chronic ML (1–3x). Specific horse anti-HuTLA was obtained after absorptions with erythocytes (3x), liver powder (2x), B-CLL (12x) and AML (6x). Only 2–5 ml of reagents were prepared and the large quantities of immunoabsorbents required precluded any therapeutic applications.

Rodt *et al.*, (1975, 1981) have absorbed a rabbit ATG with liver homogenate (2x), B-CLL (3x) and erythrocytes (2x). This kind of reagent still reacts with certain cases of non-T, non-B acute lymphoblastic leukaemia (ALL; Thiel *et al.*, 1980) but does not eliminate haemopoietic precursors in myeloid colony forming assays in vitro (CFUc) and in diffusion chamber tests (Rodt *et al.*, 1981). Finally,

Wulff and his colleagues (1981) have devised ingenious absorption protocols for bone marrow transplantation. They have demonstrated that rabbit ATG can be absorbed with continuously growing cell lines (REH, a non-T, non-B ALL line and K-562, an erythro-myeloid line) to eliminate reactivity against early myeloid and erythroid cells but leave the reactivity with lymphoid cells (T plus B lymphocytes) intact. This antiserum abolished T lymphocyte function *in vitro* but did not inhibit the CFUc assay.

## 2. ATG MAY PREVENT GRAFT VERSUS HOST DISEASE IN MAN

One of the absorbed ATG preparations (Rodt *et al.*, 1975, 1981) has been used to prevent GvHD in a very difficult group of leukaemic patients treated by bone marrow transplantation. Only 4 of the 14 patients were in full remission at the time of transplant. Eight recipients were sex-mismatched with donor bone marrow and 2 (possibly 3) of 14 patients received HLA-D incompatible grafts. In spite of these bad prognostic factors only 2 patients developed a transient skin rash but no other signs of GvHD. Thus the prevention of GvHD appears to have been successful. The bone marrow regeneration proceeded with normal speed and resulted in full engraftment in 12 cases. Engraftment was not achieved in two patients. One of these was HLA-D mismatched (which may require more than normal numbers of cells for a proper take) and died early with septicaemia. The other patient showed persistent leukaemia at autopsy, which may have prevented engraftment. Although it cannot be excluded that low levels of (opsonizing) antibodies still present in the ATG preparation could have contributed to the failure of take in these two cases, overall these results are very encouraging (Rodt *et al.*, 1981) and should be repeated in more patients who are in full remission during transplantation.

## III STANDARDIZATION OF MONOCLONAL ANTIBODIES

### A. DETAILED ANALYSIS OF THE REACTIVITY PATTERN OF SELECTED REAGENTS

The observations above have delineated the clinical uses of ATG and in addition underlined the difficulties confronting experimental biologists and physicians in obtaining reproducible observations with conventional antisera. The slow progress seen during the last 15 years in establishing ATG as a useful adjunct to immunosuppressive therapy is attributable to these problems of standardization (compare Groth, 1981 and Cosimi, 1981). Clearly, even the most thoroughly investigated ATG (ATGAM) can hardly be considered as a standard agent. The different batches admittedly show some variations in immunosuppressive action (in monkeys) and in titers against relevant (T) lymphocytes and to their subclasses as well as against other cell types (B lymphocytes, bone marrow cells, platelets, etc,; Wechter *et al.*, 1979).

Monoclonal antibodies have opened a new era in cellular immunology and in the related clinical fields. Their preparation is discussed elsewhere in this volume (chapters 1 and 21). Three important points about the analysis of monoclonal antibodies to leucocyte membrane antigens are emphasized here. First, it is an extraordinary advantage that these standard products can be analysed in several laboratories offering different approaches and that the observations can be related to each other in order to build up a comprehensive tableau about the characteristics of each reagent. The clearest example is the OKT series which, after the initial standardization by Kung *et al.*, (1980) and Reinherz and Schlossman (1980) has been studied all over the world for criteria as divergent as tissue distribution (Bhan *et al.*, 1980; Janossy *et al.*, 1980) and cross-reactivity with primate lymphocytes (Table 4·2, Cosimi *et al.*, 1981a). Second, a number of monoclonal antibodies are directed against various epitopes on the same T cell specific molecules (Table 4·3). It is interesting to note that these antibodies show an

TABLE 4·2

Sharing of T cell antigens between primates[a,b]

| Reagent | Man | Chimpanzee | Orangutan | Rhesus | Cynomolgus |
|---|---|---|---|---|---|
| OKT3 pan-peripheral T | + | + | − | − | − |
| OKT11 pan-T | + | + | + | + | + |
| OKT1 pan-T minus small subset | + | + | + | − | − |
| OKT4 inducer | + | + | − | + | + |
| OKT8 suppressor/ cytotoxic | + | + | + | + | + |
| OKT5 suppressor/ cytotoxic | + | + | + | + | + |

[a] As detected by monoclonal antibodies and flow cytometry on peripheral blood T cells (from Cosimi *et al.*, 1981a).

[b] All non-primates tested (rabbit, dog, guinea-pig) are negative.

TABLE 4·3
Monoclonal antibodies to thymocyte/T lymphocyte antigens[a]

| | | Class | Source[b] | MW[c] | Comments |
|---|---|---|---|---|---|
| Pan-T[d] | OKT11[1] | IgG$_1$ | 0 | 55·000 ) | |
| | OKT11A[1] | IgG$_2$ | 0 | 55·000 ) | E-rosette |
| | Hu Lyt3 (9·6)[2] | | NEN | 55·000 ) | receptor |
| Cortical | NA1/34 | IgG$_2$ | S | 49·000 ) | |
| thymocytes | OKT6 | IgG$_1$ | 0 | 49·000 ) | |
| Pan-peripheral | OKT3 | IgG$_2$ | 0 | 19·000 ) | |
| T | UCHT1[3] | IgG$_1$ | | 19·000 ) | mitogenic |
| | Leu-4 | IgG$_1$ | BD | 19·000 ) | |
| | MBG-6[4] | IgM | | same reactivity, not mitogenic | |
| Inducer | OKT4 | IgG$_2$ | 0 | 62·000 | |
| or | OKT4A[5] | IgG$_1$ | 0 | | |
| helper | OKT4B[5] | IgM | 0 | | |
| | OKT4C[5] | IgG$_3$ | 0 | | |
| | OKT4D[5] | IgG$_1$ | 0 | | |
| | Leu3 | IgG$_1$ | BD | 55·000 | |
| Cytotoxic- | OKT5 | IgG$_1$ | 0 | 33·000 | |
| suppressor | OKT8 | IgG$_2$ | 0 | 33·000 | |
| | OKT8A | IgG$_2$ | 0 | | |
| | Leu2a | IgG$_1$ | BD | 32·000 | |
| T cells, | OKT1 | IgG$_1$ | 0 | 66·000 | |
| some | Leu1 | IgG$_2$ | BD | 67·000 | |
| thymocytes | L17F12[6] | IgG$_2$ | | 68·000 | |
| and B-CLL | Hu Lyt2 (10·2)[7] | | NEN | 67·000 | |
| | T101[8] | | | 65·000 | |

[a]  See Kung et al., (1980), Reinherz et al., (1980) and Janossy et al., (1981) for more details about the OKT reagents. See Ledbetter et al., (1981) for Leu reagents.

[b]  Many of these reagents are commercially available from the following firms: O, Ortho; S, Seralab; BD, Beckton-Dickinson; NEN, New England Nuclear.

[c]  The monoclonal antibodies shown in each group not only have identical reactivity (see text and Fig. 4·3) but also react with antigens of similar molecular weight. A few references here are given about more recent products:
1. Verbi et al., (1982); 2. Kamoun et al., (1981); 3. Beverley et al., (1981); 4. Bastin et al., (1981); 5. Bach et al., (1981); 6. Engleman et al., (1981); 7. Martin et al., (1981); 8. Royston et al., (1980) Other potentially useful antibodies have also been described (reviewed in Boumsell and Bernard, 1981) but no detailed information about their activity on normal human bone marrow is available.

[d]  Two further monoclonal antibodies which probably react with the E-rosette receptor has been described by Bieber et al., (1981). These antibodies are immunosuppressive in primates.

identical reactivity pattern but may belong to different immunoglobulin classes (IgM, IgG) or subclasses (IgG$_1$, IgG$_2$, IgG$_3$). The (sub)class
can influence the effects of these pure reagents *in vivo* (i.e. cytolysis,
opsonization, penetration into extravascular space, etc.). Experiments
are therefore now possible, perhaps in primates, to investigate the
mechanism of anti-lymphocyte antibody mediated immunosuppression. Finally, just as the first characterization of ALG and ATG
coincided with the establishment of the basic principles of cellular
immunology, the characterization of monoclonal antibodies to T
lymphocyte subsets in man is stimulating the definition of immunoregulatory circuits and aiding the clarification of their clinical relevance
(Goldstein, *et al.*, see chapter 3; Reinherz and Schlossman, 1980). In
addition, during the last 5 years certain phenotypic and functional
characteristics of haemopoietic precursor cells have been described
(Metcalf, 1977; Greaves and Janossy, 1978) and can be rapidly applied
to the study of new reagents. It seems that the recent information
explosion has so far created clarity (and further working hypotheses)
rather than confusion.

The salient results are summarized in Fig. 4·3. These have been
obtained by cell sorter analysis and microscopic studies using double
marker methods (Reinherz *et al.*, 1980; Janossy *et al.*, 1981). Reactivity
with a number of monoclonal antibody reagents seems to be generated
during thymocyte/T cell differentiation. The two "pan-T" reagents are
OKT11 (and the equivalent OKT11A, Leu-5 and 9·6) and OKT3
(and the equivalent UCHT1, Leu-4 and the very similar MBG-6;
Table 4·3). Reactivity with OKT11 is apparently generated during the
earliest (large thymic blast) stage and includes >99% of identifiable T
lineage cells as well as a few E-rosetting cells with effector cell function
in natural killer cell assay. These antibodies react with the sheep
erythrocyte (E) receptor. (Verbi *et al.*, 1982; Kamoun *et al.*, 1981).
OKT3 is generated at a later stage, during the maturation of functional
T lymphocytes. The OKT3 population includes all cells with classical
T cell function (Kung *et al.*, 1979) and shows the typical tissue localization in the paracortical areas of lymph nodes and a few positive cells
inside the germinal centres (Fig. 4·2c). OKT1 (and the equivalent
Leu-1, T-101, L17 F12, 10·2 and A50) is another interesting "almost
pan-T" reagent which reacts with some thymocytes rather weakly but
detects the vast majority of peripheral T cells (Kung *ei al.*, 1979;
Royston *et al.*, 1980; Boumsell *et al.*, 1980; Engleman *et al.*, 1980).
Surprisingly, many T lymphocytes (effector T cells?) found in normal
parenchymal tissues such as intestinal epithelium or in virus infected
liver fail to express this marker (OKT1$^-$) while T cells in the lymph

nodes and circulating blood are predominantly OKT1$^+$ (Janossy *et al.*, 1982). OKT1 is, like OKT11 and OKT3, T cell specific, except that chronic lymphocytic leukaemia cells of B type (B-CLL) are OKT1$^+$. Intriguingly, recent double-labelling studies have revealed a few OKT1$^+$ B lymphocytes in normal lymph nodes, but not in blood or bone marrow (Caligaris-Cappio *et al.*, 1982).

Three other markers show more selective expression. OKT6, and the equivalent NA1/34, react with cortical thymocytes (McMichael *et al.*, 1979; Reinherz *et al.*, 1980) and, surprisingly, with skin Langerhans cells (Fithian *et al.*, 1981). OKT4 (and the equivalent OKT4A, OKT4B, OKT4C, OKT4D and Leu-3a) and OKT8 (and the equivalent OKT5, OKT8A and Leu-2a) react with most immature thymocytes but detect two distinct subsets of mature T lymphocytes of

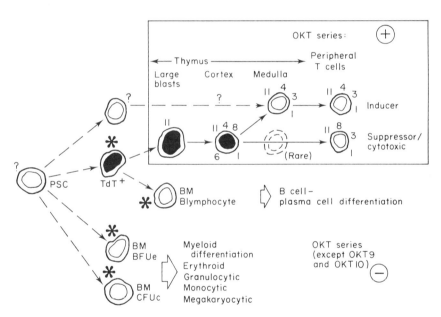

FIG. 4·3 The reactivity of OKT reagents and other corresponding monoclonal antibodies (Table 4·3) has been studied in a number of laboratories. OKT11, T1, T3, T4 and T8 are restricted to T lineage cells. All identifiable bone marrow precursor cells tested (indicated by asterisks), and presumably also the human pluripotent stem cell (PSC) which cannot be tested *in vitro*, are unreactive with these reagents. The differentiation pathways are still hypothetical (?). BM: bone marrow; BFUe: erythroid burst forming unit *in vitro*; CFUc: granulocytic-monocytic colony forming unit *in vitro*; TdT: terminal transferase enzyme present in the nucleus of putative lymphoid precursors of BM and immature thymocytes (shown by black nucleus). (For further details see Reinherz *et al.*, 1980, Janossy *et al.*, 1981, Granger *et al.*, 1981 and Hansen *et al.*, 1981).

inducer and cytotoxic-suppressor functions (Fig. 4·3; Reinherz and Schlossman, 1980 and Goldstein, see chapter 3). Many new ideas about the positive and negative regulation of immune responses are based on investigations with these two reagents.

These results do not exclude the possibility of dual (or partially overlapping) pathways for the generation of OKT8$^+$ cells (by-passing the thymic medulla) and OKT4$^+$ cells (by-passing the cortex; Goldschneider et al., 1981). Further observations are necessary in man to confirm or refute this hypothesis (Fig. 4·4).

It is not surprising that the OKT4$^+$ and OKT8$^+$ cells, which show different functions, also have different tissue distribution. The T cells inside the germinal centres are almost exclusively OKT4$^+$, while T cells in the intestinal epithelium and bone marrow are predominantly OKT8$^+$ (Poppema et al., 1981; Janossy et al., 1980.

One of the most exciting findings about these reagents is that they are T cell specific (but see qualifications of OKT6 and OKT1 above). It is easy to establish that these reagents fail to react with B lymphocytes and differentiating myeloid cells. In addition, these reagents are also negative with all identifiable bone marrow precursor cells such as TdT$^+$ putative lymphoid precursors (Fig. 4·4), BFUe (erythroid) and CFUc (granulocyticmonocytic precursor cells; Crawford et al., 1981; Hansen et al., 1981) as well as bone marrow B lymphocytes (Janossy et al., 1981). The results of cell separation experiments carried out on the cell sorter are shown in Table 4·4. These observations taken together with double labelling experiments using anti-T cell antisera, indicate that the OKT3$^+$, OKT11$^+$ and OKT1$^+$ populations in the human bone marrow are peripheral T lymphocytes and not "stem" cells (Janossy et et al., 1981).

TABLE 4·4

Granulocytic-monocytic colony forming units in vitro (CFUc) in unseparated and cell sorter separated fractions[a]

| Antibody | Fraction | CFUc $10^{-5}$ cells plated | CFUc $10^{-5}$ original marrow cells | Contribution of each population to recovered CFUc (%) |
|---|---|---|---|---|
| OKT3 | unseparated | 88 | | |
| | +[b] | 8 | 2·3 | 4 |
| | − | 86 | 53 | 96 |
| OKT11 | unseparated | 159 | | |
| | +[b] | 7 | 2 | 3 |
| | − | 109 | 59 | 97 |

[a]   Representative figures from 2–3 experiments (Crawford et al., 1981).
[b]   The percentage of OKT3$^+$, OKT11$^+$ T lymphocytes in the bone marrow is variable (3–12%).

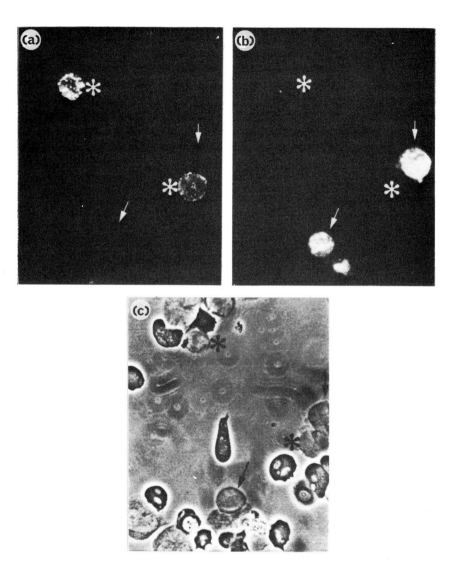

FIG. 4·4 OKT11 positive cells in bone marrow. Bone marrow cells were stained with OKT11 (membrane staining in (a) ), spun and restained for nuclear TdT (b). OKT11$^+$ cells (T lymphocytes, asterisks) are TdT$^-$. TdT$^+$ precursor cells (arrows) are OKT11$^-$ See also Table 4·4. (From Verbi et al., 1982.)

Finally OKT3, OKT11 and OKT11A were analyzed in sections of non-lymphoid tissues and were found to be unreactive with all samples studied (kidney, liver, heart, muscle, pancreas, testis, vascular endothelium throughout the body, Fig. 4·2(c). Some cytoplasmic protein (but no membrane antigen) was labelled weakly in a few brain cells with OKT11 and OKT11A but these cells are not accessible to circulating immunoglobulin. In particular, the glomerular basal membrane in kidneys was totally negative (Fig. 4·2(c) ).

In conclusion, a range of specific antibodies to T lymphocytes is now available for clinical studies (Table 4·3). Other antibodies to T cells or subsets have also been described but have not been fully analyzed on human bone marrow and other tissues (reviewed by Boumsell and Bernard, 1981).

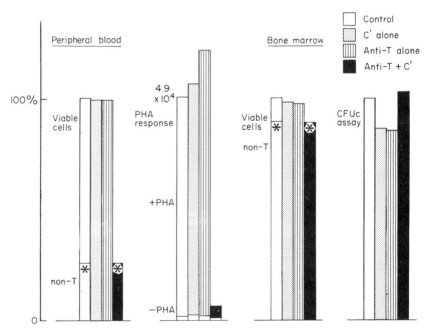

FIG. 4·5 Selection of a non-toxic, lytic complement source. Washed cells were incubated with monoclonal antibodies for 30 mins at room temperature, washed into a balanced salt solution containing $Ca^{++}$ and rabbit complement added for 45 mins at 37°C in 1:2 dilution. Phytohaemagglutinin response of peripheral blood lymphocytes *in vitro* was abolished on the addition of antibody and complement. At the same time rabbit complement (± antibody) inhibited less than 10% of recovered CFUc. Asterisk indicates the number of non-T cells in the suspension. The same observations were obtained with OKT3, MBG6 and OKT11A antibodies (from Granger *et al.*, 1981, 1982).

## B. Efficacy of Monoclonal Antibodies

One might predict that although monoclonal antibodies are convenient specific reagents they may be less effective than conventional antisera. However this prediction does not appear to be correct. Nevertheless it is likely that some monoclonal antibodies will perform poorly and others will efficiently activate the secondary mechanisms necessary for T cell removal and immunosuppression (Fig. 4·1). These selected monoclonal antibodies, used either alone or in combination with other efficient monoclonal antibodies, will probably be more effective than conventional antisera containing natural mixtures of various types of antibodies (i.e. excellent and poor "performers"). The efficacy of "triggering" secondary mechanism(s) will probably depend on a multiplicity of factors. These include the Fc part of the antibody, perhaps activation of complement as well as the way membrane associated molecules (that are recognized by monoclonal antibodies) are inserted into the lipid bilayer. These facts may determine whether or not the association of the given antigen with an antibody will lead to a firm interaction or to mere shedding and modulation of the membrane molecule. At present, we have at our disposal large numbers of specific monoclonal antibodies which can already be selected and mixed with each other if required (Table 4·3). It is important to learn more about the performance of these monoclonal antibodies in the relevant tests.

### 1. SOME MONOCLONAL ANTIBODIES ARE EFFICIENT IN COMPLEMENT (C') MEDIATED LYSIS

Murine monoclonal antibodies of $IgG_2$ subclass (but not $IgG_1$) and at least a proportion of antibodies of IgM class are effective in C' lysis (Table 4·5, Fig. 4·5). Rabbit serum is optimal as a source of C'; human, rat and guinea pig sera are inefficient. The rabbit serum needs to be used at high concentrations. Careful selection of non-toxic batches (to haemopoietic precursor cells) is, therefore, imperative (Granger *et al.*, 1981; Hansen *et al.*, 1981; Van Wauwe and Gossens, 1981).

Two important observations facilitate the clinical applications of this work. First, large amounts of erythrocytes inhibit C' action. The red cells need to be removed from the bone marrow before incubation with monoclonal antibodies and C'. This can be done, on a large scale, with the IBM cell processor using a Ficoll-Hypaque gradient. Similarly to the same procedure done on a small scale in the laboratory, this procedure depletes erythrocytes and mature polymorphs and yields a

*G. Janossy* et al.

low-volume "concentrate" of immature and differentiating haemopoietic cells together with lymphocytes. This preparation is ideally
suited for manipulations with antibodies and C' as well as for storage in
liquid nitrogen (Netzel *et al.*, 1981; Gilmore *et al.*, 1981). The method is
simpler than that of Dicke (1969) because it does not intend to remove
lymphocytes, a task to be performed by the monoclonal antibodies.
Second, a careful study involving combined analysis of cell suspensions
using both membrane fluorescence and viability showed that minute
(<5%) populations of T lymphocytes (undetectable by viability test

TABLE 4·5

Combined staining for membrane fluorescence (green, FITC) and dead cells
(red, ethidium bromide) before and after complement (C') mediated lysis
with monoclonal antibodies[a,b]

| Treatment | All cells with membrane staining (all green) | Dead cells (red) | Dead cells with membrane staining (red & green) | Viable cells with membrane staining (only green and no red) |
|---|---|---|---|---|
| OKT3 (control) | 64 | < 1 | < 1 | 64 |
| OKT11 (control) | 62 | < 1 | < 1 | 62 |
| OKT3 + C' | 11 | 32[c] | 4·5 | 6·5[d] |
| OKT11A + C' | 9 | 34[c] | 5·5 | 3·5 |
| OKT3 + OKT11A + C' | 19 | 44[c] | 19 | < 0·2[d] |

a   Mononuclear cells from peripheral blood were separated on Ficoll-Isopaque gradient. The
    population contained 65% E-rosetting cells which were also recognized by OKT11A. Similar
    observations were made with human bone marrow containing 10–18% E-rosetting OKT3[+],
    OKT11A[+] T cells. In the Table the percentages of peripheral blood cells left after C' lysis and
    recognized by membrane staining or ethidium bromide staining (nuclear positivity on dead
    cells) are shown.
b   The two monoclonal antibodies used, individually or in combination, were OKT3 and
    OKT11A (both of IgG₂ class). For membrane fluorescence the cells were labelled with goat
    anti-mouse Ig-FITC (green) second layer Ab-s. The complement mediated lysis was
    performed with specially selected rabbit complement (used in 1 : 2 dilution in Hanks solution).
    The dead cells were either totally lysed (and therefore lost for further analysis; approximately
    50–60% of lysed cells) or positively recognised by staining with ethidium bromide (EB, red).
    This staining gives identical values to the more conventional analysis of damaged dead cells
    with Tripan blue but has the extra advantage that it can be used in combination with the
    membrane fluorescence staining. Thus the cells with recognizable green membrane staining
    can be classified as dead (EB[+] red) or alive (EB[-]). From Granger *et al.*, (1982).
c   Absolute cell counts have demonstrated that 60% of dead cells were totally lysed and not
    shown here.
d   The T cells which survived the OKT3 + C' treatment formed E-rosettes. In contrast the
    surviving population after OKT3 + OKT11A + C' treatment contained no cells which could
    be identified (with combination staining) as OKT3[+] OKT11A[+] viable cells or as E-rosette
    forming cells. These surviving cells were non-T cells which failed to respond to phytohaemag-
    glutinin, a T cell mitogen.

alone, or by phytohaemagglutinin stimulation and mixed lymphocyte cultures) may escape the cytotoxic action of individual monoclonal antibodies such as OKT3 and OKT11A and C'. Nevertheless, the two antibodies act synergistically and no detectable viable (<$0·2\%$) T cells are left in blood mononuclear cell preparations or in the bone marrow after the two antibodies are used together in C' mediated cytotoxicity (Table 4·5). Thus monoclonal antibodies provide the most efficient C' mediated T cell removal system so far standardized with no apparent toxicity toward the haemopoietic cells (Granger *et al.*, 1982).

2. SOME MONOCLONAL ANTIBODIES ARE
EFFICIENT IN OPSONIZATION

The clearest demonstration of opsonizing effects (Fig. 4·1(d) ) has been obtained in a patient with T cell leukaemia (Sezary syndrome, white blood cell count $135 \times 10^9 \ l^{-1}$) following the administration of 1 mg monoclonal antibody L17F12 of IgG$_2$ class (Table 4·3; Miller *et al.*, 1981). Within 3 hours the white blood cell count (WBC) dropped to $95 \times 10^9 \ l^{-1}$ and reached a nadir of $74 \times 10^9 \ l^{-1}$ at 6 hours, a response slightly better than that seen after the leucophoresis of $4·6 \times 10^{11}$ tumour cells (equivalent to 200 to 400 g tumour mass). It is unlikely that the drop of WBC seen was a result of C' mediated cytotoxicity because serum C3 and C4 levels were unchanged during treatment and autologous serum as C' source was totally ineffective with this mono-clonal antibody. These authors have shown that $^{111}$In-labelled autolo-gous leukaemic cells (injected into the patients prior to antibody therapy) sequestered into the liver and spleen. In these organs whole body scans indicated intense radioactivity after the administration of antibody. When the WBC returned to pre-treatment levels 36 hours later the decrease of $^{111}$In specific activity in the tumour cell population indicated the influx of unlabelled "fresh" leukaemic cells and excluded the possibility that "opsonized" pre-labelled cells returned into the circulation en mass (Miller *et al.*, 1981).

The removal of 400 g tumour mass may "saturate" the capacity of the reticuloendothelial system. It is, therefore, not surprising that the elimi-nation of all circulating lymphocytes which react with the injected monoclonal antibody can be better demonstrated in patients with lower WBC counts. This has been shown in a patient with T cell lymphoma (abnormal Sezary cells: $1·1 \times 10^9 \ l^{-1}$ pre-treatment) injected with L17F12 monoclonal antibody. These abnormal T cells were immediately (within 10 minutes) removed from the circulation together with monocytes and half of the granulocytes (contributing to phagocytosis?). No changes in erythrocyte and platelet counts were observed. Similarly, eight patients were injected with OKT3 (of IgG₂ class) in order to treat acute rejection of renal allografts (see below) and the effective selective removal of all OKT3 reactive T lymphocytes from the circulation was documented in each case by flow cytometry analysis within minutes after the infusion of OKT3 antibody. This was followed by chills and fever within 1 hour. These symptoms could have been due to the sequestration and breakdown of T lymphocytes. No reactions to subsequent injections were noted at the time when the number of circulating T lymphocytes was low (Cosimi *et al.*, 1981).

Clearly more experimental work is required to analyze the exact requirements and efficacy of opsonization. A reliable assay *in vitro* would be desirable. The analysis of lymphocyte recirculation in primates, which share multiple T cell membrane markers recognized by the anti-human monoclonal antibodies (Table 4·2), could also be rewarding. After all, single injections of monoclonal antibody are unlikely to cause serious damage to the animals but can quickly reveal the inefficacy of particular antibodies and may help to establish the main criteria (Ig class or the characteristics of detected membrane antigens?) which govern potency. These kinds of experiments are quicker and simpler than the formal trials of immunosuppression, which can also be carried out simultaneously and perhaps repeated with appropriate mixtures of monoclonal antibodies. Surprises might be on the way. When OKT4 antibody (IgG₂), detecting T cells of inducer function, was evaluated as the sole immunosuppressive agent in Cynomolgus monkeys receiving heterotopic renal allografts, the number of OKT4$^+$ lymphocytes fell from normal levels of 809 ± 130 mm$^{-3}$ to a range of 200–300 mm$^{-3}$ (Cosimi *et al.*, 1981a). In some animals antibody excess was still present 48 hours after the previous injection and some of the OKT4$^+$ cells were in fact coated with monoclonal antibody of IgG₂ class but not removed by the reticuloendothelial system. Further studies are essential to establish whether there is a species difference here: OKT3 coated T cells are efficiently removed in man. Alternatively, different antibodies may act differently *in vivo* in spite of their identical Ig subclass.

3. THE "BLIND-FOLDING" EFFECT

Reinherz *et al.* (1980) and Chang *et al.* (1981) have observed that OKT3 blocks T lymphocyte function. This antibody is also mitogenic but only in the absence of human serum, which suggests that this effect does not, in all probability, occur *in vivo* (Van Wauwe *et al.* 1980). If the "blind-folding" effects of the ATG contributes to immunosuppression (Fig. 4·1(b) ) then OKT3 could be a more effective antibody than the other T cell specific reagents (Table 4·3).

4. SOME MONOCLONAL ANTIBODIES
MODULATE MEMBRANE ANTIGENS

Antibody induced loss of membrane antigen expression has been shown by Old *et al.*, (1967) in mice treated with anti TL antibody for TL-positive leukaemia. After modulation cells were no longer destroyed by anti-TL antibody. The important point is that this is a reversible phenotypic change which does not represent immunoselection. The same phenomenon has been observed in cases of non-T, non-B ALL treated with the J-5 monoclonal antibody recognizing the common ALL antigen (Ritz *et al.*, 1980). It was clearly demonstrated that cALL antigen negative leukaemic blasts developed which nevertheless were capable of rapidly regenerating cALL antigen *in vitro*. The multiplicity of membrane markers available for T lymphocyte characterization makes it feasible to analyze antigenic modulation by phenotypic studies. When the phenotype of malignant T cell lymphoma cells is established it can be demonstrated that, for example, progressively greater antigen modulation of the OKT1-like antigen takes place *in vivo* when the dose of L17F12 monoclonal antibody is increased (Miller *et al.*, 1981). The prevalent malignant population, in other respects, retains its phenotypic identity. These observations are important in three respects. First, they demonstrate a dramatic, although "unwanted", effect of monoclonal antibodies on their target cells *in vitro* and *in vivo*. Second, they indicate that experiments can be designed to analyze which antibody is likely to cause modulation and how this can be avoided by using the appropriate antibody dose or, more importantly, the suitable antibody combinations. Third, these studies introduce the concept of careful patient monitoring during treatment with mono-clonal antibodies using recently developed immunological methods (see below).

## IV CLINICAL APPLICATIONS OF MONOCLONAL ANTIBODIES

### A. TREATMENT OF PATIENTS *IN VIVO*

During the last year the first systematic studies have been initiated in animal models and in certain selected diseases (such as kidney allograft

rejection and T cell leukaemia/lymphoma) where the antibody treat-
ment of circulating T lymphocytes is likely to be beneficial for patients.
These preliminary observations are compared to those obtained with
ATG (Table 4·1).

1.  IMMUNOSUPPRESSION IN SUB-HUMAN PRIMATES

The reactivity of various monoclonal antibodies in monkeys is shown in
Table 4·2. OKT4, an antibody to inducer T cells, was evaluated as the
sole immunosuppressive agent in Cynomolgus monkeys receiving
heterotopic renal allografts (Cosimi *et al.*, 1981a). The antibody was
given intravenously on a daily or on alternate day basis for 7–14 days.
Allograft function was evaluated by creatinine determinations and
frequently by renal biopsies. The animals were monitored for lymphocyte subsets and levels of free OKT4 antibody. The main conclusions of
the study are two-fold. First the dosage of OKT4 antibody required to
achieve coating of cells plus a serum antibody excess was 0·5–1
mg kg$^{-1}$, given at 24 hour intervals. This caused no local phlebitis or
any side effects and toxicity. Second, the OKT4 antibody was effective
in significantly prolonging allograft survival in some animals to 36, 46
and 47 days (see details in Cosimi *et al.*, 1981a) but only if the antibody
was first given before transplantation and antibody excess in the circulation was maintained. (If no immunosuppression was given the kidney
was rejected within 8–11 days.) The immunosuppressive effect was
achieved in spite of the fact that OKT4 antibody was not very effective
in removing all OKT4$^+$ cells from the circulation (see above) and the
treatment did not lower the total number of T cells in the blood.

Two further monoclonal antibodies (ATM 1 and 2) capable of
blocking E-rosetting (and probably equivalent to OKT11) have also
been shown to prolong allogeneic skin graft survival in primates (Bieber
*et al.*, 1981).

2.  IMMUNOSUPPRESSION IN KIDNEY
TRANSPLANT RECIPIENTS

Encouraged by the ease of administration and lack of toxicity of monoclonal antibodies in the primate model Cosimi *et al.*, (1981b) have
evaluated immunosuppressive effects of OKT3 antibody, a pan-
peripheral T cell reagent, on acute rejection in eight cadaver donor
renal allograft recipients. These patients had been treated with azathioprine and prednisone from the time of transplantation. As was pointed
out above, when a single agent (i.e. ATG or OKT3) alone is added to

the immunosuppressive protocol at the time of acute rejection, the clinical efficacy can be readily demonstrated. The purpose of the study was to identify the most effective and least toxic combinations of conventional and OKT3 therapy (Table 4·6). The striking observation was that in every instance the rejection episode for which OKT3 therapy was instituted was reversed with steady improvement in allograft function. This was achieved in spite of the decreased doses of azathioprine and prednisone during OKT3 therapy. In addition, OKT3$^+$ cells were effectively removed from the blood (see above), and the lymphoid infiltrates in the kidneys decreased. Thus OKT3 is a more efficient opsonizing antibody in man than OKT4 proved to be in Cynomolgus monkeys.

The main problem encountered in patients 1–4 was the recurrence of rejection episodes after the cessation of OKT3 therapy while the patients were maintained on azathioprine and prednisolone. These second rejection episodes in patients 3 and 4 could not be reversed despite increased steroids, local irradiation and Actinomycin D. At that stage in patient 3 severe cytomegalovirus infection developed and she expired 3 months after transplant. Patient 4 lost his kidney. The repeated use of OKT3 in patient 4 was prevented by the development of high titers of antibody to the OKT3 reagent. Due to these complications in patients 5–8 an increased dose of OKT3 (5 mg day$^{-1}$) was administered during the acute rejection phase (Table 4·6) and at the same time the dose of other immunosuppressive drugs was decreased to a minimum. This principle has already been established with the effective ATG preparations (see above) and leads to the sparing of steroids and other drugs at a stage when they are not required and can be deleterious. Thus, after the cessation of OKT3 these drugs can be given in higher amounts to prevent the recurrence of rejection. Patients 5–8 are on these protocols and doing well.

3. TREATMENT OF T CELL LEUKAEMIA/LYMPHOMA

When patients with a large tumour burden, such as high count leukaemia or widespread lymphoma, are treated with passive immunotherapy (i.e. injection of heterologous antisera or monoclonal antibodies) it is well known that this kind of intervention offers little hope for any substantial long-term improvement (reviewed by Rosenberg and Terry, 1977). There are many reasons why serotherapy of tumours should fail (Table 4·7). The primary aim in cancer therapy is the destruction of all malignant cells, but not all malignant cells recirculate and a substantial proportion are likely to be inaccessible to

TABLE 4·6

Results of treatment of acute rejection with OKT3 monoclonal antibody[a]

| Patient[b] | Post-transplant day of rejection | Creatinine (mgml$^{-2}$) | | | Days to reversal | Total (mg) | OKT3 (days) | Daily dose (mg) |
|---|---|---|---|---|---|---|---|---|
| | | Pre-rejection | Peak | After OKT3 | | | | |
| 1 | 6 | 1·6 | 5·4 | 1·3 | 4 | 13 | (10 d) | 1–2 |
| 2 | 16 | 1·9 | 4·8 | 1·6 | 2 | 20 | (10 d) | 2 |
| 3 | 8 | 1·6 | 4·3 | 0·9 | 2 | 18 | (15 d) | 1–2 |
| 4 | 9 | 5·0 | 8·1 | 2·9 | 2 | 34 | (14 d) | 1–3 |
| 5 | 7 | 1·6 | 5·8 | 1·3 | 2 | 70 | (14 d) | 5 |
| 6 | 6 | 2·9 | 8·5 | 0·9 | 5 | 57 | (14 d) | 3–5 |
| 7 | 6 | 3·0 | 8·1 | 1·2 | 4 | 90 | (17 d) | 5 |
| 8 | 9 | 10·4 | 11·3 | 1·1 | 7 | 100 | (20 d) | 5 |

[a] From Cosimi et al., 1981b.

[b] The patients have been treated with azathioprine (A) and prednisolone (P) throughout but the doses were modified in order to find the best combinations with OKT3. In Patients 1 and 2 100 mg kg$^{-1}$ A was given on the day of transplantation (day 0) and maintained at 100–150 mg per day. P was begun at 2 mg kg$^{-1}$ per day and from day 5 it was slowly decreased to 0·8 mg kg$^{-1}$ per day (by 10 mg per day) and eventually to the 0·25 mg kg$^{-1}$ per day maintenance dose. In patients 3 and 4, during OKT3 therapy the doses of A and P were reduced to 50 mg per day and 0·6 mg kg$^{-1}$ per day, respectively, and the A increased to 100–150 mg per day after OKT3 therapy. Finally, in patients 5–8 during OKT3 therapy the doses of A and P were further reduced to 25 mg per day and 0·4 mg kg$^{-1}$ per day, respectively, but increased again to 100–150 mg per day after OKT3. The rationale of this protocol is to reverse acute rejection by OKT3 and to avoid excessive immunosuppression (and consequent viral infections) during this period. After cessation of OKT3 therapy the level of non-specific immunosuppression can be increased again to prevent the recurrence of the rejection episode. The acute rejection was reversed by OKT3 in all cases in spite of decreasing the doses of A and P.

TABLE 4·7
The effects of antibodies on "target" cells and the escape mechanisms

---

A.  Elimination of inhibition of "target" cells.
    1. Complement mediated lysis.
    2. Inhibition of function ("blind-folding").
    3. Mitogenic stimulation of cells ("sterile" activation).
    4. Altered recirculation pattern of Ab-coated cells.
    5. "Arming" of macrophages and K cells.
    6. Increased phagocytosis, by macrophages, of "opsonized" target cells.
    7. Target cell immunogenicity is increased by heterologous Ab.

B.  Escape mechanisms for target cells.
    1. Subpopulations of relevant cells are unreactive with the Ab.
    2. Antigenic modulation by Ab (the cells "shed their spoiled coat").
    3. The Ab does not reach the cells[a].
    4. The functions of cells blocked and/or the circulation patterns of Ab-coated cells
       are altered temporarily, but these cells are not killed. They "surface" again and
       regain their function.

---

[a]   The three possible reasons are: (i) the malignant cell is inaccessible for serum immunoglobulin
    (particularly if it is of IgM class); (ii) the Ab binds to free antigen released from the tumour cell
    (see Nadler *et al.*, 1980; Hamblin *et al.*, 1980), and (iii) the Ab is "neutralized" by preformed
    human antibodies to mouse Ig (Cosimi *et al.*, 1981b).

antibodies. Effective serotherapy in leukaemias and generalized lymphomas may reduce the tumour burden and lead to a more localized lymphomatous growth pattern. This has been observed as the typical course in most cases of T cell leukaemias and Sezary syndrome treated with ATG (Barrett *et al.*, 1976; Fisher *et al.*, 1978; Edelson *et al.*, 1979) and with anti-T monoclonal antibody (L17F12, Miller and Levy, 1981). These authors demonstrated that the lymphoma cells inside these regrowing deposits did in fact express the OKT1-like L17F12 antigen, and the lack of response to the antibody was not due to antigenic modulation or immunoselection. The important point, however, is that during ATG therapy serious toxicity was noted which was related to the large amount of foreign protein injected (200–1000 mg), while the monoclonal antibody given (1–20 mg) caused no side effects. It might, therefore, be ethical to attempt serotherapy using monoclonal antibodies in cases with lower tumour burden at a stage when, perhaps as a result of antibody therapy, the residual "pockets" of tumour cells inaccessible to antibody might still be or become more responsive to cytotoxic drugs.

It is also interesting that in the first case treated with L17F12 antibody important facts emerged about the efficacy of opsonization, the phenomenon of antigenic modulation (see above) as well as the release of free antigen (from the destroyed cells?) into the circulation after the monoclonal antibody therapy (Miller *et al.*, 1981). These pieces of information were then utilized in the second patient in order to optimize the protocol of antibody therapy. This patient tolerated 17 treatment courses over a 10-week period without any toxicity and showed a marked clinical response (regression of cutaneous tumours, healing in the local lesions, decrease in lymphadenopathy and increase of haemoglobin) over a 3 month period.

4. OTHER DISEASES

With the availability of large quantities of monoclonal antibodies other immunoregulatory disorders might become amenable for therapy. There are two interesting examples. First, certain haemopoietic disorders (aplastic anaemia, selective neutropenia and red cell aplasia) show, in 40–60% of cases, high numbers of T cells expressing the suppressor-cytotoxic phenotype (OKT8$^+$) in the circulating blood (Callard *et al.*, 1981, Linch *et al.*, 1981, and other functional signs of activation in the patient's bone marrow (Bacigalupo *et al.*, 1980). Second, during acute graft versus host disease there are large proportions of activated OKT8$^+$ cells, a distinct subpopulation of which has been identified in the skin lesions (Lampert *et al.*, 1981; Janossy *et al.*, 1982). It will be interesting to see whether any of these diseases respond to monoclonal antibody treatment using either pan-T reagents (such as OKT3 and OKT11), more selective anti-T cell subset antibodies (such as OKT8) or combinations of the two.

    Before any considerations are raised about long term therapy it will be necessary to establish whether or not mouse monoclonal antibodies are immunogenic in man. In animals, small doses of aggregate-free (ultracentrifuged) heterologous immunoglobulin are well known to be tolerogenic (Dresser and Gowland, 1964). Similarly, when a patient was given 17 doses of aggregate free monoclonal antibody during a 10 week period no antibody response was seen (Miller and Levy, 1981). In a previous patient only a transient response of IgM class to mouse Ig was detected (Miller *et al.*, 1981). It is nevertheless possible that the humoral immune response in these patients was compromized by their tumour and/or chemotherapy. In another 4 patients recently treated with OKT3 for the reversal of kidney rejection high levels of anti-mouse Ig antibodies developed after the completion of the 14-day course (Cosimi *et al.*, 1981b).

## B. Treatment of Bone Marrow Cells *In Vitro*

This is one of the main lines of therapeutic applications for the following reasons. Under these conditions the bone marrow (BM) cell suspensions are accessible to antibody, and can be washed to eliminate shed membrane antigens or preformed human antibodies to mouse Ig. Furthermore, the antibody mediated removal of "unwanted" cells can be amplified by incubating the BM with rabbit complement (for C' mediated cytotoxicity in vitro) or by using antibodies coupled to toxins (see chapter 7). Prior to re-infusion into the host the BM is washed and, therefore, the rabbit serum or unbound toxin-coupled monoclonal antibodies are not injected into the host. Clearly these therapeutic applications are ethically more acceptable than the injection of toxin-coupled antibodies into the patient, which may not reach their inaccessible targets but can cause serious non-specific cytopathic effects (e.g. in the liver or in macrophages, etc.). In fact a large part of monoclonal antibody standardization has been devoted to the analysis of their potential uses in human BM transplantation (see above, Granger *et al.*, 1981, 1982; Crawford *et al.*, 1981; Janossy *et al.*, 1981; Hansen *et al.*, 1981)

### 1. PREVENTION OF GRAFT VERSUS HOST DISEASE (GvHD)

Optimally one could use the combination of OKT3 and OKT11A monoclonal antibodies together with rabbit serum as C' for the removal of T lymphocytes from concentrated red cell free allogeneic donor BM (see above, and Table 4·5). These manipulations are feasible but require skill and equipment. It is unknown whether the removal of $OKT3^+$, $OKT11^+$ peripheral T lymphocytes alone would be sufficient to prevent GvHD or whether an additional antibody reactive with the so far unidentified "prothymocytes" (as suggested by Müller-Ruchholtz *et al.*, 1980) is also necessary. It is interesting to note that the heterologous ATG used by Rodt *et al.*, (1981) to prevent GvHD might contain an extra contaminating antibody against this putative prothymocyte population and also react with its leukaemic counterpart (Thiel *et al.*, 1980).

There is indirect evidence that "coating" of lymphocytes with OKT3 alone removes T cells from the circulation by opsonization (Cosimi *et al.*, 1981b). It is, therefore, reasonable to suggest that simple coating of BM T cells with OKT3 will also lead to the sequestration and elimination of infused T lymphocytes by the reticuloendothelial system *in vivo*. This hypothesis has been tested in 17 leukaemic patients who received

matched HLA-A,B,C and HLA-D compatible allogeneic BM from
their siblings (Prentice *et al.*, 1982). The patients (6–42 years of age)
were in complete remission during transplantation with the exception
of one patient (19 year old male) who did not respond to conventional
therapy. In this patient the leukaemia was eliminated with intensive
therapy which also induced total BM aplasia. The observations have
been compared with "historical" controls of the same hospital; previously the occurrence of GvHD in matched BM transplantation was
79%. The incubation of BM (65–200 ml) with 1 mg OKT3 improved
the results. T cells were "coated" with monoclonal antibody, but there
was no BM toxicity and all the transplanted BM have regenerated
normally. 82% of patients remained free of acute GvHD throughout
their course, although two patients developed small areas of lichen
planus which cleared on 10 mg prednisone given on alternative days.
Three patients, however, had acute GvHD. Two developed classical
acute GvHD from days 11, 16 and 21. In both cases this was accompanied by acute cytomegalovirus infection. The other patient, the 19
year old male mentioned above, presented with isolated liver GvHD
with additional involvement of skin and gut at day 50 which was also
irreversible.

One of the possible interpretations of these preliminary observations
is that considerable numbers of T lymphocytes are eliminated by
coating with OKT3 and opsonization *in vivo*. As a result, patients with
mild incompatibility did not develop GvHD and the incidence of
GvHD dropped. A few T cells seemed to escape, however, and in the
event of virus infection or strong incompatibility (not detected by HLA
typing) these were able to mount a fatal, although somewhat delayed,
GvHD (Prentice *et al.*, 1981). Similar findings were reported in mice
with monoclonal antibodies where, in addition, it was also demonstrated that the GvHD in the fully incompatible combination could be
prevented by antibody plus complement (Vallera *et al.*, 1981; Hoffman-
Fezer *et al.*, 1981). These results in man represent a considerable
improvement over previous results, particularly if one considers the
simplicity and low cost of the method involved. Further possible
developments are the application of rabbit C' with antibody combinations as shown above, or the incubation of BM with OKT3 followed by
treating GvHD with OKT3 *in vivo* in occassional patients who still
develop the disease.

3. "CLEANSING" OF CRYOPRESERVED REMISSION
BONE MARROW OF RESIDUAL LEUKAEMIC CELLS

This task is a logical extension of the current trend of autologous BM transplantation in leukaemia (Gorin *et al.*, 1981). When HLA matched allogeneic BM is not available, the patient's own marrow is harvested and cryopreserved during the first remission. It is unlikely, when established only on the basis of haematological criteria, that this BM is free of leukaemic or lymphoma cells, or that the few residual leukaemic cells present are selectively hampered by the transplantation process while normal BM precursor cells survive. Nevertheless, the procedure has already worked in a few patients where preserved autologous BM was used to reconstitute patients and the leukaemia/lymphoma did not relapse (Gorin *et al.*, 1981). Leukaemia/lymphoma heterogeneity recently observed with monoclonal antibodies indicates that the immunologists' task here is difficult; careful phenotyping of malignant cells and reagent selection, from a panel of well characterized antibodies will be required. This characterization needs to include the reactivity on normal haemopoietic cells (Fig. 4·3), and selected monoclonal antibodies may have to be coupled to toxins or shown to be effective in C' mediated lysis. Opsonization alone this time would probably not suffice (see corresponding animal experiments by Hoffman -Fezer *et al.*, 1981; Trigg and Poplack, 1981; Jansen *et al.*, 1981; Vallera *et al.*, 1981).

Although this approach requires such an intimate collaboration between immunologists, haematologists and oncologists which is difficult to reach, the aims are not impossible. The antibodies used in the animal experiments (with immunotoxin or C') will literally kill >99·9% of tumour cells without damaging control BM cells (Jansen *et al.*, 1981; Trigg and Poplack, 1981) and there are at least three haematological disease groups where the phenotype of malignancy is different from that of the haemopoietic precursor cells. These are:

1. Malignant disorders of the thymocyte-T cell lineage including thymic acute lymphoblastic leukaemia (Thy-ALL) and peripheral T cell leukaemia (T-CLL and cutaneous T cell lymphoma). The most appropriate monoclonal antibody in this group is OKT11A (of IgG$_2$) class (Crawford *et al.*, 1981; Janossy *et al.*, 1981a; Verbi *et al.*, 1982). Recent studies indicate that WT-1 and CALL2 may show anti Thy-ALL specificity (Tax *et al.*, 1981, Deng *et al.*, 1982.

2. Cases of non-T, non-B ALL which react well (>95% of positive blasts) with anti-ALL antiserum (Netzel *et al.*, 1981) or with the corresponding monoclonal antibodies: J-5 (IgG$_2$ class) and VIL-A1 (IgM class, both of which are lytic with C'; Ritz *et al.*, 1980; Liszka *et al.*, 1981). 1981). Netzel *et al.*, (1981) have already used this approach in two patients during the third relapse of non-T, non-B ALL resistant to

conventional therapy. Within 24 hrs after total body irradiation the BM cells collected during first remission (30 months previously) and pretreated with rabbit anti-ALL globulin were re-infused. Both patients regenerated the BM and one of them is well. Similar attempts have been made recently with J5, (Kersey et al., 1981 and unpublished).

3.    Cases of B cell malignancy including Hodgkin's disease and B cell lymphoma. B cell malignancies carry distinctive antigens detected by monoclonal antibodies (FMC-1, B-1, B-2, Tü-1) which have not yet been fully characterized on normal human BM cells (Brooks et al., 1980; Nadler et al., 1981; Ziegler et al., 1981). Two other monoclonal antibodies which have been analyzed in this respect indicate that BM precursor cells and B cells in the BM do indeed show a phenotype which is distinctly different from that of peripheral B cells and many B cell malignancies (Caligaris-Cappio et al., 1982). Again, the removal of B lymphoma cells from the BM without destroying precursor cells should be possible. This project is clinically very important.


# V  CONCLUSIONS

It is interesting to observe that the groups which have initiated the inevitable use of monoclonal antibodies in human therapy have also developed the expert technology to monitor their patients and the antibody effects by a number of criteria. These include: (i) levels of free mouse antibody, (ii) amounts of human antibodies to mouse Ig in the serum, (iii) cell population analysis by multiple markers in order to detect elimination of lymphocyte subsets and to analyze antigenic modulation, (iv) immuno-histological analysis. Some of these groups have, in addition, initiated experiments in primates in line with the best tradition of transplantation research. It is unlikely that therapeutic applications will be achieved without this detailed, basic approach.

ACKNOWLEDGEMENTS

The work from the authors laboratories was supported by the Leukaemia Research Fund of Great Britain (to G.J.), by U.S.P.H.S. Grant HL/AM-18646 (to A.B.C.) and the Ortho Pharmaceutical Corporation. We most gratefully acknowledge the contributions of our colleagues who are listed in the references.

REFERENCES

Abaza, H. M., Nolan, B., Watt, J. G. and Woodruff, M. F. A. (1966). *Transplantation* **4**, 618–622.

Bach, J. F. and Dormont, J. (1971). *Transplantation* **11**, 97–100.

Bach, M-A., Phan-Dinh-Tuy, F., Bach, J. F., Wallach, D., Biddison, W. E., Sharrow, S. O., Goldstein, G. and Kung, P. C. (1981). *J. Immunol.* **127** 980–982. ·

Bacigalupo, A., Podesta, M., Mingari, M., Moretta, L., Van Lint, M. and Marmont, A. (1980). *J. Immunol.* **125**, 1449–1453.

Balch, C. M., Dougherty, P. A., Dagg, M. K., Diethelm, A. G. and Lawton, A. R. (1977). *Clin. Immunol. Immunopathol.* **8**, 448–457.

Balner, H. (1971). *Transpl. Proc.* **3.**, 949–957.

Barrett, J. A., Bridgen, D., Roberts, J., Staughton, R., Byrom, N. and Hobbs, J. (1976) *Lancet* **i**, 940–941.

Bastin, J. M., Granger, S., Tidman, N., Janossy, G. and McMichael, A. J. (1981). *Clin. Exp. Immunol.* **46**, 597–606.

Beverley, P. C. L. and Callard, R. E. (1981). *Eur. J. Immunol.* **11**, 329–334.

Bhan, A. K., Reinherz, E. L., Poppema, S., McClusky, R. T. and Schlossman, S. F. (1980). *J. exp. Med.* **152**, 771–782.

Bieber, C. P., Howard, F. D., Pennock, J., Wong, J., Shorthouse, R. and Stinson, E. B. (1981). *Transplantation* **31**, 283–289.

Boumsell, L. and Bernard, A. (1981). *In* "Leukaemia Markers" (W. Knapp, Ed.), pp. 129–142. Academic Press, London and New York.

Boumsell, L., Coppin, H., Pham, D., Raynal, B., Lemerle, J., Dausset, J. and Bernard, A. (1980). *J. exp. Med.* **152**, 229–234.

Brent, L., Courtenay, T. and Gowland, G. (1967). *Nature* **215**, 1461–1463.

Brooks, D. A., Beckman, I., Bradley, J., McNamara, P. J., Thomas, M. E. and Zola, H. (1980) *Clin. exp. Immunol.* **39**, 477–485.

Caligaris-Cappio, F., Gobbi, M., Boffill, M. and Janossy, G. (1982) *J. Exp. Med.* **155**, 623–628.

Callard, R. E., Smith, C. M., Worman, C., Linch, D., Cawley, J. C. and Beverley, P. C. L. (1981). *Clin. exp. Immunol.* **43**, 497–505.

Cantor, H. (1972). *Progr. Bioph. Molec. Biol.* **25**, 71.

Chang, T. W., Kung, P. C., Gingras, V. P. and Goldstein, G. (1981). *Proc. natn. Acad. Sci. U.S.A.* **78**, 1805–1808.

Cosimi, A. B. (1981). *Transpl. Proc.* **13**, 462–468.

Cosimi, A. B., Burton, R. C., Kung, P.C., Colvin, R., Goldstein, G., Lifter, J., Rhodes, W. and Russell, P. S. (1981a). *Transpl. Proc.* **13**, 499–503.

Cosimi, A.B., Burton, R.C., Colvin, R. B., Goldstein, G., Delmohico, F.L., La Quaglia, M. P., Tolkoff-Rubin, N., Rubin, R. H., Herrin, J. T. and Russell, P. S. (1981). *Transplantation* **32**, 535–562.

Crawford, D. H., Francis, G. E., Wing, M. A., Edwards, A. J., Janossy, G., Hoffbrand, A. V., Prentice, H. G., Secher, D., McConnell, I., Kung, P. C. and Goldstein, G. (1981). *Br. J. Haematol.* **49** 209–217.

Deng, C., Chia, J., Terasaki, P. and Billing, R. (1982) *Lancet* **i** 10–11.

Dicke, K. A., Tridente, G. and van Bekkum, D. W. (1969). *Transplantation* **8**, 422.

Doney, K. C., Weiden, P. L., Storb, R. and Thomas, E. D. (1981). *Transplantation* **31**, 141–143.

Dresser, D. W. and Gowland, G. (1964). *Nature* **203**, 733–736.

Edelson, R., Raafat, J., Berger, C., Grossman, M., Trager, C. and Hardy, M. (1979). *Cancer Treat. Rep.* **63**, 675–680.

Engleman, E., Warnke, R., Fox, R. and Levy, R. (1981). *Proc. natn. Acad. Sci. U.S.A.* **28**, 1791–1795.

Filo, R. S., Smith, E. J. and Leapman, S. B. (1981). *Transpl. Proc.* **13**, 482–490.

Fisher, R., Kubota, T., Mandell, G., Broder, S. and Young, R. (1978). *Ann. intern. Med.* **88**, 799–800.

Fithian, E., Kung, P. C., Goldstein, G., Rubenfeld, M., Fenoglio, C. and Edelson, R. (1981). *Proc. natn. Acad. Sci. U.S.A.* **78**, 2541–2544.

Gilmore, M., Prentice, H. G., Blacklock, H., Ma, D. and Hoffbrand, A. V. (1982). *Br. J. Haematol.* **50**, 360–366.

Goldschneider, I., Ahmed, A., Bollum, F. J. and Goldstein, A. (1981). *Proc. natn. Acad. Sci. U.S.A.* **78**, 2469–2473.

Gorin, N. C., David, R., Stachowiack, J., Salmon, E., Petit, J. C., Parlier, Y., Najman, A. and Duhamel, G. (1981) *Eur. J. Cancer* **17**, 557–568.

Granger, S., Janossy, G., Tidman, N., Ashley, J., Crawford, D. H., Koubek, K., Francis, G., Prentice, H. G., Hoffbrand, A. V., Kung, P. C. and Goldstein, G. (1981). *In* "Leukaemia Markers" (W. Knapp, Ed.), pp. 419–424. Academic Press, London and New York.

Granger, S., Poulter, L. W., Francis, G., Goldstein, G. and Janossy, G. (1982). *Br. J. Haematol.* **50**, 367–374.

Grathwohl, A., Nissen, C., Osterwalder, B., Leibundgut, U., Burri, H. P., Kuospe, W. and Speck, B. Manuscript in preparation.

Gray, J. G., Monaco, A. P. and Russell, P. S. (1964). *Surg. Forum* **15**, 142.

Greaves, M. F. and Janossy, G. (1976). *In* "In Vitro Methods in Cell Mediated and Tumour Immunity" (B. R. Bloom and J. R. David, Eds), pp. 89–111. Academic Press, London and New York.

Greaves, M. F. and Janossy, G. (1978). *Biochim. biophys. Acta.* **516**, 193–230.

Greaves, M. F., Tursi, A., Playfair, J. H. L., Torrigiani, G., Samir, R. and Roitt, I. M. (1969). *Lancet* **i**, 68–72.

Groth, C. G. (1981). *Transpl. Proc.* **13**, 460–461.

Hamblin, T. J., Abdul-Ahad, A. K., Gordon, J., Stevenson, F. K. and Stevenson, G. T. (1980). *Brit. J. Cancer* **42**, 495–502.

Hansen, J. A., Martin, P. J., Kamoun, M., Torok-Strob, B., Newman, W., Nowinski, R. C. and Thomas, E. D. (1981). *Transpl. Proc.* **13**, 1133–1137.

Hoffman-Fezer, G., Thierfelder, S., Rodt, H., Kumer, U., Doxiadis, I., Stunkel, K. and Eulitz, M. (1981). *In* "Leukaemia Markers" (W. Knapp, Ed.), pp. 405–418. Academic Press, London and New York.

Ivanyi, J. (1980). *In* "Immunobiology of Bone Marrow Transplantation" (S. Thierfelder, H. Rodt, H. J. Kolb, Eds), pp. 219–237. Springer, Berlin-Heidelberg.

James, K. (1967). *Clin. exp. Immunol.* **2**, 615–622.

Janossy, G. (1981). *In* "Methods in Haematology. Leukaemic Cells" (D. Catovsky, Ed.), pp. 129–183. Churchill-Livingstone, Edinburgh and New York.

Janossy, G. and Greaves, M. F. (1972). *Clin. exp. Immunol.* **10**, 525–534.

Janossy, G., Greaves, M. F., Sutherland, R., Durrant, J. and Lewis, C. (1977). *Leukaemia Res.* **1**, 289–300.

Janossy, G., Goldstone, A. H., Capellaro, D., Greaves, M. F., Kulenkampff, J., Pippard, M. and Welsh, K. (1977). *Br. J. Haematol.* **37**, 391–402.

Janossy, G., Francis, G., Capellaro, D., Goldstone, A. H. and Greaves, M. F. (1978). *Nature* **276**, 176–178.

Janossy, G., Tidman, N., Selby, W. S., Thomas, J. A., Granger, S., Kung, P. C. and Goldstein, G. (1980) *Nature* **287**, 81–84.

Janossy, G., Tidman, N., Papageorgiou, E. S., Kung, P. C. and Goldstein, G. (1981). *J. Immunol.* **126**, 1608–1613.

Janossy, G., Montano, L., Selby, W. S., Dake, O., Panayi, G., Lampert, I., Thomas, J. A., Goldstein, G. (1982). *J. Clin. Immunol.* (in press).

Jansen, F. K., Blythman, H. E., Casellas, P., Gros, O., Gros, P., Paolucci, F., Pau, B. and Vidal, H. (1981). *In* "Leukaemia Markers" (W. Knapp, Ed.), pp. 397–401. Academic Press, London and New York.

Jonasson, O., Simmon, R. and Cohen, C. (1982). *Transplantation* (in press).

Kamoun, M., Martin, P. J., Hansen, J. A., Brown, M. A. and Nowinski, R. C. (1981). *J. exp. Med.* **153**, 207–212.

Kersey, J. H. (1981). Personal communication.

Kolb, H. J., Rieder, I., Rodt, H., Netzel, B., Grosse-Wilde, H., Scholz, S., Schäffer, E., Kolb, H. and Thierfelder, S. (1979). *Transplantation* **27**, 242–245.

Kung, P. C., Goldstein, G., Reinherz, E. L. and Schlossman, S. F. (1979). *Science* **206**, 347–351.

Kung, P. C., Talle, M. A., DeMaria, M., Butler, M., Lifter, J. and Goldstein, G. (1980). *Transpl. Proc.* **12**, 141–146.

Lampert, I. A., Thomas, J. A., Snitters, A. J., Bofill, M., Palmer, S., Gordon-Smith, E., Prentice, H. G. and Janossy, G. (1982). *Clin. Exp. Immunol.* (in press).

Lance, E. M., Medawar, P. B., and Taub, R. N. (1973). *Advances in Immunol* **17**, 1–92.

Ledbetter, J. A., Evans, R. L., Lipinski, M., Cunningham, C. R., Good, R. A. and Herzenberg, L. A. (1981). *J. exp. Med.* **153**, 310–323.

Leuchars, E., Wallis, V. J. and Davies, A. J. S. (1968). *Nature* **219**, 1325–1328.

Levey, R. H. and Medawar, P. B. (1966). *Ann. N.Y. Acad. Sci.* **129**, 164–177.

Light, J. A., Alijani, M. R., Biggers, J. A., Oddenino, K. and Reinmuth, B. (1981). *Transpl. Proc.* **13**, 475–481.

Linch, D. C., Cawley, J. C., Warman, C. P., Galvin, M. C., Roberts, B. E., Callard, R. E. and Beverley, P. C. L. (1981). *Br. J. Haematol.* **48**, 137–145.

Liszka, K., Majdic, O., Bettelheim, P. and Knapp, W. (1981). *In* "Leukaemia Markers" (W. Knapp, Ed.), pp. 61–64. Academic Press, London and New York.

Marmont, A., Peschle, C. and Sangniulti, M. (1975). *Blood* **45**, 247–261.

Martin, P. J., Hansen, J. A., Siadeck, A. W. and Nowinski, R. C. (1981). *J. Immunol.* **127**, 1920–1926.

Martin, W. J. (1969). *J. Immunol.* **103**, 979–999.

McMichael, A. J., Pilch, J. R., Galfre, G., Mason, D. Y., Fabre, J. W. and Milstein, C. (1979). *Eur. J. Immunol.* **9**, 205–210.

Metcalf, D. (1977). *In* "Hemopoietic Colonies: in vitro cloning of normal and leukaemic cells". Springer Verlag, Berlin/Heidelberg.

Miller, R. A., Maloney, D. G., McKillop, J. and Levy, R. (1981). *Blood* **58**, 78–86.

Miller, R. A. and Levy, R. (1981). *Lancet* ii, 116–229.

Milstein, C. (1981). This volume.

Monaco, A. P., Abbott, W. M., Otherson, H. B., Simmons, R. L., Wood, M. L., Flax, M. H. and Russell, P. S. (1966b) Science 153, 1264–1267.

Monaco, A. P., Wood, M. L. and Russell, P. S. (1966a) *Ann. N.Y. Acad. Sci.* **129**, 190–209.

Monaco, A. P., Wood, M. L. and Russell, P. S. (1967). *Transplantation* 5, 1106–1114.

Müller-Ruchholz, W., Wottge, H. V., and Müller-Hermelink, H. K. (1980). *In* "Immunobiology of Bone Marrow Transplantation" (S. Thierfelder, H. Rodt, H. J. Kolb, Eds), pp. 153–178. Springer Verlag, Berlin/Heidelberg.

Nadler, L. M., Ritz, J., Reinherz, E. L. and Schlossman, S. (1981). *In* "Leukaemia Markers" (W. Knapp, Ed), pp. 3–18. Academic Press, London and New York.

Nadler, L. M., Stashenko, P., Hardy, R., Kaplan, W. D., Button, L. N., Kufe, D. W., Antman, K. H. and Schlossman, S. F. (1980). *Cancer Res.* **40**, 3147–3154.

Nehlsen, S. L. (1971). *Clin. exp. Immunol.* **9**, 63–77.

Netzel, B., Haas, R. J., Rodt, H., Kolb, H. J., Belohradsky, B. and Thierfelder, S. (1980). *Transpl. Proc.* **13**, 254–256.

Nowygrod, R., Appel, G. and Hardy, M. A. (1981). *Transpl. Proc.* **13**, 469–472.

Old, L. J., Stockert, E., Boyse, E. A. and Geering, G. (1967). *Proc. Soc. exp. Biol. Med.* **124**, 63–67.

Poppema, S., Bhan, A. K., Reinherz, E. L., McCluskey, R. T. and Schlossman, S. F. (1981) *J. exp. Med.* **153**, 30–41.

Prentice, H. G., Blacklock, H. A., Janossy, G., Bradstock, K. F., Skeggs, D., Goldstein, G. and Hoffbrand, A. V. (1982). *Lancet* i. (in press).

Reinherz, E. L. and Schlossman, S. F. (1979). *J. Immunol.* **122**, 1325–1342.

Reinherz, E. L. and Schlossman, S. F. (1980). *Cell* 19, 821–827.

Reinherz, E. L. and Hussey, R. E. and Schlossman, S. F. (1980). *Eur. J. Immunol.* **10**, 758–762.

Reinherz, E. L., Kung, P. C., Goldstein, G., Levey, R. H. and Schlossman, S. F. (1980). *Proc. natn. Acad. Sci. U.S.A.* **77**, 1588–1592.

Ritz, J., Pesando, J. M., Notis-McConarty, J. and Schlossman, S. F. (1980). *J. Immunol.* **125**, 1506–1514.

Rodt, H., Thierfelder, S., and Eulitz, M. (1974). *Eur. J. Immunol.* **4**, 25–29.

Rodt, H., Thierfelder, S., Thiel, E., Götze, D., Netzel, B., Huhn, D. and Eulitz, M. (1975). *Immunogenetics* 2, 411–421.

Rodt, H., Kolb, H. J., Netzel, B., Haas, R. J., Wilms, K., Götze, C. B., Link, H. and Thierfelder, S. (1981). *Transpl. Proc.* 13 157–261.

Rosenberg, S. A. and Terry, W. D. (1977). *Adv. Cancer Res.* 25, 323–388.

Royston, I., Majda, J., Baird, S., Meserve, B. and Griffiths, (1980). *J. Immunol.* 125, 725–731.

Speck, B., Gluckman, E., Haak, H. L. and van Rood, J. J. (1977) *Lancet* ii, 1145–1148.

Starzl, T. E., Marchioro, T. L., Hutchinson, D., Porter, K. A., Cerilli, C. J. and Brettschneider, L. (1967). *Transplantation* 5 suppl. 1100.

Taub, R. N. and Lance, E. M. (1968). *Immunology* 15, 633.

Tax, W. J. M., Willem, S. H. W., Kibbelaar, M. D. A., de Groot, J., Capel, P. J. A., de Waal, R. M. W., Reekers, P., and Koene, R. A. P. (1981) *Protides Biol. Fluids* 29. (in press).

Thiel, E., Rodt, H., Huhn, D. and Thierfelder, S. (1980). *Blood* 56, 759–772.

Thierfelder, S., Rodt, H. and Netzel, B. (1977). *Transplantation* 23, 459–463.

Thierfelder, S., Rodt, H. and Thiel, E. (1977). *In* "Immunological Diagnosis of Leukemias and Lymphomas". Springer Verlag, Berlin/Heidelberg.

Transplantation Society Meeting in Santa Barbara (1967). *Transplantation* 5.

Transplantation Society Meeting in New York (1977). *Transpl. Proc.* 9.

Transplantation Society Meeting in Boston (1981). *Transpl. Proc.* 13

Trigg, M. E. and Poplack, D. G. (1981). *In* "Leukaemia Markers" (W. Knapp, Ed.), pp. 425–428, Academic Press, London and New York.

Vallera, D. A., Soderling, C-C.R., Carlson, G. J. and Kersey, J. H. (1981). *Transplantation* 31, 218–222.

Van Wauwe, J. P., De Mey, J. R. and Goossens, J. G. (1980). *J. Immunol.* 124, 2708–2713.

Van Wauwe, J. P. and Goossens, J. G. (1981). *Immunology* 42, 157–164.

Verbi, W., Greaves, M. F., Koubek, K., Janossy, G., Kung, P. C. and Goldstein, G. (1982). *Eur. J. Immunol.* 12, 81–86.

Waksman, B. H., Arbouys, S. and Arnason, B. G. (1961). *J. exp. Med.* 114, 997.

Wechter, W. J., Brodie, J. A., Morrell, R. M., Rafi, M. and Schultz, J. R. (1979a). *Transplantation* 28, 294–302.

Wechter, W. J., Nelson, J. W., Perper, R. J., Parcells, A. J., Riebe, K. W., Evans, J. S., Satoh, P. S. and Ko, H. (1979b). *Transplantation* 28, 303–307.

Winchester, R. J., Ross, G. D., Jarowski, C. I., Wang, C. Y., Halper, J. and Broxmeyer, H. E. (1977). *Proc. natn. Acad. Sci. U.S.A.* 74, 4012–4016.

Woodruff, M. F. A. (1968). *Nature* 217, 821–824.

Woodruff, M. F. A. and Anderson, N. F. (1963). *Nature* 200, 702.

Wulff, J. C., Anderson, M., Held, H., Müller-Hermelink, H. K., Schlaak, M. and Müller-Ruchholtz, W. (1981). *Transpl. proc.* 13, 230–233.

Ziegler, A., Stein, H., Müller, C. and Wernet, P. (1981). *In* "Leukaemia Markers" (W. Knapp, Ed.), pp. 113–116. Academic Press, London and New York.

# C CANCER

# 5 Definition of Human Tumour Antigens

EDWIN S. LENNOX[a] AND KAROL SIKORA[b]

a MRC Laboratory of Molecular Biology, Hills Road,
  Cambridge. CB2 2QH
b Ludwig Institute for Cancer Research, MRC Centre,
  The Medical School, Hills Road, Cambridge. CB2 2QH

## I INTRODUCTION

The use of monoclonal antibodies with their individual specificities is freeing tumour immunologists from some of the limitations of conventional serology and is giving hope that the nature of tumour antigens will at last be revealed. If we knew how antigens on tumour cells were related to those on normal cells we could develop better strategies for their clinical use in diagnosis, prognosis and therapy. The rapidly increasing number of monoclonal antibodies made with tumour cells as immunogens is allowing this comparison. We would like to focus our attention on the particular information we need to know about the cross reactions of each monoclonal antibody with normal tissue and with other tumours to make best use of it.

If malignant cells had antigens not present on any normal cell then life would be simple for the tumour immunologist. In this case, monoclonal antibodies against these antigens could be used for all the clinical applications (see Table 5·1) without danger of misdiagnosis or of causing damage to normal tissue by misdirecting antibodies coupled to toxic agents. But neither is the situation likely to be that simple nor is this extreme situation necessary for fruitful use of monoclonal antibodies in cancer.

TABLE 5·1
Uses of monoclonal antibodies in cancer

1.  Tumour diagnosis—by detection of antigen in serum
2.  Tumour localization—using labelled antibodies
3.  Targetting toxic agents to tumour—using coupled antibodies
4.  Monitoring therapeutic agents—by detection in serum as agent is administered
5.  Monitoring of intrinsic agents—by detection in serum of hormones etc.
6.  Monitoring of state of the immune and haematopoietic systems—by assaying numbers and proportions of cells of different types

Taken from Lennox, E. S. (1982). *In* "Hybridomas in Diagnosis and Treatment of Cancer" (M. S. Mitchell and H. F. Oettgen Eds). Reproduced with permission from Raven Press, New York.

In the analysis of tumour antigens the immune response of laboratory animals and of the cancer patient are used. Each sees the tumour cell surface from a different point of view and this affects the spectrum of anti tumour monoclonal antibodies produced. The argument is often made that responses of experimental animals to human tumour specific antigens would be lost amidst the responses to the large collection of normal antigens that tumour cells bear. In this situation, the argument continues, the response of the tumour patient himself will be only to tumour specific neoantigens since he is immunologically unresponsive to all of his own antigens. In conventional sera, it is true that anti tumour antibodies prepared by injection of human tumours do by and large recognize many different normal and malignant cells although occasionally tumour specific ones are claimed. Both the wide cross reactions and specific responses are difficult to interpret in view of the mixtures of antibodies that constitute conventional sera. Human immune responses to tumours are often very weak, hence characterization of the recognized antigen is difficult. Both these problems are avoided by use of monoclonal antibodies.

There are inherent difficulties in defining "tumour specific" antigens regardless of the type of antibodies used for analysis. Firstly, a tumour may anomalously express cell surface antigens, not found on the normal cell from which it derives, but that are produced by other normal cell types. This might result from the ability of tumours to make products inappropriate to their normal state of differentiation. Secondly, because most tumours result from the clonal expansion of single cells they magnify the expression of differentiation markers characteristic of the normal cell from which they derive. Such clonally expanded normal antigens may masquerade as tumour specific especially if the normal cell is only a small proportion of the normal cells of the tissue in which the tumour arises.

In model animal systems, particularly the chemically induced tumours of rodents (Baldwin, 1973), there are tumour specific trans-plantation antigens, not shared by normal tissue. However, since it has recently been suggested that these specificities are carried on envelope glycoproteins of retroviruses, similar tumour specific antigens may not occur in man (Lennox, 1980). So far the evidence for the existence of tumour specific antigens in man analogous to the tumour specific transplantation antigens in animals is circumstantial. The natural history of certain tumours, the waxing and waning of tumour masses and the occurrence of spontaneous regression suggests that there may be some host control – possibly immunological – of tumour growth (Everson and Cole, 1966). Similarly, the relationship between histological evidence of tumour infiltration by immuno-competent cells and prognosis suggests that these infiltrating cells have some controlling influence of tumour growth (Bloom *et al.*, 1970). Further circumstantial evidence comes from the increased incidence of certain malignancy in immuno-suppressed patients, although here the kinds of tumours that arise are not similar to those found in the normal population. This makes it unlikely that an effective immune response is mounted except for certain types of malignancies (Kinlen *et al.*, 1979). Serological analysis and assays of lymphocyte function of tumour patients have repeatedly shown that the immune system in man can actually recognize the tumour cell surface though at least part of this response is to antigens shared with normal tissue (Shiku *et al.*, 1976).

Monoclonal antibodies provide promising tools for exploring differences between tumour cells and their normal tissue counterparts. Once identified, unique tumour markers would have considerable clinical significance for diagnosing, localizing, monitoring and treating tumours in patients. Much effort has been exerted in the last three years in deriving monoclonal antibodies to human tumours. We discuss how

near we are to the goal of detecting tumour specific markers and how
the degree of specificity of a monoclonal antibody, that is its cross
reactions with normal tissues and with other tumours, determines the
limitations on its possible uses.

## II PRODUCTION OF MONOCLONAL ANTIBODIES TO HUMAN TUMOUR CELL SURFACES

### A. PRACTICAL CONSIDERATIONS

#### 1. CHOICE OF ANIMAL

Currently there are three systems in which anti-tumour monoclonal
antibodies can be raised; mouse, rat and human. For human tumours,
mice and rats have the obvious advantages of responding to a wide
variety of antigens and are thus the choice for an exhaustive analysis of
tumour cell surface components. This wide response may be a disadvantage because of the response to the many normal antigens expressed
on malignant material. Indeed, xenogeneic immunizations often result
in antibodies directed against histocompatibility antigens (Howard *et
al.*, 1978) and blood group substances (Voak *et al.*, 1980). However,
other xenogeneic monoclonal antibodies have been extraordinarily useful in defining antigens which distinguish sub-populations of normal
lymphocytes and haemopoietic cells and in refining the classification of
the leukaemias (Greaves *et al.*, 1981 and see chapter 6). Such antibodies
will surely be useful in human medicine both for analysis of lymphocytes
infiltrating tumours and for assessing the immune status of patients
during treatment. Indeed an anti pan-T lymphocyte antibody has
already been shown to have therapeutic effects in patients with T cell
neoplasms (Miller and Levy, 1981).

    In mice and rats there are choices of different inbred strains which
have different response characteristics. An example of this differential
response to immunization comes from attempts to raise monoclonal
antibodies to a colon carcinoma line (Voak *et al.*, 1980). Immunization
of C3H mice with HT29 colon carcinoma cells resulted in several
monoclonal antibodies that were found to be predominantly anti-blood
group substance and therefore not interesting in a search for colon
tumour specific antibodies. In subsequent experiments, rat strains that
were unresponsive to either blood group A or B antigens were used for
immunization. One of the problems in immunizing mice and rats with

human material is that antibodies specific for a single antigenic determinant in a complex mixture often predominates. By using this monoclonal antibody as an affinity reagent to deplete the predominating antigen from the mixture one can force a response to the other immunogens (Springer *et al.*, 1982) and increase the chance of finding a tumour specific antigen.

It is possible to do fusions of human lymphocytes directly from patients with tumours, either with mouse or rat myelomas, and obtain mixed species hybrids producing human monoclonal antibodies (Schlom *et al.*, 1980; Sikora and Wright, 1981) (Table 5·2). The frequency of hybridization and the quantity of human immunoglobulin produced by inter-species hybrids is considerably less than in mouse-mouse or rat-rat fusions. In addition, the preferential loss of human chromosomes in rodent-human hybrids results in frequent loss of immunoglobulin production. All of this makes for a lot of hard work. Recently, however, several human myeloma lines suitable for fusion (Table 5·3) have become available. Since there is abundant evidence

TABLE 5·2
Human monoclonal Ig production

| Lymphocyte source | Myeloma | Screening assay | Target antigen | Reference |
|---|---|---|---|---|
| Peripheral blood | TEPC-15 | human Ig | — | Schwaber and Cohen, 1974 |
| Chronic lympho-cyte leukaemia cells | NS1 | human Ig | — | Levy *et al.*, 1980 |
| Spleen | NS1 | binding RIA to influenza virus | Forssman glycolipid (influenza virus) | Nowinski *et al.*, 1980 |
| Peripheral blood | EM1500 6T6 A12 | immuno-precipitation of measles virus | measles virus nucleocapsid | Croce *et al.*, 1980 |
| Spleen (patient immunized with DNCB) | U266 AR1 | binding assay to DNCB | DNCB | Olsson and Kaplan, 1980 |
| Axillary lymph nodes | NS1 | immuno-peroxidase of tissue sections | breast carcinoma | Scholm *et al.*, 1980 |
| Intrathoracic lymph nodes | NS1 | binding assay to tumour membrane | lung carcinoma | Sikora and Wright, 1981 |

TABLE 5·3
Human myeloma lines used for fusion

| Name | Origin | Resistance | Reference |
|------|--------|-----------|-----------|
| U266 AR1 | U266 | 8 Azaguanine | Olsson and Kaplan, 1980 |
| GM1500 6TGA12 | GM1500 | 6 Thioguanine | Croce *et al.*, 1980 |
| LUD-LON HuMy2 | ARH 77 | 8 Azaguanine | Edwards *et al.*, 1981 |

that patients with cancer often have in their serum antibodies which recognize their own tumours (Shiku *et al.*, 1976; Smith *et al.*, 1976), fusion of lymphocytes from such patients should sample these responses. To do this lymphoctyes from cancer patients can be collected from several sites. Peripheral blood, while easy to sample, may not contain enough tumour specific lymphocytes in the right stage of differentiation to yield fruitful fusions. More likely to be involved in active anti-tumour response are the lymphocytes in lymph nodes draining the tumour. Such lymphocytes are easily collected in large quantities from patients with breast, lung and colorectal cancer. Another source of such lymphocytes is the tumour itself. Certain tumours, for example gliomas, are often heavily infiltrated by lymphocytes (Phillips *et al.*, 1982). Use of these lymphocytes separated from the tumour and fused to a human myeloma line may avoid responses to normal antigens and allow screening directly for neoantigens on tumour cells. This would be possible if these lymphocytes are not responding to any normal antigens and if the "new antigens" are not included in the collection of antigens to which an individual is immunologically tolerant. However, this view of the possible responses of the patients to his tumour may be too simple. The tolerant state is not only achieved in part by deletion of clones but is also maintained by complex suppression networks. The balance of this tolerant state might well be upset in the cancer patient because of the large amount of normal, possibly auto-antigenic, material shed into the circulation resulting in responses to normal antigens as to possible 'neoantigens" of the tumour cells. Thus many of the immunoglobulin products of fusions using lymphocytes harvested from tumours may well be auto-antibodies to normal cell components.

## 2. IMMUNIZATION PROTOCOLS AND CHOICE OF IMMUNOGEN

The choice of tumour derived material and the manner of administering it in xenogeneic immunizations probably has a determining effect on the antigenic determinants to which monoclonal antibodies will be

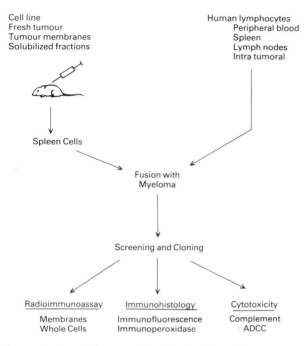

Cell line
Fresh tumour
Tumour membranes
Solubilized fractions

Human lymphocytes
Peripheral blood
Spleen
Lymph nodes
Intra tumoral

Spleen Cells

Fusion with
Myeloma

Screening and Cloning

Radioimmunoassay

Membranes
Whole Cells

Immunohistology

Immunofluorescence
Immunoperoxidase

Cytotoxicity

Complement
ADCC

FIG. 5·1 Strategies for making monoclonal antibodies to human tumour antigens.

selected. While both these parameters have varied considerably from one laboratory to another (Fig. 5·1), very little is known about how to optimize them to provide possible tumour specific monoclonal antibodies. Source of tumour material used for immunization have been *in vitro* grown lines, pieces of fresh tumour tissue, membrane preparations from fresh tissue, or fractionated solubilized components from fresh tumour cell membranes. These different immunization procedures will almost certainly result in different spectra of monoclonal antibodies. The use of *in vitro* grown cell lines has obvious advantages but may introduce a particular bias into the antibodies selected. Most cell lines are highly selected representatives of their tumour of origin. In addition, growing rapidly in tissue culture, they may express cell surface molecules related to rapid growth and not found in great abundance on tumour cells *in vitro*.

In the production of human monoclonal antibodies experimental immunization is not an option and the choices lie in the sources of lymphocytes taken for fusion (Fig. 5·1). It is too early to know whether choice of the source of lymphocytes:- peripheral blood, spleen, lymph node or the tumour itself affects the resulting specificities.

3. SCREENING METHODS

The production of monoclonal antibodies against human tumour cell surfaces requires the screening of many fusion products to find suitable immunoglobulins. Several strategies have been developed, each putting its own bias into the specificities of the monoclonal antibodies that emerge. The most common method is to immunize with a chosen tumour cell line, for example a melanoma. The fusion products are screened on that melanoma in an indirect binding assay and the activity of any positive supernatants determined on other melanomas as well as on cell lines of different types, both normal and malignant. In this way the specificity of the monoclonal antibody is characterized and its ability to distinguish tumour cells from normal cells is determined. Definition of specificity is thus limited by the kinds of assays and the number and variety of targets used. Use of cell lines gives constant sources of renewable reference material but biases the results because of the selection of that cell line and the conditions under which it grows. In addition, the normal cell counterpart of that line is usually not available for comparison.

There is an alternate strategy of immunization and screening using primary tumour material. The same membrane preparations of tumours can be used both as immunogen to immunize rodents and as antigen bound to plastic wells in a solid phase radioimmunoassay to screen the activity of resulting monoclonal antibodies. A variant of this screening procedure is the use of immuno-histological procedures on sections of normal and tumour material to assay the antibodies. In this case binding of antibody is detected either by using fluorescent or immuno-peroxidase coupled second antibody. Frozen or paraffin imbedded sections can be used and use of either will alter the activity of monoclonal antibodies and their possible cross reaction. Screening for antibodies that detect antigens on paraffin sections has the advantage of allowing retrospective surveys of material readily available from hospital pathology departments and wide comparison with normal adult and embryonic tissues. It has the disadvantage of picking up carbohydrate determinants, appearance of which is subject to enormous variation under different physiological conditions. These immuno-histological techniques can quickly show differences in monoclonal antibody specificity not detected by simple binding assays on membrane preparations or on cell lines. In addition, the recognized antigens, present even as a very minor component of adjacent normal material, may be detected. By comparing tumour samples from different patients with cancer of the same or different tissues, the specificity of the monoclonal antibody can be further defined for possible use.

Another aspect of screening is the characterization of the molecule carrying the recognized determinant, at least with regard to heat stability and size in a one-dimensional gel. This gives clues whether different monoclonals are recognizing the same molecule in different targets and whether the determinant is in the primary structure of a protein. In the production of human monoclonal antibodies screening strategies are less well worked out. One problem in screening them by indirect binding techniques and using tumour material rather than cell lines as targets is the presence of human immunoglobulin that interferes with detection of the bound Ig of the monoclonal. This can obscure binding of monoclonal antibodies that are weak either because its antigen is there in relatively small amounts or because the antibody has low affinity. This problem is avoided by using cell lines or alternatively tumour derived material can be used to detect direct binding of the human monoclonal antibodies labelled by growth of the hybrid lines with a radioactive amino acid. This is of course laborious.

With these general considerations in mind, we want to summarize briefly how matters stand with regard to specificity of monoclonal antibodies against human tumours and how this affects their uses in diagnosis and therapy. Details will be found of course in other chapters.

## B. Results with Particular Tumours

### 1. Colorectal Carcinoma

Colorectal cancer is a common problem in clinical oncology. Diagnosis is often difficult, requiring extensive endoscopic or radiological investigation. The assessment of recurrent disease following primary surgery is usually impossible until large masses of neoplastic tissue have accumulated. For the last 15 years in attempts to improve this situation much effort has been spent investigating carcino-embryonic antigen, detected by an antiserum produced in rabbits or goats after immunization with extracts from colonic cancer. This antigen, a glycoprotein with a molecular weight of 180,000 daltons, is found in several gastrointestinal tumours, some lung and breast tumours as well as in normal foetal colon (Heuman *et al.*, 1979). In patients with these tumours, the level of CEA in the serum is often markedly elevated. Considerable interest has been aroused in the possibility that the amount of CEA in the peripheral blood detected by a specific antiserum would relate to the tumour load in an individual patient, thus allowing the development of a diagnostic test and marker for monitoring progress of the disease. A major problem in the use of CEA for these purposes has been the extensive cross reaction between CEA and a variety of similar normal glycoproteins such as non-specific cross reacting antigens (NCA), biliary glycoprotein (BGP) and a glycoprotein found in washings of normal colon (NCW) (Shively and Todd, 1980). These glycoproteins share antigenic determinants with CEA and therefore confuse the serological analysis. Additionally they make difficult the comparison of results from different laboratories because varying immunization and absorption protocols yield antisera that differ in their specificities. Since several monoclonal antibodies that detect CEA have been prepared their use will hopefully lead to more precise definition of the inter-relationships among these cell surface components that cross react with conventional sera and thus yield more selective and sensitive assays for tumour related products. It is also possible that monoclonal antibodies may discriminate CEA from tumours arising in different tissues.

Several groups have now produced monoclonal antibodies to either CEA or other antigens of colorectal carcinomas by immunizing mice with either purified CEA preparations or colorectal carcinoma cell lines. Screening was done on either CEA or the immunizing cell line. Accolla and his colleagues (1980) raised 400 hybrids from mice immunized with purified CEA and found two that secreted antibodies reacting specifically with different antigenic determinants on CEA molecules. The affinities of these antibodies are relatively high and they were used for affinity purification of labelled solubilized CEA.

An anti CEA monoclonal antibody has been used to explore possible structural differences in CEA obtained from different sources (Rogers *et al.*, 1981). In comparing the binding to this antibody by CEA extracted from tumour tissue with CEA precipitated from sera of tumour bearing patients it was found that the latter is much more effective. This suggests either that serum CEA has a larger amount of molecules with the determinant recognized by this monoclonal antibody or has a different determinant from tumour CEA that is recognized with higher affinity. These differences could result from chemical modifications of CEA by extraction from the serum of cancer patients or by the predominance in the serum of CEA which has been degraded or altered in the liver.

Our own experience (Takei *et al.*, 1981) with CEA reacting monoclonal antibodies prepared both against tumour membrane preparations or purified CEA have been rather different in that they all do weakly react with normal colon mucosa. This is easy to detect in immunofluorescence on frozen sections but is usually undetectable on paraffin sections with immunoperoxidase coupled second antibody. In addition they cross react with polymorphs in peripheral blood (Karsten and Lennox, 1981) as would be expected for an anti CEA cross reaction with NCA.

Polyclonal CEA antibodies prepared in goats have been used in an attempt to localize metastatic human colorectal carcinoma (Mach *et al.*, 1980). Radiolabelling suitable antibodies with $^{131}$I and subsequent scanning of patients with a gamma camera have shown the potential of this technique. Recently a mouse monoclonal anti-CEA antibody has also been used (Mach *et al.*, 1981). It is too early to say whether there are any advantages in the monoclonal antibody over the polyclonal goat antiserum. There are several ways in which we might imagine the superiority of monoclonal antibodies for tumour localization. One is in the possibility of anti-CEA specificities that might better discriminate tumours of one tissue from another. The other is that with the availability of anti CEA monoclonal antibodies of different Ig classes and affinity, those suitable for the job might be found. For example, too high affinity may be undesirable for this may lead to its elimination by combining with CEA shed into the circulation.

Herlyn *et al.*, (1979) immunized mice with *in vitro* grown colon carcinoma cells and screened on this line by radioimmunoassay, mixed haemabsorption assays and immunofluorescence. Two hybridomas were found which secreted antibodies binding specifically to human colorectal carcinomas, either growing in culture or obtained directly from patients. These antibodies do not bind to normal colonic mucosa, other malignant cells, including melanoma, osteocytoma, myeloma or purified CEA. One of these monoclonal antibodies detecting monosialoganglioside from colorectal tumour cells was used to screen serum samples (Koprowski *et al.*, 1981). Blocking activity was found in the serum of 24 out of 32 patients with colorectal cancer but not in the serum of 38 healthy donors and 36 patients with other cancer types. This sort of observation could well lead to sensitive assays of tumour load in an individual patient.

A colorectal carcinoma specific monoclonal antibody has been used to explore the possibility of coupling diphtheria and ricin toxins to produce specific cytotoxic molecules. As discussed in chapter 7, these toxins can be separated into two functionally distinct chains, the A toxic chain and the B membrane binding chain. The A chains coupled by conventional cross-linking agents to the anti-tumour monoclonal antibody should provide a specific toxic agent. Such conjugates are cytotoxic *in vitro* for colorectal carcinoma cells but not, in the same concentration range, for a variety of other human tumour cell lines (Gilliland *et al.*, 1980). Such studies promise therapeutic possibilities. It remains for experiments to determine whether these toxin coupled antibodies can destroy tumour masses *in vivo* without doing unacceptable damage to normal tissue.

## 2. MELANOMA

Melanoma is a tumour studied frequently by immunologists. Panels of patient sera and melanoma cells, have been used to construct serological matrices defining many antigens and antibodies (Shiku *et al.*, 1976). However, the biochemical separation of the different serologically recognized antigens has been impossible because of the low titres of the sera. There are several monoclonal antibodies against a variety of human melanoma antigens. Some of these antibodies are directed against the human DR antigen and seem melanoma specific if the cells or tissue compared lack these antigens. In one study (Herlyn *et al.*, 1980), three out of six hybridoma secreted antibodies which bind to the majority of melanoma cell lines, astrocytomas, as well as to all samples of normal peripheral blood and Epstein-Barr virus transformed lymphocytes. This parallels the distribution of DR Antigens. Two of the remaining antibodies, however, detect two different antigens common to melanoma and astrocytoma cells only. In another detailed analysis of melanoma antigens (Dippold *et al.*, 1980) mice were immunized with the melanoma cell line SK-MEL 28 and 18 monoclonal antibodies derived were tested on a large panel of human cell lines from a variety of tumour types, as well as on early passages of normal tissue in culture. Serological studies, in conjunction with immunoprecipitation analysis of radio labelled cell extracts and antibody inhibition tests with solubilized antigens indicated that the 18 monoclonal antibodies detected 6 antigenic molecules. Two of them are glycoproteins with molecular sizes of 95,000 and 150,000 daltons respectively in reducing gels, and two have characteristics of glycolipid antigens. The biochemical nature of the remaining two antigenic molecules has not been determined.

In another study (Woodbury *et al.*, 1980) a monoclonal antibody was found that recognizes a protein of molecular weight 97,000 daltons in reducing gels and that extensive testing in binding assays indicated as melanoma specific with no cross reaction to normal tissues. In a later paper (Brown *et al.*, 1981), using a more sensitive assay that takes advantage of the availability of two monoclonal antibodies recognizing different determinants of the same molecule they showed cross reactions with several normal adult tissues including colon, bladder, muscle, kidney and lung (Table 5·4).

It is striking that proteins of 97,000 daltons are turning up as immunogenic molecules in several kinds of tumours including the melanomas and lymphoid tumours (Woodbury *et al.*, 1980). In two different laboratories (Trowbridge and Omary, 1981; Sutherland *et al.*, 1981) two different monoclonal antibodies were revealed as specific for transferrin receptor (a molecule of about 95,000 daltons reduced and 190,000 unreduced) the presence of which is correlated not with malignancy but with rapid growth. It is also striking as is pointed out by Sutherland *et al.* (1981) that the transferrin receptor has the same sizes in reducing and non-reducing gels as a molecule previously associated with malignancy (Bramwell and Harris, 1979) in rodent and human cells.

## 3. BREAST CANCER

Xenogeneic monoclonal antibodies have been raised against breast tumour lines, although the number of antibodies available is less than in colorectal and melanoma systems. A monoclonal antibody that may have considerable clinical use is that raised against the human oestrogen receptor (Greene *et al.*, 1980). It is known that the presence of oestrogen receptors in breast cancer tissue is an indicator of the likelihood of responses to hormone therapy. The derivation of monoclonal antibodies which can be used for immuno-histological detection of receptors would greatly increase the clinical pathologist's ability to provide information of prognostic value to the clinician.

By using lymphocytes derived from axillary lymph nodes from patients with breast cancer, and fusing with a mouse myeloma, monoclonal antibodies which bind to breast carcinoma cells have been produced (Schlom *et al.*, 1980). A human IgM monoclonal antibody produced in this way discriminates between mammary carcinoma cells and normal mammary epithelial cells by indirect immunohistological methods. This antibody also reacted with metastatic mammary carcinoma cells in lymph nodes of breast cancer patients with no binding to the normal lymphocytes or to the stroma of the same node. Thus whatever is revealed by more extensive and sensitive assays about its possible cross reactions, its specificity is sufficient for detection of invasion of lymph nodes.

TABLE 5·4

| Antigen: Monoclonal antibody | Dippold et al. (1980) | | | | | | | | Imai et al. (1980) | | | | Woodbury et al. (1980) p97 binding assay | Brown et al. (1981) p97 DD1A ng mg$^{-1}$ |
| --- | --- | --- | --- | --- | --- | --- | --- | --- | --- | --- | --- | --- | --- | --- |
| | gp95 | | gp150 | | M19 | R8 | | R24 | | | | | | |
| | 1 | 2 | 3 | 4 | 5 | 6 | 7 | 8 | 1 | 2 | 3 | 4 | | |
| Cell lines | | | | | | | | | | | | | | |
| Melanoma | ++ | ++ | ++ | ++ | ++ | ++ | ++ | ++ | ++ | ++ | ++ | ++ | ++ | 0·1–610 |
| Astrocytoma | + | + | ++ | ++ | ++ | ++ | + | + | + | + | | + | – | |
| Renal Ca. | + | + | + | + | + | + | – | – | + | + | – | – | + | 0·1 |
| Breast | – | + | – | – | – | – | – | – | – | – | – | – | + | 10·0 |
| Bladder Ca. | + | + | + | + | – | + | – | – | – | – | – | – | – | 14·0 |
| Ovary Ca. | – | – | + | – | + | – | – | – | | | | | + | |
| Colon Ca. | – | + | + | + | – | – | – | – | | | + | | | |
| Cervix Ca. | – | – | + | – | – | – | – | – | | | | | | |
| Lung Ca. | – | – | + | – | – | – | – | – | – | – | – | – | + | 3·7 |
| Teratomas | – | + | + | – | – | – | – | – | – | + | + | – | – | |
| B Cell Lines | – | + | + | + | + | – | – | – | | | | | | |
| Normal adult cells | | | | | | | | | | | | | | |
| Melanocyte | – | – | – | – | – | – | – | – | – | – | – | – | – | |
| Fibroblast | – | + | + | + | + | – | + | – | | | | | – | 2·7 |
| Brain | ± | ± | + | ± | – | + | + | – | | | | | – | 0·5 |
| Leucocyte | – | + | – | – | + | + | + | – | | | | | – | |
| Colon | | | | | | | | | | | | | – | 2·2 |
| Liver | | | | | | | | | | | | | – | 1·2 |
| Lung | | | | | | | | | | | | | – | 0·9 |

Comparison is made of the specificity of mouse anti melanoma monoclonal antibodies from three laboratories using a variety of assays. Quantitative comparison among them is not possible. Data of the last two columns reveal that in the same laboratory, a more sensitive assay (DD1A) shows the presence of the p97 antigen in normal tissue earlier scored as negative as well as a 6000 fold range in amount in melanomas.

## 4. OTHER TUMOURS

Monoclonal antibodies have been, or are being, raised against a wide variety of other human solid tumours, including gliomas, neuroblastomas, lung cancer as well as bladder, prostate and testicular tumours. In most cases only a small number of cloned defined antibodies are available for study. Even after considerable effort on the part of the investigators little is known about the chemical nature of the antigenic determinants seen by these antibodies or details of cross reactions with other tumours and normal tissue. There are many monoclonal antibodies raised against leukaemias and these are discussed in greater detail in Chapter 6. While the literature on monoclonal antibodies against normal and malignant lymphoid cells is too vast to summarize briefly, there are several generalizations that emerge which are relevant to our discussions of "specificity" of monoclonal antibodies: most monoclonal antibodies are often not absolutely specific for any particular state of differentiation and the discriminations are quantitative (Greaves, 1981); monoclonal antibodies recognizing only an antigen specific for malignant cells, and absent from normal cells have not been found (chapter 6).

## III HOW SPECIFIC SHOULD MONOCLONAL ANTIBODIES BE?

Table 5·1 lists the presently contemplated uses of monoclonal antibodies in cancer. As we discuss below each use may make different demands both with regard to cross reactions with various normal tissues and with other tumours on the degree of tumour specificity of the monoclonal antibody.

In tumour diagnosis by detection of antigen in serum, for example, the contributions of normal tissue to materials in the serum that crossreact with the monoclonal antibody are relevant only in so far as they mask the level of tumour antigen shed into the serum or cause variations in this measured level in ways irrelevant to the amount of the particular tumour to be detected. In this way the usefulness of conventional anti CEA antibodies is limited by the extent to which they cross react with normal components shed into serum and the variation in the amount of these components in apparently normal people. The monoclonal antibody that detects a glycolipid in serum of colon carcinoma patients but not normal patients (Koprowski *et al.*, 1981) is an example of one useful for diagnosis. A possibility in this application is that a panel of several monoclonal antibodies may increase the sensitivity and specificity of the assays. In using monoclonal antibodies for tumour localization, a different requirement for specificity is illustrated. For example to recognize breast or colon tumour cells in a lymph node all that is needed is lack of cross reaction with the other cells of the node by immunohistological procedures. This is achieved already by several monoclonal antibodies (Schlom *et al.*, 1980; Finan *et al.*, 1981). Detection of metastases in other tissues have similar specificity requirements. In general the demands of specificity for localization are not the most exacting for one only needs to see abnormalities. Targetting of toxic agents to tumours using the monoclonal antibodies as specific carriers has some demands in common with those for tumour localization but is more demanding, for one will want to know whether the likely damage by antibody-toxin to the normal tissue is tolerable in the particular clinical situation where it is used. Here too a panel of monoclonal antibodies might increase tumour-normal tissue discrimination.

In all these and similar applications the point that needs emphasis is that each use of a monoclonal antibody or mixture of monoclonal antibodies in diagnosis or therapy makes its own demands on specificity and brings its own set of consequences for failure to achieve the ideal specificity that the clinical use would demand. In this sense, questions raised about the specificities of monoclonal antibodies for clinical aspects of cancer will be like those asked about the use of any new therapeutic or diagnostic agent and brings us back to a familiar setting.

REFERENCES

Accolla, R. S., Carrel, S., Mach, J. P. (1980). *Proc. natn. Acad. Sci. U.S.A.* **77**, 563–566.
Baldwin, R. W. (1973). *Adv. Cancer Res.* **18**, 1–76.
Bloom, H. J., Richardson, N. W. and Field, J. R. (1970). *Br. Med. J.* **2**, 181–184.
Bramwell, M. E. and Harris, H. (1979). *Proc. R. Soc. Lond.* B. **203**, 93–99.
Brown, J. P., Woodbury, R. G., Hart, C. E., Hellstrom, I. and Hellstrom, K. E. (1981). *Proc. natn. Acad. Sci. U.S.A.* **78**, 539–543.
Croce, C. M., Linnenbach, A., Hall, W., Steplewski, Z. and Koprowski, H. (1980). *Nature* **288**, 488–489.
Dippold, W. G., Lloyd, K. O., Lucy, T. C., Ikeda, H., Oettgen, H. F. and Old, L. J. (1980). *Proc. natn. Acad. Sci. U.S.A.* **77**, 6114–6118.
Edwards, P., O'Hare, M. and Neville, M. *Eur. J. Immunol* (in press).
Everson, T. C. and Cole, W. H. (1966). *In* "Spontaneous regression of Cancer". Saunders, Philadelphia.
Finan, P. J., Grant, R.M., de Mattos, C., Takei, F., Berry, P. J., Lennox, E. S. and Bleehen, N. M. (1982). *Br. J. Cancer*. (in press).

Gilliland, D. G., Steplewski, Z., Collier, R. J., Mitchell, K. F., Chang, T. H. and Koprowski, H. (1980). *Proc. natn. Acad. Sci. U.S.A.* **77**, 4539–4543.

Greaves, M. F. (1981). *In* "Leukaemia Markers" (W. Knapp, Ed.) pp. 19–32. Academic Press, London.

Greaves, M. F., Robinson, J. B. and Delia, D. (1981). *In* "Modern trends in leukaemia IV" (R. Neth, Ed.). Verlag, Munich. (in press).

Greene, G. L., Nolan, C., Engler, J. P. and Jensen, E. V. (1980). *Proc. natn. Acad. Sci. U.S.A.* **77**, 5115–5119.

Herlyn, M., Steplewski, Z., Herlyn, D. and Koprowski, H. (1979). *Proc. natn. Acad. Sci. U.S.A.* **76**, 1438–1442.

Herlyn, M., Clark, W. H., Mastrangelo, M., Guerry, D., Elder, D. E., Larossa, P., Hamilton, R., Bondi, E., Tuthill, R., Steplewski, Z. and Koprowski, H. (1980). *Cancer Res.* **40**, 3602–3608.

Heuman, D., Candardjis, P., Carrel, S. and Mach, J.-P. (1979). *In* "Carcino-embryonic proteins" (F. G. Lehmann, Ed.). Elsevier-North Holland Bio-medical, Amsterdam.

Howard, J. C., Butcher, G. W., Galfrè, G. and Milstein, C. (1978). *Curr. Top. Microbiol. Immunol.* **81**, 54–57.

Imai, K., Molinaro, G. A. and Ferrone, S. (1980). *Transpl. Proc.* **12**, 380–383.

Karsten, U. and Lennox, E. S. (manuscript in preparation).

Kinlen, L. J., Sheh, A. G. R., Peto, J. and Doll, R. (1979). *Br. med. J.* **2**, 1461–1466.

Koprowski, H., Herlyn, M., Steplewski, Z. and Sears, H. F. (1981). *Science* **212**, 53–54.

Lennox, E. S. (1980). *In* "Progress in Immunology IV" (M. Fougereau and J. Dausset, Eds), pp. 658–667. Academic Press, London.

Levy, R., Dilley, J., Brown, S. and Bergman, Y. (1980). *In* "Monoclonal Antibodies" (R. H. Kennett, T. J. McKearn and K. B. Bechtol, Eds). pp. 137–152. Plenum Press, New York.

Mach, J.-P., Forni, M., Ritschard, J., Buchegger, F., Carrel, S., Widgren, S., Donath, A. and Alberto, P. (1980). *Onco-devl. Biol. Med.* **1**, 49–69.

Mach, J.-P., Buchegger, F., Girardet, C., Forni, M., Ritschard, J., Accolla, R. S. and Carrell, S. (1981). Serono Symposium on Tumour Markers (G. Della Porta, Ed.). (in press).

Miller, R. A. and Levy, R. (1981). *Lancet* **1**, 226–230.

Nowinski, R., Berglund, C., Lane, J., Lostrom, M., Bernstein, I., Young, W., Hakomori, S. I., Hill, L. and Cooney, M. (1980). *Science* **210**, 537–539.

Olsson, L. and Kaplan, H. (1980). *Proc. natn. Acad. Sci. U.S.A.* **77**, 5429–5431.

Phillips, J. R., Eremin, O. and Anderson, J. R. (1981) *Br. J. Cancer.* (in press).

Rogers, G. T., Rawlins, G. A. and Bagshawe, K. D. (1981). *Brit. J. Cancer* **43**, 1–4.

Schlom, J., Wunderlich, D. and Teramoto, Y. A. (1980). *Proc. natn. Acad. Sci.* **77**, 6841–6845.

Schwaber, J. and Cohen, E. P. (1974). *Proc. natn. Acad. Sci. U.S.A.* **71**, 2203–2207.

Shiku, H., Takahashi, T., Oettgen, H. and Old, L. J. (1976). *J. exp. Med.* **144**, 873–881.

Shively, J. E. and Todd, C. W. (1980). *In* "Cancer Markers" (S. Sell, Ed.), pp. 295–312. Humana Press, Clifton.

Sikora, K. and Wright, R. (1981). *Brit. J. Cancer* **43**, 696–700.

Smith, K. O., Gehle, W. P. and Newman, J. T. (1976). *Cancer* **38** 157–165.

Springer, T. (1982). *In* "Hybridomas in Diagnosis and Treatment of Cancer" (M. S. Mitchell and H. F. Oettgen, Eds). Raven Press, New York. (in press).

Sutherland, R., Delia, D., Schneider, C., Newman, R., Kemshead, J. and Greaves, M. (1981). *Proc. natn. Acad. Sci. U.S.A.* **78**, 4515–4519.

Takei, F., Alderson, T., Grant, R., Finan, P., Lennox, E. and Bleehan, N. (manuscript in preparation).

Trowbridge, I. S. and Omary, M. B. (1981). *Proc. natn. Acad. Sci. U.S.A.* **78**, 3039–3043.

Voak, D., Sacks, S., Alderson, T., Takei, F., Lennox, E., Jarvis, J., Milstein, C. and Darnborough, J. (1980). *Vox Sanguinis* **39** 134–140.

Woodbury, R. G., Brown, J. P., Yeh, M. Y., Hellstrom, I. and Hellstrom, K. E. (1980). *Proc. natn. Acad. Sci. U.S.A.* **77**, 2183–2187.

# 6 Analysis of leukaemic cells with monoclonal antibodies

M. F. GREAVES, D. DELIA, R. NEWMAN AND
L. VODINELICH

*Membrane Immunology Laboratory, Imperial Cancer Research
Fund, Lincoln's Inn Fields, London. WC2A 3PX*

# I INTRODUCTION

Immunological and enzymatic phenotypes of leukaemic cells have provided new insights into the biology of leukaemia (reviewed in Greaves and Janossy, 1978; Brouet and Seligmann, 1978; Thiel *et al.*, 1980; Thierfelder *et al.*, 1976; Knapp, 1981), as well as a basis for a prognostically relevant and biologically rational subclassification of certain leukaemias (e.g. acute lymphoblastic leukaemia (ALL) and chronic granulocytic leukaemias (CGL), in blast crisis).

Three relatively recent technical innovations are likely to greatly facilitate the further understanding of leukaemic cell properties, namely analysis and physical sorting in flow systems (e.g. fluorescence activated cell sorter (FACS) ) (Herzenberg and Herzenberg, 1978; Greaves, 1975), monoclonal antibodies produced by the hybridoma methodology as discussed in this book, and in vitro culture methods for maintaining haemopoietic stem cells (Dexter, 1979).

In this report we summarize some of our experience with monoclonal antibodies used in conjunction with FACS analysis and sorting and speculate on the possible biological and clinical significance of the data obtained. Some of the questions we have in mind are:

1.  How much heterogeneity is there within particular leukaemic subclasses, e.g. T-ALL?
2.  To what extent are individual phenotypes determined or influenced by (a) differentiation/maturation status, (b) proliferation status, and (c) malignant status? In order to approach this question we have carried out a systematic comparison of leukaemic cells with their presumed counterparts in normal or non-leukaemic tissue using various combinations of single cell markers and cell sorting (FACS), and also investigated the biochemical nature of some of the antigenic structures used as cell surface markers.
3.  Can the composite phenotype of leukaemic cells be manipulated *in vitro*, i.e. how stringent is the apparent "maturation arrest"?
4.  Which combinations of markers have immunodiagnostic potential in reproducibly identifying particular leukaemic subclasses which might otherwise remain misclassified or unclassified and inappropriately treated?
5.  Do any of the monoclonal antibodies have sufficient selectivity to be candidates for therapeutic applications?

The application of monoclonal antibodies in studies on human leukaemia and lymphoma is rapidly expanding and this chapter does not provide a comprehensive review of the field. The published proceedings of a recent conference on this subject will give the interested reader access to more information (Knapp, 1981). At this particular stage of development, it is also inevitable that there is no consistent nomenclature for monoclonal antibodies. Several have been given provisional labels that presume or imply more specificity than is established. It is already becoming clear that monoclonal antibodies raised in different laboratories (e.g. against T cells or melanoma) identify the same molecular structure though possibly via different epitopes. Rationalization of nomenclature will hopefully be forthcoming during the coming year or two and will require extensive exchange of reagents as well as detailed biochemical investigations.

## II MATERIALS AND METHODS

### A. PATIENTS AND CELLS

Leukaemic samples (heparinized blood and bone marrow, lymph node biopsies, cerebro-spinal fluid and peritoneal aspirates) were obtained from referring hospitals throughout the U.K. as part of a routine immunodiagnostic service linked principally to the Medical Research Council's UKALL trials of chemotherapy (and radiotherapy) (Greaves *et al.*, 1981c). All samples were separated on ficoll-isopaque ($1 \cdot 077$ gm cm$^{-3}$, 40 mins at 400 g and 20°C). A panel of established leukaemic cell lines were maintained as previously described (Minowada *et al.*, 1978).

### B. MONOCLONAL ANTIBODIES

The monoclonal antibodies used in this study, their laboratory of origin, apparent cellular specificity and, where known, the general biochemical features of the antigens they detect, are listed in Table 6·1.

Absorbed (but possibly polyclonal) heteroantisera used included rabbit or horse anti-thymus (Greaves and Janossy, 1976) and rabbit anti-common ALL/gp100 (Greaves *et al.*, 1975; Brown *et al.*, 1975a). All leukaemic samples were also tested with an affinity purified anti-terminal deoxynucleotidyl transferase (TdT; Bollum, 1979).

### C. IMMUNOFLUORESCENCE, FLOW CYTOFLUORIMETRY AND SORTING

Binding of murine monoclonal antibodies was assessed with

TABLE 6·1

Monoclonal antibodies used in the analysis of leukaemic cells

| Designation | Reference | Cellular/molecular specificity |
|---|---|---|
| **1. *HLA-associated*:** | | |
| W6/32 | Brodsky *et al.*, 1979 | } monomorphic HLA-ABC |
| BB7·7 | Brodsky *et al.*, 1979 | |
| BB5 | Brodsky *et al.*, 1979 | } $\beta_2$ microglobulin |
| EC3 | Brodsky *et al.*, 1979 | |
| DA2 | Brodsky *et al.*, 1979 | } monomorphic HLA-DR |
| OKIa-1 | Reinherz *et al.*, 1980b | |
| **2. *T lineage associated*:** | | |
| OKT1 | Reinherz *et al.*, 1979b | |
| | Van Agthoven *et al.*, 1981 | } Pan-T     p65–69 |
| L17F12(Leu-1)[a] | Engleman *et al.*, 1981 | (+ B-CLL) |
| T101 | Royston *et al.*, 1980 | |
| UCH-T2, UCH-T3[b] | Beverley and Callard, 1981 | |
| OKT3 | Kung *et al.*, 1979 | |
| | Van Agthoven *et al.*, 1981 | } Pan mature T     p19 |
| UCH-T1[b] | Beverley and Callard, 1981 | |
| OKT4 | Reinherz *et al.*, 1979a | "Helper"/"Inducer" |
| | Terhorst *et al.*, 1980 | subset     p62 |
| OKT6 | Reinherz *et al.*, 1980 | } Thymic cortex antigen |
| | Terhorst *et al.*, 1981 | (HTA-1)     p45–49 |
| NA134 | McMichael *et al.*, 1979 | (+p12)[c] |
| OKT8 | Reinherz *et al.*, 1980 | Suppressor/Cytotoxic |
| | Terhorst *et al.*, 1980 | subset     p30 + p32 |
| OKT11 | Verbi *et al.*, 1981 | Pan-T, E rosette |
| OKT11A⁰ | Verbi *et al.*, 1981 | receptor     p50 |
| **3. *B lineage associated*:** | | |
| FMC 1 | Brooks *et al.*, 1980 | Pan B |
| BA-1 | Abramson *et al.*, 1980 | Pan B |
| P1153/3 | Kennett and Gilbert, 1979 | Pan B/neural |
| | Greaves *et al.*, 1980c | |
| FMC 7 | Catovsky *et al.*, 1981 | B subset |
| **4. *Non-lymphoid haemopoietic lineage associated*:** | | |
| OKM-1 | Breard *et al.*, 1980 | Monocytes/granulocytes |
| MI/N1 | Kemshead *et al.*, 1981a | Granulocytes |
| TG-1 | Beverley *et al.*, 1980 | Granulocytes |
| LICR/LON/R10 | Edwards, 1980; | Erythroid cells |
| | Robinson *et al.*, 1981 | —Glycophorin |
| 1/6A | Edwards, 1980 | Erythroid cells—Band III |
| AN51 | McMichael *et al.*, 1981 | Platelets—Glycoprotein I |
| J15 | *See chapter 8 | Platelets—Glycoprotein IIb/IIIa |
| **5. *Common ALL associated*:** | | |
| J-5 | Ritz *et al.*, 1980 | gp100 |
| | Liszka *et al.*, 1981 | |
| BA-2[e] | Kersey *et al.*, 1981 | p24 |
| **6. *Pan-haemopoietic associated*:** | | |
| HeLe-1 | Beverley *et al.*, 1980 | |
| OKT10 | Reinherz *et al.*, 1980a | p40 |
| | Terhorst *et al.*, 1981 | |
| **7. *Ubiquitous, cell proliferation associated*:** | | |
| OKT9 | Reinherz *et al.*, 1980a | gp80 (dimer) |
| | Sutherland *et al.*, 1981 | Transferrin receptor |
| | Terhorst *et al.*, 1981 | |

[a]  Leu-1 designation given to reagent marketed by Becton-Dickinson.

[b]  See also Chapter by Beverley in this book.

[c]  A similar antibody (9·6) has been reported by Kamoun *et al.*, (1981).

[d]  The small polypeptide chain (approximate molecular weight 12,000) is non-covalently associated with the 45–49,000 polypeptide; whether or not the former is $\beta_2$ microglobulin is a topic of current debate (see Ziegler and Milstein, 1979; Terhorst *et al.*, 1981).

[e]  Also reacts with some other cells including activated T cells and neural crest derived tumours (see Table 6·5).

fluorochrome labelled, affinity purified IgG F(ab')₂ fragments of goat anti-mouse Ig using both fluorescence microscopy (Standard 16 Zeiss photomicroscope with epi-illuminescence) and flow cytometry (Fluorescence Activated Cell Sorter, FACS-I, Becton Dickinson, Mountain View, California, U.S.A.). Monoclonal antibodies were also titrated by indirect immunofluorescence binding to leukaemic cell lines using the FACS. Percentage cells staining (above threshold set by control reagents) and average staining intensity are quantified, the latter by determining the fluorescence "window" on the FACS at which 50% of the cells are positive (Fig. 6·1).

For intranuclear TdT staining, cytospin cell preparations were first fixed in cold methanol, then incubated with rabbit antibodies specific for TdT followed, after washing, by fluorochrome labelled goat antibodies specific for rabbit Ig. Simultaneous staining for cell surface antigens with monoclonal antibodies and for nuclear TdT with rabbit

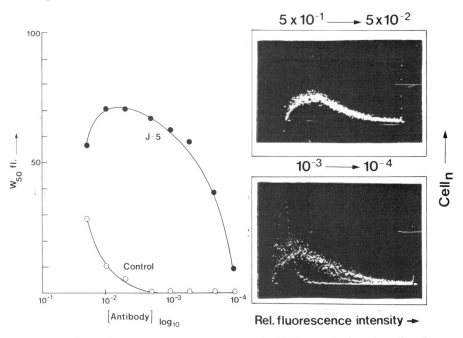

FIG. 6·1 Quantification of monoclonal antibody binding to leukaemic cells using fluorochrome labelled antibodies and the Fluorescence Activated Cell Sorter (FACS). W₅₀. Fluorescence window on FACS oscilloscope at which 50% of the cells are fluorescent (see text). FACS profiles: vertical axis, relative cell number; horizontal axis; relative fluorescence. Cells from the line Nalm-1 (pre-B, common ALL phenotype) were stained with J-5 monoclonal anti-cALL (Ritz *et al.*, 1980) followed by fluorescein-labelled anti-mouse Ig.

anti-T antibodies coupled to different fluorochromes provides a very useful approach to cellular identification and "phenotyping" in leukaemia (Janossy *et al.*, 1980a). Simultaneous staining with two different monoclonal antibodies is also possible if these are directly labelled with fluorochromes or indirectly when these are of different Ig classes, e.g. IgG₁ and IgG₂ binding detected with anti-IgG₁ and anti-IgG₂ labelled with different fluorochromes.

Using the FACS it is also now possible to investigate the relationship between cell cycle or aneuploidy and cell surface antigen expression or phenotype as defined by monoclonal antibody binding. DNA content can be analyzed by flow cytometry using DNA binding dyes as quantitative labels, e.g. propidium iodide, mithramycin (Crissman *et al.*, 1979) following cell surface labelling with fluorescein isothiocyanate labelled antibodies. Interrelating DNA content with cell surface antigen expression can be performed by cell sorting (for antigen expression) followed by DNA analysis or, with suitable FACS modifications (Roberts, 1980), by simultaneous analysis. Using these methods it has been possible to show that several antigenic determinants detected by monoclonal antibodies on leukaemic and normal cells, e.g. HLA-DR, HLA-ABC, $\beta_2$ microglobulin and the gp100 cALL antigen, increase only slightly in quantity as the cells enlarge and pass through $S_2$ $G_2$ and M (Roberts, 1980; Delia and Greaves, 1981). When the leukaemic cells contain abnormal DNA profiles, associated usually with aneuploidy, it is possible with monoclonal antibody labelling, e.g. monoclonal J-5, anti-gp100 cALL antigen in common ALL—Fig. 6·2 to demonstrate the presence of a particular antigenic determinant on the abnormal population. These dual or multi-parameter analyses incorporating monoclonal antibodies may have useful applications in leukaemia research since growth fraction, aneuploidy and cell phenotype are in some instances linked to prognosis. Furthermore, some monoclonal antibody detected cell surface structures show an important association with cell proliferation *per se* (see under Results F and Fig. 6·10.

## D. E-Rosette Test

25 $\mu$l of lymphocytes (at $10^7$ ml$^{-1}$) were mixed with 25 $\mu$l foetal calf serum (absorbed with sheep red blood cells) and 50 $\mu$l of 2% sheep red blood cells/E (pretreated with 15 U ml$^{-1}$ neuraminidase at 37°C for 30 mins). The mixture was centrifuged for 5 mins at 400 g (av) and left 1 hr at room temperature before gentle resuspension, dilution and counting.

## E. ISOLATION OF CELL SURFACE ANTIGENS

Membrane glycoproteins were labelled ($^{125}$I-lactoperoxidase or $^{35}$S-methionine) and isolated by detergent solubilization, lectin affinity chromatography, immunoprecipitation and SDS-polyacrylamide gel electrophoresis as previously described (Sutherland *et al.*, 1978; Newman *et al.*, 1981a).

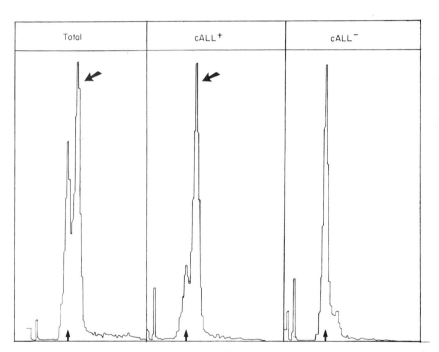

FIG. 6·2 Application of monoclonal antibody and the FACS to inter-relate DNA content and cell surface phenotype. Flow cytometry analysis of DNA content. Vertical axis, relative cell number; horizontal axis, relative DNA content. ↑ = 2N, G0/G1 positive; ↙ = abnormal peak. Bone marrow cells from an untreated patient with ALL were stained with monoclonal (J-5) anti-common ALL/gp100. Stained and unstained cells were separated on the FACS, fixed and DNA stained with mithramycin. Analysis (on the FACS) of the unseparated, DNA stained marrow revealed an abnormally high peak approximately in the position expected of S phase cells. This pattern is unusual in cALL and reflects either synchronized cells in S or more likely a substantial aneuploid (hyperdiploid) karyotype. Separation of the cALL$^+$ and cALL$^-$ cells revealed that the abnormal population is largely co-incident with the cALL$^+$ cells. (Reproduced by permission from Greaves *et al.*, 1981b).

## III RESULTS AND DISCUSSION

### A. DIFFERENTIATION LINKED PHENOTYPES OF T CELL MALIGNANCIES

Using the panel of monoclonal anti-T reagents listed in Table 6·1 in parallel with several other important markers (e.g. anti-cALL, anti-HLA-DR, anti-TdT), we have determined the composite phenotype of 82 consecutive untreated T cell malignancies (Greaves *et al.*, 1981d).

The results are summarized in Table 6·2 and Fig. 6·3 and reveal several interesting points. Firstly, there is a clear association between clinical/haematological subgroup and the maturity of T cell phenotype. Cases of T-ALL all had, with one exception, a very immature thymic phenotype, T-non Hodgkin lymphoma (T-NHL) in young patients had an "intermediate" or cortical thymic phenotype, whereas the chronic T leukaemias and cutaneous T lymphomas (Sezary) associated with

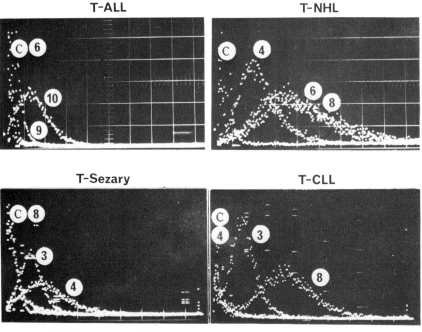

FIG. 6·3 FACS analysis of OKT monoclonal defined phenotypes in T cell leukaemias. Vertical axis, relative cell number; horizontal axis, relative fluorescence; 4 etc. OKT4 monoclonal; C, control. Normal mouse ascites IgG plus fluorescein labelled goat anti-mouse Ig. (Reproduced with permission from Greaves *et al.*, 1981d).

## TABLE 6·2

Phenotypic heterogeneity of T cell malignancy in relation to normal differentiation

| Cell type | | OKT series | | | | | | | | Others | | | Clinical diagnosis (n) |
|---|---|---|---|---|---|---|---|---|---|---|---|---|---|
| | | 1 | 3 | 4 | 6 | 8 | 9 | 10 | 11 | "T" | ER | TdT | |
| **T precursors:** Early/Pre‑thymic | 1 | +w | − | − | − | − | +/− | + | − | + | − | + | (4) ⎫ |
| | 2 | +w | − | − | − | − | +/− | + | + | + | + | + | (10) ⎬ ALL (46) |
| | 3 | +w | − | +/− | +/− | +/− | − | + | + | + | + | + | (31) ⎭ |
| Cortical thymic | 4 | +w | +/− | + | + | + | − | + | + | + | + | + | (1) |

Precursor clinical diagnoses also grouped as:

| | cNHL |
|---|---|
| (1) | ⎫ |
| (4) | ⎬ cNHL (12) |
| (7) | ⎭ |

| | |
|---|---|
| (18) | ⎫ |
| (2)[a] | ⎬ |
| (4) | ⎭ |

| Mature T | | 1 | 3 | 4 | 6 | 8 | 9 | 10 | 11 | "T" | ER | TdT | Sezary | CLL | PLL | Lympho‑blastic lymphoma |
|---|---|---|---|---|---|---|---|---|---|---|---|---|---|---|---|---|
| "Inducer/Helper" T | 5 | + | + | + | − | − | − | − | + | + | + | − | 7 | 2 | 6 | 3 |
| "Suppressor" T | 6 | + | + | − | − | + | − | − | + | + | + | − | 0 | 4 | 2[a]  /  0 | 0 |

[a] 2 cases of T prolymphocytic leukaemia (T‑PLL) were reactive with both OKT4 and OKT8 (see text).

−, <5% cells staining (or rosetting); +, >25% cells staining (or rosetting); +w, weak staining on all cells; +/−, variable expression; "T", rabbit or horse anti‑T; ER, sheep erythrocyte rosettes; cNHL, childhood non‑Hodgkin lymphoma. (from Greaves et al., 1981d) much older aged patients were invariably of either mature "helper" or, in a few cases of T-chronic lymphocytic leukaemia (T-CLL), a mature "suppressor" phenotype. A detailed scrutiny of the data reveals more heterogeneity of phenotype than can be accommodated within the framework of the supposed normal differentiation sequence, e.g. lack of TdT or E rosette formation or OKT1 or OKT3 in some individual samples when the rest of the composite phenotype anticipates its presence, as well as unexpected "double" staining with OKT4 and OKT8 in two patients with prolymphocytic leukaemia (PLL) (Fig. 6·4).

The consistent combination of strong staining for both HLA-ABC

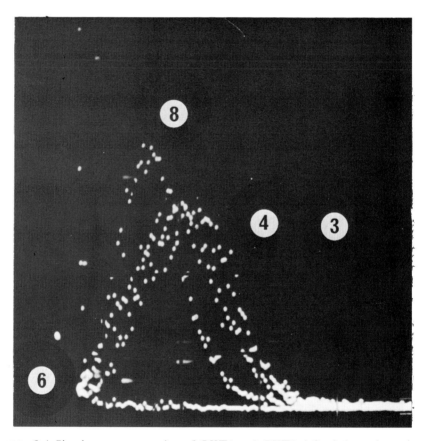

FIG. 6·4 Simultaneous expression of OKT4 and OKT8 defined determinants on T-PLL cells. Vertical axis, relative cell number; horizontal axis, relative fluorescence; 3, OKT3 etc. Note OKT6 gives no staining. Composite phenotype of this case (patient S.A., 49, ♂) was OKT1$^+$, OKT3$^+$, OKT4$^+$, OKT6$^-$, OKT8$^+$, OKT9$^-$, OKT10$^-$, OKT11A$^+$, DR$^-$, cALL (gp100)$^-$, TdT$^-$, Ig$^-$. (Reproduced with permission from Greaves *et al.*, 1981d).

and TdT on most T-ALL (Bradstock *et al.*, 1980; Greaves, 1980; Greaves, *et al.*, 1981d) is surprising since normal thymic TdT positive cells have very low levels of HLA until they mature to the $TdT^-$ stage (Brown *et al.*, 1979; Bradstock *et al.*, 1980). This observation implies a possible asynchrony of gene expression but needs re-evaluating if T-ALL do not correspond to the $TdT^+$ cortical thymocytes but rather to their immature and numerically infrequent precursors. HLA-ABC reactivity is indeed low on those $TdT^+$ NHL with a typical cortical thymic phenotype (Group 4, Table 6·2). Nevertheless, HLA expression and/or some of the "incomplete" phenotypes mentioned above may reflect the existence of some minor alterations in gene expression in T malignancy. Another possible "abnormality" of cell surface antigen expression concerns the common ALL antigen. This antigen was previously reported as being present on approximately 10% of T-ALL (Roberts *et al.*, 1978; Janossy *et al.*, 1980b) and on several T cell lines (Minowada *et al.*, 1978; Janossy *et al.*, 1978a). In the series of 82 T malignancies listed above 15 cases were positive with the monoclonal anti-cALL reagent, J-5; these had the phenotypes distributed between all 4 thymic categories (Table 6·2) although reactivity was most frequently observed in T-NHL with a cortical thymocyte phenotype. 7 out of 12 T-ALL/NHL cell lines tested were also J-5 positive (Greaves *et al.*, 1981). Since anti-cALL binding to any normal thymocytes is rare it is possible that in this circumstance the cALL antigen expression is a manifestation of leukaemia; this antigen is nonetheless a normal gene product of lymphoid cells (see below).

Despite these caveats we conclude that T leukaemic phenotypes reflect primarily a pattern of normal gene expression "appropriate" for a level of maturation arrest of the dominant subclone. Although this does not necessarily identify the "target" cell for the disease it is likely that T-ALL and T-NHL are derived from a malignant transformation of a T lineage committed progenitor or stem cell whereas T-CLL, T-PLL and T-Sezary are probably the result of clonal selection of immunocompetent (and perhaps immunoactivated) mature T cells (Greaves, *et al.*, 1981d; Greaves *et al.*, 1981a). If the latter were instead derived from a T stem cell or multipotential stem cell then, by analogy with CGL (Greaves and Janossy, 1978), we would expect to see their inevitable progression into acute leukaemia with an associated immature phenotype. This rarely, if ever, occurs.

Other groups have also reported detailed studies on the heterogeneity of T cell leukaemias as identified with monoclonal antibodies. Thus, Reinherz *et al.* (1980a) first used the OKT series of antibodies to document the predominant immature thymic phenotypes

expressed in T-ALL. Bradstock *et al.* (1980) similarly suggested that
T-ALL had a very early or immature thymic phenotype based on their
observations with the monoclonal antibody NA134 (McMichael *et al.*,
1979). Kung *et al.* (1981) and Boumsell *et al.* (1981) reported that
leukaemic T cells in Sezary syndrome had $OKT4^+/OKT8^-$ "helper"/
"inducer" phenotypes.

Monoclonal antibodies OKT11 and OKT11A have given consistently concordant results with E (sheep) rosettes. One interpretation of
such data is that these antibodies are directed against the receptor for
sheep erythrocytes on T cells. This possibility was tested by screening
all the OKT series of monoclonals for their capacity of block rosette
formation. Only OKT11 and OKT11A had the capacity to block sheep
erythrocyte binding to normal or leukaemic T cells (Fig. 6·5; Verbi *et
al.*, 1981). Kamoun *et al.* (1981) have recently reported another monoclonal anti-T antibody (9·6) which also blocks E-rosette formation.
Both 9·6 and OKT11A appear to precipitate a single polypeptide with
an apparent molecular weight in SDS-polyacrylamide gel electrophoresis of 50,000.

Observations of T leukaemias and normal T cells also indicate
similarities between various monoclonals. Thus, NA134 and OKT6
show concordant binding (Greaves *et al.*, 1981d) and appear to pre-
cipiate a similar P45−49 polypeptide which may be associated with a
P12 $\beta_2$ microglobulin-like protein (McMichael *et al.*, 1979; Terhorst *et
al.*, 1981). OKT1, T101, UCH-T2 and P17F12 in our hands also give
concordant reactivity and all four precipitate a similar polypeptide with
an approximate molecular weight of 65−69,000.


### B.  Non-T ALL and Early B Cell Differentiation

Application of monoclonal antibodies and other cell markers to a large
series of non-T ALL indicates a probable B cell lineage affiliation of null
ALL and common (c) ALL (Fig. 6·6; Greaves *et al.*, 1980c, 1981;
Kersey *et al.*, 1981). Note that several markers are shared exclusively
(within the haemopoietic system) by $\mu^-$ ALL and mature B cells. No
unique marker shared exclusively by cALL and the T cell lineage has
been described so far. The majority of non-T, non-B (excluding pre-B)
ALL have re-arranged Ig heavy chain genes (Korsmeyer, 1981) which
provides genetic evidence for commitment to the B cell lineage prior to
detectable Ig ($\mu$ chain) synthesis.

Several years ago we reported the serological characteristics of the
cell surface antigen associated with most cases of non-T, non-B acute

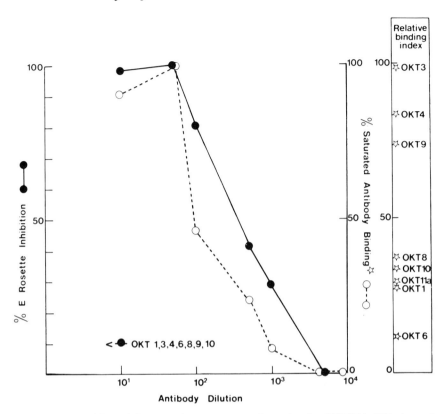

FIG. 6·5 Inhibition of sheep erythrocyte rosette formation by OKT11A. Dilutions of OKT11A were added to T cells (T-ALL cell line) at room temperature for 30 minutes prior to E rosette assay. Other monoclonals were added at saturating concentrations. All samples were also tested for binding using fluorescein labelled anti-mouse Ig and FACS analysis. Relative binding was quantified by determining the window at which 50% of the cells in any sample were fluorescent (cf. Fig. 6·1). Relative binding index = window giving 50% cells positive at saturating concentrations (1:10) of all antibodies used. (Reproduced with permission from Verbi *et al.*, 1982.)

lymphoblastic leukaemia (= the common ALL antigen) (Greaves *et al.*, 1975; Brown, 1975a, b; Roberts *et al.*, 1978). This antigen defines the subclass of ALL with the best prognosis (Chessells *et al.*, 1977; Greaves *et al.*, 1981c). 8 or 9 other groups have produced essentially similar sera (e.g. Billing *et al.*, 1978; Borella *et al.*, 1977; Pesando *et al.*, 1979), one of which is a monoclonal antibody (Ritz *et al.*, 1980). Several of these reagents from other laboratories, including monoclonal J-5 (Ritz *et al.*, 1980) have been assessed in our laboratory and found to have completely concordant reactivity with our own antibodies. Monoclonal J-5

Phenotypic Sequence in

NON-T ALL

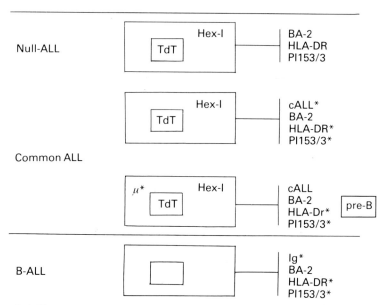

FIG. 6·6 Phenotypic subgroups and putative differentiation sequence in non-T ALL as determined by monoclonal antibodies and other markers. *Marker invariably present (marker usually but not invariably present in those not labelled*); $\mu$, cytoplasmic $\mu$ heavy chain of immunoglobulin; Hex-I, hexosaminidase I (lysosomal) isoenzyme; TdT, nuclear terminal deoxynucleotidyl transferase. Note that these leukaemias are unreactive with T cell specific monoclonals (OKT3, 4, 6, 8, 11, 11A) as well as other monoclonals specific for non-lymphoid cells (Table 6·1). (Reproduced with permission from Greaves *et al.*, 1981a).

is now routinely used in our laboratory for differential diagnosis of common ALL and during 1980 was applied to more than 1000 haemopoietic malignancies (Table 6·3; Greaves, 1981a).

Unfortunately, the key question of precise specificity of anti-cALL antisera has become muddled and confusing. Our studies provide what we believe to be compelling evidence that the cALL associated antigen is not leukaemia specific but is a normal differentiation antigen of lymphocyte progenitors which are normally restricted to bone marrow. Two serial monitoring studies on paediatric and adult ALL patients with anti-ALL failed to provide a clear predictive test for relapse because of this association with normal cells; this was particularly evident with respect to "false-positives" in post-chemotherapy associated lymphocytosis (Greaves *et al.*, 1980a, b).

TABLE 6·3
Selective reactivity of monoclonal J-5, anti-cALL (g100)
with haemopoietic malignancies (1137 consecutive cases:
March–December 1980)

| Diagnosis* | n. positive/negative (relapsed) |
|---|---|
| Non-T, non-B ALL | 374(53)/61(26) = 86% |
| T-ALL/T-NHL[a] | 17(2)/60(0) |
| B-ALL[0] | 0/12(1) |
| AML, AMML, AMonL, APML | 3(0)[b]/323(16) |
| CGL | 0/27 |
| CGL blast crisis—TdT[+] | 19/3 |
| —TdT[-] | 0/62 |
| Erythroleukaemia | 0/12 |
| B lymphoma[c], B-CLL, B-PLL myeloma, plasma cell leukaemia | 1/81 |
| "AUL"—TdT[+] | 6/1 |
| —TdT[-] | 0/6 |
| Acute megakaryoblastic leukaemia | 0/6 |
| Others | 7[d]/57[e] |

[a]  In children. [0]All TdT[-] $\kappa$ or $\lambda$ restricted.
[b]  Although diagnosed and treated as AML, these 3 cases contained a mixed population with 20–65% cALL[+]/TdT[+] cells. Another 12 cases diagnosed as AML had 15–75% cells cALL[-]/TdT[+] and were presumably also mixed lymphoid-myeloid leukaemia.
[c]  Disseminated, monoclonal ($\kappa/\lambda$) B cells in blood.
[d]  4 cases of non-Hodgkin lymphoma in children, all TdT[+], non-T, non-B. 2 cases of "lymphoproliferative disorders" and 1 case of "glandular fever".
[e]  Includes 7 cases of neuroblastoma disseminated to the marrow.
*  AML, acute myeloid leukaemia; AMML, acute myelomonocytic leukaemia; AMonL, acute monocytic leukaemia; APML, acute promyelocytic leukaemia; AUL, acute undifferentiated leukaemia. Other abbreviations as in text.
Taken from Greaves, 1981a.

The key observations are, however, that:

1.  The majority of terminal deoxynucleotidyl transferase (TdT) lymphoid cells in normal paediatric bone marrow are cALL antigen positive when tested with either rabbit (Janossy *et al.*, 1979) or monoclonal (J-5) antisera (Greaves *et al.*, 1981e).
2.  When tested with a panel of monoclonal antibodies the majority of

TdT positive cells in paediatric marrow have the same composite "non-T, non-B lymphoid" phenotype as seen in cALL itself (Table 6·4; Greaves *et al.*, 1981e).

3. A molecule with the same general biochemical characteristics as the cALL antigen (Table 6·5; Fig. 6·7) can be isolated from normal bone marrow using rabbit antisera or monoclonal (J-5) antibody (Newman *et al.*, 1981a, b).

TABLE 6·4

Monoclonal antibody defined, cell surface phenotype of TdT positive cells in normal bone marrow

| | |
|---|---|
| 1. Positive[a] | W6/32, PA2·6 (HLA-ABC) |
| | DA2, OKIa-1 (HLA-DR) |
| | J-5 (gp100, cALL antigen) |
| | BA-2 (p24 ALL antigen) |
| | PI153/3 (neural/ALL antigen) |
| | OKT10 (pan haemopoietic) |
| 2. Negative[b] | OKT1, 3, 4, 6, 8, 11, 11A, L17F12, NA134 |
| | OKT9 |
| | OKM-1 |
| | LICR/LON/R10 |
| | 1/6A |
| | AN51 |

[a]  45–95% of TdT⁺ cells stained. A minimum of 3 normal or regenerating paediatric bone marrows tested with each antibody.
[b]  <5% TdT⁺ cells stained.

Since both rabbit and monoclonal anti-gp100 cALL reagents have already been used immunotherapeutically *in vivo* (Ritz, *et al.*, 1981; Ritz, J. and Schlossman, S., personal communication) or *in vitro* (for autologous marrow transplants—ref. Netzel *et al.*, 1980) the question of the precise specificity of these antibodies is not solely an academic issue. Lack of absolute leukaemia specificity does not, however, exclude the possible value of such therapeutic applications since even a potentially lethal deficit due to a total elimination of normal lymphocyte progenitors by anti-ALL might be salvaged by replenishment from a cALL antigen negative stem cell pool. At present, we do not know that the gp100 cALL antigen is present on stem cells (it is, however, undetectable on granulocytic and erythrocytic committed progenitor cells).

One lesson to be learned from this exercise seems clear and has a broad relevance to "cancer associated" antigens (Greaves, 1979a, b). Since the majority (if not all) of acute leukaemias and malignant carcinoma probably derive from infrequent tissue progenitors or stem

TABLE 6·5

Biochemical features and cellular distribution of 4 ALL-associated cell surface antigens identified by monoclonal antibodies

| | cALL associated antigen (gp100) J-5 | ALL associated antigen (p24) BA-2 | T-ALL and cell proliferation associated antigen (gp90) OKT9 | HLA-DR/Ia antigens DA-2, OKIa-1 |
|---|---|---|---|---|
| Protein/M. W. | Single polypeptide 100K | Single polypeptide 24K | 2 disulphide bond linked polypeptides of 90K | Cell surface: 2 non covalently linked polypeptides, 28K, 33K + intracellular 30K polypeptide. |
| Glycosylated | + | −[a] | + | − |
| pI | 5·2 | 7·3 | 5·0 | $\alpha \sim 5$[b] $\beta \sim 7$[b] |
| Peripheral or Integral (hydrophobic) and Transmembrane (t) | P | P | $I_t$ | $I_t$ |
| Cellular distribution: | | | | |
| (a) Leukaemia/cancer | cALL T-NHL, some T-ALL CGL-BC, "AUL" | Most cALL Some null ALL CGL-BC, "AUL" some T-ALL and B-CLL; neural crest der. tumours | Ubiquitous on proliferating cells[a] | Non-T ALL, AML, B-CLL, B lymphoma, rare T leukaemias, melanoma. |
| (b) Normal | TdT+ cells in marrow Kidney tubules Some epithelia[c] | TdT+ cells in marrow. Weakly on myeloid cells(?) Activated T cells. | Proliferating cells and placenta. | B cells, some monoblasts, activated T cells. Haemopoietic progenitor cells including BFU-E, CFU-GM, TdT+ cells. Some epithelial cells. |

[a] May have small amounts of $O$-glycosidically linked oligosaccharide.
[b] Mean pI of several spots. $\beta$ chain spots vary according to DRw type.
[c] Metzgar et al., 1981.

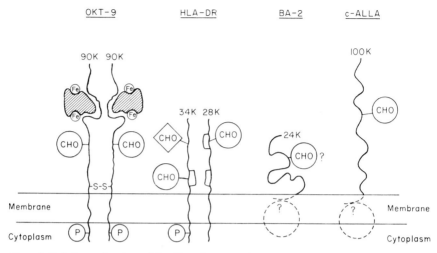

FIG. 6·7 Schematic view of 4 cell surface proteins of acute lymphoblastic leukaemia detected by monoclonal antibodies. CHO, carbohydrate; S-S, disulphide bonds, P, phosphorylation site; Fe, iron-saturated transferrin (i.e. each 90K polypeptide of the transferrin receptor binds one molecule of transferrin and each molecule of transferrin has two iron binding sites (Schneider *et al.*, 1982).

cells we should anticipate the expression of normal "early" differentiation antigens with pseudo-tumour specificity. Whether such antigens would normally tolerize the host or, in cancer/leukaemia, evoke an immunological response is an interesting point for speculation. The existence of such antigens need not necessarily compromise attempts at immunotherapy; indeed they might provide an ideal "target" in tumours of non vital organs (e.g. mammary carcinoma).

Two other monoclonal anti-common ALL reagents have recently been reported. Monoclonal BA-2 (Kersey *et al.*, 1981) does not show complete concordance of binding with J-5 or rabbit anti-cALL and binds to a different polypeptide (Fig. 6·7; Kersey *et al.*, 1981; Newman *et al.*, 1981b) which has a broader spectrum of cellular expression than the gp100 cALL associated antigen, though it includes the TdT positive cell in normal bone marrow. Monoclonal 12A1 shows a very similar if not identical pattern of reactivity to J-5 and rabbit antibodies to the gp100/cALL antigen (Liszka *et al.*, 1981) and may precipitate the same structure (W. Knapp, personal communication). Table 6·5 (and Fig. 6·7) compares the biochemical features and pattern of cellular distribution of 4 membrane antigens present in the various subtypes of ALL.

A final comment on this topic concerns the relevance of gp100 positive cells in normal bone marrow to the cellular origins of ALL. We assume that this cell either provides the major target cell population for common ALL or is a dominant position of maturation arrest in a leukaemia (ALL) induced in an "earlier" haemopoietic progenitor cell. Since ALL only very rarely transforms intra-clonally to AML and never (in >150 cases analyzed) to T-ALL, we conclude that common ALL is probably a malignant transformation of B lineage committed precursors or stem cells. This perspective contrasts significantly with the explanation for the presence of cALL (including pre-B) phenotypes in Ph[1] positive and Ph[1] negative CGL (Janossy *et al.*, 1977, 1978b; Greaves, 1981b; Greaves *et al.*, 1979c); here it is most likely that we are looking at an indicator of maturation arrest (of the dominant subclone) in a leukaemia derived from a pluripotential stem cell (Janossy *et al.*, 1976; Fialkow *et al.*, 1978; Greaves, 1981b).

## C. Detection of Erythroid Lineage Leukaemias with Monoclonal Antibodies specific for Erythroid Membrane Proteins Glycophorin and Band III

Andersson *et al.* (1979a, 1980) have suggested that glycophorin may provide a useful marker for immature erythroleukaemias diagnosed "incorrectly" as AML (M-1) or even ALL. The availability of monoclonal antibodies to glycophorin as well as band III (Edwards, 1980) (Table 6·1) prompted an investigation of the expression of these antigenic determinants during normal erythroid differentiation and in acute leukaemia. Neither the band III or glycophorin determinants detected by the monoclonal antibodies used were detectable by FACS analysis and sorting on BFU-E or CFU-E (Robinson *et al.*, 1981; Greaves *et al.*, 1981f). Glycophorin was detected (weakly) on the earliest morphologically recognizable erythroid cells (basophilic pronormoblasts) but anti-band III binding was only seen on enucleated erythrocytes. This latter observation should be interpreted with caution, since the exposure or expression of antigenic determinant involved may be controlled in part at least by glycosylation changes during maturation (P. Edwards, personal communication). However, rabbit anti-glycophorin (a gift from Dr. L. Andersson) also fails to bind to BFU-E and CFU-E (Sieff, Bicknell and Greaves, unpublished observations) suggesting the glycophorin is first expressed at a post-CFU-E of erythroid ontogeny.

These data indicate that acute leukaemias originating in pluripotential stem cells, myeloid and/or erythroid progenitors/stem cells and with a very early maturation arrest, i.e. at the BFU-E/CFU-E equivalent level, would probably not be readily detectable by the LICR/LON/R10 anti-glycophorin. We have screened a large series of acute leukaemias for reactivity with this monoclonal antibody (Table 6·6). 12 cases of unequivocal erythroleukaemia gave positive staining on a variable proportion of cells as did two cases of erythroid blast crisis of CML. A small number of acute leukaemias which were not diagnosed as erythroleukaemias were also glycophorin⁺ (Table 6·6) including two Ph¹ positive CGL in blast crisis, two ALL and one "AUL" whose

TABLE 6·6
Glycophorin positive leukaemias not diagnosed as erythroleukaemia

| Number positive (number tested) | Leukaemia | Phenotype |
|---|---|---|
| 2 (157)[a] | ALL | 2 ALL/AUL? (no ALL markers) |
| 2 (33)[b] | Ph¹ CGL blast crisis | "Myeloid" |
| 1 | AUL/megakaryoblastic | Mixed megakary./Glyco⁺ |
| 4 (105) | AML | Mixed? 17–30% Glyco⁺ |

[a]  Includes 54 in relapse (41 cALL, 8 null ALL and 5 T-ALL).
[b]  One of these cases became overtly erythroblastic 6 weeks later. (from Greaves, 1981a).

blast cell population consisted of two cell types (on three repeated occasions), one glycophorin positive and one positive with an anti-platelet antibody, AN51 (see Table 6·1). We assume this latter leukaemia to originate from a common erythroid-platelet progenitor cell. One of the two glycophorin positive cases of CGL blast crisis evolved to an overt erythroleukaemia 6 weeks following our tests. We also find that the Ph¹ positive cell line K562 (Lozzio and Lozzio, 1979a) is reactive with monoclonal anti-glycophorin which confirms the controversial suggestion that this line has erythroid developmental potential (Andersson *et al.*, 1979b; see also Lozzio and Lozzio, 1979b). Neither K562 or erythroleukaemias react with monoclonal anti-band III which is a very "late" gene product in the erythroid series. In contrast to the results of Andersson and colleagues we have found very few cases of ALL in relapse or AML that were clearly glycophorin positive (Table 6·6).

## D. Monoclonal Anti-Platelet (Glycoprotein I) as a Probe for Megakaryoblastic Leukaemias

Malignant transformation of platelet precursors is probably relatively rare although some cases are recorded. Breton-Gorius and colleagues have suggested, however, that a considerable proportion of pluripotential stem cell leukaemias—Ph[1] chromosome positive CGL in blast crisis—may have a dominant subclone in maturation arrest at the small megakaryoblast level of differentiation (as detected by platelet peroxidase staining by E.M.) (Breton-Gorius *et al.*, 1978). This observation has so far not been confirmed by another laboratory (D. Catovsky, personal communication) and we felt it important to investigate this point particularly since one implication of Breton-Gorius' work was that blast crises that we regard as cALL-like might be megakaryoblastic. We found that 5 out of 8 "possible" Ph[1] negative megakaryoblastic leukaemias had between 20 and 68% of cells weakly positive with monoclonal AN51 which is specific for glycoprotein I of human platelets and megakaryocytes (McMichael *et al.*, 1981, chapter 8). Only one other acute leukaemia investigated (out of 60 tested to date) had a major AN51[+] population and this was the "AUL" patient referred to above who had a glycophorin positive population present also. Four cases of CGL blast crisis (out of 16 tested so far) did, however, have a minor (5–16%) AN51[+] population including one case which was considered to be erythroblastic (with glycophorin[+] cells). AN51 may, however, like anti-glycophorin monoclonal LICR/LON/R10, be an inadequate probe for detecting very early platelet precursors if, as is quite possible, it binds to a determinant whose expression is correlated with maturation in the platelet lineage. We could therefore be underestimating the involvement of both erythroid and platelet precursors in acute leukaemias.

## E. Modulation of Leukaemic Cell Phenotype *In Vitro*

Since the phenotype of leukaemic cells reflects the apparent imposition of maturation arrest it is of some interest to determine whether maturation is inducible. Extensive studies with Friend virus erythroleukaemia (Harrison, 1977) and rat myeloid leukaemia cell lines (Sachs, 1978) indicate that leukaemic cells may retain the competence for differentiation. Fewer studies have been carried out with human leukaemic cell lines although HL-60, a promyelocytic cell line, can be induced to mature with DMSO or phorbol esters (Collins *et al.*, 1978; Gallagher *et al.*, 1979) and K562, a line derived from PH[1] positive blast crisis of CGL (Lozzio and Lozzio, 1979a), synthesizes embryonic haemoglobin when cultured with butyric acid or haemin (Andersson *et al.*, 1979b; Rutherford *et al.*, 1981). We have confirmed the inducibility of these latter two lines and documented the maturation-linked changes in monoclonal antibody defined phenotype that occur (Boss *et al.*, 1980; Delia *et al.*, 1981).

13 T-ALL/T-NHL cell lines have been assessed for their OK monoclonal defined phenotypes in relation to other markers (Greaves *et al.*, 1981d). Although they all appear to have an immature T phenotype it is considerably more difficult to place these lines (all of which are aneuploid and come from patients in relapse) in a normal maturation sequence than uncultured T leukaemias.

We have screened a number of known maturation inducers including DMSO, butyric acid, retinoic acid and TPA against these cell lines and find that only TPA is able to induce phenotypic changes. Nagasawa and Mak (1980) have similarly recently reported that TPA induces an increase in E rosettes and a loss of TdT activity in the T cell line MOLT-4. We succeeded in modulating the OKT defined phenotype in 7 lines to date as well as in two fresh T-ALL (Delia *et al.*, 1982). Fig. 6·8 summarizes the reproducible phenotypic alterations induced in the cell line HPB-ALL and Fig. 6·9 illustrates some of these changes as documented using the FACS. This pattern of modulation appears to mimic normal T cell differentiation and it is particularly interesting that cells with simultaneous expression of OKT4 and OKT8 defined determinants become restricted to OKT8 positivity through the selective loss of the OKT4 binding determinant. Loss of the peanut lectin binding site ($\beta$-D-galactosyl(1-3)-N-acetyl-D-galactosamine) is attributable to its masking with sialic acid residues and associated increase (3–5x) in sialotransferase activity. Several of these induced alterations in membrane antigen expression have been confirmed biochemically, e.g. increase in the OKT1/p65 molecule, decrease in OKT9/gp90 molecule, decrease in lectin binding glycoproteins.

So far we have not been able to induce any phenotypic modulation of T cell lines with the synthetic pentapeptide (thymopoietin) TP5 (Goldstein, 1977). Some cell lines also appear to be resistant to induction by TPA. We interpret these data to indicate that despite their aneuploid and highly malignant nature (having outlived their donors by several years!), some T-ALL cells at least are still capable of relatively normal differentiation if a presumed regulatory defect is bypassed with "abnormal" inducers. Those inducible lines may provide an ideal model system for investigating the molecular biology of T cell differentiation. The possible binary option of $OKT4^+$ or $OKT5/8^+$ phenotypes for the cortical thymocyte leukaemia equivalent may in particular provide an especially useful system to analyze the basis of the genetic decision making process in differentiation.

The antigenic changes observed with HL-60, K562 and T-ALL cell lines all parallel those observed in normal maturation and are accompanied by decrease or slowing in cell cycling. These provide further support for the view that maturation arrest in leukaemia may be a reversible regulatory defect which "uncouples" maturation and proliferation (Sachs, 1980; Greaves, 1979a).

Some of the monoclonal antibody defined T cell associated determinants studied can also be induced by activating normal T cells that are normally antigen negative. Thus more than 90% of circulating T cells are $OKT9^-/OKT10^-$ but become positive when activated by lectins or calcium ionophore plus TPA (Terhorst *et al.*, 1981; Greaves *et al.*, 1981b; Sutherland *et al.*, 1981).

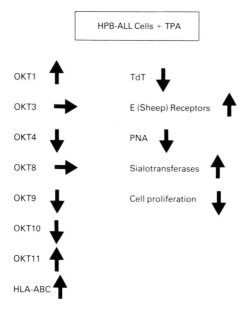

FIG. 6·8 Summary of phenotypic alteration inducible in T-ALL cell line HPB-ALL by phorbol ester (TPA). (Reproduced by permission from Greaves *et al.*, 1981b).

↑  increased expression
→  unaltered expression
↓  decreased expression.

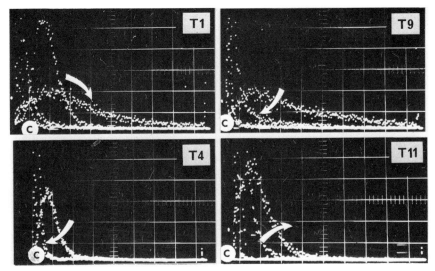

FIG. 6·9 FACS analysis of phenotypic modulation of HPB-ALL by phorbol ester (TPA). Axes as in Fig. 6·4; C, control. Arrows indicate direction of modulation, i.e. OKT1 increases, OKT9 decreases, OKT4 is lost. (Reproduced by permission from Greaves *et al.*, 1981b).

## F. MONOCLONAL OKT9 IDENTIFIES THE UBIQUITOUS PROLIFERATION-LINKED RECEPTOR FOR TRANSFERRIN

The observations of cell lines and normal T cells suggested a possible relationship of OKT9 binding to proliferation status. This possibility has been investigated in detail (Sutherland *et al.*, 1981).

Reinherz *et al.* (1980a) used OKT9 as an early thymocyte marker. We confirmed that this monoclonal antibody does indeed react preferentially with T-ALL (Greaves *et al.*, 1981b; Sutherland *et al.*, 1981) but it does not identify a T cell specific differentiation antigen. Serological and biochemical analyses have clearly shown that OKT9 defines a structure associated with proliferation on a wide spectrum of normal and malignant cell types (Table 6·7) (Sutherland *et al.*, 1981; Greaves *et al.*, 1981b). Expression of the OKT9 defined determinant correlates with the cycling fraction in T-ALL (Fig. 6·10) as well as with the dividing cells in foetal thymus, foetal liver and normal adult bone marrow. Synthesis of the antigen can be induced on normal resting cells by PHA (blood T cells) or by ionomycin ionophore plus TPA on paediatric thymocytes. Leukaemic cell lines (e.g. HL-60, HPB-ALL) induced to mature, lose OKT9 binding capacity concomitantly with

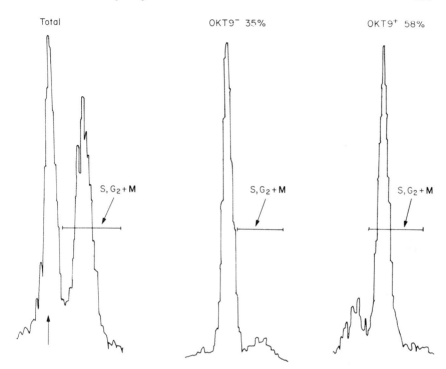

Total        OKT9⁻ 35%        OKT9⁺ 58%

FIG. 6·10 Association of OKT9 binding with proliferating fraction in uncultured T-ALL. DNA content cell cycle analysis by flow cytometry (FACS). Vertical axis, relative cell number; horizontal axis, relative DNA content. Vertical arrow marks G0/G1 position (= 2N), horizontal bar marks S, $G_2$+M fraction (= 4N). Cells from a case of T-ALL in relapse were stained with OKT9, and some cells separated on the FACS into positive and negative cells before staining DNA with mithramycin. (from Sutherland *et al.*, 1981.)

the appearance of other maturation associated determinants (e.g. OKM-1, Fig. 6·11) and either exit from the cell cycle (HL-60) or a slowing down of proliferation rate (T-ALL). The density of the OKT9 detected antigen varies only minimally throughout the cell cycle (data not shown) and our current view is that this structure is not strictly speaking a cell cycle/proliferation antigen but rather a determinant on a structure whose expression is regulated by active growth and/or metabolism.

The structure carrying the OKT9 determinant has been isolated from T-ALL, neuroblastoma, pancreatic carcinoma and melanoma (Table 6·5; Fig. 6·7). Its biochemical characteristics are essentially identical to those described by Omary *et al.* (1980) using monoclonal antibody B3/25. Judd *et al.* (1980) have also described a rabbit antibody

TABLE 6·7
Cell types reactive with OKT9

---

1. *Normal cells*:
   Foetal thymus, foetal liver (normoblasts).
   Adult bone marrow (myelocytes, normoblasts, some BFU-E, CFU-E).
2. *Normal cells in culture*:
   Myoblasts, mammary fibroblasts, epithelial cells.
3. *Normal cells activated in vitro*:
   Blood T cells (PHA).
   Paediatric thymocytes (ionomycin + TPA).
4. *Normal cells in culture "transformed" by viruses*:
   EBV—B cell lines.
5. *Uncultured leukaemic cells*:
   Many T-ALL, some AML, and erythroleukaemias.
6. *Established tumour cell lines*:
   Neuroblastoma, pancreatic carcinoma, colon carcinoma, bladder carcinoma,
   teratocarcinoma, oat cell carcinoma, melanoma.
7. *Established leukaemic cell lines*:
   cALL (4), B-lymphoma (2), erythroid (1), myeloid (2), T-ALL (12).

---

See Sutherland *et al.*, (1981).

which precipitates a similar if not identical structure. These biochemical features are strikingly similar to those of the transferrin receptor isolated from reticulocytes, placenta, kidney or T-ALL cell lines (see Sutherland *et al.*, 1981); furthermore, expression of transferrin receptors is known to be coupled or associated with proliferation or growth rates (Larrick and Cresswell, 1979). Studies with leukaemic cell lines and normal cells reveal that transferrin binding can be regulated in parallel to OKT9 binding (Fig. 6·11). Definitive evidence that OKT9 does indeed detect the transferrin receptor comes from the observation that this antibody can coprecipitate iodinated transferrin bound to its membrane receptors although it does not bind to transferrin itself or inhibit the binding of transferrin to its receptor (Sutherland *et al.*, 1981). The monoclonal B3/25 described by Omary *et al.* (1980) also appears to be directed against the transferrin receptor (Trowbridge and Omary, 1981).

The availability of monoclonal antibodies against transferrin receptors provides the opportunity for further study of this important iron delivery system. Since transferrin usually binds with reasonable affinity across mammalian species barriers and receptor mutants would be difficult to obtain for an "obligatory" structure, it has not so far been possible to use transferrin binding to human-mouse somatic cell hybrids to chromosomally map the genes controlling this receptor.

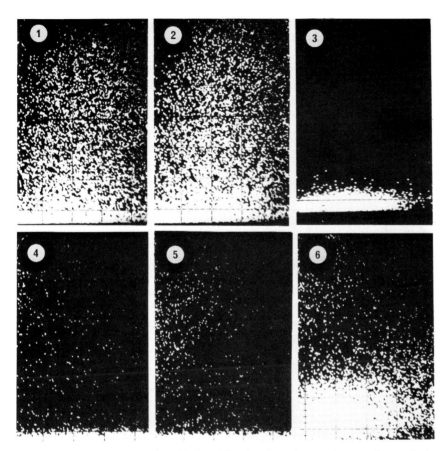

FIG. 6·11 Modulation of the OKT9 defined cell surface antigen and transferrin receptors on HL-60 cells by retinoic acid. Fluorescence Activated Cell Sorter (FACS-I) analysis. Vertical axis, relative fluorescence intensity; horizontal axis, relative light scattering (cell size). 1, 2, 3: uninduced HL-60 (promyelocytic leukaemia) cells. 4, 5, 6: HL-60 cells induced to mature by retinoic acid ($10^{-7}$M/5 days). 1, 4: staining with OKT9. 2, 5: staining for transferrin receptors (transferrin plus rabbit anti-transferrin). 3, 6: staining with monoclonal antibody OKM-1—a cell surface antigen marker for mature granulocytic and monocytic cells (Breard *et al.*, 1980). (from Sutherland *et al.*, 1981.)

OKT9 antibody, however, does not bind to mouse transferrin receptors and it has therefore been possible to "map" the transferrin receptor via its OKT9 binding determinant. The latter appears to segregate in human-mouse hybrids with chromosome 3 which we therefore presume carries either structural or regulatory genes for assembling the transferrin receptor (Goodfellow *et al.*, 1982).

## G. How Specific are Anti-T Monoclonals for the T Cell Lineage?

The remarkably broad pattern of reactivity with OKT9 raises the issue of whether other monoclonal defined antigens which have a restricted expression within the T lineage are necessarily T cell specific. Of the series investigated in depth, OKT11 and OKT11A appear to be as T specific as E rosettes (no non-T leukaemias positive out of >80 investigated to date), and are indeed probably directed against sheep erythrocyte receptor (see above). The argument for exclusive T specificity here is, however, clearly circular since we have no irrefutable gene product which is both exclusive to T cells and expressed on all T cells (cf. Ig in B cells). Some E rosette$^+$/OKT11$^+$ cells, e.g. some but not all T$\gamma$ cells (cf. Reinherz *et al.*, 1980b), may indeed not be T cells.

OKT6, like NA134, appears to be specific for cortical thymocytes within the lymphoid lineages. However, the antigen it defines is not restricted to T cells and is present on some neuroblastoma (Fig. 6·12; Greaves *et al.*, 1981b) as well as on Langerhans cells in the skin (P. Kung and G. Janossy, personal communication). The former is one example of a number of intriguing cross reactions in humans between haemopoietic cells and neural tissue as defined by monoclonal antibodies (Greaves *et al.*, 1980c; Kemshead *et al.*, 1981a, b). However, other OKT monoclonals, with the exception of OKT9 (see above), do not bind to the neuroblastoma lines we have available or to non-T cell haemopoietic cell lines. OKT3, OKT4, OKT5/8 and similar monoclonal antibodies may therefore define structures unique to T cell subsets; at present, however, their possible presence on other cell types (e.g. epithelia) has not been rigorously examined.

OKT10 is not at all specific for T cells. We, like Reinherz *et al.* (1980a), do see preferential reactivity of immature (thymic) T cells and their corresponding leukaemias but the majority of acute myeloid leukaemias are also positive as are >90% of common ALL (including the pre-B subclass) and some mature B-ALL (Greaves *et al.*, 1981b). OKT1 also appears to recognize an antigen which is not exclusive to T cells at least as evidenced by reactivity with some B-CLL. Monoclonal antibodies L17F12 (Engleman *et al.*, 1981), T101 (Royston *et al.*, 1980) and UCH-2 (P. Beverley, personal communication) in our hands shows the same pattern of pan-T plus B-CLL reactivity as OKT1 and all 4 antibodies precipitate a p65–69 polypeptide. These observations indicate that a full appreciation of the specificity of putative cell type directed monoclonals requires binding tests and biochemical analyses on a broad spectrum of haemopoietic and non-haemopoietic lineages.

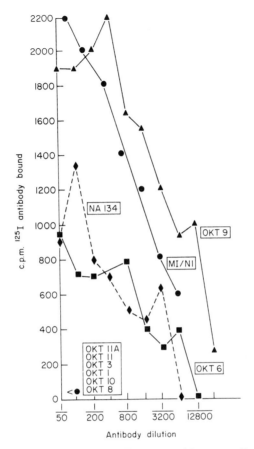

FIG. 6·12 Binding of monoclonal antibodies to neuroblastoma cells. Monoclonal antibody titrated against fixed number of neuroblastoma cells (cell line CHP 100) followed by $^{125}$I labelled goat anti-mouse Ig. MI/N1 = monoclonal anti-neuroblastoma antibody (Kemshead *et al.*, 1981a).

## H. Clinical Potential of Monoclonal Antibodies in Haemopoietic Malignancies

Experiments with monoclonal antibody provide some insight into the basic biology of haemopoietic malignancy differentiation. Some more direct or practical applications to patient management can also be considered. These include differential diagnosis, serial monitoring and immunotherapy. Monoclonal antibodies are used routinely in the I.C.R.F. laboratories for differential diagnosis of subtypes of ALL (Fig. 6·13 Greaves *et al.*, 1981c; Greaves, 1981a), CGL blast crisis and

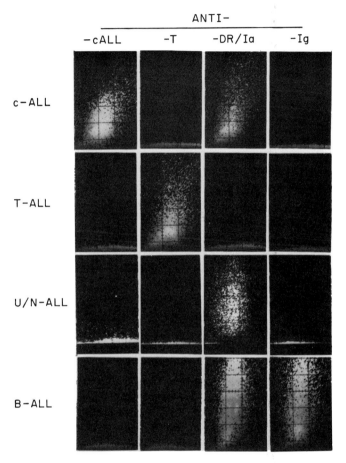

FIG. 6·13  4 subclasses of ALL detected by monoclonal antibodies and flow cytometry (FACS). Fluorescence activated cell sorter (FACS) analysis. Vertical axis, relative fluorescence; horizontal axis, relative cell size (light scatter). 10,000 cells screened for each test. cALL, common acute lymphoblastic leukaemia; U/N-ALL, unclassified or null ALL; anti-cALL = monoclonal J-5; anti-T = monoclonal NA134; anti-DR/ Ia = monoclonal DA-2; anti-Ig = "conventional" antibody/F(ab′)₂ against human immunoglobulin.(Reproduced by permission from *Cancer Res.* **41**.)

non-Hodgkin lymphoma. Monoclonal antibodies to kappa and lambda Ig light chains are replacing conventional sera for monoclonality assays in cases referred as possible B cell malignancies. OKM-1 (Breard *et al.*, 1980) is used to confirm monocytic involvement in acute leukaemia but as yet we have no ideal monoclonal antibody which has selective anti-myeloblast reactivity. Several different anti-myeloid monoclonal antibodies are, however, currently being screened for such activity.

Monoclonal antibody FMC7 is useful for distinguishing B-PLL from B-CLL since only the former is reactive (Catovsky *et al.*, 1981).

Sensitive detection of residual or re-emerging leukaemic cells would be of considerable value to physicians treating patients with leukaemia or lymphoma. Unfortunately, to date no unequivocally leukaemia or lymphoma specific antigens have been detected with either conventional or monoclonal reagents. Claims to the contrary should be evaluated very critically since they have in the past almost invariably reflected inadequate controls. Nadler *et al.* (1980) have recently reported a very interesting monoclonal antibody (Ab89) which appears to react with a subset (~10%) of B-CLL and non-Hodgkin lymphoma but not with normal B cells. Paradoxically the best example we have of tumour specific antigens in humans are in fact normally expressed gene products—idiotypic determinants of immunoglobulin variable regions (Greaves and Janossy, 1978). Since these determinants have a clonal distribution they can provide unique markers for monitoring or possibly treating B cell (or T cell?) malignancy (Stevenson *et al.*, 1977; Lampson and Levy, 1979). Similar patient-specific determinants might exist in other leukaemias as well as solid tumours (Old, 1981). Fortunately, absolute leukaemia specificity may not be required for some practical applications. For example, since cell differentiation is associated with topographical compartmentalization of cells, monoclonal antibodies or other probes detecting differentiation-linked features may have an operational leukaemic specificity when applied to certain tissues. Good examples of this are the detection of cells expressing the cALL/gp100 antigen (Greaves *et al.*, 1980b) or terminal deoxynucleotidyl transferase (Thomas *et al.*, 1981) in cerebro-spinal fluid or testicular biopsies, and the detection of cells of thymic phenotype in the bone marrow in T-ALL patients (Bradstock *et al.*, 1981). It remains to be shown that serial tests of this kind, which now include monoclonal antibodies, can lead to a therapeutic impact and improved survival.

Finally, monoclonal antibodies have a potential in therapy, e.g. for targeting of drugs, toxin or radio-isotope *in vivo*, or cell selection *in vitro* prior to allogeneic or autologous marrow transplantation. These topics are dealt with in chapters 4 and 7.

ACKNOWLEDGEMENTS

This work was supported by the Imperial Cancer Research Fund. We are grateful to those colleagues listed in Table 6·1 who made monoclonal antibodies available. We thank those physicians and

haematologists who referred leukaemic samples, and J. Riggs for typing
the manuscript.

REFERENCES

Abramson, C. S., Kersey, J. H. and LeBien, T. W. (1981). *J. Immunol.* **126**,
  83–88.
Andersson, L. C., Gahmberg, C. G., Teerenhovi, L. and Vuopio, P. (1979a).
  *Int. J. Cancer* **23**, 717–720.
Andersson, L. C., Jokinen, M. and Gahmberg, C. G. (1979b). *Nature* **278**,
  364–365.
Andersson, L. C., Wegelius, R., Borgström, G. H. and Gahmberg, C. G.
  (1980). *Scand. J. Haematol.* **24**, 115–121.
Beverley, P. C. L. and Callard, R. E. (1981). *In* "XXIX Ann. Coll. Protides of
  the Biological Fluids". pp. 653–658
Beverley, P. C. L., Linch, D. and Delia, D. (1980). *Nature* **287**, 332–333.
Billing, R., Minowada, J., Cline, M., Clark, B. and Lee, K. (1978). *J. natn.
  Cancer Inst.* **61**, 423–429.
Bollum, F. (1979). *Blood* **54**, 1203–1215.
Borella, L., Sen, L. and Casper, J. T. (1977). *J. Immunol.* **118**, 309–315.
Boss, M. A., Greaves, M. F. and Teich, N. (1981). *Eur. J. Immunol.* **11**,
  136–140.
Boumsell, L., Bernard, A., Reinherz, E. L., Nadler, L. M., Ritz, J., Coppin,
  H., Richard, Y., Dubertret, L., Valensi, F., Degos, L., Lemerie, J.,
  Flandrin, G., Dausset, J. and Schlossman, S. F. (1981). *Blood* **57**, 526–530.
Bradstock, K. F., Janossy, G., Pizzolo, G., Hoffbrand, A. V., McMichael, A.,
  Pilch, J. R., Milstein, C., Beverley, P. and Bollum, F. J. (1980). *J. natn.
  Cancer Inst.* **65**, 33–42.
Bradstock, K. F., Janossy, G., Hoffbrand, A. V., Ganeshaguru, K., Llewellin,
  P., Prentice, H. G. and Bollum, F. J. (1981). *Br. J. Haematol.* **47**, 121–131.
Breard, J., Reinherz, E. L., Kung, P. C., Goldstein, G. and Schlossman, S. F.
  (1980). *J. Immunol.* **124**, 1943–1948.
Breton-Gorius, J., Reyes, F., Vernant, J. P., Tulliez, M. and Dreyfus, B.
  (1978). *Br. J. Haematol.* **39**, 295–303.
Brodsky, F. M., Parham, P., Barnstable, C. J., Crumpton, M. J. and Bodmer,
  W. F. (1979). *Immunological Rev.* **47**, 3–61.
Brooks, D. A., Beckman, I., Bradley, J., McNamara, P. J., Thomas, M. E.,
  and Zola, H. (1980). *Clin. exp. Immunol.* **39**, 477–485.
Brouet, J. C. and Seligmann, M. (1978). *Cancer* **42**, 817–827.
Brown, G., Capellaro, D. and Greaves, M. F. (1975a). *J. Natn. Cancer Inst.* **55**,
  1281–1289.
Brown, G., Hogg, N. and Greaves, M.F. (1975b). *Nature,* **258**, 454–456.
Brown, G., Biberfield, P., Christensson, B. and Mason, D. Y. (1979). *Eur. J.
  Immunol.* **9**, 272–275.

Catovsky, D., Cherchi, M., Brooks, D., Bradley, J. and Zola, H. (1981) *Blood*
58, 406–408.

Chessells, J. M., Hardisty, R. M., Rapson, N. T. and Greaves, M. F. (1977).
*Lancet* ii 1307–1309.

Collins, S. J., Ruscetti, F. W., Gallagher, R. E. and Gallo, R. C. (1978). *Proc.
natn. Acad. Sci. U.S.A.* 75, 2458–2462.

Crissman, H. A., Stevenson, A. P., Kissane, R. J. and Tobey, R. A. (1979). *In*
"Flow Cytometry and Sorting" (M. R. Melamed, P. F. Mullaney and M. L.
Mendelsohn, Eds), pp. 243–262. Wiley, New York.

Delia, D., Newman, R., Greaves, M. F., Goldstein, G. and Kung, P. (1981). *In*
"Leukaemia Markers" (W. Knapp, Ed.). p. 293–297. Academic Press.
London and New York.

Dexter, T. M. (1979). *Clinics in Haematology* 8, 453–468.

Edwards, P. A. W. (1980). *Biochem. Soc. Transact.* 8, 334–335.

Engleman, E. G., Warnke, R., Foz, R. I., Dilley, J., Benike, C. J. and Levy, R.
(1981). *Proc. natn. Acad. Sci. U.S.A.* 78, 1791–1795.

Fialkow, P. J., Denman, A. M., Singer, J., Jacobson, R. J. and Lowenthal,
M. N. (1978). *In* "Differentation of Normal and Neoplastic Hemopoietic
Cells' (B. Clarkson, P. A. Marks, J. E. Till, Eds), pp. 131–144. Cold Spring
Harbor Publ.

Gallagher, R., Collins, S., Trujillo, J., McCredie, K., Ahearn, M., Tsai, S.,
Metzgar, R., Auklakh, G., Ting, R., Ruscetti, F. and Gallo, R. (1979). *Blood*
54, 713–733.

Goldstein, G. (1977). *In* "Progress in Immunology" T. E. Mandel, C. Cheers,
C. S. Hosking, I. F. C. McKenzie and G. J. V. Nossal, Eds), pp. 390. North
Holland, Amsterdam.

Goodfellow, P. N., Banting, G., Sutherland, D. R., Greaves, M. F. and
Solomon, E. (1982) *Somatic Cell Genetics* (in press).

Greaves, M. F. (1975). *Prog. Haematol.* 9, 255–303.

Greaves, M. F. (1979a). *In* "Tumour Markers" (E. Boelsma, T. Rümke, Eds),
pp. 201–211. Elsevier, Amsterdam.

Greaves, M. F. (1979b). *In* "Essays in Biochemistry" (P. N. Campbell and
R. D. Marshall, Eds), Vol. 15, pp. 78–124. Academic Press, London and
New York.

Greaves, M. F. (1980). *In* "Advances in Comparative Leukemia Research
1979" (D. S. Yohn, B. A. Lapin, J. R. Blakeslee, Eds), pp. 235–242.
Elsevier/North Holland Inc., Amsterdam.

Greaves, M. F. (1981a). *In* "Leukaemia Markers" (W. Knapp, Ed.),
Academic Press, New York pp. 19–32.

Greaves, M. F. (1981b). *In* "Chronic Granulocytic Leukaemia" (M. T. Shaw,
Ed.) pp. 16–47. W. B. Saunders Publ.

Greaves, M. F. and Janossy, G. (1976). *In* "In vitro Methods in Cell
Mediated and Tumour Immunity" (B. R. Bloom, J. David, Eds), pp.
89–104. Academic Press, London and New York.

Greaves, M. F. and Janossy, G. (1978). *Biochim. Biophys. Acta* 516, 193–230.

162

Greaves, M. F., Brown, G., Rapson, N. and Lister, T. A. (1975). *Clin. Immunol. Immunopathol.* **4**, 67–84.

Greaves, M. F., Verbi, W., Reeves, B. R., Drysdale, H. C., Jones, L., Sacker, L. S. and Samaratunga, I. (1979c). *Leukemia Res.* **3**, 181–191.

Greaves, M. F., Delia, D., Janossy, G., Rapson, N., Chessells, J., Woods, M. and Prentice, G. (1980a). *Leukemia Res.* **4**, 15–32.

Greaves, M. F., Paxton, A., Janossy, G., Pain, C., Johnson, S. and Lister, T. A. (1980b). *Leukemia Res.* **4**, 1–14.

Greaves, M. F., Verbi, W., Kemshead, J. and Kennett, R. (1980c). *Blood*, **56**, 1141–1144.

Greaves, M. F., Delia, D., Robinson, J., Sutherland, R. and Newman, R. (1981a). *Blood Cells* **7**, 257–280.

Greaves, M. F., Delia, D., Sutherland, R., Rao, J., Verbi, W., Kemshead, J., Robinson, J., Hariri, G., Goldstein, G. and Kung, P. (1981b). *Int. J. Immunopharmacol.* **3**, 283–300.

Greaves, M. F., Janossy, G., Peto, J. and Kay, H. (1981c). *Brit. J. Haematol.* **48**, 179–197.

Greaves, M. F., Rao, J., Hariri, G., Verbi, W., Catovsky, D., Kung, P. and Goldstein, G. (1981d). *Leukemia Res.* **5**, 281–299.

Greaves, M. F., Robinson, J. B. Delia, D., Ritz, J., Schlossman, S., Sieff, C., Goldstein, G., Kung, P., Bollum, F. and Edwards, P. (1981e) *In* "Modern Trends in Human Leukemia IV" (R. Neth, Ed.), pp. 296–304. Springer-Verlag, Munich.

Greaves, M. F., Robinson, J., Delia, D., Sutherland, R., Newman, R. and Sieff, C. (1981f). *In* "Cell Interactions in Haematopoietic Differentiation" (R. Porter, Ed.), pp. 109–121. Ciba Foundation Symp.

Harrison, P. R. (1977). *Int. Rev. Biochem.* **15**, 227–267.

Herzenberg, L. A. and Herzenberg, L. A. (1978). *In* "Handbook of Experimental Immunology" (D. M. Weir, Ed.) Vol. 3, pp. 1–21. Blackwell, Oxford.

Janossy, G., Roberts, M. and Greaves, M. F. (1976). *Lancet*, **ii**, 1058–1061.

Janossy, G., Greaves, M. F., Sutherland, R., Durrant, J. and Lewis, C. (1977). *Leukemia Res.* **1**, 289–300.

Janossy, G., Greaves, M. F., Capellaro, D., Minowada, J. and Rosenfeld, C. (1978a). *In* "Protides of the Biological Fluids" (H. Peeters, Ed.) Vol. 25 pp. 591–600. Pergamon Press, Oxford.

Janossy, G., Woodruff, R. K., Paxton, A., Greaves, M. F., Capellaro, D., Kirk, B., Innes, E. M., Eden, O. B., Lewis, C., Catovsky, D. and Hoffbrand, A. V. (1978b). *Blood* **51**, 861–877.

Janossy, G., Bollum, F., Bradstock, K., Rapson, N. and Greaves, M. F. (1979). *J. Immunol.* **123**, 1525–1529.

Janossy, G., Bollum, F. J., Bradstock, K. F. and Ashley, J. (1980a). *Blood* **56**, 430–441.

Janossy, G., Hoffbrand, A. V., Greaves, M. F., Ganeshaguru, K., Pain, C., Bradstock, K., Prentice, H. G. and Kay, H. E. M. (1980b). *Brit. J. Haematol.* **44**, 221–234.

Judd, W., Poodry, C. A. and Strominger, J. L. (1980). *J. exp. Med.* **152**, 1430–1435.

Kamoun, M., Martin, P. J., Hansen, J. A., Brown, M. A., Siadak, A. W. and Nowinski, R. C. (1981). *J. exp. Med.* **153**, 207–212.

Kemshead, J. T., Bicknell, D. and Greaves, M. F. (1981). *Paediatric Res.* 1282–1286.

Kemshead, J. T., Fritschy, J., Asser, U., Sutherland, R. and Greaves, M. (1982). *Hybridoma* **1**, 109–123.

Kennett, R. H. and Gilbert, F. (1979). *Science* **203**, 1120–1121.

Kersey, J. H., LeBien, T. W., Abramson, C. S., Newman, R., Sutherland, R. and Greaves, M. (1981). *J. exp. Med.* **153**, 726–731.

Knapp, W. (Ed.) (1981). "Leukaemia Markers". Academic Press, London and New York.

Korsmeyer, S. (1981). *In* "Leukaemia Markers" (W. Knapp, Ed.) pp. 85–99. Academic Press, London, New York.

Kung, P. C., Goldstein, G., Reinherz, E. L. and Schlossman, S. F. (1979). *Science* **206**, 347–349.

Kung, P. C., Berger, C. L., Goldstein, G., LoGerfo, P. and Edelson, R. L. (1981). *Blood* **57**, 261–266.

Lampson, L. A. and Levy, R. (1979). *J. natn. Cancer Inst.* **62**, 217–219.

Larrick, J. W. and Cresswell, P. (1979). *J. Supramolec. Struct.* **11**, 579–586.

Liszka, K., Majdic, O., Bettelheim, P. and Knapp, W. (1981). *In* "Leukaemia Markers" (W. Knapp, Ed.) pp. 61–64. Academic Press, London and New York.

Lozzio, B. B. and Lozzio, C. B. (1979a) *Leukemia Res.* **3**, 363–370.

Lozzio, B. B. and Lozzio, C. B. (1979b) *Int. J. Cancer* **24**, 513.

McMichael, A. J., Pilch, J. R., Galfre, G., Mason, D. Y., Fabre, J. W. and Milstein, C. (1979). *Eur. J. Immunol.* **9**, 205–210.

McMichael, A. J., Rust, N. A., Pilch, J. R., Solchynsky, R., Morton, J., Mason, D. Y., Ruan, C., Tobelem, G. and Caen, J. (1981). *Brit. J. Haematol.* **49**, 501–509.

Metzgar, R. S., Borowitz, M. J., Jones, N. H. and Dowell, B. L. (1981). *J. exp. Med.* **154**, 1249–1254.

Minowada, J., Janossy, G., Greaves, M. F., Tsubota, T., Srivastava, B. I. S., Morikawa, S. and Tatsumi, E. (1978). *J. natn. Cancer Inst.* **60**, 1269–1277.

Nadler, L. M., Stashenko, P., Hardy, R. and Schlossman, S. F. (1980). *J. Immunol.* **125**, 570–577.

Nagasawa, K. and Mak, T. W. (1980). *Proc. natn. Acad. Sci. U.S.A.* **77**, 2964–2968.

Netzel, B., Rodt, H., Haas, R. J., Kolb, H. J. and Thierfelder, S. (1980). *Lancet* **i**, 1330–1332.

Newman, R. A., Sutherland, R. and Greaves, M. F. (1981a). *J. Immunol.* **126**, 2024–2030.

Newman, R. A., Sutherland, D. R., Greaves, M. F., Ritz, J. and Kersey, H. (1981b). *In* "Leukaemia Markers" (W. Knapp, Ed.) pp. 69–72. Academic Press, London and New York.

164

Old, L. J. (1981). *Cancer Res.* **41**, 361–375.
Omary, M. B., Trowbridge, I. S. and Minowada, J. (1980). *Nature* **286**, 888–891.
Pesando, J. M., Ritz, J., Lazarus, H., Baseman Costello, S., Sallan, S. and Schlossman, S. F. (1979). *Blood* **54**, 1240–1248.
Reinherz, E. L., Kung, P. C., Goldstein, G. and Schlossman, S. F. (1979a). *J. Immunol.* **123**, 2894–2896.
Reinherz, E. L., Kung, P. C., Goldstein, G. and Schlossman, S. F. (1979b). *J. Immunol.* **123**, 1312–1317.
Reinherz, E. L., Kung, P. C., Goldstein, G., Levey, R. H. and Schlossman, S. F. (1980a). *Proc. natn. Acad. Sci. U.S.A.* **77**, 1588–1592.
Reinherz, E. L., Moretta, L., Roper, M., Breard, J. M., Mingari, M. C., Cooper, M. D. and Schlossman, S. F. (1980b). *J. exp. Med.* **151**, 969–974.
Ritz, J., Pesando, J. M., Notis-McConarty, J., Lazarus, H. and Schlossman, S. F. (1980). *Nature* **283**, 583–585.
Ritz, J., Pesando, J. M., Sallan, S. E., Clavell, L. A., Notis-McConarty, J., Rosenthal, P. and Schlossman, S. F. (1981). *Blood* **58**, 141–152.
Roberts, M. (1980). Ph.D. Thesis, London University.
Roberts, M., Greaves, M. F., Janossy, G., Sutherland, R. and Pain, C. (1978). *Leukemia Res.* **2**, 105–114.
Robinson, J., Sieff, C., Delia, D., Edwards, P. A. W. and Greaves, M. F. (1981). *Nature* **289**, 68–71.
Royston, I., Majda, J. A., Baird, S. M., Meserve, B. L. and Griffiths, J. C. (1980). *J. Immunol.* **125**, 725–731.
Rutherford, T., Clegg, J. B., Higgs, D. R., Jones, D. W., Thompson, J. and Weatherall, D. J. (1981). *Proc. natn. Acad. Sci. U.S.A.* **78**, 348–352.
Sachs, L. (1978). *Nature* **274**, 535–539.
Sachs, L. (1980). *Proc. natn. Acad. Sci. U.S.A.* **77**, 6152–6156.
Schneider, C., Sutherland, R., Newman, R. and Greaves, M. (1982). *J. Biol. Chem.* (in press).
Stevenson, G. T., Elliott, E. V. and Stevenson, F. K. (1977). *Fed. Proc.* **36**, 2268–2271.
Sutherland, R., Smart, J., Niaudet, P. and Greaves, M. F. (1978). *Leukemia Res.* **2**, 115–126.
Sutherland, R., Delia, D., Schneider, C., Newman, R., Kemshead, J. and Greaves, M. (1981). *Proc. natn. Acad. Sci. U.S.A.* **78**, 4515–4519.
Terhorst, C., van Agthoven, A., Reinherz, E. and Schlossman, S. (1980). *Science* **209**, 520–521.
Terhorst, C., van Agthoven, A., LeClair, K., Snow, P., Reinherz, E. and Schlossman, S. (1981). *Cell* **23**, 771–780.
Thiel, E., Rodt, H., Huhn, D., Netzel, B., Grosse-Wilde, H., Ganeshaguru, K. and Thierfelder, S. (1980). *Blood* **56**, 759–772.
Thierfelder, S., Rodt, H. and Thiel, E. (Eds) (1976). *In* "Immunological Diagnosis of Leukemias and Lymphomas". Springer-Verlag, Berlin.
Thomas, J. A., Janossy, G., Bollum, F. J. and Eden, O. B. Submitted for publication.

Trowbridge, I. S. and Omary, M. B. (1981). *Proc. natn. Acad. Sci. U.S.A.* **78**, 3039–3043.

Van Agthoven, A., Terhorst, C., Reinherz, E. and Schlossman, S. (1981). *Eur. J. Immunol.* **11**, 18–21.

Verbi, W., Greaves, M. F., Koubek, K., Janossy, G., Stein, H., Kung, P. and Goldstein, G. (1982). *Eur. J. Immunol.* **12**, 81–86.

Ziegler, A. and Milstein, C. (1979). *Nature* **279**, 243–244.

# 7 Monoclonal Antibody-Toxin Conjugates: aiming the magic bullet

PHILIP E. THORPE,[a] D. C. EDWARDS,[b]
A. J. S. DAVIES[b] AND W. C. J. ROSS[b]

[a] *Drug Targeting Laboratory, Imperial Cancer Research Fund,
Lincoln's Inn Fields, London. WC2A 3PX*
[b] *Divisions of Biology and Chemistry, Chester Beatty Research Institute,
Institute of Cancer Research, Fulham Road,
London. SW3 6JB*

# I INTRODUCTION

Paul Ehrlich conceived the notion of bifunctional chemotherapeutic molecules which would be selective in their cytotoxic action. He envisaged that the complexes would comprise a "haptophore", to provide anchorage specifically to the target cell, and a "toxophore" to bring about the cell's destruction. They would thus, in his view, resemble the antibodies, then newly discovered by Behring, which "in the manner of magic bullets, seek out the enemy" (Ehrlich, 1913).

In the light of contemporary knowledge, the haptophore or carrier molecule could be a lectin, a hormone, or an antibody molecule. Lectins are known to bind to carbohydrate sequences such as are found on the glycoproteins and glycolipids of cell surfaces and some may prove to possess useful cell-recognition properties. The specificity of binding of polypeptide hormones to their physiological target tissue may also prove useful as a means of delivering drugs to neoplasias arising in these tissues. It is the antibody, however, that is the most attractive choice of carrier molecule since desired specificities can be elicited by immunizing appropriate hosts with the target tissue itself. The present review will concentrate upon the use of antibodies as carriers for drugs and mainly ignore the possibilities presented by lectins and polypeptide hormones which have been reviewed elsewhere (Olsnes and Pihl, 1982a).

Several therapeutic applications of antibody-drug conjugates can be envisaged. Cytotoxic agents, could, for example, be coupled to anti-lymphocyte antibodies to provide specific immunosuppressive agents, to antibodies against tumour-associated antigens to generate anti-cancer agents, or to anti-parasite antibodies to combat parasitic infections.

The class of the antibody employed may be tailored to its particular application. IgM antibodies on account of their large molecular size tend to be retained within the bloodstream and may therefore be the most suitable class of immunoglobulin for attacking intravascular targets. Conversely, the use of the smaller $F(ab')_2$ or $Fab'$ fragments of IgG may be preferable for the delivery of drugs to targets outside the bloodstream since they should have optimal diffusion properties. The added bonus could be that, lacking the Fc-portion, they should be free from interaction with polymorphonuclear cells, B-lymphocytes, macrophages and other cells with Fc-receptors.

The toxophore or cytotoxic moiety could, in principle, be any of a great number of cell poisons since it need not have pre-existing selectivity for the target cell. Many cytotoxic drugs of low molecular weight, including chlorambucil, methotrexate, daunomycin and other established anti-cancer drugs, have been linked to antibodies and the conjugates have been claimed to exhibit some selectivity of cytotoxic action upon cells which express the appropriate antigens (reviewed by Ghose and Blair, 1978; and O'Neill, 1979). Rather more promising as toxophores, however, are the extremely potent macromolecular cytotoxins of bacterial or plant origin such as diphtheria toxin, abrin and ricin. Their use maximizes the chance of killing targets like cancer cells which probably do not have on their surface a high density of specific antigens. In addition access for the conjugate may be restricted by poor vascularisation and inefficient extravasation within solid tumour masses.

Diphtheria toxin, the exotoxin secreted by *Corynebacterium diphtheriae*, and the plant toxins, abrin, from the seeds of *Abrus precatorius* and ricin, from *Ricinus communis*, are all so potent that it has been judged that just one molecule needs to penetrate a cell to kill it (Yamaizumi *et al.*, 1978; Eiklid *et al.*, 1980). Other toxins such as exotoxin A secreted by *Pseudomonas aeruginosa* and modeccin from the roots of *Adenia digitata* show comparable activity. Some of the properties of these toxins are presented in Table 7·1. Such toxins comprise two polypeptide chains, A and B, neither of which separately is highly toxic to cells or whole animals. The B-chains bind to receptors, which are found on the plasma membrane of most cell types, and the A-chain penetrates the cell membrane and completes the lethal action by inhibiting protein synthesis. In the instance of diphtheria toxin it is known that the mechanism of inhibition of protein synthesis is enzymic. This is very likely to be so for the other toxins.

Part of this review will concern attempts to confer cell type specificity upon intact toxins by linking them to antibodies. The remainder will consider conjugates in which the B-chain of the toxin has been dispensed with entirely and the A-chain linked directly to the antibody molecule.

## II THE TOXINS AND OTHER RIBOSOME-DAMAGING PROTEINS

### A. Diphtheria Toxin

Diphtheria toxin is transcribed by *Corynebacterium diphtheriae* from structural genes carried by the DNA corynephage $\beta^{tox+}$ (Gill *et al.*, 1972; Murphy *et al.*, 1974). It is synthesized as a single polypeptide

TABLE 7·1
Properties of the toxins

| Toxin | [a]$LD_{50}$ $\mu$g Kg$^{-1}$ | Intact Mr | Subunit Mr | Receptor | Interaction with cell surface | | | Mechanism of inhibition of protein synthesis | Reviewed by |
|---|---|---|---|---|---|---|---|---|---|
| | | | | | Cell type examined | Number of binding sites | Apparent Affinity (Ka) at 37°C M$^{-1}$ | | |
| Diphtheria toxin | 0·1 (guinea pig) | 62,000 | A 21,145 B 39,000 | ? glyco-protein | HeLa Vero | 4,000 1-2 × 10$^5$ | 1 × 10$^8$ 9 × 10$^8$ | ADP-ribosylation of EF-2 | Pappenheimer, 1977 Gill, 1978 Collier, 1977 |
| Abrin | 0·5 (mouse) | 65,000 | A 30,000 B 35,000 | galactose | HeLa BHK | 3 × 10$^7$ 9 × 10$^6$ | 1·5 ×10$^7$ to 1·2 × 10$^8$ 3·3 × 10$^7$ | Damage to 60S ribosomal subunit | Olsnes and Pihl, 1977 Gill, 1978 Olsnes and Pihl, 1982b |
| Ricin | 2·6 (mouse) | 62,047 | A 31,422 B 30,625 | galactose | HeLa BHK | 3 × 10$^7$ 9 × 10$^6$ | 2·0 × 10$^7$ 2·1 × 10$^7$ | Damage to 60S ribosomal subunit | Olsnes and Pihl, 1977 Gill, 1978 Olsnes and Pihl, 1982b |
| Modeccin | 0·9 (rat) | 63,000 (57,000?) | A 28,000 (26,000?) B 38,000 (31,000?) | galactose | HeLa S3 | 1-2 × 10$^5$ | 10$^8$ | Damage to 60S ribosomal subunit | Olsnes, 1978 Barbieri et al. 1980a |
| Pseudomonas aeruginosa exotoxin A | 4·8 (mouse) | 66,000 (72,000?) | A 26,000? B 40,000? | | | | | ADP-ribosylation of EF-2 | Collier, 1977 |

a  Intraperitoneal administration.

chain containing two disulphide bridges. The intact molecule is readily cleaved by bacterial and mammalian proteases at an arginine-rich exposed loop of the molecule to generate "nicked" toxin which consists of two polypeptide chains joined by a disulphide bond (Gill and Dinius, 1971; Drazin *et al.*, 1971).

Little is known about the receptor molecule which is involved in the first step of the cytotoxic process except that it is (*a*) sparsely distributed even on highly sensitive cells (see Table 7·1), (*b*) probably a glycoprotein (Draper *et al.*, 1978; Proia *et al.*, 1979) and (*c*) needs divalent cations to interact with the toxin B-chain (Duncan and Groman, 1969; Chang and Neville, 1978). Mice and rats are resistant to diphtheria toxin, either because they lack specific receptors on their cell surfaces, as was indicated by the studies of Boquet and Pappenheimer (1976) and Proia *et al.* (1979) or, as Chang and Neville (1978) suggested, because they have no device for transporting the A-chain into the cytosol.

The mechanism by which the A-chain is translocated into the cell is obscure. Boquet and Pappenheimer (1976) have suggested that the sizeable hydrophobic region, which is known to be situated within the B-chain (Lambotte *et al.*, 1980), could, possibly in association with that part of the receptor which lies within the membrane, insert into the lipophilic core of the membrane to form a channel through which the A-chain can pass. There is evidence that the cellular compartment from which A-chain penetration to the cytosol occurs is the phagolysosome since chloroquine, ammonium chloride and other amines which raise lysosomal pH (Ohkuma and Poole, 1978) inhibit the toxicity of diphtheria toxin (Kim and Groman, 1965). It has been proposed that lysosomal enzymes may be needed to cleave off a hydrophilic segment of the B-chain to expose the hydrophobic domain (Pappenheimer, 1979). However it has recently been demonstrated by Sandvig and Olsnes (1980) and Draper and Simon (1980) that cells exposed to diphtheria toxin at low pH are killed rapidly, without the usual lag phase, and in a manner insusceptible to antagonism by chloroquine, suggesting that diphtheria toxin can readily penetrate cell membranes in the acid conditions which would normally prevail in the lysosomes.

The final step in the cytotoxic process is that the A-chain catalyses the transfer of ADP ribose from $NAD^+$ (Kandel *et al.*, 1974) to a novel amino acid called "diphthamide" in elongation factor 2 (Van Ness *et al.*, 1980).

$$NAD^+ + EF\text{-}2 \rightleftharpoons ADP\text{-}ribosyl\text{-}EF2 + nicotinamide + H^+.$$

The ADP-ribosyl EF-2, although still able to bind to ribosomes in the presence of GTP, cannot participate in the translocation of peptidyl t-RNA from the A-site to the P-site of the ribosomes (reviewed by Gill, 1978) and thus protein synthesis ceases.


## B. Abrin and Ricin

Abrin and ricin are glycoproteins which, although extracted from the seeds of unrelated plants, have very similar structures and mechanisms of action (see Olsnes and Pihl, 1977; Olsnes and Pihl, 1982b) and, like nicked diphtheria toxin, both toxins comprise two polypeptide chains, A and B, linked by a disulphide bond.

Abrin and ricin seem to bind via their B-chains to any carbohydrate moiety on cell surface glycoproteins or glycolipids that terminates in non-reducing galactose. In addition ricin binds to oligosaccharides in which penultimate galactose is attached through C6 to sialic acid (Baenziger and Fiete, 1979). Thus the number of receptors for the toxins is very high, ranging from $10^6$ for human erythrocytes to $3 \times 10^7$ for HeLa cells (Sandvig *et al.*, 1976). However, of these receptors few may be able to mediate the penetration of the toxin A-chains through cell membranes.

Galactose or lactose can competitively antagonize the binding of the toxins to cell surface glycoproteins and reduce toxicity (Olsnes *et al.*, 1974b). The affinity of interaction of these blocking sugars with the toxins, (Ka around $10^4 M^{-1}$) is much lower than that of the cell surface receptors ($3 \times 10^8 M^{-1}$ at 0°C for HeLa cells) and so high concentrations of sugars are required (Sandvig *et al.*, 1976).

The mechanism by which the A-piece of abrin and ricin penetrate cell membranes to reach the cytosol also has not been elucidated. There is a temperature-dependent time lag between application of the toxins to cells and the onset of inhibition of protein synthesis which is consonant with the view that endocytosis is obligatory (Olsnes *et al.*, 1976; Sandvig and Olsnes, 1979). One possible mechanism is that hydrophobic regions on the A or B chains, either independently or in association with the cell receptor, insert into the lipid membrane and form a channel through which the A-chain unfolds. Alternatively, as was suggested by Olsnes *et al.* (1974a), it may be that abrin and ricin are fortuitously transported into the cell in mistake for some other physiologically important macromolecule. Interestingly, there is some indication that the chemical modification of mannose on ricin A and B chains destroys its toxic properties without affecting cell-binding or A-chain effectiveness, hinting that carbohydrate may act as a signal for operation of the translocation mechanism (Simeral *et al.*, 1980).

The A-chain of abrin and ricin inactivates the 60S subunit of the ribosome. Although precise details are lacking, the action is probably enzymic because one A-chain molecule can inactivate 1500 ribosomes per minute in reticulocyte lysates (Olsnes *et al.*, 1975). Ricin-treated ribosomes display damage in their binding site for EF-2 suggesting that a protein or RNA molecule at this site may be modified by the toxins (Montanaro *et al.*, 1975; Nolan *et al.*, 1976).

### C. Non-toxic Proteins with A-chain-like Properties

Several plants have been found to contain proteins which inactivate isolated eukaryotic ribosomes apparently by the same mechanism as, and with similar potency to, the A-chains of abrin, ricin and modeccin. Inhibitors have been purified from the leaves of *Phytolacca americana* (Obrig *et al.*, 1973; Irvin, 1975) and of *Dianthus caryophyllus* (Stirpe *et al.*, 1981), from wheat germ (Stewart *et al.*, 1977; Roberts and Stewart, 1979) and from the seeds of *Gelonium multiflorum* (Stirpe *et al.*, 1980), *Momordica charantia* (Barbieri *et al.*, 1980b) and probably also from *Croton tiglium* and *Jatropha curcas* (Stirpe *et al.*, 1976). All are single chain polypeptides which seem not to bind to cells which may account for the low toxicity to cultured cells and animals.

## III CHEMISTRY OF THE COVALENT LINKAGE OF ANTIBODIES AND TOXINS OR TOXIN A-CHAINS

### A. Conjugates with Intact Toxins

The chemists attempting to devise a method for linking intact toxins covalently to antibodies had to satisfy the following constraints:

1. The antibody in conjugated form should retain its antigen-binding capacity.
2. The linkage should be stable in tissue culture and, if the conjugate is intended for therapy, in animals.
3. Non-disulphide cross-links between A- and B-chains of the toxins should be avoided since these are believed to prohibit the liberation of the A-chain from the conjugate and deny it access to its site of action in the cytosol.

4.  Polymerization of toxin, antibody or conjugate to form large molecular complexes with poor diffusion qualities in animals should be minimal if it is intended to attack a target cell or tissue outside the bloodstream.

In much of the early work with antibody-toxin conjugates simple homobifunctional coupling agents were employed such as glutaraldehyde (Moolten *et al.*, 1972, 1975a, b, 1976), diethylmalonimidate (Philpott *et al.*, 1973) and difluorodinitrophenylsulphone (Samagh and Gregory, 1972). These suffered from problems of polymerization of the conjugate and from inactivation of the toxin most likely due to the introduction of non-reducible bonds between its A- and B-chains.

More recently heterobifunctional coupling agents have been preferred and these come closer to meeting the above conditions. One such reagent, developed in our laboratory, is the mixed anhydride derivative of chlorambucil formed by its reaction with butyl chloroformate. The coupling is carried out in two stages. In the first stage, amino acids with primary amino groups in the antibody are reacted with the mixed anhydride part of the coupling agent to yield a primary conjugate of chlorambucil and antibody. This reaction is performed at 4°C at which the chloroethylamino groups of chlorambucil are relatively unreactive. To complete the conjugation, toxin is added in at least a four-fold molar excess and the temperature raised to 25°C to activate the chloroethylamino groups which can then react with amino groups (at pH 9) in the toxin. The component of conjugate comprising one molecule each of antibody and toxin can then be purified by chromatography (Thorpe *et al.*, 1978; Ross *et al.*, 1980). In a further development the use of the N-hydroxysuccinimide ester of chlorambucil has been found advantageous, this having better solubility and permitting more reproducible conjugation conditions (Edwards *et al.*, 1982a). Both reagents avoid polymerization and intrachain reaction in the toxin component, although antibody-antibody coupling can still occur.

Another coupling procedure, described by Olsnes and Pihl (1982a), is to oxidise the sugar groups of abrin or ricin, mainly or entirely associated with the B-chain, into aldehydes which can then be used to react with amino groups in the antibody component. Toxin homopolymer formation can be prevented by reductive methylation of its amino groups.

The "SPDP" reagent, a commercially available heterobifunctional coupling agent developed by Carlsson *et al.* (1978), has been used by Edwards *et al.* (1982b) to link ricin and anti-mouse lymphocyte globulin and by Thorpe *et al.* (1981b) to link gelonin and monoclonal anti-Thy

1.1 antibody. This reagent causes minimal homopolymer formation in the toxin and immunoglobulin components. A disulphide group is introduced into one of the proteins to be coupled and a sulphydryl group into the other; these then react together to form a conjugate with the two proteins linked by a disulphide bond.

The heterobifunctional reagent, n-maleimido benzoyl-N-hydro-xysuccinimide ester has also been used successfully to link ricin and immunoglobulin (Youle and Neville, 1980).

## B. Conjugates with Toxin A-chains

Most workers have chosen to emulate the natural construction of the toxins and employ a disulphide bond to link together the A-chain and the antibody. Several different methods for generating the disulphide linkage have been devised (reviewed by Olsnes and Pihl, 1982a).

Usually a disulphide group is introduced in the antibody component which on mixing with the A-chain reacts with its free SH-group by a thiol-disulphide interchange reaction:

$$\text{Antibody-SSX} + \text{HS-A-chain} \rightarrow \text{Antibody-SS-A-chain} + \text{XSH}$$

Cystamine plus a carbodiimide (Gilliland *et al.*, 1980), 3-(2-pyridyl-dithio) propionic acid plus a carbodiimide (Jansen *et al.*, 1980; Pau *et al.*, 1980; Blythman *et al.*, 1981) and methyl 3-mercaptopropionimidate plus Ellman's reagent (Miyazaki *et al.*, 1980) have all been used for introducing the disulphide group into intact antibodies. Raso and Griffin (1980) and Masuho and Hara (1980) used Ellman's reagent to convert the sulphydryl group on Fab′ monomers of their antibodies into a disulphide group. Masuho *et al.* (1979) preferred to activate the SH-group of diphtheria toxin A-chain by converting it to an S-sulphonate group and reacted this with the free sulphydryl group on Fab′ monomers of the antibody.

A second method, such as used by Krolick *et al.* (1980) is to insert a sulphydryl group into the antibody and rely upon oxidation-induced disulphide coupling with the A-chain:

$$\text{Antibody-SH} + \text{HS-A-chain} \overset{[O]}{\rightleftharpoons} \text{Antibody-SS-A-chain} + H_2O$$

This type of reaction, although it can be catalyzed by heavy metal ions and o-phenanthroline (Uchida *et al.*, 1978a), tends to be inefficient and suffers from the generation of homopolymers.

# IV CONJUGATES OF ANTIBODIES WITH INTACT TOXINS

The objective when preparing conjugates of antibodies with intact toxins is to modify the binding patterns of toxins to cells so that they attach to and kill designated target cells. As will be seen, considerable selectivity of cytotoxic effect can often be gained simply by attaching the toxin to an antibody molecule. Two factors cooperate to produce this improvement in selectivity. Firstly, the avidity of interaction of bivalent antibody with antigens upon the target cell surface may exceed that of the toxin moiety for its receptor so that the conjugate preferentially binds to the target cell. Secondly, the bulky immunoglobulin molecule seems to hinder the freedom with which the toxin moiety can bind to its receptor on non-target cells and thus the non-specific toxicity of the toxin in the conjugate both in relation to cells in tissue culture and to animals is somewhat reduced.

## A. CONJUGATES WITH DIPHTHERIA TOXIN

Moolten and Cooperband in 1970 pioneered this field of research when they showed that monkey kidney cells bearing new antigens induced by infection with mumps virus could be lysed selectively in tissue culture by diphtheria toxin conjugated to an antibody against mumps virus. Although a control conjugate of toxin linked to normal guinea pig globulin was not included, the authors did show that uninfected and infected cells were equally sensitive to native diphtheria toxin.

Therapy in animals was also first attempted by Moolten and his colleagues in 1972. They created an artificial tumour-associated antigen by attaching dinitrophenyl groups to hamster sarcoma cells and then used affinity-purified antidinitrophenyl antibodies coupled covalently to diphtheria toxin to attack the modified tumour cells implanted subcutaneously in hamsters. Treatment with the conjugate delayed the appearance of tumours and prolonged the lifespan of the animals, and, when used against a small tumour burden of $3 \times 10^2$ cells, also reduced tumour incidence. Using a similar approach, Philpott *et al.* (1973) showed that rabbit anti-trinitrophenyl antibody conjugated to diphtheria toxin was selectively toxic to trinitrophenol-coated HeLa cells whilst sparing unsubstituted cells. The immunological specificity of the effect upon coated cells was confirmed by the ability of the free hapten competitively to inhibit the toxic effect of the conjugate.

Samagh and Gregory (1972) tried to use chicken antilactate dehydrogenase antibody, which had previously been reported to bind to and accumulate in malignant but not normal cells, as a carrier with which to deliver diphtheria toxin selectively to cultured tumour cells. They found that diphtheria toxin was more toxic to Ehrlich tumour cells and less toxic to "normal" murine kidney cells in tissue culture after its linkage to the antibody.

In a further study in 1975(a), Moolten and his coworkers covalently coupled diphtheria toxin to immunopurified rabbit and hamster antibodies against SV40-induced antigens and produced conjugates which displayed a 1·7 to 2·2-fold greater "specific toxicity" for SV40-transformed tumour cells *in vitro* than a conjugate with normal immunoglobulin. In spite of this small differential, a single injection of the conjugates partially protected hamsters from a concurrent challenge with SV40-transformed fibrosarcoma cells. Repeated treatment with the conjugates, although ineffective against established fibrosarcomas, cured 20–56% of hamsters with established transplants of an SV40-induced lymphoma.

Using the novel coupling method detailed above designed to minimize damage to the toxin component of the conjugate, Thorpe *et al.* (1978) and Ross *et al.* (1980) linked diphtheria toxin to horse anti-human lymphocyte globulin (AHLG) and to F(ab')$_2$ fragments derived from it. The conjugates were over one thousand times more effective at inhibiting protein synthesis by the human lymphoblastoid cells, Daudi and CLA4, in tissue culture than was free diphtheria toxin. By contrast, conjugates with normal horse IgG (NIgG) were fifty to one hundred-fold less potent than the free toxin. In a control experiment it was shown that when antibody and toxin were applied simultaneously to the cells but not in chemically coupled form, no enhancement of toxicity occurred. This, together with the observations that the specific cytotoxic effects of AHLG-toxin could be abrogated by diphtheria antitoxin or by pretreating the cells with non-conjugated antibody contributed to our interpretation that the antibody moiety had facilitated the binding of a lethal quantity of toxin to the lymphoblastoid cells. In Fig. 7·1. it is shown that AHLG-toxin is about a thousand times more effective at inhibiting protein synthesis by CLA4 cells than non-conjugated antibody in the presence of guinea pig complement.

The dramatic increase in the toxicity of diphtheria toxin to human lymphoblastoid cells after its linkage to the antibody owes much to the natural resistance of these cells to the toxin. Hitherto the only other toxin-resistant cells known to derive from toxin-sensitive species were rabbit reticulocytes (Collier, 1977) and intentionally selected variants

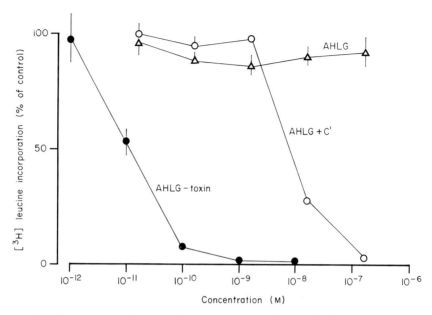

FIG. 7·1 A comparison between the cytotoxic effects of AHLG-toxin and AHLG plus complement. Human lymphoblastoid cells, CLA4, were incubated for one hour either with anti-human lymphocyte globulin (AHLG) conjugated to diphtheria toxin (●) or with AHLG followed by 10% v/v fresh (O) or heat-inactivated (△) guinea pig serum. The capacity of the cells to incorporate [³H] leucine into protein was measured one day later.

of HeLa (Venter and Kaplan, 1976; Moehring and Moehring, 1972) and Chinese hamster ovary (Moehring and Moehring, 1977) cell lines. The most plausible explanation for the resistance of the human lymphoblastoid cells is that their cell surface receptors for the toxin are either unusually sparse or cryptic; the attachment of the toxin to an antibody thus restores its ability to bind and kill.

Interestingly, murine spleen cells which, in common with other normal cells from this species, are insensitive to diphtheria toxin were not killed by the toxin coupled to anti-mouse lymphocyte globulin, even though the conjugate did bind to them (Ross *et al.*, 1980). This suggests that mouse cells, perhaps in addition to lacking receptors for diphtheria toxin, are deficient in a mechanism for transporting the A-chain across cell membranes into the cytosol.

Monoclonal antibodies can also function as delivery vehicles for diphtheria toxin. This is not self-evident since endocytosis of the toxin seems obligatory for the expression of its lethal action and many IgG

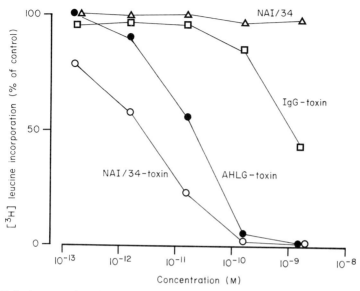

FIG. 7·2 A comparison between the cytotoxic effects upon MOLT4 human lympho-blastoid cells of diphtheria toxin conjugated to monoclonal anti-human thymocyte antibody, NA1/34 (O), to polyclonal anti-human lymphocyte globulin, AHLG (●), or to normal mouse IgG (□). The cells were incubated with the conjugates or with NA1/34 alone (△) for 24 hours and were then pulsed with [³H] leucine to measure their capacity to synthesize protein. The monoclonal antibody was kindly provided by Dr. C. Milstein.

monoclonal antibodies do not stimulate capping and endocytosis (Roser and Howard, unpublished observations). A conjugate of diphtheria toxin and the monoclonal antibody, NA1/34, which recognizes the HTA1 antigen on human thymocytes (McMichael *et al.*, 1979), proved to be an extremely potent and specific inhibitor of protein synthesis by the thymic leukaemia cell line, MOLT4. It was about ten-times more effective than a comparable conjugate with polyclonal AHLG (Fig. 7·2).

## B. Conjugates with Abrin

An investigation into the immunosuppressive properties of abrin coupled to horse anti-mouse lymphocyte globulin (AMLG) has been carried out by Edwards *et al.* (1981). The conjugate was about twice as effective as a similar conjugate with NIgG at suppressing the ability of mice to produce specific IgM-antibody forming cells following an im-

TABLE 7·2
The effect of anti-lymphocyte antibodies conjugated to abrin upon the
immune response of mice to sheep erythrocytes

|  | PFC$_{50}$[a] (moles) | LD$_{50}$ (moles) | Therapeutic index[b] |
|---|---|---|---|
| AMLG | $2 \times 10^{-8}$ | | |
| Abrin | $1·8 \times 10^{-13}$ | $4·3 \times 10^{-13}$ | 2·4 |
| AMLG-abrin | $4·1 \times 10^{-13}$ | $7·8 \times 10^{-12}$ | 19 |
| Normal IgG-abrin | $1·4 \times 10^{-12}$ | $8·1 \times 10^{-12}$ | 5·8 |
| anti Thy1·1 F(ab')$_2$-abrin | $3·8 \times 10^{-12}$ | $1·1 \times 10^{-11}$ | 2·8 |
| Normal F(ab')$_2$-abrin | $4·6 \times 10^{-12}$ | $1·1 \times 10^{-11}$ | 2·4 |

[a]  PFC$_{50}$ = dose which halves the production of specific antibody-forming cells in the spleens of
      mice responding to an immunological challenge with sheep erythrocytes.
[b]  Therapeutic Index = ratio LD$_{50}$ : PFC$_{50}$

munological challenge with sheep erythrocytes. The differential
between the immunosuppressive potencies of AMLG-abrin and NIgG-
abrin matched that observed for inhibition of protein synthesis in tissue
culture. Antibody alone was only immunosuppressive when injected in
quantities 50,000 times greater than that in the conjugate.

This work has been repeated using an improved conjugation and
isolation procedure and a differential of some fourfold between AMLG-
abrin and NIgG-abrin was established. It was a feature of this work that
the conjugates were much less toxic to mice than the free toxin and this
in turn led to considerable improvements in therapeutic index (Table
7·2). It was also found that the conjugate more readily suppressed the
generation of IgG-plaque forming cells after immunization with sheep
erythrocytes than IgM-plaque forming cells (Edwards *et al.*, 1982a).

The F(ab')$_2$ fragment of a monoclonal anti Thy 1·1 antibody coupled
to abrin was found to suppress skin allograft rejection by AKR mice to a
significantly greater extent than a conjugate containing normal F(ab')$_2$,
but showed no superiority in its ability to inhibit the generation of
IgM-plaque forming cells (Table 7·2) (Thorpe *et al.*, unpublished
results). Thus it appears that the immunosuppressive action of anti Thy
1·1-abrin is principally directed against T-lymphocytes.

In a further study, Edwards *et al.* (1982b) compared the immunosuppressive effects of conjugates of AMLG and abrin linked together by
two different methods. The first method of linkage employed the N-
hydroxysuccinimide ester of chlorambucil whereas the second used the

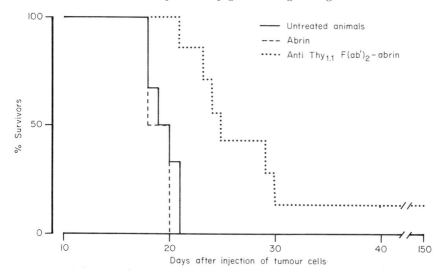

FIG. 7·3 Prolongation of survival of immunologically-deprived CBA mice bearing a Thy 1·1 +ve lymphoma following the administration of the F(ab')₂ fragment of monoclonal anti Thy 1·1 antibody conjugated to abrin. The mice received an intra-peritoneal injection of $10^5$ AKR-A tumour cells and on each of the following four days were treated with either $4 \times 10^{-13}$ moles of the conjugate or with $4 \times 10^{-12}$ of abrin. The antibody alone was ineffective.

SPDP reagent which introduces a disulphide link between the two proteins (Carlsson *et al.*, 1978). Although the differential between AMLG-abrin and NIgG-abrin was the same for both methods of linkage when tested against murine spleen cells in tissue culture, the AMLG-SS-abrin conjugate was much inferior to the chlorambucil-linked conjugate at immunosuppressing mice, as judged by a direct plaque assay. It was suggested that the disulphide-bonded materials dissociate in animals.

The anti-tumour activity of abrin coupled to monoclonal anti Thy 1·1 F(ab')₂ has been evaluated using as the target the Thy 1·1-expressing lymphoma, AKR-A, growing in immunologically-deficient CBA mice. Intraperitoneal administration of a total dose of 100 ng abrin linked to the antibody to mice which previously had received $10^5$ AKR-A cells (also intraperitoneally) prolonged the median survival time of the animals by 5·5 days (Fig. 7·3), and cured 50% of mice which had received $10^3$ tumour cells (Thorpe *et al.*, unpublished results). Since 10 lymphoma cells will grow progressively and kill, it was judged that the conjugate had eradicated about 99% of the tumour cells. Neither antibody alone, nor a control conjugate with normal F(ab')₂ afforded as good protection.

It was clear from these studies that, although some selectivity of action upon cells engaged in the immune response or upon lymphoma cells had been conferred upon abrin by its attachment to antibodies, the abrin moiety of the conjugate had retained part of its ability to bind to and kill cells non-specifically. This was evident from the immuno-suppressive action of normal IgG linked to abrin, its toxicity to cells in tissue culture, and from the fact that the conjugates were overtly poisonous to animals.

One way of abrogating the non-specific toxicity of antibody-abrin conjugates to cells in tissue culture is competitively to antagonize, with excess free galactose or lactose, the interaction between the abrin moiety and the galactose-containing receptor molecule (Thorpe *et al.*, 1981a). In the absence of galactose, AHLG-abrin is only about ten times more toxic to Daudi cells than the control conjugate containing normal immunoglobulin and both conjugates are less potent than free abrin. However, in the presence of excess free sugar the toxic actions of abrin and NIgG-abrin are abolished whereas that of AHLG-abrin is virtually unimpaired (Fig. 7·4). This finding has an important implication in that it may well be possible chemically to modify abrin to destroy its cell-surface recognition properties and then by linking the modified molecule to an antibody provide a new means of attaching to and killing cells with a specificity determined solely by the antibody.

## C. Conjugates with Ricin

The first conjugates of ricin and antibodies were linked non-covalently. Refsnes and Munthe-Kaas (1976) showed that complexes consisting of ricin and antibodies directed against the ricin B-chain weakly inhibited protein synthesis by Kupffer cells and peritoneal macrophages after binding to their Fc-receptors. Raso and Griffin (1979) used hybrid antibodies with dual specificities, one for the A-chain of ricin and the other for human IgG, to encourage ricin to bind to and kill human lymphoid cells in tissue culture.

A true covalent conjugate of monoclonal anti Thy 1·2 antibody and ricin was formed by Youle and Neville (1980) with a thioether linkage. On a molar basis the conjugate was as toxic as ricin itself to murine leukaemia cells, EL4, which expressed the Thy 1·2 antigen. Lactose antagonized the toxicity of the conjugate to cells lacking the Thy 1·2 antigen, such as HeLa and AKR thymic leukaemia cells, but did not attenuate that for EL4 cells.

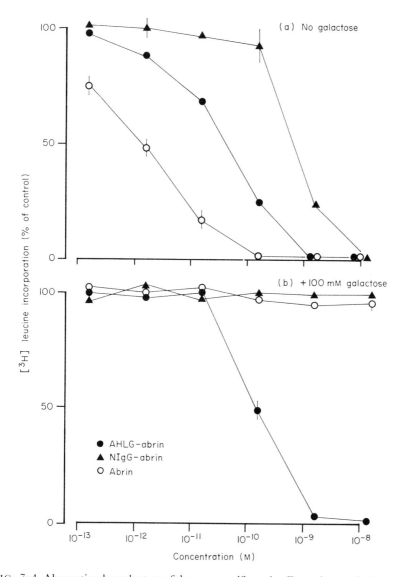

FIG. 7·4 Abrogation by galactose of the non-specific toxic effects of an antibody-abrin conjugate. Daudi lymphoblastoid cells were incubated for one hour, in the presence (b) or absence (a) of 100mM galactose, with abrin alone (O) or with abrin conjugated to normal horse IgG (▲) or to anti-human lymphocyte globulin, AHLG (●). The capacity of the cells to incorporate [³H] leucine was measured one day later. (Reproduced by permission of Blackwell Scientific Publications Ltd.) From Thorpe, P. E. (1981). *Clin. exp. Immunol.* **43**, 195–200.

## V. CONJUGATES OF ANTIBODIES WITH TOXIN A-CHAINS OR A-CHAIN-LIKE INHIBITORS

A particularly attractive idea for generating potent and selective cell poisons is to link the A-chain derived from a toxin to a new cell-binding entity such as an antibody molecule. In dispensing entirely with the B-chain of the toxin, the problem of non-specific binding that was observed with conjugates containing intact toxins is solved and the conjugates are thus not poisonous to animals. The drawback is that the B-chain, besides its role in cell binding, may mediate the penetration of the A-chain through cell membranes, a function which may be replaced inefficiently or not at all by the antibody molecule.

A related approach is to couple to antibodies one of the naturally-occurring plant A-chain-like molecules described earlier. So far only gelonin, the inhibitor from *Gelonium multiflorum*, has been utilized.

### A. CONJUGATES WITH TOXIN A-CHAINS

Fab' fragments from rabbit antibodies against the murine leukaemia L1210 were linked by Masuho *et al.* (1979) through a disulphide bond to the A-chain from diphtheria toxin. The conjugate at a concentration of $0 \cdot 5 \, \mu g \, ml^{-1}$ reduced the number of trypan blue dye-excluding L1210 cells in tissue culture to $5 \cdot 5\%$ of the number observed untreated cultures. Native diphtheria toxin, its A-chain and a conjugate with an irrelevant IgG (anti DNP) were virtually without effect, as was anti-L1210 Fab' admixed with non-conjugated A-chain. In a later study comparable results were obtained with a conjugate of ricin A-chain linked to anti-L1210 Fab' (Masuho and Hara, 1980). Although the combination of the A-chains with the fragment of an antibody molecule seems to have provided them with a means of attaching to and killing cells, it is clear that the conjugates lacked the potency normally attributable to native ricin or to diphtheria toxin when used against cells from species sensitive to the toxin.

Raso and Griffin (1980) also prepared Fab' fragments from an antibody, this time raised against and immunopurified upon human IgG, and coupled them to ricin A-chain. In tissue culture the conjugate was entirely selective and produced inhibition of protein synthesis, impedance of growth, as well as lysis only of those human cells which possessed surface immunoglobulin determinants. The potency of effect upon the Ig-bearing lymphoblastoid line, Daudi, was about one-fiftieth of that of native ricin. Similar results were also obtained by Miyazaki *et al.* (1980) who showed that a conjugate of rabbit anti-mouse IgG and ricin A-chain could exert selective toxic effects upon murine B-lymphocytes, albeit with a potency only one-thousandth that of intact ricin.

Gilliland and Collier (1980) coupled the A-chain from diphtheria toxin to immunopurified antibodies against the lectin, concanavalin A, and showed that the conjugate was only toxic to murine 3T3 cells and chinese hamster ovary cells that had been coated with concanavalin A. The potency of the cytotoxic effect was, however, rather weak.

Monoclonal B-lymphoid cell neoplasias often express cell surface immunoglobulin with a single idiotypic sequence which can function as a tumour-specific marker. Krolick *et al.* (1980) coupled immunopurified rabbit antibodies against the idiotype of the immunoglobulin expressed by the murine lymphoid tumour, $BCL_1$, to ricin A-chain. The conjugate at a concentration of $0 \cdot 25$ $\mu$g ml$^{-1}$ inhibited protein synthesis by the $BCL_1$ cells in tissue culture by 70% whereas little or no effect was exerted upon normal BALB/c spleen cells or upon two unrelated lymphoid tumour lines. In the same study selective cytotoxic effects were also reported using ricin A-chain linked to affinity-purified rabbit antibodies against the $\mu$-chain of $BCL_1$ immunoglobulin or to hybridoma antibodies to two of the allotypes of IgD.

The first attempt at generating cytotoxic agents specific for a human tumour was described by Gilliland *et al.* (1980). The monoclonal antibody 1083-17-1A against a colorectal carcinoma tumour-associated antigen was linked by a disulphide bond to the A-chains from diphtheria toxin or from ricin. The conjugates, although a thousand times less potent than the native toxins, specifically inhibited the protein synthesis and growth of two different colorectal carcinoma cell lines and were without effect upon human melanoma cell lines, embryonal and normal lung fibroblasts and lung carcinoma cells. The expression of the cytotoxic effects of the conjugates correlated with their ability to bind to the cells.

The therapeutic value of ricin A-chain coupled to antitumour antibodies in the treatment of cancer in mice has been assessed by Jansen and his colleagues. Immunopurified rabbit antibodies to dinitrophenyl-BSA were linked by a disulphide bond to the A-chain and were administered intraperitoneally to nude mice which one hour previously had received an intraperitoneal injection of hapten-coated HeLa cells. The treatment significantly reduced tumour incidence and growth. Twenty-five days after their inoculation with the tumour cells 14/15 of the untreated animals but only 1/15 of the conjugate recipients had discernable tumours (Jansen *et al.*, 1980). Similarly, monoclonal anti Thy $1 \cdot 2$ antibodies (IgM) linked to the A-chain when administered to

BALB/c mice which had previously received $6 \times 10^5$ Thy 1·2-positive
WEHI-7 leukaemic cells prolonged their median survival times by nine
days. No protection, however, was afforded against a larger inoculum
of $2·4 \times 10^6$ leukaemic cells (Blythman *et al.*, 1981). In tissue culture
the conjugates exhibited highly potent and almost completely selective
cytotoxicity for tumour cells which either bore the Thy 1·2 determinant
or which had been modified by the attachment of dinitrophenyl groups.


B. CONJUGATES WITH GELONIN

Following on from a study by Stirpe *et al.* (1980) in which it was shown
that gelonin could acquire cytotoxic activity by its linkage to concanavalin A, gelonin was conjugated by a disulphide bond to monoclonal anti Thy 1·1 antibody (Thorpe *et al.*, 1981b). The results were
remarkable. The conjugate inhibited those Thy 1·1-bearing T-lympho
cytes from AKR mice which will respond to phytohaemagglutinin and
concanavalin A in tissue culture with a potency which matched that of
abrin and exceeded that of ricin (Fig. 7·5). The conjugate exerted little
or no effect upon B-lymphocytes or Thy 1·2-expressing T-lymphocytes
from CBA mice. An enigmatic finding was that two Thy 1·1-positive
AKR lymphoma cell lines, AKR-A and BW5147, were far less sensitive
to the conjugate than the normal T-lymphocytes. Nevertheless, when
injected at dose levels corresponding to less than one-fiftieth of the
minimal lethal dose for free gelonin, the conjugate prolonged by one
week the median survival time of CBA mice carrying an AKR-A
tumour allograft (Fig. 7·6).


VI THERAPEUTIC APPLICATIONS OF
ANTIBODIES CONJUGATED TO TOXINS OR
TO TOXIN FRAGMENTS

A. THE DESTRUCTION OF LYMPHOCYTES OR MALIGNANT
CELLS IN BONE MARROW GRAFTS

A major obstacle to the extension of bone-marrow grafting has proved
to be the sometimes-lethal graft-versus-host reactions which can arise.
It is supposed that these reactions are caused by T-lymphocyte contamination of the transplanted marrow. Selective destruction of the
T-lymphocytes may well be possible by treating the marrow prior to
transfer with anti-lymphocyte antibodies conjugated to toxins or to

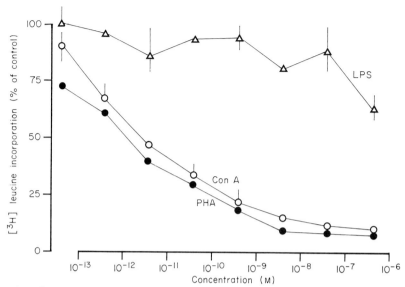

FIG. 7·5 Potent inhibition of AKR T-cells by monoclonal anti-Thy 1·1 antibody conjugated to gelonin. AKR spleen cells were incubated for one hour with anti Thy 1·1-gelonin (Mr > 200,000). One day later cultures either received the B-cell mitogen, bacterial lipopolysaccharide (△), or one of the T-cell mitogens, concanavalin A (O) or phytohaemagglutinin (●). The [$^3$H] leucine incorporation stimulated by the mitogens was measured after a further 24 hour period.

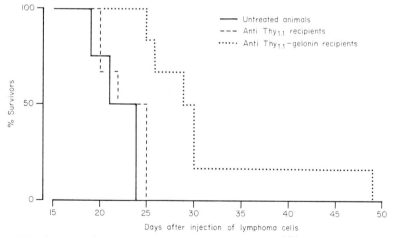

FIG. 7·6 Prolongation of survival of immunologically-deprived CBA mice bearing a Thy 1·1 +ve lymphoma, following the administration of monoclonal anti Thy 1·1 antibody conjugated to gelonin. The mice received an intraperitoneal injection of $10^5$ AKR-A tumour cells and one day later were treated with $6·7 \times 10^{-10}$ moles of anti Thy 1·1 antibody alone (--) or of the conjugate (··).

toxin A-chains. The studies of Mason (1981) in the rat have shown that both "helper" T-cells and "suppressor" or cytotoxic T-cell precursors (distinguished by their reactions with monoclonal antibodies W3/25 and MRC OX8 respectively) can give rise to graft-versus-host disease on transfer to irradiated F₁ recipients. In man the OKT3 antibody recognizes both of these major peripheral T-cell subsets (Reinherz and Schlossman, 1980) and would therefore be a good candidate for conjugation to toxins for attempts to rid human marrow of T-lymphocytes.

It may be feasible also to use antibody-toxin conjugates to destroy leukaemic or other malignant cells in autologous marrow prior to its injection back into the irradiated patient. The antibody must recognize an antigenic determinant which is present on malignant cells but absent from pluripotential stem cells which are needed for regeneration of the blood tissues. It may be envisaged that such antigens will be difficult to find upon leukaemias which derive from lesions early in the differentiation from the stem cell. One monoclonal antibody which could be useful is J-5, described by Ritz *et al.* (1980), which binds to leukaemic cells from many patients with non-T-cell-ALL and from some patients with CML (see chapter 6). Similarly the removal of neuroblastoma cells from bone marrow grafts in man may be possible using conjugates of the monoclonal antibody A2B5 which was raised against chick neural retina cells by Eisenbarth *et al.* (1979) and has since been found apparently to discriminate between neuroblastoma cells and haemopoietic cells in human bone marrow (Kemshead *et al.*, 1981).

## B. Immunosuppression

It is foreseeable that antibody-toxin conjugates will find extensive application in immunosuppression. This is because lymphoid cells or their subsets seem to express unique antigens and seem freely accessible for interaction with antibodies, as attested to by studies in which radiolabelled antilymphocyte antibodies have been found to localize specifically within the lymphoid tissues (Houston *et al.*, 1980). The generalized suppression of T-cell function in man for the prevention of allograft rejection and certain hypersensitivity responses may be possible using conjugates with monoclonal antibodies like OKT3 which, as mentioned earlier, binds to all recirculating T-lymphocytes in man. Further, it may be possible to suppress selected aspects of the immune response using antibodies such as OKT4 which recognizes "helper" T-cells in man or OKT5 which recognizes "suppressor" or cytotoxic T-cells (reviewed by Reinherz and Schlossman, 1980). Even more refined immunosuppression may be possible through recognition of the antigen receptor upon specific clones of T and B-lymphocytes, using conjugates with either anti-idiotypic antibodies or with the antigen itself, leading to the induction of specific tolerance through clonal deletion.

## C. Chemotherapy of Cancer

It is still not clear whether there exist in man antigens which are sufficiently tumour-specific to provide a target for therapy with anti-body-toxin conjugates. There have been several reports of monoclonal antibodies which show specificity for human malignant cells, including melanomas (Koprowski *et al.*, 1978; Dippold *et al.*, 1980; Herlyn *et al.*, 1980), colorectal carcinomas (Herlyn *et al.*, 1979), lymphomas (Nadler *et al.*, 1980), non-T-cell ALL (Ritz *et al.*, 1980) and leiomyosarcoma cells (Deng *et al.*, 1981). However, most of these antibodies have now been shown to react with some normal cell types (see chapter 5). This need not be too serious a problem. It may be that the normal but not the malignant cells are protected by anatomical barriers. Further, a degree of interaction of antibody-toxin conjugates with normal tissues not essential to life may be tolerable. Indeed, if an antibody can be found which recognizes normal epithelial cells from "expendable" organs like the breast or prostate, it may be feasible to destroy tumours arising in such organs along with the normal epithelium.

Although radiolabelled antibodies to antigens associated with cancer cells clearly do localize within solid tumours both in man (Mach *et al.*, 1980) and in mice (Reif, 1971; Mach *et al.*, 1974; Moshakis *et al.*, 1981), the proportion of the injected antibody actually found associated with the tumours is invariably small. Although hard to ascertain, this may be a consequence of poor vascularization of large tumour masses. It could transpire, therefore, that the principal use of antibody-toxin conjugates will be for destroying metastatic tumour deposits after surgical removal or radiological annihilation of the primary malignant mass.

## D. Chemotherapy of Parasitic Disease

Protozoan parasites, such as malaria or *Trypanosoma cruzi*, whose surface coats have stable antigenic expression and whose development cycle in the mammalian host includes an extracellular stage could feasibly be attacked with specific antibodies conjugated to cytotoxic agents. Likewise filarial worms and schistosomes are promising targets, although the latter have a tendency to disguise themselves by incorporating host blood group antigens and other host glycoproteins into their outer coats (Smithers, 1976).

It is not known whether protozoan and metazoan parasites are susceptible to toxins; if not, drugs acting directly upon the cell surface, or intracellularly-acting drugs of low molecular weight may have to be utilized.

## VII THE CURRENT STATUS OF ANTIBODY-TOXIN CONJUGATES AS MAGIC BULLETS

The selective destruction of a cell type *in vitro* can usually be achieved using an appropriate specific antibody conjugated to a toxin or to a toxin A-chain. This has application both for the scientist who might wish to study the effects of removing a particular cell type from a mixed population and for the clinician who is contemplating the removal of lymphocytes or malignant cells from bone marrow grafts. Some re-appraisal of the various studies reviewed above may help to clarify the question of which cytotoxic entity should be used for *in vitro* work— intact toxins, A-chains or gelonin.

Conjugates of antibodies with intact toxins have in our laboratories and those of others nearly always yielded highly potent cytotoxic agents (summarized in Table 7·3). For tissue culture work, excellent selectivity of cytotoxic action can normally be achieved with conjugates containing abrin or ricin when galactose or lactose is included in the culture competitively to antagonize the non-specific toxic effects of the conjugate.

Conjugates with A-chains or A-chain-like molecules such as gelonin have the advantage that the risk of incurring non-specific toxic effects is minimal but suffer from the disadvantage that the potency of their cytotoxic action upon target cells is variable and largely unpredictable (summarized in Table 7·4). Diphtheria toxin A-chain seldom seems to yield highly potent conjugates, regardless of whether it is linked to antibodies, lectins (Gilliland *et al.*, 1978; Uchida *et al.*, 1978a; Uchida *et al.*, 1980), hormones (Chang *et al.*, 1977; Miskimins *et al.*, 1979), epidermal growth factor (Cawley *et al.*, 1980b) or to the fibroblast-binding small molecule, monophosphopentamannose (Youle *et al.*, 1979). Ricin A-chain, on the other hand, when attached through a disulphide bridge to carrier molecules, can sometimes mediate selective cytotoxic effects with a potency rivalling that of the native toxin. This result was seen with Blythman's anti-Thy 1·1 monoclonal antibodies and with conjugates which used lectins (Yamaguchi *et al.*, 1979; Uchida *et al.*, 1980), asialofetuin (Cawley *et al.*, 1980a) and epidermal growth factor (Cawley *et al.*, 1980b) as the carriers. Gelonin, likewise, can acquire extremely potent and specific cytotoxic properties by its linkage to monoclonal anti Thy 1·1 antibody.

The reason why ricin A-chain and gelonin but not the A-chain from diphtheria toxin should sometimes yield extremely potent conjugates is unknown. It could be that gelonin and ricin A-chain have a signal molecule, such as carbohydrate, which is recognized by a cellular device for transporting macromolecules across cell membranes. Alternatively, hydrophobic regions, known to be present in the A-chain of ricin but lacking in that of the bacterial toxin, may be required for membrane penetration.

On other occasions ricin A-chain and gelonin when linked to carrier molecules have yielded rather feeble cytotoxic agents. Oeltmann and Heath (1979) failed to inhibit Leydig cells with ricin A-chain coupled to a subunit of human chorionic gonadotrophin. Similarly Stirpe *et al.* (1980) observed only weak toxic effects upon HeLa cells using gelonin conjugated to concanavalin A, as did Thorpe *et al.* (1981b) using anti Thy 1·1-gelonin against AKR lymphoma cells. The resistance of such cells may arise because their receptors for the carrier moiety either are shed or fail to associate efficiently with a mechanism for transporting the inhibitors through cell membranes.

The state of the art as far as therapy in animals is concerned is much more primitive. Intact toxins coupled to specific antibodies do show some selectivity of action upon target cells in animals but their use is problematical because the toxin moiety retains much of its capacity to bind non-specifically to cells. Thus the conjugates are poisonous to animals and this limits their therapeutic value. A solution to this problem might be to utilise toxins which have been modified chemically to reduce their capacity to bind to cells.

Conjugates of antibodies with toxin A-chains or gelonin, outstandingly specific in tissue culture systems, have so far not lived up to their potential in animals. Even when attacking tiny numbers of tumour cells growing in the peritoneal cavity of mice by the administration of near-lethal doses of conjugates into this same site, the results have been relatively unimpressive. Indeed, it is difficult to avoid concluding that factors must operate in the animal to negate the cytocidal action of these conjugates. The dissociation of the disulphide bond introduced between the A-chain and the antibody is one possible explanation.

## TABLE 7·3
### Summary of cytotoxic effects of antibodies conjugated to intact toxins

| Toxic moiety | Antibody moiety | Test cells | Toxicity to cells with appropriate antigens | | Specificity factor $\frac{Y}{X}$ | Toxicity to cells lacking appropriate antigens | | Selectivity factor $\frac{Z}{X}$ | Reference |
|---|---|---|---|---|---|---|---|---|---|
| | | | (X) $ID_{50}$ (M) Antibody-toxin | (Y) $ID_{50}$ (M) Normal IgG-toxin | | Test cells | (Z) $ID_{50}$ (M) Antibody-toxin | | |
| Diphtheria Toxin | anti-human lymphocyte | CLA4 | $1·6 \times 10^{-11}$ | $>1·6 \times 10^{-8}$ | $>1000$ | | | | Thorpe et al., 1978 |
| | anti-human lymphocyte | Daudi | $8 \times 10^{-12}$ | $>1·6 \times 10^{-8}$ | $>2000$ | human fibroblasts | $1·6 \times 10^{-9}$ | 200 | Ross et al., 1980 |
| | anti-human lymphocyte F(ab')$_2$ | MOLT4 | $1·5 \times 10^{-11}$ | $1·1 \times 10^{-9}$ | 73 | | | | Present work |
| | anti-human lymphocyte | Daudi | $8 \times 10^{-11}$ | $>1·6 \times 10^{-8}$ | $>200$ | human fibroblasts | $1·6 \times 10^{-9}$ | 20 | Ross et al., 1980 |
| | monoclonal anti-human thymocyte NA1/34 | MOLT4 | $2·5 \times 10^{-12}$ | $1·1 \times 10^{-9}$ | 440 | | | | Present work |
| | anti-mouse lymphocyte | murine T-lymphocytes | $>1·6 \times 10^{-8}$ | $>1·6 \times 10^{-8}$ | | | | | Ross et al., 1980 |
| Abrin | anti-human lymphocyte | Daudi | $5 \times 10^{-11}$ | $6·3 \times 10^{-10}$ | 12 | | | | Thorpe et al., 1981 |
| | anti-human lymphocyte | Daudi +galactose | $1·2 \times 10^{-10}$ | $>1·6 \times 10^{-8}$ | $>133$ | | | | Thorpe et al., 1981 |

| | | | | | | | | |
|---|---|---|---|---|---|---|---|---|
| | anti-mouse lymphocyte F(ab')$_2$ | murine T-lymphocytes | $1 \cdot 5 \times 10^{-12}$ | $1 \cdot 5 \times 10^{-11}$ | 10 | | | Edwards et al., 1981 |
| | monoclonal anti-Thy·2 F(ab')$_2$ | AKR T-lymphocytes | $2 \cdot 4 \times 10^{-11}$ | $4 \cdot 9 \times 10^{-11}$ | 2 | human fibroblasts | $3 \cdot 0 \times 10^{-10}$ | 12 | Thorpe et al., (unpublished) |
| | monoclonal anti-Thy·1 F(ab')$_2$ | AKR-A lymphoma | $9 \cdot 7 \times 10^{-12}$ | $2 \cdot 4 \times 10^{-10}$ | 25 | human fibroblasts | $3 \cdot 0 \times 10^{-10}$ | 31 | Thorpe et al., (unpublished) |
| | monoclonal anti-Thy·1 | BW5147 lymphoma | $2 \cdot 4 \times 10^{-11}$ | $2 \cdot 4 \times 10^{-9}$ | 100 | human fibroblasts | $3 \cdot 0 \times 10^{-10}$ | 12 | Thorpe et al., (unpublished) |
| Ricin | monoclonal anti-Thy·2 | EL4 +lactose | $1 \cdot 4 \times 10^{-10}$ | | | AKR T-cell leukaemia | $9 \cdot 5 \times 10^{-8}$ | 700 | Youle and Neville, 1980 |
| | monoclonal anti-Thy·1 | AKR T-lymphocytes | $1 \cdot 5 \times 10^{-11}$ | $6 \cdot 1 \times 10^{-10}$ | 41 | | | | Thorpe et al., (unpublished) |
| | anti-mouse lymphocyte | murine T-lymphocytes | $9 \cdot 7 \times 10^{-11}$ | $9 \cdot 7 \times 10^{-11}$ | 1 | | | | Thorpe et al., (unpublished) |
| | anti-mouse lymphocyte | murine T-lymphocytes + lactose | $1 \cdot 5 \times 10^{-9}$ | $1 \cdot 5 \times 10^{-8}$ | 10 | | | | Thorpe et al., (unpublished) |

(i) antibodies are polyclonal unless stated otherwise.

(ii) ID$_{50}$ = concentration of conjugate needed to inhibit by 50% the observed cellular function (usually protein synthesis).

(iii) "Specificity factor" compares the potency of cytotoxic action of an antibody-toxin conjugate with that of a conjugate with normal immunoglobulin upon cells bearing the appropriate antigen.

(iv) "Selectivity factor" indicates the extent to which an antibody-toxin conjugate can exert selective cytotoxic effects upon an antigen-bearing as opposed to an antigen-lacking cell type.

## TABLE 7·4

### Summary of cytotoxic effects of antibodies conjugated to toxin A-chains or to gelonin

| Toxic moiety | Antibody moiety | Toxicity to cells with appropriate antigens | | | | Toxicity to cells lacking appropriate antigens | | Selectivity factor $\frac{Z}{X}$ | Reference |
| --- | --- | --- | --- | --- | --- | --- | --- | --- | --- |
| | | Test cells | (X) ID$_{50}$ (M) Antibody-toxin | (Y) ID$_{50}$ (M) Normal IgG-toxin | Specificity factor $\frac{Y}{X}$ | Test cells | (Z) ID$_{50}$ (M) Antibody-toxin | | |
| Diphtheria toxin A-chain | Fab' anti-L1210 | L1210 | $\sim 8 \times 10^{-9}$ | $> 8 \times 10^{-7}$ | $> 100$ | | | | Masuho et al., 1979 |
| | anti-Con A | Con A-coated 3T3 | $2 \times 10^{-9}$ | $> 3 \times 10^{-8}$ | $> 15$ | 3T3 | $> 3 \times 10^{-8}$ | $> 15$ | Gilliland and Collier, 1980 |
| | anti-Con A | Con A-coated CHO | $5 \times 10^{-9}$ | $> 3 \times 10^{-8}$ | $> 6$ | | | | Gilliland and Collier, 1980 |
| | monoclonal anti-colorectal carcinoma | SW 1116 colorectal | $10^{-9}$ | | | WM 56 melanoma | $> 10^{-7}$ | $> 100$ | Gilliland et al., 1980 |
| | monoclonal anti-Thy1 | AKR T-lymphocytes | $4 \times 10^{-8}$ | | | AKR B-lymphocytes | $4 \times 10^{-7}$ | $10$ | Thorpe et al., (unpublished) |
| | monoclonal anti-Thy1 | AKR lymphomas | $1 \times 10^{-7}$ | | | | | | Thorpe et al., (unpublished) |
| Ricin A-chain | anti-DNP | TNP-coated HeLa | $10^{-8} - 10^{-9}$ | | | HeLa | $2 \times 10^{-6}$ | $\sim 500$ | Jansen et al., 1980 |
| | monoclonal anti-colorectal carcinoma | SW 1116 colorectal | $10^{-9}$ | | | WM 56 melanoma | $> 10^{-7}$ | $> 100$ | Gilliland et al., 1980 |
| | anti-mouse $\mu$ chain | murine B-lymphocytes | $< 5 \times 10^{-9}$ | $> 5 \times 10^{-8}$ | $> 10$ | | | | Krolick et al., 1980 |
| | monoclonal anti-$\delta^b$ allotype | C57BL/6 B-lymphocytes | $< 2 \times 10^{-9}$ | | | BALB/c B-lymphocytes | $> 5 \times 10^{-9}$ | $> 2 \cdot 5$ | Krolick et al., 1980 |

| Antibody | Target cell | $ID_{50}$ | | Second cell | $ID_{50}$ | | Reference |
|---|---|---|---|---|---|---|---|
| monoclonal anti-$\delta^a$ allotype | BALB/c B-lymphocytes | $<2 \times 10^{-9}$ | | C57BL/6 B-lymphocytes | $>5 \times 10^{-9}$ | $>2.5$ | Krolick et al., 1980 |
| anti-BCL$_1$ idiotype | BCL$_1$ | $<1.4 \times 10^{-9}$ | $>2$ | BALB/c B-lymphocytes | $>5 \times 10^{-9}$ | $>4$ | Krolick et al., 1980 |
| Fab' anti-human immunoglobulin | Daudi | $2.5 \times 10^{-9}$ | | CEM | $>2 \times 10^{-7}$ | $>80$ | Raso and Griffin, 1980 |
| Fab' anti-L1210 | L1210 | $\sim 5 \times 10^{-9}$ | $>100$ | | | | Masuho and Hara, 1980 |
| anti-mouse IgG | murine B-lymphocytes | $\sim 2 \times 10^{-8}$ | | murine T-lymphocytes | $>10^{-7}$ | $>5$ | Miyazaki et al., 1980 |
| monoclonal IgM anti-Thy1.2 | WEHI-7 leukaemia | $10^{-10}$ | 5000 | BC-3A | $5 \times 10^{-7}$ | 5000 | Blythman et al., 1981 |
| monoclonal anti-rat T-lymphocyte W3/25 | rat T-lymphocytes | $>10^{-8}$ | | rat B-lymphocytes | $>10^{-8}$ | | Thorpe et al., (unpublished) |
| Gelonin | | | | | | | |
| monoclonal anti-Thy1.1 | AKR T-lymphocytes | $4 \times 10^{-10}$ to $10^{-12}$ | | AKR B-lymphocytes | $>3 \times 10^{-7}$ | $>1000$ to $300,000$ | Thorpe et al., 1981 |
| monoclonal anti-Thy1.1 | AKR-A lymphoma | 2 to $13 \times 10^{-7}$ | | | | | Thorpe et al., 1981 |
| monoclonal anti-Thy1.1 | BW5147 lymphoma | 6 to $15 \times 10^{-7}$ | | | | | Thorpe et al., 1981 |

Notes  (i) antibodies are polyclonal unless stated otherwise.

(ii) $ID_{50}$ = concentration of conjugate needed to inhibit by 50% the observed cellular function (usually protein synthesis).

(iii) "Specificity factor" compares the potency of cytotoxic action of an antibody-A-chain conjugate with that of a conjugate with normal immunoglobulin upon cells bearing the appropriate antigens.

(iv) "Selectivity factor" indicates the extent to which an antibody-A-chain conjugate can exert selective cytotoxic effects upon an antigen-bearing as opposed to an antigen-lacking cell type.

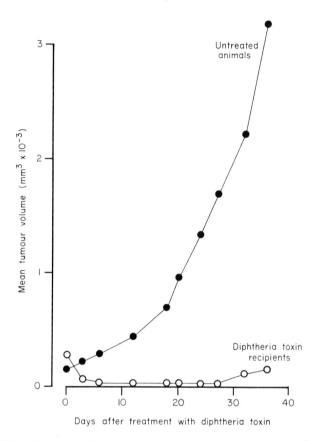

FIG. 7·7 The anti-tumour effect of a single intravenous injection of 1 μg of diphtheria toxin (o) into immunologically-deprived CBA mice bearing xenografts of the human colonic carcinoma, LOVO. Thirty six days after their treatment with the toxin 2/7 mice had palpable tumours.

Another is that ricin A-chain and gelonin have mannose and N-acetyl glucosamine-containing side chains which potentially could be recognized by specific receptors for these sugars on sinusoidal cells in the liver and elsewhere in the reticuloendothelial system (reviewed by Neufeld and Ashwell, 1980) leading to the rapid removal of the conjugates from free circulation.

In the clinical situation there are sure to be other problems. Neutralizing antibodies against the toxin moiety, or the antibody, if xenogeneic, or its idiotype, if syngeneic, are likely to develop but this could be countered either by the implementation of immunosuppressive regimens or by switching monoclonal antibodies or toxins. Antigen-shedding by certain types of tumour cells may neutralize the antigen-recognition properties of the conjugate before it reaches the target. This may not be as problematical as often assumed since radiolabelled antibodies to carcinoembryonic antigen clearly do localize upon human colonic carcinomas in man and animals even in the presence of secreted soluble antigen.

Let us take encouragement from the experiment described in Fig. 7· 7. A single injection of l$\mu$g of diphtheria toxin was sufficient to cause marked or complete regression of large human colonic carcinomas in immunologically-deprived mice. Similar results have been reported by Reid *et al.* (1978) for several other human tumour xenografts. These demonstrate that the toxin, at least in non-conjugated form, is able to permeate solid tumour masses and, most probably through the recognition of specific receptors on the human cells which are lacking in the mouse, binds selectively to and kills the tumour.

It is this result that we seek to mimic using antibody molecules to confer upon a toxin (or toxin fragment) selectivity of binding to designated target cells.

ACKNOWLEDGEMENT

We thank Marjorie Butt for her time and care in typing the manuscript.

REFERENCES

Baenziger, J. U. and Fiete, D. (1979). *J. biol. Chem.* **254**, 9795–9799.
Barbieri, L., Zamboni, M., Montanaro, L., Sperti, S. and Stirpe, F. (1980a). *Biochem. J.* **185**, 203–210.
Barbieri, L., Zamboni, M., Lorenzoni, E., Montanaro, L., Sperti, S. and Stirpe, F. (1980b). *Biochem. J.* **186**, 443–452.
Blythman, H. E., Casellas, P., Gros, O., Gros, P., Jansen, F. K., Paolucci, F., Pau, B. and Vidal, H. (1981). *Nature* **290**, 145–146.
Boquet, P. and Pappenheimer, A. M. (1976). *J. biol. Chem.* **251**, 5770–5778.
Carlsson, J., Drevin, D. and Axen, R. (1978). *Biochem. J.* **173**, 727–737.
Cawley, D. B., Simpson, D. L. and Herschman, H. R. (1980a). *Fed. Proc.* **1015**, 1798.
Cawley, D. B., Herschman, H. R., Gilliland, D. G. and Collier, R. J. (1980b). *Cell* **22**, 563–570.
Chang, T. and Neville, D. M., Jr. (1978). *J. biol. Chem.* **253**, 6866–6871.
Chang, T., Dazord, A. and Neville, D. M. (1977). *J. biol. Chem.* **252**, 1515–1522.

Collier, R. J. (1977). *In* "Receptors and Recognition, Series B,: The Specificity and action of animal, bacterial and plant toxins" (P. Cuatrecasas, Ed.), pp. 67–98. Chapman and Hall, London.

Deng, C., Terasaki, P. I., El-Awar, N., Billing, R., Cicciarelli, J. and Lagasse, L. (1981). *Lancet* i, 403–405.

Dippold, W. G., Lloyd, K. O., Li, L.T.C., Ikeda, H., Oettgen, H. F. and Old, L. J. (1980). *Proc. natn. Acad. Sci. U.S.A.* **77**, 6114–6118.

Draper, R. K. and Simon, M. I. (1980). *J. Cell Biol.* **87**, 849–854.

Draper, R. K., Chin, D., and Simon, M. I. (1978). *Proc. natn. Acad. Sci. U.S.A.* **75**, 261–265.

Drazin, R., Kandel, J. and Collier, R. J. (1971). *J. biol. Chem.* **246**, 1504–1510.

Duncan, J. L. and Groman, N. B. (1969). *J. Bacteriol.* **98**, 963–969.

Edwards, D. C., Smith, A., Ross, W. C. J., Cumber, A. J., Thorpe, P. E. and Davies, A. J. S. (1981). *Experientia* **37**, 256–257.

Edwards, D. C., Brown, A., Cumber, A. J., Smith, A., Ross, W. C. J., Thorpe, P. E. and Davies, A. J. S. (1982a). *Biochem. Biophys. Acta* (in press).

Edwards, D. C., Ross, W. C. J., Cumber, A. J., Smith, A., Thorpe, P. E., Brown, A., Williams, R. H. and Davies, A. J. S. (1982b). (submitted for publication.)

Ehrlich, P. (1913). "Chemotherapy", Proc. 17th Int. Congr. Med. (1913) 1914. *In* "The Collected Papers of Paul Ehrlich" (1960) (F. Himmelweit, Ed.) Vol. III, p. 510. Pergamon Press, Oxford.

Eiklid, K., Olsnes, S. and Pihl, A. (1980). *Expl. Cell Res.* **126**, 321–326.

Eisenbarth, G. S., Walsh, F. S. and Nirenberg, M. (1979). *Proc. natn. Acad. Sci. U.S.A.* **76**, 4913–4917.

Gasperi-Campani, A., Barbieri, L., Lorenzoni, E., Montanaro, L., Sperti, S., Bonetti, E. and Stirpe, F. (1978). *Biochem. J.* **174**, 491–496.

Ghose, T. and Blair, A. H. (1978). *J. natn. Cancer Inst.* **61**, 657–676.

Gill, D. M. (1978). *In* "Bacterial Toxins and Cell Membranes" (J. Jeljaszewicz and T. Wadstrom, Eds), pp. 291–332. Academic Press, London and New York.

Gill, D. M. and Dinius, L. L. (1971). *J. biol. Chem.* **246**, 1485–1491.

Gill, D. M., Uchida, T. and Singer, R. A. (1972). *Virology* **50**, 664–668.

Gilliland, D. G. and Collier, R. J. (1980). *Cancer Res.* **40**, 3564–3569.

Gilliland, D. G., Collier, R. J., Moehring, J. M. and Moehring, T. J. (1978). *Proc. natn. Acad. Sci. U.S.A.* **75**, 5319–5323.

Gilliland, D. G., Steplewski, Z., Collier, R. J., Mitchell, K. F., Chang, T. H. and Koprowski, H. (1980). *Proc. natn. Acad. Sci. U.S.A.* **77**, 4539–4543.

Herlyn, M., Steplewski, Z., Herlyn, D. and Koprowski, H. (1979). *Proc. natn. Acad. Sci. U.S.A.* **76**, 1438–1442.

Herlyn, M., Clark, W. H., Mastrangelo, M. J. Guerry, D., Elder, D. E., La Rossa, D., Hamilton, R., Bondi, E., Tuthill, R., Steplewski, Z. and Koprowski, H. (1980). *Cancer Res.* **40**, 3602–3609.

Houston, L. L., Nowinski, R. C. and Bernstein, I. D. (1980). *J. Immunol.* **125**, 837–843.

Irvin, J. D. (1975). *Arch. Biochem. Biophys.* **169**, 522–528.

Jansen, F. K., Blythman, H. E., Carriere, D., Casellas, P., Diaz, J., Gros, P., Hennequin, J. R., Paolucci, F., Pau, B., Poucelet, P., Richer, G., Salhi, S. L., Vidal, H. and Voisin, G. A. (1980). *Immunol. Letters* **2**, 97–102.

Kandel, J., Collier, R. J. and Chung, D. W. (1974). *J. biol. Chem.* **249**, 2088–2097.

Kemshead, J. T., Walsh, F., Pritchard, J. and Greaves, M. (1981). *Int. J. Cancer* **27**, 447–452.

Kim, K. and Groman, N. B. (1965). *J. Bacteriol.* **90**, 1552–1556.

Koprowski, H., Steplewski, Z., Herlyn, D. and Herlyn, M. (1978). *Proc. natn. Acad. Sci. U.S.A.* **75**, 3405–3409.

Krolick, K. A., Villemez, C., Isakson, P., Uhr, J. W. and Vitetta, E. S. (1980). *Proc. natn. Acad. Sci. U.S.A.* **77**, 5419–5423.

Lambotte, P., Falmagne, P., Capiau, C., Zanen, J., Ruysschaert, J. and Dirkx, J. (1980). *J. Cell Biol.* **87**, 837–840.

McMichael, A. J., Pilch, J. R., Galfre, G., Mason, D. Y., Fabre, J. W. and Milstein, C. (1979). *Eur. J. Immunol.* **9**, 205–210.

Mach, J. P., Carrel, S., Merenda, C., Sordat, B. and Cerrotini, J. C. (1974). *Nature* **248**, 704–706.

Mach, J. P., Carrel, S., Forni, M., Ritschard, J., Donath, A. and Alberto, P. (1980). *New Engl. J. Med.* **303**, 5–10.

Mason, D. W. (1981). Transplantation, (in press).

Masuho, Y. and Hara, T. (1980). *Gann* **71**, 759–765.

Masuho, Y., Hara, T. and Teruhisa, N. (1979). *Biochem. biophys. Res. Commun.* **90**, 320–326.

Miskimins, W. K. and Shimizu, N. (1979). *Biochem. biophys. Res. Commun.* **91**, 143–151.

Miyazaki, H., Beppu, M., Terao, T. and Osawa, T. (1980). *Gann* **71**, 766–774.

Moehring, T. J. and Moehring, J. M. (1972). *Infect. Immunol.* **6**, 487–492.

Moehring, T. J. and Moehring, J. M. (1977). *Cell* **11**, 447–454.

Montanaro, L., Sperti, S., Mattioli, A., Testoni, G. and Stirpe, F. (1975). *Biochem. J.* **146**, 127–131.

Moolten, F. L. and Cooperband, S. R. (1970). *Science* **169**, 68–70.

Moolten, F. L., Capparell, N. J. and Cooperband, S. R. (1972). *J. natn. Cancer Inst.* **49**, 1057–1062.

Moolten, F. L., Capparell, N. J., Zajdel, S. H. and Cooperband, S. R. (1975a). *J. natn. Cancer Inst.* **55**, 473–477.

Moolten, F. L., Capparell, N. J. and Zajdel, S. H. (1975b). *J. natn. Cancer Inst.* **55**, 709–712.

Moolten, F. L., Zajdel, S. and Cooperband, S. (1976). *Ann. N. Y. Acad. Sci.* **277**, 690–699.

Moshakis, V., Bailey, M. J., Ormerod, M. G., Westwood, J. H. and Neville, A. M. (1981). *Br. J. Cancer* **43**, 575–581.

Murphy, J. R., Pappenheimer, A. M, Jr. and de Borms, S. T. (1974). *Proc. natn. Acad. Sci. U.S.A.* **71**, 11–15.

Nadler, L. M., Stashenko, P., Hardy, R., Kaplan, W. D., Button, L. N., Kufe,

D. W., Antmann, K. H. and Schlossman, S. F. (1980). *Cancer Res.* **40**, 3147–3154.

Neufeld, E. F. and Ashwell, G. (1980). *In* "The Biochemistry of Glycoproteins and Proteoglycans" (W. J. Lennarz, Ed.), pp. 241–266. Plenum Publishing Corporation.

Nolan, R. D., Grasmuk, H. and Drews, J. (1976). *Eur. J. Biochem.* **64**, 69–75.

Obrig, T. G., Irvin, J. D. and Hardesty, B. (1973). *Arch. Biochem. Biophys.* **155**, 278–289.

Oeltmann, T. N. and Heath, E. C. (1979). *J. biol. Chem.* **254**, 1028–1032.

Ohkuma, S. and Poole, B. (1978). *Proc. natn. Acad. Sci. U.S.A.* **75**, 3327–3331.

Olsnes, S. (1978). *In* "Transport of Macromolecules in Cellular Systems" (S. C. Silverstein, Ed.), pp. 103–116. Dahlem Konferenzen. Abakon Verlagsgesellschaft, Berlin.

Olsnes, S. and Pihl, A. (1977). *In* "Receptors and Recognition, Series B: The specificity and action of animal, bacterial and plant toxins" (P. Cuatrecasas, Ed.), pp. 131–173. Chapman and Hall, London.

Olsnes, S. and Pihl, A. (1982a). "Chimaeric Toxins". *In* "Pharmacology of Bacterial Toxins" (J. Drew and F. Dorner, Eds), Pergamon Press. (in press).

Olsnes, S. and Pihl, A. (1982b). *In* "The Molecular Actions of Toxins and Viruses" (S. van Heyningen and P. Cohen, Eds). Elsevier/North Holland, Amsterdam. (in press).

Olsnes, S., Refsnes, K. and Pihl, A. (1974a). *Nature* **249**, 627–631.

Olsnes, S., Saltvedt, E. and Pihl, A. (1974b). *J. Biol. Chem.* **249**, 803–810.

Olsnes, S., Fernandex-Puentes, C., Carrasco, L. and Vazquez, D. (1975). *Eur. J. Biochem.* **54**, 499–503.

Olsnes, S., Sandvig, K., Refsnes, K. and Pihl, A. (1976). *J. biol. Chem.* **257**, 3985–3992.

O'Neill, G. J. (1979). "The Use of Antibodies as Drug Carriers" *In* "Drug Carriers in Biology and Medicine" (G. Gregoriadis, Ed.). Academic Press, London.

Pappenheimer, A. M. (1977). *Ann. Rev. Biochem.* **46**, 69–94.

Pappenheimer, A. M. (1979). *Microbiology* 1979, 187–192.

Pau, B., Blythman, H., Casellas, P., Gros, O., Gros, P., Paolucci, F., Jansen, F. K., Vidal, H. and Voisin, G. A. (1980). *In* "Protides of the Biological Fluids" Colloquium 28, Brussels. Pergamon Press, Oxford.

Philpott, G. W., Bower, R. J. and Parker, C. W. (1973). Surgery **73**, 928–935.

Proia, R. L., Hart, D. A., Holmes, R. K., Holmes, K. V. and Eidels, L. (1979). *Proc. natn. Acad. Sci. U.S.A.* **76**, 685–689.

Raso, V. and Griffin, T. (1979). *Proc. Am. Ass. Cancer Res.* **20**, 207.

Raso, V. and Griffin, T. (1980). *J. Immunol.* **125**, 2610–2616.

Refsnes, K. and Munthe-Kaas, A. C. (1976). *J. exp. Med.* **143**, 1464–1474.

Reid, L. M., Colburn, P., Sato, G. and Kaplan, N. O. (1978). *In* "Proceedings of the Symposium on the Use of Athymic (Nude) Mice in Cancer Research" (D. P. Houchens and A. A. Ovejara, Eds), pp. 123–131. Gustav Fischer, New York.

Reif, A. E. (1971). *Cancer* **27**, 1433–1439.
Reinherz, E. L. and Schlossman, S. F. (1980). *Cell* **19**, 821–827.
Ritz, J., Pesando, J. M., Notis-McConarty, J., Lazarus, H. and Schlossman, S. F. (1980). *Nature* **283**, 583–585.
Roberts, K. and Stewart, T. S. (1979). *Biochemistry* **18**, 2615–2621.
Ross, W. C. J., Thorpe, P. E., Cumber, A. J., Edwards, D. C., Hinson C. A. and Davies, A. J. S. (1980). *Eur. J. Biochem.* **104**, 381–390.
Samagh, B. S. and Gregory, K. F. (1972). *Biochim. Biophys. Acta.* **273**, 188–198.
Sandvig, K. and Olsnes, S. (1979). *Expl. Cell. Res.* **121**, 15–25.
Sandvig, K. and Olsnes, S. (1980). *J. Cell Biol.* **87**, 828–832.
Sandvig, K., Olsnes, S. and Pihl, A. (1976). *J. biol. Chem.* **251**, 3977–3984.
Simeral, L. S., Kapmeyer, W., MacConnell, W. P. and Kaplan, N. O. (1980). *J. biol. Chem.* **255**, 11098–11101.
Smithers, S. R. (1976). *In* "Immunology of Parasitic Infections" (S. Cohen and E. Sadun, Eds), pp. 296–332. Blackwell Scientific Publications, U.K.
Stewart, T. S., Hruby, D. E., Sharma, O. K. and Roberts, W. K. (1977). *Biochim. Biophys. Acta* **479**, 31–38.
Stirpe, F., Pession-Brizzi, A., Lorenzoni, E., Strocchi, P., Montanaro, L. and Sperti, S. (1976). *Biochem. J.* **156**, 1–6.
Stirpe, F., Olsnes, S. and Pihl, A. (1980). *J. biol. Chem.* **255**, 6947–6953.
Stirpe, F., Williams, D. G., Onyon, L. J., Legg, R. F. and Stevens, W. A. (1981). *Biochem. J.* **195**, 399–405.
Thorpe, P. E., Ross, W. C. J., Cumber, A. J., Hinson, C. A., Edwards, D. C. and Davies, A. J. S. (1978). *Nature* **271**, 752–755.
Thorpe, P. E., Cumber, A. J., Williams, N., Edwards, D. C., Ross, W. C. J. and Davies, A. J. S. (1981a). *Clin. exp. Immunol.* **43**, 195–200.
Thorpe, P. E., Brown, A. N. F., Ross, W. C. J., Cumber, A. J., Detre, S. I., Edwards, D. C., Davies, A. J. S. and Stirpe, F. (1981b). *Eur. J. Biochem.* **116**, 447–454.
Uchida, T., Yamaizumi, M., Mekada, E., Okada, Y., Tsuda, M., Kurokawa, T. and Sugino, Y. (1978a). *J. biol. Chem.* **253**, 6307–6310.
Uchida, T., Yamaizumi, M. and Okada, Y. (1978b). *Biochem. biophys. Res. Commun.* **81**, 268–273.
Uchida, T., Mekada, E. and Okada, Y. (1980). *J. biol. Chem.* **255**, 6687–6693.
Van Ness, B. G., Howard, J. B. and Bodley, J. W. (1980). *J. biol. Chem.* **255**, 10710–10716.
Venter, B. R. and Kaplan, N. O. (1976). *Cancer Res.* **36**, 4590–4594.
Yamaizumi, M., Mekada, E., Uchida, T. and Okada, Y. (1978). *Cell* **15**, 245–250.
Yamaguchi, T., Kato, R., Beppu, M., Tarao, T., Inoue, Y., Ikawa, Y. and Osawa, T. (1979). *J. natn. Cancer Inst.* **62**, 1387–1395.
Youle, R. J. and Neville, D. M. (1980). *Proc. natn. Acad. Sci. U.S.A.* **77**, 5483–5486.
Youle, R. J., Murray, G. J. and Neville, D. M. (1979). *Proc. natn. Acad. Sci. U.S.A.* **76**, 5559–5562.

# D  HAEMATOLOGY

# 8 Studies with Monoclonal Antibodies on Normal and Diseased Platelets

Gerard Tobelem, Changgeng Ruan,
Andrew McMichael,[a] Nelly Kieffer and
J. P. Caen

*Unite 150 INSERM, Department of Haemostasis and
Thrombosis, Hopital Saint Louis, 2 Place du
Dr. A. Fournier, 75475 Paris Cedex 10, France*
[a] *The Nuffield Department of Medicine, John Radcliffe Hospital,
Headington, Oxford. OX3 9DU*

# I INTRODUCTION

The interactions between platelets and the blood vessel wall are of importance in the maintenance of a balance between haemorrhage and thrombosis.

Exposure of normal platelets to vascular subendothelial structures results, within a matter of seconds, in the formation of a haemostatic plug. The sequence of reactions leading to this includes the following: adhesion of platelets to the exposed connective tissue; prostaglandin metabolism; contraction of the platelet actomyosin fibrils and platelet secretion; aggregation; participation in the coagulation mechanism; and finally, clot retraction. Platelets have a complex machinery to subserve these many functions, with the cell membrane playing a key role. It is within the platelet membrane that messages are received and platelet functions initiated.

The plasma membrane of platelets, with its outer carbohydrate rich coat or glycocalyx, contains specific glycoproteins which are essential for both adhesion and aggregation. This cell surface also carries receptor sites and transducing mechanisms for a range of stimulating agents.

In this chapter we shall describe our approach to the elucidation of the basic pathways responsible for the different aspects of platelet function. The first stage was to investigate the nature of the inherited molecular defects which cause specific abnormalities of platelet function. A similar approach was largely responsible for uncovering the molecular basis of blood coagulation. The genetic abnormalities of platelet function comprise a complex family of hereditary disorders, of which two form the basis of this discussion. In the Bernard Soulier syndrome there is a defective mechanism of platelet adhesion and in Glanzmann's thrombasthenia there is impaired platelet aggregation. We describe the specific biochemical abnormalities found in the platelets in each of these syndromes and the abnormalities in platelet function found in von Willebrand disease. The second stage of the investigation was to study the effect on platelet function of alloantibodies to components of platelet membrane, generated by patients when treated with, and immunized by, normal platelets. The third stage is the confirmatory and additional information being gained by using monoclonal antibodies specific for platelet antigens such as those missing in Bernard Soulier disease, Glanzmann's thrombasthenia and for von Willebrand factor.

# II FACTORS PLAYING A ROLE IN THE PLATELET-VESSEL WALL INTERACTIONS

The review of these factors is not intended to be exhaustive and because our orientation is directed towards the role of membranes in platelet function, only the interactions between platelet membrane, vascular subendothelium and von Willebrand factor are considered.

## A. The Vessel Wall

The intimal part of the vessel wall consists of a vascular endothelium and subendothelium.

### 1. THE VASCULAR ENDOTHELIUM

The vascular endothelium is made of a single layer of flattened, polygonal and elongated cells. An important feature of intact normal vascular endothelium is that it does not promote platelet adherence or activate the coagulation system (Thorgeirsson and Robertson, 1978). Although this nonthrombogenic property of the vascular endothelium has been known for a long time, its nature is still poorly understood. The discovery of prostacyclin ($PGI_2$) has permitted a reappraisal of endothelial and platelet physiology (Moncada *et al.*, 1976). $PGI_2$, an unstable prostaglandin synthesized mainly by endothelial cells, is the most potent known inhibitor of platelet aggregation *in vitro* and prevents thrombus formation *in vivo*. Continuous synthesis of $PGI_2$ by endothelial cells could explain their nonthrombogenic property (Moncada *et al.*, 1978).

### 2. THE VASCULAR SUBENDOTHELIUM

The subendothelium is made of several macromolecular components: collagen, basement membrane, microfibrils, fibronectin and elastin (Stemerman, 1974). The most important functional property of the subendothelium is that it is thrombogenic.

The interaction between human blood platelets and subendothelium has been extensively evaluated by Baumgartner and Muggli (1976) in an experimental model that involved deendothelialization of rabbit aorta. The subendothelium promotes platelet adherence and platelet aggregation resulting in platelet thrombi formation *in vitro*. The factors involved in this thrombogenesis include subendothelial components, platelets and other blood cells, plasma factors, particularly von Willebrand factor, and blood flow. The exact nature of the macro-molecule(s) responsible for the adhesion of platelets is still under investigation.

Collagen type I can induce platelet adhesion and aggregation *in vitro* (Fauvel *et al.*, 1978) but as this type of collagen is mainly localized beyond the internal elastic lamina, it is not accessible to the platelets *in vivo*. Collagen type III which is localized in the subendothelium, could be responsible for platelet adhesion *in vivo*. Purified collagen type III induces adhesion and aggregation of platelets (Legrand *et al.*, 1978; Fauvel and Legrand, 1980). This property seems to be mediated by a small part of the molecule, possibly a sequence of nine amino acids (Legrand *et al.*, 1980). Collagenase resistant arterial microfibrils are also able to interact with platelets (Stemerman *et al.*, 1971) and there-fore could respresent a second thrombogenic structure in the vessel wall (Caen and Levy-Toledano, 1973a). This has recently been confirmed with microfibrils purified from human placenta, which could induce adhesion-aggregation of human platelets *in vitro* (Legrand *et al.*, 1980).

## B. THE PLATELET MEMBRANE

The platelet membrane contains lipids and proteins (Barber and Jamieson, 1980). Carbohydrate is distributed among the glycoproteins and glycolipids. A number of proteins have been identified by gel electrophoresis of solubilized platelet membranes (Phillips and Agin, 1977a). Three major groups of glycoproteins were identified initially and termed glycoproteins I, II and III with molecular weights of, around 150,000, 130,000 and 100,000 respectively (Phillips, 1972). More sophisticated techniques have since shown that there are several individual glycoproteins within each of these groups (Phillips and Agin, 1977b; Nurden and Caen, 1978; Clemetson *et al.*, 1979). Specific func-tions have been assigned to some of these glycoproteins (Nurden and Caen, 1979) and are described below.

### 1. PLATELET MEMBRANE GLYCOPROTEIN I

The glycoprotein I complex consists of at least two different glycopro-tein components, glycoprotein Ia and glycoprotein Ib (Phillips and Agin, 1977b). The latter has a molecular weight of approximately 150,000 (Nurden and Caen, 1979). It consists of 60% carbohydrate and readily stains with Periodic Acid Schiff reagent (PAS) although it is only weakly iodinated by lactoperoxidase (Okumura and Jamieson, 1976). Glycoprotein Ib, which is very rich in sialic acid (Nurden and Caen, 1975), seems to be amphiphillic and is located in the membrane. Another form of glycoprotein I seems to be hydrophilic and is located, in part, in the glycocalyx; this form has been called glycocalicin or glycoprotein Is. When normal platelets are solubilized in the absence of EDTA, glycocalicin can be readily identified by polyacrylamide gel electrophoresis, probably because it is released from the glycoprotein I complex by a platelet calcium dependant protease. The glycoprotein I complex is very susceptible to digestion by chymotrypsin and trypsin, which release a macroglycopeptide with a molecular weight of 120,000 (Okumura and Jamieson, 1976).

Nurden and Caen (1975) were the first to propose that glycoprotein I could play an essential role in adhesion of platelets to subendothelium and aggregation induced *in vitro* by the antibiotic ristocetin. The glycoprotein I complex also seems to be involved in the binding of factor VIII/Willebrand factor (Ruan *et al.*, 1981a), as a receptor for quinidine or quinine dependant antibodies (Kunicki *et al.*, 1978), as a binding site for thrombin (Okumura and Jamieson, 1976) and as a receptor for the Fc fragment of immunoglobulins (Moore *et al.*, 1978).Some of these functions of glycoprotein I will be discussed later in this chapter.

## 2. PLATELET MEMBRANE GLYCOPROTEIN COMPLEX IIb/IIIa

The glycoprotein II complex contains at least three different glycoproteins, IIa, IIb and IIc. Glycoprotein IIb stains most readily with PAS; its apparent molecular weight in SDS polyacrylamide gel electrophoresis is approximately 135,000 daltons. Its isoelectric point is 4·8 to 5·1.

Glycoprotein III contains at least two different glycoproteins, IIIa and IIIb. Glycoprotein IIIa stains strongest with PAS; its apparent molecular weight is approximately 116,000. Its isoelectric point is 5·0 to 5·3.

Using a cross immuno electrophoresis technique with rabbit anti human platelet antiserum, platelet proteins and glycoproteins can be precisely identified (Fig. 8·1). The most pronounced precipitin line, band 16, corresponds to the complex glycoprotein IIb/IIIa. SDS polyacrylamide gel electrophoresis of this band reveals the two components and this result suggests that they are closely associated (Hagen *et al.*, 1980).

Nurden and Caen (1975) were the first to postulate that glycoprotein

(a)                          (b)

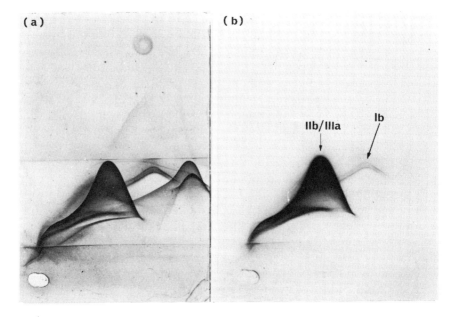

FIG. 8·1. Autoradiography of platelet proteins and Glycoproteins by cross immunoelectrophoresis. Control platelets have been iodinated by $^{125}$I with lactoperoxy-
dase and solubilized in Triton X100. Electrophoresis in the first dimension is performed
in 1% agarose gel in presence of triton X100. Immunoelectrophoresis in the second
dimension is performed in 1% agarose gel in presence of Triton X100 and rabbit anti
human platelet immunoglobulins. Immunoplate (a) is stained with coomassie blue.
Immunoplate (b) is an autoradiograph.

IIb/IIIa could play a role in platelet aggregation. A platelet alloantigen, PLA¹, seems to be associated with this glycoprotein complex
(Kunicki and Aster, 1979). Recently, it has been suggested that
glycoprotein IIb/IIIa could be a binding site for fibrinogen (Marguerie
*et al.*, 1979).

## C. VON WILLEBRAND FACTOR (MEYER, 1980)

Factor VIII/von Willebrand factor (FVIII/WF) is a high molecular
weight glycoprotein complex which is characterized by two biological
functions: procoagulant activity, called VIII coagulant activity or VIII
C; and ristocetin cofactor activity which is necessary for the aggregation
of normal platelets in the presence of the antibiotic and is called VIII R
CO.

FVIII/WF is also defined by two specific antigenic determinants: human anti VIII C antibodies identify an antigenic determinant called VIII CAg; heterologous (rabbit) anti FVIII/WF antisera identify an antigenic epitope called VIII RAg.

The relationship between these entities is still the subject of controversy. There is much evidence suggesting that they are associated as a complex of at least two molecules; factor VIII which includes VIII C and VIII CAg and von Willebrand factor which comprises VIII RCO and VIII RAg. There are several ways of separating factor VIII from von Willebrand factor.

Evidence has recently been obtained that factor VIII/WF in plasma is not a homogeneous entity but consists of a continuous series of molecular forms covering a wide range of molecular weight. This was demonstrated by SDS Agarose electrophoresis and the most recent structural model is compatible with a series of polymers in which the basic unit is a dimer of 230,000 molecular weight subunits.

Until recently, little was known about the synthesis and linkage of the various components of FVIII/WF. Von Willebrand factor seems to be synthesized by megakaryocytes and endothelial cells, under the control of autosomal genes. This protein contains ristocetin cofactor activity and VIII related antigen (VIII RAg) but no VIII coagulant activity (VIII C) or VIII coagulant activity (VIII CAg). Factor VIII seems to be under the control of X linked genes and contains VIII C and VIII CAg; the site of its synthesis is not known.

Abnormalities of FVIII/WF are found in inherited bleeding disorders. In haemophilia A, there is a decreased level or absence of Factor VIII which results in abnormal plasma coagulation. In von Willebrand disease there is a partial or complete deficiency in von Willebrand factor and defective adhesion of platelets to subendothelium.

## III PLATELET ADHESION

Platelet adhesion is the initial event in the platelet-vessel wall interactions that lead up to thrombus formation. Our current view of this important step has been obtained from studies of congenital platelet disorders and with both human and monoclonal antibodies to platelet membrane proteins.

## A. THE PLATELET MEMBRANE GLYCOPROTEIN I AND PLATELET ADHESION

### 1. THE BERNARD SOULIER SYNDROME

(a) *Defect in platelet adhesion*

The Bernard Soulier syndrome which is inherited as an autosomal recessive trait, is characterized by a severe muco-cutaneous bleeding tendency, a prolonged bleeding time and morphologically enlarged platelets on blood smears (Bernard and Soulier, 1948). The long bleeding time, in the face of a normal or slightly decreased platelet count, has only recently been explained; the giant Bernard Soulier platelets show defective adhesion to rabbit aorta subendothelium (Weiss *et al.*, 1974) (Table 8·1). Adhesion of Bernard Soulier platelets to human vascular subendothelium has not been measured, but it seems probable that the same defect will be found.

Purified human collagen, type I and type III, has been tested *in vitro* for its capacity to induce adhesion-aggregation of Bernard Soulier platelets (Caen *et al.*, 1976; Tobelem *et al.*, unpublished results). Their reactivity with both collagen type I and type III was normal. This fact does not support the view that collagen has a potent role in the thrombogenic property of subendothelium. Other purified components of human subendothelium have not yet been tested with Bernard Soulier platelets.

(b) *Defect in platelet membrane glycoprotein I*

In 1969 Gröttum and Solum found that the platelets in Bernard Soulier syndrome were deficient in sialic acid. Nurden and Caen (1975) demonstrated a defect in platelet membrane glycoprotein I by SDS

TABLE 8·1

| | | Area (%) of subendothelium[a] | |
| | Naked | Adherent platelets | Thrombi |
|---|---|---|---|
| Healthy controls (7) | 53·2 ± 13·1 | 45·9 ± 13·9 | 0·9 ± 1·1 |
| BSS1 | 92·0 ± 3·7 | 6·1 ± 3·5 | 1·8 ± 1·0 |
| BSS2 | 98·6 ± 0·4 | 1·3 ± 0·5 | 0·1 ± 0·1 |

[a]  Rabbit aorta subendothelium was exposed to platelets from either normal platelets (× 7) or BSS (2 patients) platelets according to the technique described by Baumgartner and Muggli (1976). Results are expressed as a percentage of the total surface of exposed subendothelium.

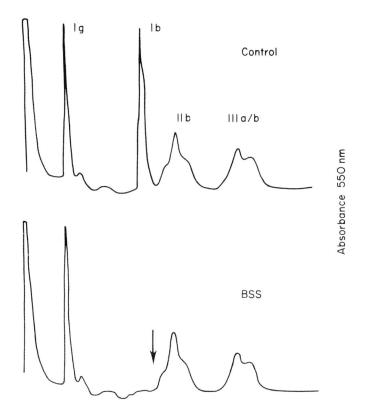

FIG. 8·2. SDS polyacrylamide gel electrophoresis of platelets. Platelets from control or from Bernard Soulier patients (BSS) have been solubilized in SDS at 100°C in presence of N-ethyl Maleimide. Polyacrylamide gel electrophoresis has been performed with SDS in unreduced condition. Major glycoproteins are stained with PAS. Glycoprotein Ib is absent in BSS platelet.

polyacrylamide gel electrophoresis of membrane from Bernard Soulier platelets (Fig. 8·2). This abnormality has been confirmed by other techniques (Nurden *et al.*, 1981). Cross immunelectrophoresis with rabbit anti human platelet antiserum showed that Bernard Soulier platelets were deficient in one specific precipitin line, band 13, which corresponds to glycoprotein Ib (Hagen *et al.*, 1980). The deficiency in glycoprotein Ib is therefore well established.

    The decreased adhesion to subendothelium and the defect in platelet membrane glycoprotein I in Bernard Soulier platelets are probably related (Caen *et al.*, 1976), indicating that glycoprotein I could be specifically implicated in adhesion.

(c) *Other abnormalities in Bernard Soulier platelets*

Bernard Soulier platelets have a reduced survival time in the circulation (Caen *et al.*, 1973b) which has been related to the sialic acid deficiency. Decreased binding of factor XI to Bernard Soulier platelets has been reported (Walsh *et al.*, 1975), possibly explaining the abnormal prothrombin consumption originally described by Bernard and Soulier (1948).

Kunicki *et al.* (1978) found that Bernard Soulier platelets were not lysed by drug dependent antibodies in the presence of the corresponding drugs, suggesting that Bernard Soulier platelets were deficient in a drug dependant antibody receptor.

Zucker *et al.* (1977) reported that Bernard Soulier platelets seemed unable to bind plasma Factor VIII/von Willebrand factor. This was confirmed in a direct binding assay using $I^{125}$-factor VIII/von Willebrand factor (Moake *et al.*, 1980), when the platelets of three Bernard Soulier patients bound less than 20% of factor compared to controls. In a study of five different Bernard Soulier patients, we have recently demonstrated that the binding was decreased (Table 8·2); the mean value for the five patients was 39·4% of the control (Ruan *et al.*, 1981b).

Freeze fracture studies of the plasma membrane of Bernard Soulier platelets showed abnormalities of the particles, suggesting that glycoprotein Ib could play a role in their formation (Chevalier *et al.*, 1979).

A comparison between the shape of control and Bernard Soulier platelets suggested that the giant size of Bernard Soulier platelets results from abnormal behaviour during preparation of the blood smear. This abnormality is also likely to be secondary to the glycoprotein Ib defect (Frojmovic *et al.*, 1978).

2. ROLE OF PLATELET MEMBRANE GLYCOPROTEIN I

(a) *Role in adhesion*

Since Bernard Soulier platelets have a decreased adhesion to subendothelium and since they are deficient in platelet membrane glycoprotein Ib, it has been postulated that glycoprotein Ib could be a specific membrane site responsible for the adhesion mechanism (Nurden and Caen, 1975). However, direct evidence for such a function for glycoprotein Ib still does not exist.

The antibiotic ristocetin aggregates normal, but not Bernard Soulier, platelets *in vitro* (Caen and Levy-Toledano, 1973a). Ristocetin-induced

TABLE 8·2
Binding of $^{125}$I-factor VIII/Willebrand factor to control or
Bernard Soulier platelets

| | Fresh washed platelets Ristocetin 1 mg ml$^{-1}$ | Fixed platelets Ristocetin 1 mg ml$^{-1}$ | Ristocetin 0·5 mg ml$^{-1}$ |
|---|---|---|---|
| Control n = 10 | 35·1 ± 3·8 | 34·7 ± 3·2 | 30·9 ± 2·5 |
| BSS 1 | 10·2 | 13·7 | 7·2 |
| 2 | 12·3 | 13·7 | 5·8 |
| 3 | 11·8 | 14·7 | 6·9 |
| 4 | 17·9 | 14·8 | 5·0 |
| 5 | 9·2 | 11·5 | 2·9 |

For each sample to $2 \times 10^7$ platelets were added 0·5 mg of $^{125}$I-factor VIII/Willebrand factor in presence of ristocetin at a final concentration of 1 mg ml$^{-1}$ or 0·5 mg ml$^{-1}$ for 30 minutes at room temperature without stirring. Results are expressed in percentage of the $^{125}$I-factor VIII/Willebrand added.

aggregation of control platelets requires normal plasma Factor VIII/von Willebrand factor (Howard and Firkin, 1971) which binds to the platelet membrane, (Zucker et al., 1977). Ristocetin probably represents an *in vitro* counterpart of components of the subendothelium, ristocetin-induced aggregation *in vitro* corresponding to platelet adhesion to subendothelium *in vivo*. Platelet membrane glycoprotein Ib seems to be necessary for ristocetin-induced platelet aggregation. Digestion of normal platelets with chymotrypsin, which releases a macroglycopeptide from glycoprotein Ib, resulted in inhibition of ristocetin-induced aggregation. Digestion with neuraminidase did not affect ristocetin-induced aggregation suggesting that sialic acid is not involved. Neuraminidase treated platelets, however, have a reduced life span when reinjected into the circulation (Greenberg et al., 1975).

Platelet membrane glycoprotein Ib could be a receptor for plasma factor VIII/von Willebrand factor (Ruan et al., 1981a). Binding sites for factor VIII/von Willebrand factor, like glycoprotein Ib (Okumura and Jamieson, 1976), seem to be susceptible to enzymatic digestion by chymotrypsin (Green and Muller, 1978; Schneider et al., 1979). The binding of plasma factor VIII/von Willebrand factor to Bernard Soulier platelets was decreased in the presence of ristocetin (Zucker et al., 1977; Moake et al., 1980; Ruan et al., 1981b). Liposomes coated with a preparation enriched in glycoprotein Ib were agglutinated by ristocetin in the presence of factor VIII/von Willebrand factor (Sie et al., 1980).

Plasma VIII/von Willebrand factor thus seems to bind to platelet membrane glycoprotein Ib which allows ristocetin induced platelet aggregation or subendothelium induced platelet adhesion.

(b) *Other roles*

Since Bernard Soulier platelets are deficient in a drug dependant antibody receptor, it has been suggested that glycoprotein Ib could also serve this function. Using enzymatic digestion, it has been shown that the drug dependant antibody receptor could be a structural part of the glycoprotein I complex, which is resistant to protease digestion. Glycoprotein Ib, purified from Triton X100 solubilized normal platelets, by a wheatgerm agglutinin column, induced the drug dependant antibody receptor activity. However, glycocalicin, the soluble part of the glycoprotein I complex, did not contain such activity (Kunicki *et al.*, 1981a).

Moore *et al.*, (1978) suggested that a membrane component of the glycoprotein I complex either functions as a platelet Fc receptor or is closely associated with such a receptor. However, this platelet Fc receptor, unlike the major components of the glycoprotein I complex, is resistant to protease digestion (Pfueller *et al.*, 1977). The Fc receptor, therefore, may be an additional membrane component, or perhaps a part of the glycoprotein I complex which is situated more deeply in the membrane where it is protected from enzymatic digestion.

Glycocalicin appears to carry a thrombin binding site (Okumura and Jamieson, 1976) and it has recently been proposed that the glycoprotein I complex is a high affinity thrombin receptor (Ganguly and Gould, 1979); another thrombin receptor site has been identified on glycoprotein V (Phillips and Agin, 1977b). Jamieson and Okumura (1978) have claimed that Bernard Soulier platelets also have a partial defect in thrombin binding and thrombin induced aggregation, but we have not been able to confirm this last finding. Moreover, Kao *et al.* (1979) showed that human thrombin did not compete with factor VIII/von Willebrand factor for binding sites on the platelet. The role of the glycoprotein I complex in the binding of thrombin is therefore still controversial.

## B. Human Alloantibody to Glycoprotein I

### 1. IMMUNOLOGICAL STUDIES

(a) *Case history of the patient*

The Bernard Soulier patient whose clinical findings were reported in the first description of the syndrome (Bernard and Soulier, 1948) developed an anti platelet antibody following several platelet infusions for bleeding episodes (Tobelem *et al.*, 1976; Degos *et al.*, 1977). Serum samples were obtained shortly after an infusion of $5 \times 10^{11}$ platelets.

## (b)  *Agglutination and complement fixation tests*

The anti platelet antibody from the patient was shown to be an IgG. Unlike most anti platelet antibodies it did not activate the complement system. The thromboagglutination test was invariably positive, however, on 50 samples of normal human platelets, regardless of HLA, PLA[1], KOa, KOb and ABO type. The intensity of agglutination was directly related to the concentration of added antibody. No agglutination was observed with a final dilution greater than 1 in 40.

Further studies with this antibody showed that it could activate platelets by inducing ADP and serotonin release and thromboxane synthesis (Tobelem *et al.*, 1979).

## (c)  *Specificity of the antibody*

No agglutination at any dilation was observed when the antibody was added to platelet rich plasma from six different Bernard Soulier patients. Using the agglutination assay with platelet rich plasma from families of two of these patients, we were able to distinguish between the normal and heterozygous state.

After treatment of control platelets with chymotrypsin or neuraminidase, the binding of the antibody was inhibited, suggesting that both the macroglycopeptide and the carbohydrate contributed to the antigen (Fig. 8·3).

The molecular weight of the molecule bearing the antigenic determinant reacting with the patient's antibody was determined using indirect immunoprecipitation of $^{125}I$ labelled soluble platelet antigens. SDS polyacrylamide gel electrophoresis revealed a single radioactive peak which accounted for 0·5% of the total proteins precipitable by trichloroacetic acid. The molecular weight of this molecule was 150,000.

These results indicated, therefore, that the antigen recognized by this antibody was glycoprotein I. This conclusion was based on its molecular weight of 150,000, its susceptibility to chymotrypsin and neuraminidase digestion, and absence from Bernard Soulier platelets.

## 2. EFFECT ON PLATELET FUNCTIONS

### (a)  *Effect of platelet aggregation*

This antibody was a strong inhibitor of the aggregation of normal platelets which is induced by ristocetin. In contrast, aggregations triggered by ADP, human collagen type I or type III, or thrombin (human or bovine) were not inhibited by the antibody. This antibody, therefore,

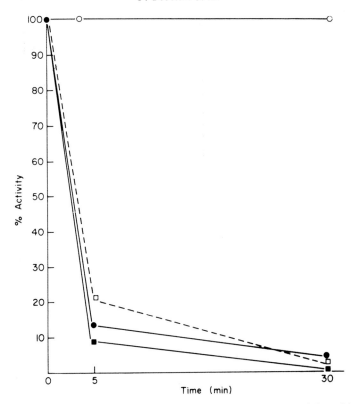

FIG. 8·3 Effect of enzymatic digestion of control platelets on reactivity with monoclonal (AN51) or human alloantibody (IgG P.) to Glycoprotein I. ●———● % of
AN51 activity after chymotrypsin. O———O % of AN51 activity after Neuraminidase.
■———■ % of IgG P. activity after chymotrypsin. □———□ % of IgG P. activity
after Neuraminidase.

confirmed that glycoprotein I is involved in ristocetin induced aggregation but not that induced by collagen or thrombin.

## (b)  *Effect on platelet adhesion*

In the presence of the antibody, the adhesion of control platelets to
rabbit aorta subendothelium was markedly decreased (Caen *et al.*,
1977). This confirmed that glycoprotein I plays an essential part in the
adhesion of platelets to subendothelium.

## (c)  *Effect on the binding of factor VIII/von Willebrand factor to platelets*

The antibody inhibited, the ristocetin induced binding of purified
human [125]I factor VIII/von Willebrand factor to formalinized washed

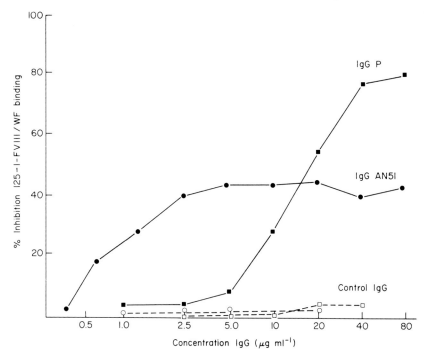

FIG. 8·4 Effect of monoclonal antibody (IgG AN51) or human alloantibody (IgG P.) to Glycoprotein I on the binding of $^{125}$I-factor VIII/ Willebrand factor to control platelets. (control IgG from human O— — —O or from mouse □— — —□ were without effect).

platelets by 80% (Fig. 8·4). The inhibition was dose dependant, and a final concentration of 80 $\mu$gml$^{-1}$ of antibody was needed to obtain maximal effect (Ruan *et al.*, 1981 in preparation).

The studies with this antibody to glycoprotein I confirmed, therefore, that a major part of factor VIII/von Willebrand factor binds to platelet glycoprotein I.

## C. MONOCLONAL ANTIBODY TO GLYCOPROTEIN I

### 1. IMMUNOLOGICAL STUDIES (McMichael *et al.*, 1981)

#### (a) *The AN51 antibody*

The hybrid myeloma clone AN51 was selected from a fusion of spleen cells from a mouse that had been immunized with human platelets and lymphocytes, with the cell P3-NS1/1Ag4·1. The cell line has remained stable for over two years. The antibody, AN51, was specific for human platelets.

## (b)  *Tissue distribution of AN51 antigen*

AN51 was shown initially to bind to platelets but not to peripheral blood mononuclear cells. Immunoperoxidase staining revealed that the antigen was evenly distributed on the surface of the platelets. Binding was also detectable on a small subpopulation of bone marrow cells which have been shown to be mature megakaryocytes (Vainchenker *et al.*, 1981 in preparation). AN51 antibody was tested, by immunofluorescence , on several human tissues and found to be negative on all. It was concluded, therefore, that the antigen recognized by AN51 is restricted in its distribution to the surface of platelets and mature megakaryocytes.

## (c)  *Specificity of AN51*

AN51 antibody bound to the platelets of over 30 normal blood donors tested, including one negative for the PLA[1] antigen. When Bernard Soulier platelets from six different patients were tested in a radiobinding assay with AN51, no binding was found. Decreased binding was observed with platelets from heterozygous relatives of Bernard Soulier syndrome patients.

Binding measurements of AN51, under saturating conditions, indicated that $1 \cdot 6 \times 10^4$ molecules of AN51 bound to each normal platelet, giving an estimate of the number of antigenic sites present.

When normal platelets were treated with chymotrypsin, the binding of AN51 was dramatically reduced, while it was not affected after neuraminidase digestion of platelets (Fig. 8·3).

When control platelets were radioiodinated by the iodosulphanilic acid method and lysed with 5% Nonidet P40, SDS polyacrylamide gel electrophoresis of the antigen precipitated by AN51 revealed a single peak of 150,000 daltons.

When Triton X100 solubilized platelets were tested by cross immunoelectrophoresis, with a rabbit anti human platelet antiserum in the upper gel and $I^{125}$-AN51 F(ab)$_2$ fragment in an intermediate gel, a single radioactive precipitin line was revealed by autoradiography. This line, band 13, corresponded to that previously identified as glycoprotein Ib. No radioactive precipitin line was observed when Bernard Soulier platelets were tested.

Thus, AN51 antibody is a monoclonal anti platelet antibody which recognizes an antigen expressed only on platelets and megakaryocytes. The antigen is missing in Bernard Soulier platelets and is susceptible to chymotrypsin digestion. The molecular weight of the antigen is 150,000. This evidence, together with the cross immunoelectrophoresis result shows that AN51 is specific for glycoprotein Ib.

While the human alloantibody to glycoprotein I appeared to recognize a sugar residue because its binding was affected by neuraminidase treatment of the platelets, AN51 binding was not affected by this treatment. AN51, therefore, probably recognizes a different epitope. Competitive binding studies between the human antiserum and AN51 confirmed this conclusion because neither reagent significantly inhibited binding of the other.

## 2. EFFECT ON PLATELET FUNCTIONS (Ruan *et al.*,1981)

### (a) *Effect on platelet aggregation*

AN51 induced *in vitro* a Bernard Soulier like defect in normal platelet function. ADP, thrombin and arachidonic acid induced aggregations were not modified by the presence of the antibody. Aggregations induced by collagens type I or type III, were slightly modified at the highest concentrations of AN51. Ristocetin and bovine factor VIII induced aggregations were strongly inhibited (Table 8·3).

The adhesion-aggregation of normal platelets induced by purified placenta microfibrils (Legrand *et al.*, 1980) was completely inhibited by AN51.

Since ristocetin and bovine factor VIII induced aggregations were inhibited by AN51, while the other inducers (ADP, thrombin or arachidonic acid) were still effective, the distinction between the surface structures involved in these different aggregations can be confirmed.

TABLE 8·3

Effect of monoclonal antibody to Glycoprotein I (IgG AN51) on the aggregation of control platelets induced by different agents

| Inducers (final concentrations) | Control PRP in presence of different final concentrations of IgG AN51 ($\mu$g ml$^{-1}$) | | | |
|---|---|---|---|---|
| | 0 | 2·5 | 5 | 10 |
| Ristocetin (1·2 mg ml$^{-1}$) | 100 | 50 | 15 | 0 |
| Bovine FVIII (0·75 U ml$^{-1}$) | 100 | 50 | 25 | 0 |
| Porcine FVIII (0·1 U ml$^{-1}$) | 100 | 40 | 15 | 0 |
| Microfibrils (62·5 $\mu$g ml$^{-1}$) | 100 | 45 | 10 | 0 |
| Collagen | 100 | 100 | 100 | 90 |
| ADP (2 $\mu$M$^{-1}$) | 100 | 100 | 100 | 100 |
| Thrombin (0·15 U ml$^{-1}$) | 100 | 100 | 100 | 100 |
| Arachidonic acid (100 $\mu$g ml$^{-1}$) | 100 | 100 | 100 | 100 |

The lack of inhibition of thrombin induced aggregation argues against a role of glycoprotein I in a platelet membrane-thrombin interaction. Platelet membrane-collagen interactions also seem to be glycoprotein I-independant. Microfibrils, another component of the subendothelium, could act on platelet membrane through glycoprotein I.

### (b)  *Effect on adhesion*

AN51 strongly inhibited platelet deposition on control rabbit aorta subendothelium. The still persistent adhesion of platelets to collagenase treated segments was also inhibited by the antibody (Table 8·4).

These experiments confirm the role of glycoprotein I in platelet adhesion to subendothelium and suggest that non collagenic material from subendothelium could be responsible for thrombogenicity.

### (c)  *Effect on the binding of factor VIII/von Willebrand factor to platelet*

The binding of [125]I-factor VIII/von Willebrand factor to human platelets was inhibited by AN51. At low concentrations of antibody $(0·125$ to $2$ $\mu g$ $ml^{-1})$ this inhibition was dose dependant. At high concentrations a plateau of about 40% inhibition was reached (Fig. 8·4). This could mean that only a part of platelet bound factor VIII/von Willebrand factor interacts with glycoprotein Ib and that this part is mainly, if not totally, responsible for the platelet aggregation induced by ristocetin. Another explanation could be that the epitope on glycoprotein Ib seen by AN51 is not the actual binding site but that AN51 antibody interferes with factor VIII/von Willebrand factor binding by steric hindrance.

TABLE 8·4

Platelet adhesion to rabbit aorta subendothelium

| Shear rate $(s^{-1})$ Treatment of vessel segment | 810 | |
|---|---|---|
| | Control | Collagenase |
| PRP incubated in buffer | 100 | 100 |
| PRP incubated in control ascites 1:1500 | 100 | 100 |
| PRP incubated in AN51 Ascites 1:1500 | 11 | 16 |
| 1:3000 | 45 | 35 |
| 1:10 000 | 100 | 76 |

Subendothelium has been tested withou⋅ treatment (control) or after collagenase digestion (collagenase). Platelet rich plasma (PRP) has been incubated in buffer, in control ascites (without antiplatelet antibody) or in AN51 ascites at different dilutions.

The results are expressed in %.

## D. VON WILLEBRAND FACTOR AND
## PLATELET ADHESION

### 1. VON WILLEBRAND DISEASE (Meyer, 1980)

In von Willebrand disease, the bleeding time is prolonged, VIII C (coagulant activity) and VIII CAg (alloantigen) are normal or decreased, VIII RCO (ristocetin cofactor) and VIII RAg (xeno-antigen) are absent or decreased, according to the severity of the disease. Von Willebrand disease represents a heterogeneous group of patients with different types of factor defects. Two main types of the disease have been defined:-

Type I is characterized by reduced levels of FVIII RAg and FVIII RCO and normal electrophoretic mobility of VIII RAg. In this type, the number and position of factor VIII/von Willebrand factor bands on SDS-agarose electrophoresis gels is similar to that seen with normal plasma, although the total area of the bands is decreased.

Type II is characterized by a lack of FVIII RCO, and variable amounts of RAg which shows abnormal electrophoretic migration. There is a consistent absence of the high molecular weight bands and the smallest molecular weight band is increased in concentration relative to normal. This suggests that there is a polymerization defect in factor VIII/von Willebrand factor with accumulation of the small forms. As with Type I von Willebrand disease, there are abnormal platelet-vessel wall interactions.

### 2. FACTOR VIII/VON WILLEBRAND FACTOR
### AND GLYCOPROTEIN I

#### (a) *Factor VIII/Von Willebrand factor and platelet adhesion*

Factor VIII RAg, which is present in human vascular wall, is synthesized and secreted by endothelial cells in culture (Jaffe *et al.*, 1973). Exogenous factor VIII/von Willebrand factor can bind to arterial subendothelium (Sakariassen *et al.*, 1979) and this binding precedes the increased platelet adhesion and enhances platelet spreading.

Platelet adhesion to subendothelium is decreased in von Willebrand disease, particularly to the high shear rates which prevail in microvasculature (Weiss *et al.*, 1978). Adhesion is inhibited by antibody to human factor VIII/von Willebrand factor (Baumgartner *et al.*, 1980). Plasma factor VIII/von Willebrand factor seems, therefore, to act as a cofactor in platelet adhesion.

The inhibition of platelet adhesion to subendothelium observed in the presence of AN51 could be related to the inhibition of the binding of factor VIII/von Willebrand factor to the platelets.

(b) *Study of the binding sites on platelet for factor VIII/ Willebrand factor*

Platelets contain a large quantity of factor VIII/ RAg (about 25% of the circulating antigen). Several fractions have been recognized: the first can be removed by washing and can be localized on binding sites (Nachman and Jaffe, 1975); a second fraction is unmovable and may originate from the canaliculi of the megakaryocyte; a third fraction is localized in the intracellular $\alpha$ granules and can be released by collagen or thrombin (Zucker *et al.*, 1979). Plasma factor VIII/von Willebrand factor binds to the platelet membrane in the presence of ristocetin (Zucker *et al.*, 1977). Binding characteristics fulfill the criteria of high affinity, saturability and specificity (Keo *et al.*, 1978). Ristocetin increases the estimated number of factor VIII/von Willebrand factor binding sites of both high and low affinity. Factor VIII/von Willebrand factor binding sites appear to be distinct from those of ristocetin (Schneider Trip *et al.*, 1979; Morisato and Gralnick, 1980). The binding sites of factor VIII/von Willebrand factor seem, like glycoprotein I, to be susceptible to chymotrypsin digestion (Green and Muller, 1978; Schneider Trip *et al.*, 1979).

Bernard Soulier platelets failed to bind plasma factor VIII/von Willebrand plasma in the presence of ristocetin (Zucker *et al.*, 1977; Moake *et al.*, 1980). In five different Bernard Soulier patients, we have confirmed that there is a decrease in binding but under our experimental conditions it was less than previously reported (Ruan *et al.*, 1981b).

As described above, alloantibody and AN51 monoclonal antibody inhibit the binding of factor VIII/von Willebrand factor to normal platelets. 80% inhibition was the maximun achieved using the alloantibody (Fig. 8·4).

In the presence of both antibodies, at limiting concentrations, an additive inhibitory effect on the binding was observed. Since these antibodies probably recognized different epitopes on glycoprotein I, this might mean that more than one binding site for factor VIII/von Willebrand factor exists on glycoprotein I. However, in the presence of both antibodies, maximum inhibition was still 80%, suggesting that other binding sites for factor VIII/von Willebrand factor, which are independant of glycoprotein I, may exist on normal platelets (Ruan *et al.*, 1981 in preparation). The reduced binding to the Bernard Soulier platelets was not appreciably inhibited by the human alloantibody or monoclonal antibody to glycoprotein I, and can therefore be considered

TABLE 8·5
Inhibition of the binding of $^{125}$I-factor
VIII/Willebrand factor to the fixed platelets of control
or 5 Bernard Soulier patients (BSS) by allo human
antibody (IgG P.) or monoclonal antibody (AN51) to
glycoprotein I

| | % Inhibition of the binding by | |
| | IgGP | AN51 |
| Fixed platelets | $(50\,\mu g\,ml^{-1})$ | $(5\,\mu g\,ml^{-1})$ |
| --- | --- | --- |
| Control n = 6 | 76·9 | 40·9 |
| BSS     VN | 0·2 | |
| AN | 15·4 | 9·6 |
| AH | 0 | 0 |
| MP | 7·9 | 12·4 |
| BR | 17·9 | 12·2 |

to be glycoprotein I independant (Table 8·5). Because these glycoprotein I independant binding sites are normally present on Bernard Soulier platelets, this could explain why these platelets reacted positively with a peroxidase coupled antibody specific for factor VIII/von Willebrand factor (Caen *et al.*, 1976). Using drug dependant antibody or aggregated control human IgG we were able to inhibit part of the binding of factor VIII/von Willebrand factor to control platelets.

These findings suggest a hypothesis to explain the distribution and role of the different fractions of factor VIII/von Willebrand factor bound to platelets. The major part of the factor binds to glycoprotein I and this binding seems to be responsible for the ristocetin and vessel wall interactions. This binding is absent in Bernard Soulier platelets and is inhibited totally by human alloantibody and partially by AN51. These binding sites are closely associated with those for drug dependant antibodies and for the Fc fragment of IgG. Other unknown binding sites, independant of glycoprotein I, may exist on normal and Bernard Soulier platelets but their function is unknown.

3. MONOCLONAL ANTIBODIES TO FACTOR VIII/VON
WILLEBRAND FACTOR

Monoclonal antibodies to factor VIII/von Willebrand factor have been obtained recently (Meyer *et al.*, 1980). None of the seven hybridoma antibodies blocked VIII C (procoagulant activity) or VIII RCO (ristocetin cofactor) activity. The availability of these stable hybridomas which are continually producing antibody to the (presumed) VIII RAg determinant should allow more rigorous characterization and quantitation of factor VIII and its biological activities.

## IV PLATELET AGGREGATION

Platelet aggregation is the result of platelet-platelet interactions and leads to the formation of thrombi. Congenital platelet disorders and both human and monoclonal antibodies to platelet membrane have facilitated the study of the underlying mechanism.

### A. The Platelet Membrane Glyoprotein IIb/IIIa Complex and Platelet Aggregation

#### 1. THROMBASTHENIA OF GLANZMANN

(a) *Defect in platelet aggregation*

Thrombasthenia is a platelet disorder, inherited as an autosomal recessive trait, which is characterized by a severe mucocutaneous bleeding tendency, a prolonged bleeding time and a normal platelet count (Caen *et al.*, 1966). Platelets cannot be aggregated in thrombasthenia, whatever the inducing agent, and clot retraction is absent or substantially decreased (Caen, 1972). Two main types of thrombasthenia have been described: type I with an absence of clot retraction and with a total defect of platelet fibrinogen; type II with decreased clot retraction and a partial defect of platelet fibrinogen (Caen 1972).

(b) *Defect in platelet membrane glycoprotein IIb/IIIa complex*

A defect in platelet membrane glycoprotein II was first shown by Nurden and Caen (1974). This abnormality has since been confirmed and shown to be a defect of glycoprotein IIb/IIIa (Phillips and Poh Agin, 1977c; Nurden and Caen, 1977) (Fig. 8·5). By cross immunoelectrophoresis using rabbit antihuman platelet antiserum, it was shown that the thrombasthenic platelets were deficient in band 16, which represents the glycoprotein IIb/IIIa complex (Hagen *et al.*, 1980). The defect was total in thrombasthenia type I and only partial in type II.

The abnormal function of thrombasthenic platelets and the defect in platelet membrane glycoprotein IIb/IIIa have been related by Caen and Nurden (1975) who proposed that this glycoprotein could be implicated in platelet aggregation.

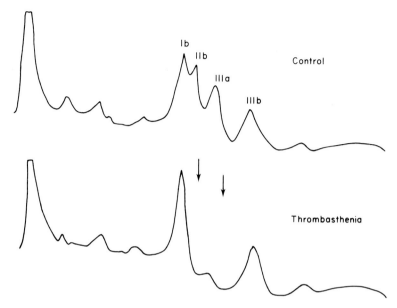

FIG. 8·5 SDS polyacrylamide gel electrophoresis of platelets. Platelet membranes from control on thrombasthenia have been isolated and solubilized in SDS. Polyacrylamide gel electrophoresis has been performed with SDS in presence of 2 mercaptoethanol. Major glycoproteins are stained with PAS. Glycoprotein IIb/IIIa are absent in thrombasthenia.

## (c) *Other abnormalities in thrombasthenic patients*

The defect in platelet fibrinogen has been confirmed in thrombasthenia type I; thrombasthenia type II platelets contain between 30 and 50% of the normal level of platelet fibrinogen (Kunicki *et al.*, 1981b).

Thrombasthenic platelets are PLA[1] negative and it has been shown that this antigenic determinant is part of glycoprotein IIIa (Kunicki and Aster, 1979). In platelets from heterozygous relatives of thrombasthenic patients, glycoprotein IIb/IIIa and PLA[1] antigen are reduced in quantity (Kunicki, *et al.*,1981b).

Specific binding of exogenous fibrinogen to thrombasthenic type I platelets has been found to be reduced. In type II patients the binding was reduced but less markedly so (Lee *et al.*, 1981).

## 2. ROLE OF PLATELET MEMBRANE GLYCOPROTEIN IIb/IIIa COMPLEX

What then, is the role of this glycoprotein complex in the haemostatic mechanism? Two observations make it clear that it is not required for the initial reaction of ADP with the platelet membrane: thrombasthenic platelets possess normal ADP membrane receptors (Legrand and Caen, 1976) and undergo a normal shape change, with sphering and filopodial formation in response to ADP (Zucker *et al.*, 1966). It has been shown by several groups (Marguerie *et al.*, 1980; Mustard *et al.*, 1979; Peerschke *et al.*, 1979) however, that this initial reaction with ADP induces, in the presence of calcium, a receptor for plasma fibrinogen on the membrane of normal but not thrombasthenic platelets. If this receptor proves to be related to the glycoprotein IIb/IIIa complex, it will provide a molecular basis for both aggregation and for clot retraction through the attachment of fibrinogen and actin respectively to the external and cytoplasmic aspects of the glycoprotein.

The readiness with which it is iodinated by lactoperoxidase suggests that the glycoprotein IIb/IIIa complex is well exposed on the platelet surface and is in a good external position to participate in platelet-platelet interactions.

## B. Human Alloantibody to Glycoprotein IIb/IIIa Complex

### 1. IMMUNOLOGICAL STUDIES (Degos *et al.*, 1975)

#### (a) *Case history*

A patient with the classical features of thrombasthenic and intestinal bleeding received a transfusion of $2 \times 10^{10}$ platelets from his sister. Serum from the patient was studied 15 days later when an IgG anti platelet antibody was found.

#### (b) *Complement fixation test*

When platelets from 350 healthy unrelated individuals were tested in a complement fixation reaction in the presence of the IgG antibody, the results were invariably positive regardless of the HLA type and PLA[1]-PLE[1] group. Negative results were obtained with platelets of thrombasthenic patients. In a quantitative fixation test, platelets from presumed heterozygous relations of the patients, showed a reactivity pattern midway between that of patients and normal individuals.

#### (c) *Study of the antigen*

Initially, an indirect immunoprecipitation technique using [125]I solubilized normal platelets, patient's IgG antibody and rabbit anti-human IgG, showed a single peak with a molecular weight of 120,000.

More sensitive techniques distinguished two peaks with molecular weights of 135,000 and 115,000.

In the cross immunoelectrophoresis technique with solubilized normal platelets and IgG antibody in the intermediate gel, band 16 (GP IIb/IIIa) was retained (Hagen *et al.*, 1980). When the patient's IgG was put in the upper gel, only band 16 was observed. With thrombasthenia type I platelets, this band was absent and with thrombasthenia type II platelets it was reduced to between 10 and 15% of normal. Using platelets from heterozygotes, it was found to be about half normal.

When the band 16, produced from the patient's IgG and $^{125}$I solubilized normal platelets, was isolated free from the immunoelectrophoresis gel, solubilized in SDS and then analysed by SDS polyacrylamide gel electrophoresis, two radioactive peaks were found with molecular weights corresponding to glycoprotein IIb/IIIa.

This human anti platelet alloantibody seemed, therefore, to be directed against an antigenic component of the glycoprotein IIa/IIb complex which is absent in thrombasthenic patients.

## 2. EFFECT ON PLATELET FUNCTIONS

### (a) *Effect on platelet aggregation and clot retraction*

ADP, collagen, epinephrine and thrombin induced aggregations were strongly inhibited by the human antibody while ristocetin induced aggregation was not influenced (Levy-Toledano *et al.*, 1978).

The shape change induced by ADP was not modified in the presence of the antibody. Clot retraction was inhibited by the antibody.

### (b) *Effect on platelet-subendothelium interactions*

The adhesion of control platelets to rabbit aorta subendothelium was not inhibited in the presence of antibody, but aggregation and thrombi formation were not observed (Caen *et al.*, 1977).

### (c) *Effect on ADP binding*

Preincubation of control platelet membranes with increasing concentrations of the IgG antibody did not modify the subsequent binding of $^{14}$C-ADP (Levy-Toledano *et al.*, 1978).

### (d) *Effect on fibrinogen binding*

The binding of fibrinogen, induced by ADP, to platelet membranes was inhibited by the IgG antibody (Lee *et al.*, 1981).

This antibody to the glycoprotein IIb/IIIa complex therefore induced a thrombasthenic-like abnormality in normal platelets.

## C.  MONOCLONAL ANTIBODIES TO GLYCOPROTEIN IIb/IIIa COMPLEX

1. ANTIBODY J15 (Keiffer *et al.*, 1982 in preparation)

In a similar experiment to that which generated the AN51 antibody, we obtained an IgM reagent which reacts with normal platelets in the complement fixation test. PLA[1] negative platelets reacted normally with J15. In a radiobinding assay, no reactivity was shown with platelets from three patients with thrombasthenia type I and from one patient with thrombasthenia type II (Fig. 8·6).

J15 inhibited clot retraction. Platelet aggregation induced by ADP, thrombin and the ionophore A28187 was inhibited by J15 when tested with washed platelets.

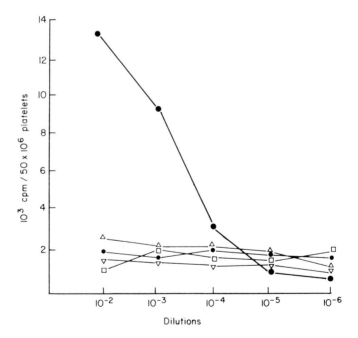

FIG. 8·.6 Radiobinding assay with J15. (●————●) Mean value of the binding obtained with 10 control platelets (△————△) (•————•) (▽————▽) (□————□) Binding obtained with 4 different thrombasthenia.

Fibrinogen binding to control platelets in the presence of ADP was decreased by J15.

This antibody seems, therefore, to recognize a platelet surface antigen absent from thrombasthenic patients but present on PLA[1] negative platelets. The antigen seems to be implicated in clot retraction, fibrinogen binding, and platelet aggregation. Further investigation, particularly biochemical evidence, is needed to determine the exact nature of the antigen which seems to be, functionally, a part of the glycoprotein IIb/IIIa complex.

## 2. THE ANTIBODY Tab

A monoclonal antibody to human platelets has been described by McEver *et al.*, (1980). This antibody, Tab, bound to a protein on normal but not thrombasthenic platelets. The protein has been isolated from Triton X100 solubilized normal platelet membranes by affinity chromatography on Tab-sepharose and shown to be a complex of glycoprotein IIb/IIIa. There was also a faint band of protein with a molecular weight of 43,000, which may represent actin associated with this glycoprotein.

By a direct binding assay with [125]I-Tab it was found that platelets bound $39,000 \pm 4,600$ Tab molecules/platelet. Platelets from obligate heterozygotes for thrombasthenia bound $24,000 \pm 5,800$ Tab molecules/platelet. PLA[1] negative subjects bound Tab normally.

Tab, unlike J15, did not inhibit either ADP or thrombin induced aggregation of normal platelets.

Our studies with thrombasthenic platelets are aimed at defining the role of the glycoprotein IIb/IIIa complex in platelet function. Using human alloantibody, the molecular defect in thrombasthenic platelets has been confirmed and the understanding of the functions of the glycoprotein IIb/IIIa complex has been increased. Preliminary work with monoclonal antibodies to the glycoprotein IIb/IIIa complex has added to this understanding of the molecular and functional defects. The following questions remain to be answered, however. What is the exact role of glycoprotein IIb/IIIa in platelet aggregation and clot retraction? What is the role of the intraplatelet fibrinogen? Is the glycoprotein IIb/IIIa complex the binding site for plasma fibrinogen during platelet aggregation? Is the PLA[1] antigen supported by glycoprotein IIb/IIIa complex or only bound to these glycoproteins? What is the relationship between glycoprotein IIb/IIIa and actin?

# V CONCLUSION

Platelets play a key role in haemostasis and arterial thrombosis and it seems probable that they participate in the development of athersclerosis. Platelets could also be involved in metastasis formation, inflammation and some immunological conflicts. These different roles underline the importance of these cells. We have attempted to show how congenital platelet disorders make useful models for the study of the basic mechanisms of platelet function and how antibodies to platelet membranes have become useful experimental tools.

Studies with monoclonal antibodies to platelets are just beginning and with their obvious advantages, it seems reasonable to expect that development of research in this field will rapidly advance our understanding of platelet physiology and pathology.

We are now planning to obtain a more complete library of monoclonal antibodies, specific for the different antigenic epitopes of platelets, and to use these to study the structure-function relationships of platelet antigens. The monoclonal antibodies will also facilitate purification of different platelet antigens (see chapter 22). These reagents will be useful in the diagnosis of haemorrhagic platelet disorders and may be useful in identifying heterozygotes. Their main value could be in studies of thrombosis. Diagnosis of a prethrombotic state, for example, could be based on the detection of very mild degrees of platelet activation, which would release platelet components into the blood stream. Very small quantities of these platelet antigens could be measured in plasma using monoclonal antibodies and so allow early diagnosis and new therapeutic opportunities.

REFERENCES

Barber, A. J. and Jamieson, G. A. (1970). *J. Biol. Chem.* **245**, 6359–6365.
Baumgartner, H. R. and Muggli, R. (1976). *In* "Platelets in Biology and Pathology" (J. L. Gordon, Ed.), pp. 23–60. Elsevier/North Holland, Amsterdam.
Baumgartner, H. R., Tschopp, T. B. and Meyer, D. (1980). *Br. J. Haematol.* **44**, 127–139.
Bernard, J. and Soulier, J. P. (1948). *Sem. Hop. Paris.* **24**, 217–223.
Caen, J. P. (1972). *Clin. Haematol.* **1**, 383–392.
Caen, J. P. and Levy-Toledano, S. (1973a). *Nature New Biol.* **244**, 159–160.
Caen, J. P., Castaldi, P. A., Le Clerc, J. C., Inceman, S., Larrieu, M. J., Probst, M. and Bernard, J. (1966). *Am. J. Med.* **41**, 21–27.
Caen, J. P., Levy-Toledano, S., Sultan, Y. and Bernard, J. (1973b). *Nouv. Rev. Fr. Hemat.* **13**, 595–602.

Caen, J. P., Nurden, A. T., Jeanneau, C., Michel, H., Tobelem, G., Levy-Toledano, S., Sultan, Y., Valensi, F. and Bernard, J. (1976). *J. Lab. clin. Med.* **87**, 586–596.

Caen, J. P., Michel, H., Tobelem, G., Bodevin, E. and Levy-Toledano, S. (1977). *Experientia* **33**, 91–93.

Chevalier, J., Nurden, A. T., Thiery, J. M., Savariau, E. and Caen, J. P. (1979). *J. Lab. clin. Med.* **94**, 232–245.

Clemetson, K. J., Capitanio, A. and Luscher, E. F. (1979). *Biochim, biophys. Acta.* **553**, 11–24.

Degos, L., Dautigny, A., Brouet, J. C., Colombani, M., Ardaillou, N., Caen, J. P., and Colombani, J. (1975). *J. clin, Invest.* **56**, 236–240.

Degos, L., Tobelem, G., Lethielleux, P., Levy-Toledano, S., Caen, J. P. and Colombani, J. (1977). *Blood* **50**, 899–903.

Fauvel, F. and LeGrand, Y. (1980). *Thrombos. Res.* **17**, 285–287.

Fauvel, F., LeGrand, Y., Caen, J. P. (1978). *Thrombos. Res.* **12**, 273–285.

Fauvel, F., LeGrand, Y., Bentz, R., Fietzek, P. P., Kuhn, K., and Caen, J. P. (1978). *Thrombos. Res.* **12**, 841–850.

Frojmovic, M. M., Milton, J. G., Caen, J. P., and Tobelem, G. (1978). *J. Lab. clin. Med.* **91**, 109–116.

Ganguly, P. and Gould, N. L. (1979). *Br. J. Haematol.* **42**, 137–145.

Green, D. and Muller, M. P. (1978). *Thromb. Haemost.* **39**, 689–694.

Greenberg, J., Packham, M. A., Cazenave, J. P., Reimers, H. J. and Mustard, J. F. (1975). *Lab. Invest.* **32**, 476–484.

Grottum, K. A. and Solum, N. O. (1969). *Br. J. Haematol.* **16**, 277–290.

Hagen, I., Nurden, A., Bjerrum, O. J., Solum, N. O. and Caen, J. P. (1980). *J. clin. Invest.* **65**, 722–731.

Howard, M. A. and Firkin, B. G. (1971). *Thromb. Diath. Haemorrh.* **26**, 362–369.

Jaffe, E., Hoyer, L. W. and Nachman, R. L. (1973). *J. clin. Invest.* **52**, 2757–2764.

Jamieson, G. A. and Okumura. T. (1978). *J. clin. Invest.* **61**, 861–864.

Kao, K. J., Pizzo, S. V. and Mac Kee, P. A. (1979). *J. clin. Invest.* **63**, 656–664.

Kunicki, T. and Aster, R. M. (1979). *Molec. Immunol.* **16**, 353–360.

Kunicki, T. J., Johnson, M. M. and Aster, R. H. (1978). *J. clin. Invest.* **62**, 716–719.

Kunicki, T. J., Johnson, M. M. and Aster, R. H. (1978). *J. clin. Invest.* **62**, 716–719.

Kunicki, T. J., Russell, N., Nurden, A. T., Aster, R. M. and Caen, J. P. (1981a). *J. immunol.* (in press).

Kunicki, T. J., Pidard, D., Cazenave, J. P., Nurden, A. T. and Caen, J. P. (1981b). *J. clin. Invest.* (in press).

Lee, H., Nurden, A. T., Thomardis, A. and Caen, J. P. (1981). *Br. J. Haematol.* (in press).

Legrand, C. and Caen, J. P. (1976). *Haemostasis* **5**, 231–238.

Legrand, Y., Fauvel, F., Gutman, N., Muh, J. P., Tobelem, G., Souchon, H., Karniguian, A. and Caen, J. P. (1980). *Thrombos. Res.* **19**, 737–739.

Legrand, Y., Karniguian, A., Le Francier, P., Fauvel, F. and Caen, J. P. (1980). *Biochem. biophys. Res. Comm.* **96**, 1579–1585.

Levy-Toledano, S., Tobelem, G., Legrand, C., Bredoux, R., Degos, L., Nurden, A. T. and Caen, J. P . (1978). *Blood* **51**, 1065–1071.

McEver, R. P., Baenziger, N. L. and Majerus, P. W. (1980). *J. clin. Invest.* **66**, 1311–1318.

McMichael, A. J., Rust, N. A., Pilch, J. R., Solchynsky, R., Morton, J., Mason, D. Y., Ruan, C., Tobelem, G. and Caen, J. P. (1981). *Br. J. Haematol.* (in press).

Marguerie, G. A. and Plow, E. F. (1980). *J. biol. Chem.* **254**, 5357–5363.

Marguerie, G. A., Plow, E. F. and Edgington, T. S. (1979). *Fed. Proc.* **38**, 1207.

Meyer, D. (1980). *In* "The regulation of coagulation" (Mann and Taylor Eds), pp. 297–308. Elsevier/North Holland, Amsterdam.

Meyer, D., Obert, B., Zimmerman, T., and Edgington, T. American Heart Association, 53rd scientific sessions, Nov., 1980, Miami.

Moake, J. L. Olson, J. D., Troll, J. M., Tang, S. S., Funicella, T. and Peterson, D. M. (1980). *Thrombos. Res.* **19**, 21–27.

Moncada, S., Cryzlewski, R. J., Bunting, S. and Vane, J. R. (1976). *Nature* **261**, 663–665.

Moncada, S., Korbut, R., Bunting, S. and Vane, J. R. (1978). *Nature* **273**, 767–768.

Moore, A., Ross, G. D. and Nachman, R. L. (1978). *J. clin. Invest.* **62**, 1053–1060.

Morisato, D. K. and Gralnick, H. R. (1980). *Blood* **55**, 9–15.

Mustard, J. F., Kinlough Rathbone, R. L., Perry, D. W. and Pat, K. R. M. (1979). *Blood* **54**, 987–993.

Nachman, R. L. and Jaffe, E. A. (1975). *J. exp. Med.* **141**, 1101–1113.

Nurden, A. T. and Caen, J. P. (1974). *Br. J. Haematol.* **28**, 252–260.

Nurden, A. T. and Caen, J. P . (1975). *Nature* **255**, 720–722.

Nurden, A. and Caen, J. (1978). *Br. J. Haematol.* **38**, 155–160.

Nurden, A. T. and Caen, J. P. (1979). *Sem. Hematol.* **16**, 234–250.

Nurden, A. T., Dupuis, D., Kunicki, T. J. and Caen, J. P. (1981). *J. clin. Invest.* (in press).

Okumura, T. and Jamieson, G. A. (1976). *J. biol. Chem.* **25**, 5944–5949.

Peerschke, E. I., Grant, R. A. and Zucker, M. B. (1979). *Thromb. Haemost.* **42**, 358.

Pfueller, S. L., Jenkins, C. S. P. and Luscher, E. F. (1977). *Biochim. biophys. Acta* **465**, 614–626.

Phillips, D. R. (1972). *Biochemistry* **11**, 4582–4588.

Phillips, D. R. and Agin, P. P. (1977a). *J. biol. Chem.* **252**, 2121–2126.

Phillips, D. R. and Agin, P. P. (1977b). *Biochem. biophys. Res. Commun.* **75**, 940–947.

Phillips, D. R. and Agin, P. P. (1977c). *J. clin Invest.* **60**, 535–545.

Ruan, C., Tobelem, G., Mc Michael, A., Drouet, L., Legrand, Y., Degos, L., Kieffer, N., Lee, H. and Caen, J. P. (1981a). *Br. J. Haematol.* (in press).

Ruan, C., Tobelem, G. and Caen, J. P. (1981b). *Nouv. Rev. Fr. Hematol.* **23** (in press).
Sakariassen, K. S., Bolhuis, P. A. and Sixma, J. J. (1979). *Nature* **279**, 636–637.
Schneider Trip, M. F., Jenkins, C. S. P., Kahle, L. H., Jturk, A. and Ten Cate, J. W. (1979). *Br. J. Haematol.* **43**, 99–112.
Sie, P., Gillois, M., Boneu, B., Chap, H., Bierme, R. and Douste Blazy, L. (1980). *Biochem. biophys. Res. Commun.* **97**, 133–138.
Stemerman, M. B. (1974). *Prog. Hemostasis Thromb.* **2**, 1–47.
Stemerman, M. B., Baumgartner, H. R., Spaet, T. H. (1971). *Lab. Invest.* **24**, 179–191.
Thorgeirsson, G. and Robertson, A. L. (1978). *Am. J. Pathol.* **93**, 801–848.
Tobelem, G., Levy-Toledano, S., Bredoux, R., Michel, H., Nurden, A., Degos, L. and Caen, J. P. (1976). *Nature* **263**, 427–429.
Tobelem, G., Levy-Toledano, S., Nurden, A. T., Degos, L. and Caen, J. P. (1979). *Br. J. Haematol.* **41**, 427–436.
Walsh, P. N., Mills, D. C. B., Pareti, F. I., Stewart, G. J., Mac Farlane, D. E., Johnson, M. M. and Egan, J. J. (1975). *Br. J. Hematol.* **29**, 639–655.
Weiss, H. J., Tschopp, T. B., Baumgartner, H. R., Sussman, I. I., Johnson, M. M. and Egan, J. J. (1974). *Aur. J. Med.* **57**, 920–931.
Weiss, H. J., Turitto, V. T. and Baumgartner, H. R. (1978). *J. Lab. clin. Med.* **92**, 750–764.
Zucker, M. B., Pert, J. H. and Hilgartner, M. W. (1966). *Blood* **28**, 524–534.
Zucker, M. B., Kian, S. J. A., Mc Pherson, J. and Grant, R. A. (1977). *Br. J. Haematol.* **35**, 535–549.
Zucker, M. B., Broekman, M. J. and Kaplan, K. L. (1979). *J. Lab. clin. Med.* **94**, 675–682.

# 9 Characterization of Human Blood Group Alloantigens

D. J. ANSTEE

*South Western Regional Transfusion Centre, Southmead Road,*
*Bristol. BS10 5ND*

## I INTRODUCTION

There are numerous inherited antigens on the surface of the human erythrocyte. Most of these antigens were first recognized by serological analysis of the specificity of haemagglutinating antibodies produced as the result of transfusion or pregnancy. Those antigens which are genetically linked are grouped together to form blood group systems. The antigens are of considerable clinical importance at the level of the blood bank where avoiding transfusion of antigen incompatible blood and early detection and prevention of haemolytic disease of the newborn are of paramount importance.

The ABH and Ii antigens are carbohydrate antigens and are present on both glycolipids and the major surface glycoproteins band 3 and band 4·5 (Hakomori, 1981). The antigens $P_1$, P and $P^k$ are also carbohydrate and located on glycolipids (Marcus, 1981). The MN and Ss antigens are exclusively located on the major erythrocyte sialoglycoproteins $\alpha$ (glycophorin A) and $\delta$ (glycophorin B) respectively; $\delta$ carries N antigen (denoted 'N') in addition to S and s. The structure of these antigens is determined by amino acid substitutions in the polypeptide chains of the glycoproteins although carbohydrate structures comprise part of the M and N antigens and probably also the S and s antigens (Furthmayr, 1978; Dahr *et al.*, 1980a,b; Anstee, 1981). Detailed structural information concerning erythrocyte antigens is thus confined to abundant antigens (known to be greater than $10^5$ sites per cell in the case of ABH, Ii and MN antigens, (Hughes-Jones, 1977; Gahmberg *et al.*, 1979) which are either totally carbohydrate in nature (ABH, $P_1$, P, $P^k$, Ii) or which have carbohydrate as a part of their structure (MNSs) Table 9·1. The only exception is the rare antigen $M^g$, an allele of M and N which has recently been shown to result from an amino acid substitution at position 4 of the carbohydrate free amino terminus of sialoglycoprotein $\alpha$ (Table 9·1, Dahr *et al.*, 1981; Furthmayr *et al.*, 1981).

Despite the clinical importance of antigens of the other major blood group systems (particularly the Rhesus blood group system) there is little or no information concerning their structure or function. The development by Kohler and Milstein of the hybridoma technique offers immense possibilities for the further characterization of these important erythrocyte antigens and may also result in the improvement of practical blood bank techniques for detecting them—techniques which have changed little since the introduction of the double antibody agglutination test of Coombs, Mourant and Race in 1945. It is the purpose of this short review to outline the strategy we have utilized in order to define the specificity of anti-erythrocyte monoclonal antibodies, to describe our results so far, and to comment on the possibilities that the hybridoma technique offers for increasing our understanding of the structure and function of erythrocyte antigens and improving the technology of blood banking.

## II STRATEGY

Serological analysis of the diversity of antigenic expression within the major human blood group systems has resulted in the discovery of

## TABLE 9·1

### Erythrocyte blood group antigens of defined structure

| Blood group system | Antigen | Immunodominant structure | Membrane location |
|---|---|---|---|
| ABO | A | GalNAcα(1-3) Galβ(1-4) GlcNAcβ(1-3) Galβ(1-4) – – – – –<br>  $\mid$α(1-2)<br>  Fuc | glycolipid and glycoprotein (predominantly band 3 and band 4·5) |
|  | B | Galα(1-3) Galβ(1-4) GlcNAcβ(1-3) Galβ(1-4) – – – – –<br>  $\mid$α(1-2)<br>  Fuc |  |
|  | H | Galβ(1-4) GlcNAcβ(1-3) Galβ(1-4) – – – –<br>  $\mid$α(1-2)<br>  Fuc |  |
| Ii | I | Galβ(1-4) GlcNAcβ1<br>  $\diagdown$ 6) Galβ(1-4) GlcNAcβ(1-3) Gal – – – – –<br>  $\diagup$ 3)<br>  Galβ(1-4) GlcNAcβ1 | glycolipid and glycoprotein (predominantly band 3 and band 4·5) |
|  | i | Galβ(1-4) GlcNAcβ(1-3) Galβ(1-4) GlcNAcβ(1-3) Gal – – – – – |  |
| P | P₁ | Galα(1-4) Galβ(1-4) GlcNAcβ(1-3) Galβ(1-4) Glc-Cer | glycolipid |
|  | P | GalNAcβ(1-3) Galα(1-4) Galβ(1-4) Glc-Cer |  |
|  | Pᵏ | Galα(1-4) Galβ(1-4) Glc-Cer |  |

MNSs[a]

| Antigen | 1 | 2 | 3 | 4 | 5 | | Membrane location |
|---|---|---|---|---|---|---|---|
| M | Ser | Ser[b] | Th[b]r | Th[b]r | Gly | – | erythrocyte sialoglycoprotein α (Glycophorin A) |
| N | Leu | Se[b]r | Th[b]r | Th[b]r | Glu | – |  |
| Mg | Leu | Ser | Thr | Asn | Glu | – |  |

| Antigen | 27 | 28 | 29 | 30 | 31 | | Membrane location |
|---|---|---|---|---|---|---|---|
| S | Gly | Glu | Met | Gly | Gln | – | erythrocyte sialoglycoprotein δ (Glycophorin B) |
| s | Gly | Glu | Thr | Gly | Gln | – |  |

a Numbers indicate the position of amino acids relative to the amino terminus of the polypeptide chain.

b Indicates the position of O-glycosidically linked oligosaccharides of the type: NeuNAcα(2-3) Galβ(1-3) GalNAc– – – – –
  α(2-6)$\mid$
  NeuNAc

several "null" phenotypes, indeed "null" types are known for most of the major blood group systems (Allen, 1976). Cells with these "null' phenotypes may lack all surface antigens associated with a particular blood group system (Table 9·2). Of course, the absence of a group of antigens does not necessarily mean that the membrane component(s) which carries the antigens is also absent. However, it is not unreasonable to suppose that immunization of mice with human erythrocytes will produce antibodies against a wide variety of surface components and that some of these antibodies will recognize surface antigens which are deficient or absent on one or other of the null type cells. If monoclonal antibodies are produced which demonstrate such specificity then it should be possible to prepare sufficiently large quantities of antibody to isolate (by affinity chromatography in detergents, see chapter 22) the appropriate native membrane component from normal cells and to characterize the molecule. It is clear (Table 9·2) that by far the most attractive candidates for such an approach are the antigens of the Rhesus and Kell blood group systems. The Rhesus antigens, especially Rh(D) are of immense clinical importance and their total absence (in RhNULL cells, Table 9·2) results in a defective red cell. The McLeod phenotype in which there is a very weak expression of most antigens of the Kell blood group system also results in a defective red cell. The Fy(a-b-) phenotype is refractory to the malarial parasites (*Plasmodium vivax* and *P. knowlesi*; Miller *et al.*, 1975) and thus elucidation of the membrane component(s) which expresses the Duffy antigens would be of considerable value in clarifying this interaction. Monoclonal antibodies to the major erythrocyte sialoglycoprotein $\alpha$ may be of value for investigating the interaction of *P. falciparum* with red cell surfaces, since En(a-) red cells are somewhat refractory to this parasite (Miller *et al.*, 1977).


### III RESULTS

Eight monoclonal antibodies LICR LON R1·3, R2, R6A, R7, R10, R18, R20·16 and R 23 from mouse hybridomas raised to normal human (group 0 Rh (D+)) erythrocytes (Edwards, 1980) were tested with a panel of cells expressing the null phenotypes listed in Table 9·2 (Anstee and Edwards, 1982).

A. MONOCLONAL ANTIBODIES SPECIFIC FOR
ERYTHROCYTE SIALOGLYCOPROTEINS

Three of the monoclonal antibodies (R10, R18 and R23) agglutinated all of the null-type cells except for those of type En(a-). En(a-) erythrocytes have a total deficiency of the major blood group MN active sialoglycoprotein $\alpha$ (Tanner and Anstee, 1976, Gahmberg *et al.*, 1976, Dahr *et al.*, 1976). This result therefore suggests that the antibodies have an anti-$\alpha$ specificity, a conclusion supported by the fact that the antibodies were completely inhibited by purified $\alpha$ (Anstee and Edwards, 1982). In fact R10 and R18 specifically precipitate $\alpha$ from detergent solubilized erythrocyte membranes (Edwards, 1980). Sialoglycoprotein $\alpha$ has two trypsin sensitive sites on intact erythrocytes (Tomita *et al.*, 1978). Unlike R18, R10 and R23 did not agglutinate trypsin-treated normal erythrocytes. The conclusion that R10 and R18 have different specificities was further supported by their different reactivity with erythrocytes from the higher apes. While R18 is relatively specific for human red cells R10 reacted strongly with erythrocytes from man, chimpanzee, gorilla and orang-utan (Anstee and Edwards, 1982). It was possible to show that another antibody (R1·3) was also specific for erythrocyte sialoglycoproteins. R1·3 reacted with all the null-type cells although only weakly with En(a-) erythrocytes. It did not agglutinate neuraminidase-treated normal erythrocytes suggesting involvement of sialic acid in its recognition site. R1·3 was inhibited by purified $\alpha$. Since it is known that sialoglycoproteins $\alpha$ and $\delta$ have identical amino-acid sequences from the amino-terminus to residue 26 (with the exception of positions 1 and 5 when $\alpha$ expresses blood group M activity; (Furthmayr, 1978, Dahr *et al.*, 1980a, b) it seemed possible that this antibody was reacting with the common amino-terminal portion of $\alpha$ and $\delta$. This possibility became likely when it was shown that trypsin-treated S-s-erythrocytes (S-s-erythrocytes lack $\delta$; Dahr *et al.*, 1975, Anstee *et al.*,1979) were not agglutinated by R1·3. Thus by using defined null-type erythrocytes it was possible to recognize four monoclonal antibodies with specificities directed towards the erythrocyte sialoglycoproteins and to provisionally assign them to three distinct antigenic determinants (Fig. 9·1).

Monoclonal antibody R18 has already proved valuable for the analysis of the composition of hybrid sialoglycoprotein molecules. When used in conjunction with a polyclonal rabbit antibody (I16) rendered specific for the intracellular (and/or intramembranous) portion of $\alpha$ by absorption with intact erythrocytes, it was possible to demonstrate that the abnormal sialoglycoprotein of homozygous

TABLE 9·2

Erythrocytes with null phenotypes found useful for defining the specificity of monoclonal anti-erythrocyte antibodies

| Blood group system | Name of null phenotype | Characteristics of null phenotype | Reference |
|---|---|---|---|
| MNSs | En(a-) | Absence of major erythrocyte sialoglycoprotein $\alpha$ (glycophorin A) and Wr$^b$ antigen. En(a-) erythrocytes are somewhat refractory to invasion by *Plasmodium falciparum*. No known functional defect. | Tanner and Anstee (1976), Miller *et al.* (1977) |
| | S-s-U- | Absence of sialoglycoprotein $\delta$ (glycophorin B). No known functional defect. | Dahr *et al.* (1975) |
| | Homozygous Miltenberger Class V | Absence of sialoglycoproteins $\alpha$ and $\delta$. Absence of Wr$^b$ antigen. Presence of abnormal sialoglycoprotein $(\alpha\text{-}\delta)^{\text{MiV}}$. No known functional defect. | Vengelen-Tyler *et al.* (1981) |
| Rhesus | Rh$_{\text{NULL}}$ | Total absence of all antigens of the Rhesus Blood Group System. Two types are known, type 1 results from homozygosity for a recessive gene at the Rh locus, type 2 results from homozygosity for a recessive gene which is not at the Rh locus but which prevents the occurrence of antigens of the Rhesus blood group system at the erythrocyte surface. Individuals with this phenotype usually have a mild anaemia with reticulocytosis and abnormally shaped erythrocytes (stomatocytes) which have reduced *in vivo* survival and increased osmotic fragility. | Race and Sanger (1975), Sturgeon (1970), Boettcher and Watts (1978) |

| | | Reference |
| --- | --- | --- |
| | Rh$_{MOD}$ | Similar to Rh$_{NULL}$ (type 2 above), but some Rhesus antigens can be detected on the erythrocytes. Clinical symptoms the same as those of Rh$_{NULL}$. | Chown et al. (1972) |
| | Homozygous -D- | Only Rhesus antigens D, G and Rh29 present on erythrocyte surface. No known functional defect. | Issitt and Issitt (1975) |
| Kell | Ko | Lacks all antigens related to Kell blood group system except Kx. No known functional defect. | Marsh et al. (1975) |
| | McLeod | Very weak expression of most common Kell antigens. Total absence of Kx antigen. Kx antigen is present on normal erythrocytes, neutrophils and monocytes and its absence from neutrophils is associated with Chronic Granulomatous Disease. The Kx antigen appears to be the product of an X-linked gene. A significant proportion of erythrocytes expressing the McLeod phenotype have abnormal shape (acanthocytes) and a reduced in vivo survival. | Marsh et al. (1975), Galey et al. (1978) |
| Duffy | Fy(a-b-) | Fy(a-b-) erythrocytes are refractory to invasion by Plasmodium vivax and P. knowlesi. The phenotype is common in West African populations. No known functional defect. | Miller et al. (1975) |
| Lutheran | Lu(a-b-) | Lacks all antigens of the Lutheran blood group system. Two types known, type 1 results from homozygosity for a recessive gene at the Lutheran locus, type 2 is inherited as an autosomal dominant characteristic. Type 2 (called the In(Lu) phenotype) also results in very weak P₁, i and Auberger antigens on the erythrocyte surface. No known functional defect. | Crawford et al. (1974) |

Miltenberger Class V cells is an α-δ hybrid with its amino-terminus derived from α (R18 positive) and its carboxy-terminus derived from a δ variant (I16 negative) while the abnormal sialoglycoprotein of Ph erythrocytes is a δ-α hybrid with its amino-terminus derived from δ (R18 negative) and its carboxy-terminus derived from α (I16 positive). These results demonstrated that the genes for α and δ are closely associated in the order, α, δ on the same chromosome (Mawby *et al.*, 1981).

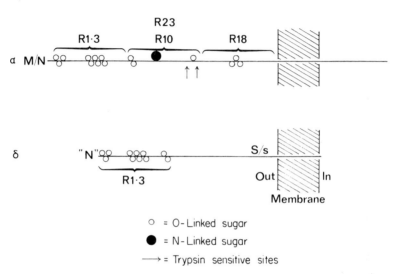

FIG. 9·1 The specificity of anti-sialoglycoprotein monoclonals.

## B. MONOCLONAL ANTIBODIES WITH A SPECIFICITY ASSOCIATED WITH THE RHESUS BLOOD GROUP SYSTEM

Perhaps the most exciting observation to come from the initial investigation of monoclonal antibodies produced to human erythrocytes was the discovery that antibodies R6A and R20·16 show a specificity associated with the Rhesus blood group system. Monoclonal antibody R6A failed to react with RhNULL erythrocytes while antibody R20·16 reacted only weakly with these cells (Anstee and Edwards, 1982). R6A also gave weaker than normal reactions with RhMOD and homozygous-D-cells when the double antibody method was used (Daniels, G. L., and Tippett, P., personal communication).

## C.  Monoclonal Antibodies R7 and R2

Antibody R7 failed to agglutinate En(a-) erythrocytes, Miltenberger Class V erythrocytes and Wr(a+b−) erythrocytes. Since each of these cells lacks the antigen denoted $Wr^b$ this antibody would be serologically characterized as anti-$Wr^b$ (Anstee and Edwards, 1982). The chemical nature of the $Wr^b$ antigen is unknown. It was not possible to determine the specificity of antibody R2 using the panel of null-type cells; however, it failed to agglutinate pronase-treated erythrocytes.

## D.  Other Antibody Specificities

The antibodies described in the previous section were prepared by growing hybrids as clones on soft agar immediately after fusion (Edwards, 1980). There was no pre-selection of hybrids in an attempt to obtain antibodies of a particular specificity. In another series of fusions using spleen cells from mice immunized with intact erythrocytes the fused cells were plated into forty-eight wells and those wells which contained haemagglutinating activity were screened for specificity using the panel of null-type erythrocytes (Judson, Donaldson and Anstee, unpublished). In four fusions from mice immunized with either normal group O or normal group $A_1B$ erythrocytes 28 culture supernatants containing strong haemagglutinating antibody were obtained, 11 supernatants did not show specificity with the null cell panel (7 of these behaved like antibody R2 in that the did not agglutinate pronase-treated cells) 9 supernatants had the specificity of antibody $R1·3$, 3 the specificity of R7, 2 the specificity of $R20·16$, 2 failed to agglutinate En(a-) erythrocytes and were therefore probably anti-$\alpha$ and one did not agglutinate Ko cells or cells of the McLeod phenotype. Thus with the notable exception of the well containing antibody which failed to agglutinate Ko or McLeod phenotype cells and therefore may have a specificity directed at some feature of the Kell blood group system all the other antibody specificities detected were the same or similar to those described previously (Anstee and Edwards, 1982). This experience led us to try different approaches in the hope of obtaining new specificities. A fusion using spleen cells from a mouse immunized with homozygous Miltenberger Class V cells (which lack the $Wr^b$ antigen; Table 9·2) produced four supernatants which showed much stronger reactivity with adult ii erythrocytes than with other cells, 2 supernatants which failed to agglutinate McLeod phenotype cells and 1 which failed to agglutinate Lu(a-b-) erythrocytes of the In Lu type

(Table 9·2). An attempt to produce new specificities by immunizing with pronase-treated RNULL cells resulted in 48 positive culture supernatants all of which showed the specificity of antibody R7! These early results indicate that monoclonal antibodies to less abundant erythrocyte antigens may be made more easily by immunizing with erythrocytes which lack the potent antigen recognized by antibody R7 (Wr$^b$). The rare En(a-) erythrocytes which lack receptors for antibodies R10 and R18 as well as R7 may be useful in this context.


## IV  MONOCLONAL ANTI-ERYTHROCYTE ANTIBODIES IN ROUTINE BLOOD BANKING

If monoclonal antibodies are to have a great impact on routine blood banking it will be necessary to produce antibodies which are specific for polymorphic antigens of the major blood group systems. Our experience so far suggests that such antibodies are unlikely to result from immunization of mice with intact erythrocytes. Analogous results have been obtained by some workers attempting to produce anti-HLA specificities with intact lymphocytes but there has been some success from immunizations with purified HLA glycoprotein (Brodsky *et al.*, 1979, and see chapter 14).

Anti-A and anti-B blood grouping reagents have already been prepared (Voak *et al.*, 1980; Sacks and Lennox, 1981). The anti-A reagent was prepared from mice immunized with tissue culture cells from a human group A colon carcinoma case while the anti-B was prepared by immunizing a mouse (selected because it had anti-B in its serum) with purified blood group B active glycoprotein. ABH, I and i active glycoproteins are easily available from human and animal body fluids (Watkins, 1974; Wood *et al.*, 1980). A blood group P$_1$ active glycoprotein is available from hydatid cyst fluid (Cory *et al.*, 1974) and also from turtle dove mucoid (François Gérard *et al.*, 1980). The blood group MN and Ss active sialoglycoproteins ($\alpha$, $\delta$) of the human red cell membrane are easily obtained (Anstee and Tanner, 1974). Thus purified sources of the abundant, well characterized red cell antigens are easily obtained. Alternative sources of antigens of other major blood group systems (Rhesus, Kell, Duffy, Kidd, Lutheran) are not available although there is some evidence that bacterial infection may stimulate anti-Kell production and so it may be possible to obtain bacterial sources of Kell antigen (Marsh *et al.*, 1976). It should be possible to use monoclonal antibodies, like R6A above, to purify, by affinity chromatography, the components on which blood group antigens are expressed (see chapter 22). It would then be possible to immunize mice with the purified blood group active components and perhaps obtain useful reagents for blood typing. Alternatively, it may be possible to utilize a human hybridoma system if it proves feasible to fuse antibody producing cells from the peripheral blood of immunized donors. Human anti-D has been produced in culture by transforming anti-D secreting lymphocytes from the peripheral blood of immunized human donors with EB-virus. The lymphocyte population is enriched in anti-D producing cells by rosetting with D+ erythrocytes prior to EB-virus transformation (Koskimies, 1980; Boylston *et al.*, 1980). If the transformed antibody producing cells can be cloned this may provide a useful source of blood grouping reagent. The feasibility of fusing EB-virus transformed antibody producing cells with human myelomas should also be explored. Stable man-mouse hybridomas secreting human anti-Forsman antibody have been reported by Nowinski *et al.* (1980) using human splenic lymphocytes and mouse myeloma cells. A hybridoma producing human anti-D would be of tremendous value not simply as a source of blood grouping reagent but also as a prophylactic agent for suppression of Rhesus immunization as a result of pregnancy. Large quantities of anti-D are required for the prevention of haemolytic disease of the newborn due to Rhesus immunization. At present this antibody is produced in male volunteers or obtained by plasmapheresis of females previously stimulated by pregnancy (Mollison, 1979).

If it proves possible to produce in culture a complete range of monoclonal blood grouping reagents then this will open the way for the development of new blood typing methods and allow greater standardization between laboratories.

## V CONCLUSION

The hybridoma technique developed by Kohler and Milstein provides a powerful new approach for determining the structure and function of important human erythrocyte antigens and the membrane components on which they are carried since by utilizing monoclonal antibody affinity chromatography in detergents it should be possible to isolate these components in a native form. Purified membrane components expressing blood group antigen activity could be used to produce monoclonal antibodies to the antigens themselves. The availability of standardized blood grouping reagents in unlimited quantity could have an immense impact on the technology of blood banking.

REFERENCES

Allen, F. H. (1976). *Am. J. clin. Path.* **66**, 467–474.
Anstee, D. J. (1981). *Sem. Haematol.* **18**, 63–71.
Anstee, D. J. and Edwards, P. A. W. (1982) *Eur. J. Immunol.* in press.
Anstee, D. J. and Tanner, M. J. A. (1974). *Biochem. J.* **138**, 381–386.
Anstee, D. J., Mawby, W. J. and Tanner, M. J. A. (1979). *Biochem. J.* **183**, 193–203.
Boettcher, B. and Watts, S. (1978). *Vox Sang.* **34**, 339–342.
Boylston, A. W., Gardner, B., Anderson, R. L. and Hughes-Jones, N. C. (1980). *Scand. J. Immunol.* **12**, 355–358.
Brodsky, F. M., Parham, P., Barnstable, C. J., Crumpton, M. J. and Bodmer, W. F. (1979). *Immunol. Rev.* **47**, 3–62.
Chown, B., Lewis, M., Kaita, H. and Lowen, B. (1972). *Amer J. hum. Genet.* **24**, 623–637.
Cory, H. J., Yates, A. D., Donald, A. S. R., Watkins, W. M . and Morgan, W. T. J . (1974). *Biochem. biophys. Res. Commun.* **61**, 1289–1296.
Crawford, M. N., Tippett, P. and Sanger, R. (1974). *Vox Sang.* **26**, 283–287.
Dahr, W., Uhlenbruck, G., Issitt, P. D. and Allen, F. H. (1975). *J. Immunogenet.* **2**, 249–251.
Dahr, W., Uhlenbruck, G., Leikola, J., Wagstaff, W. and Landfried, K. (1976). *J. Immunogenet.* **3**, 329–346.
Dahr, W., Gielen, W., Beyreuther, K. and Kruger, J. (1980a). *Hoppe-Seyler's. Z. Physiol. Chem.* **361**, 145–152.
Dahr, W., Beyreuther, K., Steinbach, H., Gielen, W. and Kruger, J. (1980b). *Hoppe-Seyler's. Z. Physiol. Chem.* **361**, 895–906.
Dahr, W., Beyreuther, K., Gallasch, E., Kruger, J. and Mavel, P. (1981). *Hope-Seyler's. Z. Physiol. Chem.* **362**, 81–85.
Edwards, P. A. W. (1980). *Biochem. Soc. Trans.* **8**, 334.
François-Gérard, C., Brocteur, J. and Andre, A. (1980). *Vox Sang.* **39**, 141–148.
Furthmayr, H. (1978). *Nature.* **271**, 519–524.
Furthmayr, H., Metaxas, M. N. and Metaxas-Buhler, M. (1981). *Proc. natn. Acad. Sci.* **78**, 631–635.
Gahmberg, C. G., Myllyla, G., Leikola, J. and Nordling, S. (1976). *J. biol. Chem.* **251**, 6108–6116.
Gahmberg, C. G., Jokinen, M., and Andersson, L. C. (1979). *J. biol. Chem.* **254**, 7442–7448.
Galey, W. R., Evan, A. P., Van Nice, P. S., Dail, W. G., Wimer, B. M. and Cooper, R. A. (1978). *Vox Sang.* **34**, 152–161.
Hakomori, S. (1981). *Sem. Haematol.* **18**, 39–62.
Hughes-Jones, N. C. (1977). *In* "Handbook Series in Clinical Laboratory Science, Section D : Blood Banking" (Greenwalt, T. J. and Steane, E. A. Eds), Vol. I pp. 493–498. Cleveland, C.R.C.
Issitt, P. D., and Issitt, C. H. (1975). *In* "Applied Blood Group Serology" 2nd edn., pp. 139–140. Spectra Biologicals, California.

Koskimies, S. (1980). *Scand. J. Immunol.* **11**, 73–76.

Marcus, D. M., Kundu, S. K., and Susuki, A. (1981). *Sem. Haematol.* **18**, 63–71.

Marsh, W. L., Øyen, R., Nichols, M. E., and Allen, F. A. (1975). *Br. J. Haematol.* **29**, 247–262.

Marsh, W. L., Thayer, R. S., Deere, W. L., Schmelter, S. E., Freed, P. J., Øyen, R. and Nichols, M. E. (1976). *Transfusion. Philadelphia.* **16**, 529–531.

Mawby, W. J., Anstee, D. J., and Tanner, M. J. A. (1981). *Nature* **291**, 161–162.

Miller, L. H., Mason, S. J., Dvorak, J. A., McGinniss, M. H., and Rothman, I. K. (1975). *Science* **189** 561–562.

Miller, L. H., Haynes, J. D., McAuliffe, F. M., Shiroishi, T., Durocher, J. R. and McGinniss, M. A. (1977). *J. exp. Med.* **146**, 277–281.

Mollison, P. L. (1979). *In* "Blood Transfusion in Clinical Medicine" (6th edn.) pp. 339–352. Blackwell, Oxford.

Nowinski, R., Berglund, C., Lane, J., Lostrum, M., Bernstein, I., Young, W., Hakomori, S., Hill, L. and Cooney, M. (1980). *Science* **210**, 537–539.

Race, R. R. and Sanger, R. (1975). *In* "Blood Groups in Man." pp. 220–227. Blackwell, Oxford.

Sacks, S. and Lennox, E. S. (1981). *Vox Sang.* **40**, 99–104.

Sturgeon, P. (1970). *Blood* **36**, 310–320.

Tanner, M. J. A. and Anstee, D. J. (1976). *Biochem. J.* **153**, 271–277.

Tomita, M., Furthmayr, H. and Marchesi, V. T. (1978). *Biochemistry* **17**, 4756–4776.

Voak, D., Sacks, S. H., Alderson, T., Takei, F., Lennox, E. S., Jarvis, J., Milstein, C. and Darnborough, J. (1980). *Vox Sang.* **39**, 134–140.

Vengelen-Tyler, V., Anstee, D. J., Issitt, P. D., Pavone, B. G., Ferguson, S. J., Mawby, W. J., Tanner, M. J. A., Blajchman, M. A. and Lorque, P. (1981). *Transfusion. Philadelphia.* **21**, 1–15.

Watkins, W. M. (1974). *In* "The Red Blood Cell" (Surgenor, Ed.) 2nd edn. pp. 293–360. Academic Press, New York and London.

Wood, E., Hounsell, E. F., Langhorne, J. and Feizi, T. (1980). *Biochem. J.* **187**, 711–718.

E   MICROBIOLOGY

# 10 Characterization, Structure and Variant Analysis of Viruses with Particular Reference to Influenza

WALTER GERHARD[a] AND ALAN P. KENDAL[b]

a   *The Wistar Institute of Anatomy and Biology, 36th Street at Spruce, Philadelphia, PA 19104. U.S.A.*
b   *World Health Organization Collaborating Center for Influenza, Viral Diseases Division, Center for Infectious Diseases, Centers for Disease Control, Atlanta, GA 30333. U.S.A.*

## I INTRODUCTION

Although many virus families contain several genera and species which have distinctive antigenic specificities, usually the virus properties, when tested by serologic procedures, appear quite stable with only limited variation detected. Influenza A, and to a lesser extent influenza B viruses, however, continually evolve new antigenic variants. This poses unique problems for the efficient diagnosis and control of influenza. Elucidation of the mechanisms by which antigenic variation occurs in influenza viruses has been a long-standing problem in virology, and accordingly it was natural that analysis of influenza viruses should be one of the first subjects of intensive study with monoclonal antibodies. Reflecting this, influenza viruses are the major object of discussion in this review, for which no apology is needed in view of the strong likelihood that the methods and concepts developed with influenza are quite relevant to analysis of other viruses.

The influenza virus genus comprises influenza virus A and B species which exhibit no immunological cross-reactions with each other except for those mediated by host antigens incorporated into virions. Within the influenza A species, subtypes of virus are recognized that differ in their hemagglutinin (HA) and neuraminidase (NA) antigens but cross-react with each other through their type-specific nucloprotein (NP) and matrix protein antigens. The antigenic evolution of influenza virus occurs predominantly in the viral HA and, to a lesser extent, the NA molecules. Operationally, two types of phenomena are distinguished: *antigenic shift* refers to extensive changes observed when a serologically distinct HA or NA subtype (e.g., H1, H2, H3 or N1 and N2) is introduced into the pool of epidemic human influenza A virus strains. This has happened in the past at irregular intervals: probably in 1918 when virus believed to be of H1N1 antigenic composition caused that year's pandemic, in 1957 with the introduction of "Asian" (H2N2) influenza, in 1968 with "Hong Kong" (H3N2) influenza and again in 1977 with the reappearance of H1N1 "Russian"influenza. Since immunity to the viral surface antigens, in particular to the HA molecule, is a major factor in the determination of susceptibility to infection by influenza virus, a shift in the HA molecule has led, in general, to a worldwide (pandemic) spread of the new influenza virus subtype. Once the human population has developed immunity against the new virus subtype, viruses with minor antigenic changes begin to arise. This phenomenon, called *antigenic drift* (which also occurs with influenza B viruses), is thought to result from the selection of spontaneously mutant viruses which circumvent the preexisting anti-viral immunity of the human population as a result of the modification in their HA or NA antigens. The modifications do not result in a complete alteration of antigenic specificity, but change a portion of the antigenic determinants so that some cross-reaction with earlier strains remains (Table 10·1). Various explanations for antigenic drift of influenza HA and NA antigens have been proposed. For instance, drift might be the result of hypermutability of the influenza virus HA and NA genes. Alternatively,

TABLE 10·1
Antigenic drift detected in epidemic strains of influenza A(H3N2)
virus with heterogeneous animal sera

| Antigen | Hemagglutination-inhibition titer with ferret sera | | | | | |
| --- | --- | --- | --- | --- | --- | --- |
| | A/Hong Kong/8/68 | A/England/42/72 | A/Port Chalmers/1/73 | A/Victoria/3/75 | A/Texas/1/77 | A/Bangkok/1/79 |
| A/Hong Kong/8/68 | *2560* | 640 | 160 | 40 | 40 | 20 |
| A/England/42/72 | 640 | *640* | 640 | 80 | 80 | 20 |
| A/Port Chalmers/1/73 | 40 | 40 | *1280* | 80 | 40 | 20 |
| A/Victoria/3/75 | 20 | 40 | 80 | *640* | 80 | 20 |
| A/Texas/1/77 | <20 | <20 | 160 | 80 | *2560* | 320 |
| A/Bangkok/1/79 | 20 | 20 | 20 | 20 | 320 | *1280* |

the antigenic structure of the HA and NA molecules might be formed or
controlled by a few crucial amino acid residues; as a result, a single
mutation in a crucial residue might be sufficient to induce epidemiologically relevant antigenic drift, whereas many mutations might be required to change the antigenic structure of "stable" viruses.

The application of monoclonal antibodies in examining these alternative hypotheses, as well as their potential use in diagnosis and control
of influenza are described. As an additional example of the new
knowledge about the antigenic relationships between viruses that has
been gained with monoclonal antibodies, recent progress in comparing
Lyssaviruses (including rabies) is given. Because of the exponential rate
of increase in reports of application of hybridoma antibodies in other
virus systems, we have chosen to exclude other viruses from this review
except in passing where comparisons are helpful in interpreting results
with influenza

# II DETERMINATION OF THE RATE OF OCCURRENCE OF ANTIGENIC VARIANT VIRUSES

Many previous studies have shown that the infectivity of influenza virus can be neutralized *in vitro* by antisera directed against the HA molecule. However, when individual monoclonal anti-HA antibodies were used instead of anti-HA antisera, viral infectivity could not be neutralized completely (Gerhard and Webster, 1978). This is exemplified in Table 10·2 which shows the infectivity titration of a plaque-cloned influenza virus (strain A/PR/8/34) in the absence and presence of anti-HA hybridoma antibodies. It is evident that the monoclonal antibody failed to abrogate completely virus multiplication at high input virus dose. This was not due to an insufficient concentration of anti-HA hybridoma antibody, because non-neutralized virus almost always had reduced reactivity with the hybridoma antibody with which the parental virus was treated, whereas many other monoclonal anti-HA antibodies reacted, in general, equally well with the parental and the non-neutralized virus. From this one could conclude that the non-neutralized virus fraction represented antigenic variants of the parental virus in which the HA-epitope[a] recognized by the selecting antibody had been modified in such a way as to prevent the monoclonal anti-HA antibody from neutralizing the antigenic variant. Thus, from the ratio of the TCID50 (= virus dose at which 50% of the tissue culture units become infected) in the presence of a monoclonal antibody versus the TCID50 in the absence of antibody one could estimate the prevalence of antigenic variants present in a given virus inoculum. This, therefore, provides an estimate of the rate at which antigenic changes occurred, as a result of spontaneously arising mutations in the HA gene, in the course of virus replication.

Using different influenza virus strains and different anti-HA hybridoma antibodies, the prevalence of antigenic variants has been found to be in the range of $10^{-4}$ to $10^{-8}$ (Yewdell *et al.*, 1979; Webster and Laver, 1980; Lubeck *et al.*, 1980; Nakajima and Kendal, 1981), although it is usually of the order of $10^{-5}$ to $10^{-6}$. This wide range of variant frequencies may have several explanations. Firstly, the proportion of a variant present in a virus seed grown from a single infectious virion may depend on whether that variant arose early or late in the course of virus replication. Clearly, the earlier a given variant arises the more progeny it will be able to generate. Therefore, accurate estimates of the inherent variant frequencies are best obtained by averaging the prevalence of variants detected in many independently grown virus

[a] The structure of the antigen with which the combining site of a monoclonal antibody interacts is termed *epitope* (Jerne, 1974). Individual epitopes may overlap to various extents. Antigenic regions that are topologically discrete and show little or no overlap among each other are termed *antigenic sites* (Atassi and Smith, 1978). Each antigenic site may represent a cluster of largely overlapping epitopes (Yewdell and Gerhard, 1981a).

TABLE 10·2

Determination of the variant virus frequency by titration of virus in the presence and absence of anti-HA antibody

| Antibody | % cultures showing virus growth | | | | | | | | | | TCID 50[a] (log 10) | Frequency of variants |
|---|---|---|---|---|---|---|---|---|---|---|---|---|
| | Dilution of virus inoculum (log 10) | | | | | | | | | | | |
| | −1 | −1·5 | −2 | −3 | −4 | −5 | −6 | −7 | −8 | −9 | | |
| No antibody | nd | nd | nd | 100 | 100 | 87 | 100 | 100 | 25 | 0 | 7·46 | |
| H2-4B3 (α-HA) | 91 | 66 | 16 | 0 | | | | | | | 1·40 | $10^{-6·06}$ |
| H9-D3 (α-HA) | 41 | 33 | 0 | 0 | | | | | | | 0·91 | $10^{-6·55}$ |

Plaque cloned influenza virus A/PR/8/34 (allantoic fluid) was titrated for virus infectivity in the allantois on shell culture system as previously described (Yewdell et al., 1979). Eight to twelve replicate cultures were inoculated at each virus dilution. The cultures were assayed for virus growth by HA titration after three days incubation.

[a] TCID 50 is the virus dose at which 50% of the tissue culture units become infected.

seeds (with the assumption that the mutation does not increase the efficiency of replication of the variant). Secondly, individual epitopes of influenza virus HA molecules might exhibit inherently different mutabilities. For example, the total number of residue changes at different amino acid positions of the HA polypeptide, through which an epitope can be modified sufficiently to permit the mutant virus to escape neutralization, might vary from epitope to epitope. Thus, assuming that each codon in the HA gene has the same inherent mutation rate, an epitope that is modified (directly or indirectly via conformational changes) by amino acid substitutions at any of 30 different sequence positions would change roughly 10 times more frequently than an epitope that can be modified only by mutations at three different amino acid positions. Thirdly, individual anti-HA antibodies may be more or less efficient in neutralization assays at detecting antigenic changes in the corresponding HA epitope, perhaps as a result of their avidity.

To determine whether the observed frequency of antigenic variation in the HA molecules of influenza virus can explain the propensity of influenza to undergo antigenic drift in nature, the frequency of antigenic variants of other viruses grown in the presence of monoclonal antibodies has been determined. Using the same experimental protocol as applied for influenza virus, antigenic variation in the HA-NA molecule of parainfluenza type 1 virus was found to occur at roughly the same frequency as in the HA molecule of influenza virus (Yewdell and Gerhard, 1981b). Yet, there is no evidence that parainfluenza viruses undergo antigenic drift in nature, at least not to the extent seen with influenza. Additionally, using monoclonal antibodies directed against the glycoprotein of rabies virus (Wiktor and Koprowski, 1980) or vesicular stomatitis virus (Portner *et al.*, 1980), antigenic variants were shown to occur among these viruses at a frequency similar to influenza, despite the fact that neither rabies nor vesicular stomatitis virus show marked antigenic drift in nature. These observations suggest that antigenic drift of influenza virus in nature is not a consequence of hypermutability of the HA molecule.

## III THE STRUCTURAL AND ANTIGENIC PROPERTIES OF THE HA MOLECULE OF INFLUENZA VARIANT VIRUSES

To investigate the structural changes that are responsible for the antigenic modifications of variant influenza viruses selected with monoclonal anti-HA antibodies, the HA molecules of several wild type (parental) and their variant viruses prepared as described above have been compared by peptide mapping and amino acid sequencing (Laver *et al.*, 1979a,b; Webster and Laver, 1980; Moss *et al.*, 1980). These studies showed that the antigenic modifications exhibited by virus variants selected in the presence of a single monoclonal antibody resulted from mutations in the HA gene which, in general, changed a single amino acid residue. This has led to identification of amino acid residues that are involved (directly or indirectly, e.g., by conformational mechanisms) in the formation of the protein structures recognized by anti-HA antibodies that have neutralizing activity. In conjunction with knowledge of the three-dimensional structure of the HA molecule of influenza virus A/Hong Kong/68 (H3) (Wilson *et al.*, 1981) it became evident that amino acid changes, found in variants selected *in vitro* with monoclonal antibodies, as well as many of the changes found among epidemic virus strains that had evolved from the A/Hong Kong/68 strain, clustered into four regions of the protein (Wiley *et al.*, 1981). Three of these regions represent external loop structures of the protein and each probably constitutes a major antigenic site of the HA molecule, which can be recognized by virus-neutralizing antibodies. The fourth region is localized in the interface area between subunits of the HA trimer and might have a complex role in determining antigenic specificity. Thus, the interface region might affect antigenic specificity by direct binding of antibodies to areas that are accessible as a result of a certain freedom of movement between subunits, as well as affecting one or several of the other antigenic sites by changing the interactions between subunits.

A consistent picture of the organization of antigenic sites within the HA molecule was obtained also from comparative antigenic analysis of a large panel of mutant viruses selected from influenza virus A/PR/8/34 in the presence of 12 different monoclonal anti-HA antibodies (Gerhard *et al.*, 1981). This approach is exemplified in Table 10·3 which shows the reactivity in radioimmunoassay of 12 anti-HA antibodies with the PR8 mutant viruses selected in their presence. Based on this analysis, the various mutant virus sets and antibodies could be assembled into four major groups designated Sa, Sb, Ca and Cb. Each of these groups is characterized by the fact that the antigenic changes exhibited by several mutant viruses within a given group reduced the binding capacity of the antibodies within the corresponding antibody group but had no or very little effect on the binding of antibodies belonging to a different group. Thus, each of these groups apparently delineates an area of the HA molecule which is able to undergo independent antigenic altera-

TABLE 10·3

Delineation of four antigenic sites on the HA molecule of A/PR/8/34 by antigenic analysis of *in vitro* selected mutant viruses

| | PR8-Mutant viruses | | | | | | | | | | |
| | Sa | | | Sb | | Ca | | | | Cb | | |
| Antibodies | CV (4) | KV (2) | PV (5) | EV (3) | BV (6) | TV (3) | NV (3) | DV (2) | SV (2) | RV (3) | LV (3) | AV (4) |
|---|---|---|---|---|---|---|---|---|---|---|---|---|
| Sa1 (C) | 0 | 1/0 | 0 | + | + | + | + | + | + | + | + | + |
| Sa6 (K) | +/0 | 0 | +/0 | + | + | + | + | + | + | + | + | + |
| Sa4 (P) | +/0 | 0 | 0 | + | + | + | + | + | + | + | + | + |
| Sb6 (E) | + | + | (+) | 0 | +/0 | + | + | + | + | + | + | + |
| Sb7 (B) | + | + | + | 0 | 0 | (+) | + | + | + | + | + | + |
| Ca10 (T) | + | + | + | + | + | 0 | +/0 | +/0 | +/0 | + | + | + |
| Ca1 (N) | + | + | + | + | +/0 | (+) | 0 | + | (+) | + | + | + |
| Ca4 (D) | + | + | + | (+) | + | 0 | +/0 | 0 | +/0 | + | + | + |
| Ca6 (S) | + | + | + | (+) | + | 0 | + | + | 0 | (+) | + | + |
| Cb5 (R) | + | + | + | + | + | + | + | + | + | 0 | +/0 | +/0 |
| Cb13 (L) | + | + | + | + | + | + | + | + | + | +/0 | 0 | 0 |
| Cb14 (A) | + | + | + | + | + | + | + | + | + | 0 | 0 | 0 |

Twelve sets of mutant viruses were selected from A/PR/8/34 in the presence of 12 monoclonal antibodies. Each set of mutant viruses and the antibody used for its selection is designated by the same capital letter, e.g., the CV mutant viruses were selected in the presence of antibody Sa1 (C), etc. The number in parenthesis indicates the number of antigenically unique mutant viruses within each set (see also Gerhard *et al.*, 1981). All mutant viruses were then analyzed in RIA for their capacity to react with the monoclonal antibodies. The plus (+) signs indicate that antibodies react equally well with each virus of a mutant set as with the parental virus PR8. This shows that none of the antigenic changes exhibited by the given mutant viruses modified detectably the epitope recognized by these antibodies. The other signs indicate strongly reduced reactivity of the antibodies with at least one (+/0) or all (0) viruses within a mutant set or [(+)] slightly reduced binding with a single variant within a mutant virus set.

tions, presumably because they represent topologically distinct structures (antigenic sites) of the HA molecule. Further support for this general "map" comes from competitive binding assays with monoclonal antibodies which demonstrate that some antibodies can bind additively to the HA molecule whereas others compete either because they are directed at the same antigenic site, or because they interfere through conformational or steric mechanisms (Lubeck and Gerhard, 1981; Breschkin *et al.*, 1981).

It is evident from the above antigenic map that any given single point mutation changes the total antigenicity of the HA molecule only to a small extent, i.e., it may prevent a variable fraction of the antibodies directed to one site from binding to the mutant virus but has little or no effect of the binding of antibodies directed to the other sites on the HA

TABLE 10·4

HI titer of anti-PR8 antisera and anti-HA hybridoma ascitic fluids
against parental virus and some selected PR8-mutant viruses

| | HI titer[a] | | | | |
| | Antisera[b] | | Hybridoma ascitic fluids[c] | | |
| Virus[d] | 1° BALB/c | 2° BALB/c | H2-4B3 | H2-6C4 | H2-4C2 |
|---|---|---|---|---|---|
| PR8 (parental) | 1050 | 1580 | 155000 | 404000 | 2950 |
| Sa CV2 | 1200 | 1580 | <2800 | 498000 | 3890 |
| Sa KV2 | 850 | 1200 | | | |
| Sa PV1 | 910 | 1200 | <2800 | 267000 | 3890 |
| Sb EV2 | 460 | 1·120 | 166000 | <4200 | 2240 |
| Sb BV2 | <280 | 420 | 83000[e] | 48000 | 1480[e] |
| Sb BV11 | 1050 | 1580 | 110000 | <4200 | 4170 |
| Sb BV13 | <280 | <280 | 48000[e] | 116000 | 1290[e] |
| Ca NV7 | 1200 | 2090 | | | |
| Ca DV4 | 600 | 1580 | | | |
| Ca SV5 | 1280 | 2240 | 309000 | 498000 | 4170 |
| Cb RV1 | 1050 | 1580 | 102000 | 233000 | 790 |
| Cb LV1 | 1200 | 2240 | 145000 | 465000 | <70 |
| Cb AV1 | 1120 | 2090 | | | |

[a]  HI-titer is given as the reciprocal of the antibody dilution inhibiting 3 out of 4 agglutinating
    doses of the virus.
[b]  Antisera obtained from a pool of 10 BALB/c mice 14 days after primary (1°) and 9 days
    after booster inoculation (2°) of purified parental virus A/PR/8/34.
[c]  Ascitic fluid from BALB/c mice inoculated intraperitoneally with hybridoma cells.
[d]  All viruses (except PR8, parental) were shown by analysis with monoclonal antibodies in
    RIA to be antigenic variants.
[e]  The slightly (2-4-fold compared to parental virus) reduced HI-titer of monoclonal anti-
    bodies, directed against sites other than Sb, with these viruses suggests that they are
    adsorptive variants.

molecule. Consequently, an antiserum that contains antibodies
directed against each of the four sites on the HA molecule would be
expected to react practically to the same extent with the parental virus
and any one of the single point mutants derived from the parental virus.
Table 10·4 shows that this is, with rare exception, indeed the case.
Thus, compared to the parental virus, pooled primary and secondary
BALB/c anti-PR8 antisera do not exhibit significantly different HI-
titers against most of the single point PR8-mutant viruses, which is in
marked contrast to the large reduction in HI-titers seen with
appropriate monoclonal antibodies. Analogous observations were
made also with single point mutants of influenza virus A/Memphis/71
(Laver *et al.*, 1979b) and with laboratory variants selected from rabies
virus (Wiktor and Koprowski, 1978).

There are, however, some notable exceptions where antiparental virus antisera were found to exhibit significantly reduced HI-titers against single point mutant viruses. For example, Webster and Laver (1980) observed that a laboratory mutant virus of A/Memphis/71 (in which the glycine at position 144 was substituted by aspartic acid), could be clearly differentiated from the parental virus in HI tests and in Ouchterlony double diffusion by a rabbit anti-parental virus antiserum. Interestingly, the same residue change was observed also among naturally occurring epidemic virus strains of the Hong Kong subtype (Laver *et al.*, 1980).

An attempt to delineate the relative significance of different epitopes in the HA of naturally occurring H1N1 strains was undertaken by Nakajima and Kendal (1981) who selected *in vitro* mutants of A/USSR/90/77 virus in the presence of individual monoclonal antibodies that had previously been used to screen natural isolates (see below). In all cases when variants were selected that had lost the ability to react with one monoclonal antibody (#264), the degree of antigenic change resulting was sufficient that it could be detected not only with the monoclonal antibody but also with heterogeneous ferret antisera. Since many natural variants exhibited a change in the epitope recognized by this antibody, the results supported the view that changes in the epitope recognized by antibody 264 might indeed be associated with epidemiologically significant antigenic drift. Furthermore, one *in vitro* variant selected with monoclonal antibody 264 resembled a field strain, A/Lackland/3/78, in its ferret serum HI reaction pattern.

Results with A/PR/8/34 also indicate that some variants (in the Sb group) exhibiting point mutations have slightly reduced reactivity with BALB/c sera to the parental virus in HI-test (Table 10·4). In this case, however, it seems that the mutations induced a generally decreased susceptibility of the variants to inhibition in the HI test, i.e., the variants may be adsorptive mutants (Fazekas de St. Groth, 1978) that bind more avidly than the parental virus to red blood cells.

These results all suggest that it is conceivable for certain point mutations in critical areas to induce relatively large, epidemiologically relevant antigenic or biologic modifications. The corollary to this is that the humoral immune response *in vivo* may often be of restricted specificity, i.e., it may be directed predominantly against a single antigenic site on the HA molecule.

The production of a restricted immune response may be crucial in the generation of antigenic drift in nature. This is because the presence of four independently mutating antigenic sites on the HA molecule will usually preclude the selection of variants containing alterations in more than one antigenic site of the HA molecule. For example, the A/PR/8/ 34 virus sample used in the experiment shown in Table 10·5, contained $10^{2·16}$ and $10^{2·06}$ infectious virus variants with an alteration in the Sa and Sb site, respectively and, therefore, could not be neutralized completely by individual antibodies directed to these sites. However, no variant able to escape neutralization by both of these antibodies was observed. This is not surprising since the appropriate double point mutant would be expected to occur at a frequency of $10^{-10·78}$ (= product of single point mutant frequencies). Obviously, the frequency of a variant having mutations in all four sites of the HA molecule would be negligably small (e.g., $10^{-20}$ if the average frequency of a single point mutation is $10^{-5}$).

TABLE 10·5

Neutralization of A/PR/8/34 by two monoclonal antibodies directed against different sites on the HA molecule

| Treatment of virus inoculum | Observed TCID50[a] | Frequency of variants | |
|---|---|---|---|
| | | observed | expected |
| None | $10^{7·50}$ | | |
| H2-4B3 (anti-Sa) | $10^{2·16}$ | $10^{-5·34}$ | |
| H2-6C4 (anti-Sb) | $10^{2·06}$ | $10^{-5·44}$ | |
| H2-4B3 + H2-6C4 | $<10^{0·44}$ | $<10^{-7·06}$ | $\sim 10^{-10·78}$ |

Samples of the same cloned virus seed were titrated without further treatment or after incubation with hybridoma antibody, for residual virus infectivity in the allantois on shell culture system as described by Yewdell *et al.* (1979).
[a]   TCID50 is the virus dose at which 50% of the tissue culture units become infected.

Extrapolation to the evolution of new epidemic virus strains, there-fore, suggests that this will be favoured under circumstances where a point mutation causes a major antigenic change and where the host, in which such a mutant arises, possesses antibody restricted largely to the site containing the critical change. Repetitions of this process in subse-quent hosts, leading ultimately to the emergence of a variant with point mutations in most or all of the antigenic sites, might thereby occur, as is proposed to be necessary for development of full epidemic potential by influenza A(H3N2) viruses (Wiley *et al.*, 1981).

# IV VARIATION IN NATURE DETECTED WITH MONOCLONAL ANTIBODIES, AND RELEVANCE TO VIRUS EPIDEMIOLOGY

Studies of natural variation in viruses detected with monoclonal antibodies, thus far reported, are primarily limited to influenza and rabies viruses, although it is to be anticipated that interesting results also will shortly be obtained using monoclonal antibodies to compare the relationships of other viral agents where questions arise about the epidemiological relationship of temporally and geographically separated outbreaks. Hybridoma antibodies specific for the H1 and H3 subtype HAs and to the type A nucleoprotein have been particularly well studied for their ability to distinguish natural variation among influenza viruses.

Much work has been done, for example, identifying the antigenic determinants shared between the HAs of A/PR/8/34 and H1N1 viruses isolated between 1931 to 1957 (Gerhard et al., 1981). Retrospective analysis with monoclonal antibodies of the extent of variation in the four antigenic sites on the HA during natural variation within the H1N1 virus suggests that the rates of variation differed between the sites. Epitopes within the Ca and Cb sites underwent much less variation (drift) than epitopes within the Sa and Sb sites. Most monoclonal antibodies reactive with the Sa and Sb sites of A/PR/8/34 failed to react with any other H1 strain, which is the basis for the designation of these sites as specific sites Sa and Sb. In contrast, monoclonal antibodies directed at epitopes within the Ca and Cb (cross-reactive) sites often (but not always) reacted with several H1N1 virus strains, sometimes including strains isolated 20 years apart (Gerhard et al., 1981). To test whether the low extent of drift in the cross-reactive sites resulted from a hypomutability of the corresponding HA structures, the frequency of antigenic variants arising in vitro in the specific and cross-reactive sites of the HA molecule of influenza virus A/PR/8/34 was determined (Gerhard et al., 1981). Antigenic variants arose, under experimental conditions, at the same frequency in both specific and cross-reactive sites, which did not support the idea of an inherent hypomutability of the Ca and Cb sites. Rather, assuming that antigenic drift in nature results from the selection of spontaneously arising mutant viruses that are less efficiently neutralized by preexisting antiviral immune mechanisms, the selection pressure may have been lower for antigenic variation in the Ca and Cb sites as opposed to the Sa and Sb sites. In agreement with this notion is the low HI- and virus-neutralizing potency (virus neutralization titer/mg antibody per ml) of antibodies directed against site Cb (Russ *et al.*, 1981). On the other hand, antibodies directed against site Ca exhibit, on the average, a high HI- and virus-neutralizing potency (Russ *et al.*, 1981) and it seems possible that the low extent of drift in the latter site resulted from a low immune response of humans to this site (Gerhard *et al.*, 1981).

Because relatively little can be done to relate results of monoclonal antibody analysis to the epidemiology of H1N1 viruses circulating before 1957, attention has also been directed towards analyzing variation in H1N1 viruses that have been prevalent since 1977. Webster *et al.* (1979) studied antigenic drift in H1N1 viruses by means of hybridoma antibodies specific for the HA of A/USSR/90/77 viruses. A set of five monoclonal antibodies specific for different epitopes were used. One question being addressed in this study was the overall relationship of the A/USSR/90/77 HA to that of the isolates from 1949/1950, known on the basis of reactions with heterogeneous antisera to be very closely related to each other. The results of the monoclonal antibody analysis were completely consistent with the belief that the HA of A/USSR/90/ 77 virus showed high genetic homology with that of H1 virus from 1949/1950.

Additionally, the study with H1N1 viruses included a variety of strains isolated from within the same epidemic of H1N1 influenza during 1977–1978. These viruses are presumed to have all derived from a common precursor virus which represented the first re-introduction of H1N1 strains into the human population in 1977. Using the five monoclonal antibodies to A/USSR/90/77 HA, four reaction patterns were detected amongst the naturally circulating H1N1 viruses from 1977– 1978. Many viruses resembled the original A/USSR/90/77 reference strain. A number of other isolates, however, were found to all exhibit a change at one epitope recognized by antibody 264. Viruses were also identified with changes in one or two other epitopes. Subsequently, viruses with a change at the epitope 264 became the predominant H1N1 strains circulating in the world and by 1980 had totally displaced the original USSR-like strains (Nakajima *et al.*, 1981).

Analysis of the evolution of the H1 HA of the A/USSR/90/77 virus was monitored with the monoclonal antibodies in parallel with traditional testing with ferret sera for several years. By 1981, approximately 18 variants distinguishable with ferret sera, monoclonal antibodies or both sets of reagents had been identified (Kendal *et al.*, 1981). Comparison of the HI test results obtained with ferret sera and monoclonal antibodies suggested that in many cases the change in epitopes recognized by monoclonal antibodies was not epidemiologically relevant and could be considered to represent "background noise." This is not surprising in view of the fact that, as described above, variation detectable by monoclonal antibodies occurs at a frequency of approximately $10^{-5}$, which is biologically significant for a virus that produces more than $10^5$ infectious particles in each infectious event. Two of the changes detected by monoclonal antibodies, however, did appear to be correlated with epidemiological events. One of these was the above mentioned loss of reactivity with monoclonal antibody 264, first detected in viruses which circulated in 1978 and which subsequently became "fixed" in all epidemic strains. A second change comparable to this was observed in 1980 when viruses from outbreaks were first identified that had lost the ability to react with monoclonal antibody 110, in addition to monoclonal antibody 264. These viruses were themselves not homogeneous when tested with ferret sera and monoclonal antibodies, but since early 1980 it has become apparent that the prevalent strains of influenza A (H1N1) all share the characteristics of failing to react with monoclonal antibodies 264 and 110 regardless of other differences that can be detected between them (Table 10·6).

TABLE 10·6

Changes in epidemic strains of influenza A(H1N1) viruses that have become "fixed", 1978–1981

| Year first detected | Variation detected in epidemic strain by antibody | | | | | Reference epidemic strain |
|---|---|---|---|---|---|---|
| | W18 | 22 | 70 | 110 | 264 | |
| 1978 | − | − | − | − | + | A/Brazil/11/78[a] |
| 1980 | − | − | − | + | + | A/England/333/80[a] |

[a] A proportion of epidemic isolates from different regions also exhibited reduced reactivity with antibody W18, believed to bind within the same determinant as antibody 264 (Kendal *et al.*, 1981).

These findings cannot, however, be interpreted to mean that changes in the epitopes recognized by antibodies 264 and 110 by themselves result in a sufficient antigenic change in the virus as to be responsible for the virus' epidemic potential. As judged by HI tests with heterogeneous animal sera the reference strains representing the isolates first seen to lack the ability to react with antibody 264 (A/Brazil/11/78) and subsequently to additionally lose the ability to react with antibody 110 (A/England/333/80) themselves show relatively small antigenic drift from their precursor epidemic strains (Table 10·7). Other variants identified at about the same time have showed far greater divergence from preceeding epidemic strains when tested with heterogeneous anti-sera yet failed to become predominant (Nakajima *et al.*, 1981). One explanation that may be proposed for this finding is that changes in the epitopes recognized by antibodies 264 and 110 exert their effect on the virus epidemiology not by altering antigenicity but by altering a func-tional property of the influenza HA which gives the virus an epidemiological advantage. Unlike the H3 HA discussed above, no information is currently available about the changes in the sequence or structure of the influenza H1 HA associated with the changes detected by monoclonal antibodies. The antibodies 264 and 110 were shown, however, to be directed at different antigenic sites on the A/USSR/90/77 HA (Nakajima and Kendal, 1981), and, as discussed in a preceeding section, the site recognized by antibody 264 demonstrably contributed to the dominant antigenic specificity of the HA.

TABLE 10·7

Antigenic variation between epidemic strains showing sequential change in hemagglutinin epitopes, tested with heterogenous animal sera

| Antigen | Ferret serum | | |
|---|---|---|---|
|  | A/USSR/77 | A/Brazil/78 | A/England/80 |
| A/USSR/90/77 | 320 | 320 | 640 |
| A/Brazil/11/78 | 80 | 640 | 640 |
| A/England/333/80 | 80 | 320 | 640 |

In the case of monoclonal antibody 110, however, mutants selected to exhibit change in the epitope recognized by this antibody were indistin-guishable from the A/USSR/77 precursor when tested with heterogene-ous ferret sera. This epitope therefore appears to participate very little in the overall antigenic specificity of the HA and is a candidate for a mutational event affecting biological properties other than antigenicity, which may have contributed to the epidemic spread of viruses related to A/England/333/80. It should be emphasized that such a view is highly speculative, but nevertheless it is important to recognize that antigenic changes detected with monoclonal antibodies may in some cases be "markers" for biological properties. A precedent for this exists in the case of A/New Jersey/76 virus where minor antigenic change was associated with altered replication characteristics (Kilbourne, 1978).

Analysis of the H3 HA with monoclonal antibodies has been largely done for the purpose of selecting variants *in vitro* to compare with reference strains representing epidemiologically important variants (Webster and Laver, 1980) and to determine the site of amino acid changes discussed above. Sleigh *et al.* (1981) independently compared a small number of reference strains of H3N2 influenza viruses isolated from 1968–1975 using a panel of monoclonal antibodies believed to have about six different reaction specificities. Results of both sets of studies are consistent with the notion that after about 1972 the epidemic strains of H3N2 virus had substantially reduced reactivities with nearly all monoclonal antibodies prepared using early A/Hong Kong/68-like viruses.

Analysis of reference strains only may provide misleading evidence about the epidemiologic significance of changes detected with monoclonal antibodies. Influenza A (H3N2) strains from within recent epidemics have been compared, and results were similar to those observed with H1N1 virus in that considerable heterogeneity is detected among those natural isolates (personal communication, R. G. Webster and J. J. Skehel) consistent with results of ferret serum analyses (WHO, (1980). *Wkly. Epid. Rec.* **55**, p. 73). Analogous results were obtained when variation among influenza B viruses was studied with monoclonal antibodies in that the heterogeneity of isolates within epidemics detected with ferret sera (WHO, (1980). *Wkly. Epid. Rec.* **55**, p. 73) was reflected in differences observed with monoclonal antibodies (Webster and Berton, 1981).

Considerable variation has been observed also in influenza NA which was studied with five monoclonal antibodies. Although one antibody detected a conserved epitope on the NA of viruses isolated from 1946–1957, in view of the small number of antibodies included in this analysis, it is premature to make a general conclusion regarding the significance of this finding. Perhaps, the conserved NA epitope represents only a minor portion of the total antigenicity of the NA molecule which happens to be recognized by one of the randomly selected monoclonal anti-NA antibodies. This possibility illustrates that results obtained with monoclonal antibodies should always be evaluated in the context of the total antigenicity as delineated with heterogeneous antisera.

Comparison of the antigenic specificity of the nucleoprotein (NP) of type A influenza viruses using hybridoma antibodies was reported by Van Wyke *et al.*, 1980. A set of five monoclonal antibodies was obtained which when tested in radioimmunoassay with the NP of different influenza viruses had individual reaction patterns even though NP is a type-specific antigen. One of the antibodies reacted with all of the type A influenza NP examined, including those from man, swine, horse and various avian species, whereas the other four antibodies failed to react with several of the large number of viruses tested. Evidence for antigenic variation in the NP detected with monoclonal antibodies is consistent with previous results obtained using absorbed hyperimmune antisera (Schild *et al.*, 1979). However, the sensitivity level for detection of variation in the NP was greater when monoclonal antibodies were used.

Six groupings of influenza A viruses were identified based on the NP monoclonal antibody reaction patterns, and the variation in the NP did not correlate with the variation in the HA or NA subtype antigens. As in the case of many changes in the HA and NA antigens detected by monoclonal antibodies, it is possible that some of the changes occurring in the NP reflect either random mutations which are of no biologic significance ("noise") or alternatively, the antigenic changes are coincidentally associated with (i.e., represent antigenic markers for) biological changes that have advantages for the survival of the virus. Many of the NP groupings determined by analysis with monoclonal antibodies included viruses from different animal species. The results therefore fail to point out a species specific structure of the NP of influenza viruses that affects the virus' host range. Currently there is also no way to relate antigenic markers in NP with epidemic potential in man.

Large-scale studies of the antigenic divergence of viruses using monoclonal antibodies have also been done for proteins of rabies and rabies-related viruses (Lyssaviruses) (Wiktor and Koprowski, 1978). In two studies the specific antigenic variation in the nucleocapsids and glycoproteins of these viruses have been described. Using 21 hybridoma antibodies, the nucleocapsids of rabies and rabies related viruses were classified into eight groups having unique reaction patterns (Flamand *et al.*, 1980a). Eleven of 21 hybridoma antibodies reacted with fixed or attenuated strains of rabies virus but failed to react with three rabies-related viruses studied; and four of the fixed strains of rabies could not be differentiated from each other. Twenty-five hybridomas were available for testing the glycoprotein antigens of these viruses and were classified into 14 groups having distinct reaction patterns (Flamand *et al.*, 1980b). As with antibodies specific for the Lyssavirus NP, a majority of antibodies reacted with the fixed strains of rabies virus but failed to react with rabies-related virus, although a small number were found that cross-reacted with all viruses tested. Some of the hybridoma antibodies exhibited extremely fine specificity in that they reacted with only one or two out of the total number of eight virus strains tested. The antibodies were used to compare, by fluorescent antibody staining of infected animal brain sections, street viruses isolated in different regions of the world. They identified previously undetected variation among these viruses and between street viruses and attenuated strains used for vaccine production (Wiktor *et al.*, 1980). The significance of these changes for vaccine efficacy is currently under evaluation. As monoclonal antibodies against other viruses are used it is likely that previously undetected variation will come to attention and require interpretation. The explosion of information about the antigenic variation made possible by monoclonal antibodies will likely test the abilities of many investigators to sift out the significant from the non-significant observations.

## V APPLICATION OF MONOCLONAL ANTIBODIES FOR VIRUS DIAGNOSIS AND CONTROL

Diagnosis of viral infections is currently done by a variety of procedures, including inhibition of a biological activity such as hemagglutination or infectivity, or by direct detection of viral antigens using immunological staining procedures or immunoassays. Monoclonal antibodies offer the potential to provide reproducible reagents of high specificity that would reliably differentiate virus isolates. Possible disadvantages in the use of monoclonal antibodies however, include the fact that natural variation among viral antigens may result in monoclonal antibodies prepared against a reference strain having reduced, or no, reactivity against certain wild isolates.

To overcome the problem of natural variation in different epitopes among field isolates, it may be necessary to use as reagents a panel of monoclonal antibodies, or alternatively a pool of monoclonal antibodies, so as to maximize chances that several of the antibodies used will retain the abilities to react with field isolates. Practical drawbacks exist to either of these approaches. If a panel of monoclonal antibodies is used, this significantly increases the total amount of work involved in identifying a virus compared to the use of a single heterogeneous antiserum. Use of pools of monoclonal antibodies may result in the reagents having variable potency depending upon the proportion of antibodies constituting the pool which react with individual field isolates. Furthermore, the potency of monoclonal antibodies for detection of viruses may be lower than obtainable with heterogeneous antisera if several antigens within the virus are capable of reaction but monoclonal antibodies specific for a single antigen are used. This is less likely to be the case in assays involving only a single virus antigen (e.g., inhibition of biological activity) than in immunometric procedures where many antigens can react (e.g., RIA, ELISA). Finally, monospecificity of the antibodies would be expected to decrease the level of reaction obtained when the amount of antigen is limiting.

Examples of several of these situations have been observed in studies with influenza virus. The above mentioned panel of five monoclonal antibodies specific for A/USSR/90/77 HA failed to react with a proportion of influenza A H1N1 isolates during 1980, although the variants nevertheless still reacted with heterogeneous animal sera to A/USSR/90/77 or related viruses (Kendal *et al.*, 1981, and Table 10·8).

TABLE 10·8

Hemagglutination inhibition reactions with heterogeneous ferret sera of sporadically identified influenza A(H1N1) variants exhibiting reduced reactivity with 80 to 100% of a panel of five monoclonal antibodies

| | Ferret sera | | | A/USSR/77 monoclonal antibody | | | | |
|---|---|---|---|---|---|---|---|---|
| Antigen | A/USSR/77 | A/Wash. DC/102/80 | A/Lerwick/80 | W18 | 22 | 70 | 110 | 264 |
| A/USSR/90/77 | *320* | 320 | 320 | 1,600 | 3,200 | 12,800 | 1,600 | 3,200 |
| A/Washington DC/102/80 | 80 | *640* | 320 | 100 | 800 | <400 | <100 | <100 |
| A/Lerwich/61694/80 | 160 | 1,280 | *1,280* | 200 | <100 | <400 | <100 | <100 |

A pool of monoclonal antibodies specific for influenza HA has been compared with heterogeneous antisera specific for HA, NP or all virus components in an immunoassay to detect viral antigen produced in tissue culture. The sensitivity of detection of antigen was considerably lower using this monoclonal antibody pool than using the hyperimmune sera (Table 10·9). As shown in Table 10·10, individual monoclonal anti-HA antibodies vary drastically with respect to their sensitivity of detecting viral antigen, probably as a result of differences in their avidities. Thus, for maximum utility in diagnostic work, it will be essential to select those antibodies which have the highest stability and avidity, and which, when incorporated into a pool, will contribute in an additive fashion to the total reaction detected (Lubeck and Gerhard, 1981; Breschkin *et al.*, 1981). If this is achieved it is probable that

TABLE 10·9

Comparison of sensitivity of reaction of monoclonal antibody and
heterogeneous antibody in immunofluorometric assay with influenza virus

| FITC-conjugate | | Sensitivity of reaction[a] | |
|---|---|---|---|
| Source antibody | Specificity | Maximum fluorescence intensity[b] | Minimum virus detected[c] |
| Hyperimmune rabbit serum | Whole virion | >0·30 | 1/128 |
| Hyperimmune goat serum | Ribonucleoprotein | 0·28 | 1/128 |
| Hyperimmune goat serum | Hemagglutinin | 0·25 | 1/128 |
| Monoclonal pool[d], mouse ascites | Hemagglutinin | 0·06 | 1/8 |

[a] FITC-conjugated antibody at optimal dilution was reacted with influenza A/Brazil/11/78 (H1N1) virus and soluble antigens bound to solid phase latex beads, and fluorescence intensity determined in a fluorometer.
[b] Determined with undiluted virus antigen.
[c] Maximum dilution of virus antigen yielding a fluorescence intensity of twice background.
[d] Contains three IgG antibodies reactive with different antigenic sites on A/Brazil/11/78 HA and having avidities ranging from about $3\text{-}30 \times 10^{-11} \, M^{-1}$.

monoclonal antibodies can be a valuable adjunct or perhaps an alternative to antisera in viral diagnosis. Advantages of monoclonal antibodies need to be objectively examined, however, under field conditions before the reagents are adopted for use as a replacement for heterogeneous animal sera in viral diagnostic tests.

Examples of use of monoclonal antibodies in virus diagnosis include studies by Wiktor *et al.* (1980) who found monoclonal antibodies useful

TABLE 10·10

Ability of anti-HA hybridoma antibodies to detect limiting quantities
of viral antigen

| Antibody | Number of hemagglutinating units of influenza virus A/PR/8/34 detected by RIA | | | | | | | |
|---|---|---|---|---|---|---|---|---|
| | 4 | 2 | 1 | 1/2 | 1/4 | 1/8 | 1/16 | 1/64 |
| H35-C10-2 | + | + | + | − | | | | |
| H36-55-4 | + | + | + | + | − | | | |
| H35-C7-2 | + | + | + | + | + | − | | |
| H36-18-2 | + | + | + | + | + | + | + | − |

Constant amounts of monoclonal antibodies were incubated with decreasing quantities of purified influenza virus adsorbed to radioimmunoassay plates. The amount of bound antibody was then determined using $^{125}$I-labeled rabbit anti-mouse immunoglobulin. The antibodies are all of the IgG2a class and were used at concentrations that gave similar amounts of bound antibody at the highest antigen concentration.

for fluorescent antibody (FA) staining of brain smears from rabies infected animals, and Richman *et al.* (1981) have used monoclonal antibodies to identify influenza viruses growing in tissue culture cells infected with clinical specimens. Advantages over use of heterogeneous sera in the latter example were not described. However, Wands *et al.* (1981) showed that the detection of hepatitis B surface antigen (HBsAg) in human sera could be improved by using an anti-HBsAg hybridoma antibody of high avidity.

One of the hopes that may be held out for application of monoclonal antibodies would be the ability to detect antigenic changes within viral molecules that were of epidemiological or clinical interest. Should knowledge of the structure of viral proteins increase to the level where certain epitopes can be recognized as being of critical significance, then analysis with monoclonal antibodies would offer new opportunities to make prognostications about the impact of virus isolates based on laboratory antigenic analysis.

The potential to use monoclonal antibodies in therapy of viral infections based on diagnostic tests identifying the specific antigenic structure of epidemic viruses is also tantilizing. Production of human monoclonal antibodies which react specifically with viral proteins has become possible (Croce *et al.*, 1980). Monoclonal antibodies might thus be used in the future to analyze viral isolates so as to determine an appropriate immunotherapeutic regime. Even in this vision of the "biotechnological age", it is necessary to recall the intrinsic biological variability of viral antigens. The use of a single monoclonal antibody for therapy would likely result in selection of a mutant no longer reactive with that antibody. There is a certain irony in the prospect of mixing antibodies that have been prepared with great effort so far as to be monoclonal, in order to obtain polyclonal pools most useful for diagnostic or therapeutic purposes. Nevertheless, the irony of the situation should not be permitted to obscure its rationality.

## VI SUMMARY

The knowledge of the antigenicity and antigenic variability of influenza virus hemagglutinin (HA) has been greatly enhanced by the use of monoclonal antibodies. With these reagents, four antigenic sites have been delineated on the HA molecule of influenza virus A/PR/8/34 on the operational basis that each site can undergo independent antigenic alterations. This is consistent with the finding that the amino acid residue changes, observed among naturally occurring epidemic virus strains of the H3N2 subtype, cluster into four topographically discreet regions of the three-dimensional structure of the H3 HA molecule.

Variant viruses that exhibit antigenic alterations in individual epitopes of the HA molecule could readily be selected *in vitro* by means of monoclonal anti-HA antibodies. With few exceptions, these antigenic variants were shown to represent point mutants resulting from single base changes in the HA gene. The mutants arise spontaneously in the course of virus replication at an average frequency of about one variant per epitope and per $10^5$ virus progeny. This is comparable to the frequency of antigenic variation occurring in the glycoproteins of all other viruses studied so far with monoclonal antibodies and indicates that antigenic drift seen with influenza viruses in nature is not the result of an inherent hypermutability of the HA molecule.

Probably not all variation that occurs naturally is of epidemiological significance and many changes detected by monoclonal antibodies may represent "background noise." Some antigenic changes, however, may be "markers" for sequence variation which affect the epidemiologic potential of the virus variant. Therefore, when monoclonal antibodies are used to compare field isolates of viruses, a major problem is to determine the significance of differences that can be detected with these highly specific reagents.

Analysis of virus variants selected *in vitro* with monoclonal antibodies suggests that emergence of new epidemic strains may be initiated by the occurrence, perhaps in an individual possessing antibodies of restricted specificity directed predominantly at one antigenic site, of a virus variant bearing a point mutation in a critical locus that significantly alters the antigenic specificity of that site. Repetition of this event in sequentially infected individuals may permit accumulation of multiple point mutations that result ultimately in the emergence of epidemiologically significant variants that would otherwise arise at an exceptionally low frequency within a single individual. The four antigenic sites in the HA may vary in their *natural* mutation rate, reflecting different evolutionary pressures, although they exhibit *in vitro* similar frequency of variation when selective pressure is applied with monoclonal antibodies.

Evaluation of hybridoma antibodies in virus diagnosis is still at an early stage. Probably panels or pools of antibodies are needed in many cases to provide information superior to that obtainable with heterogeneous antisera, and the composition of the panels or pools must be optimized for the specific purpose. Sensitivity of reactions might be lower with monoclonal antibodies than with heterogeneous sera if antigen is limiting. Optimal results are likely to depend on use of monoclonal antibodies of high avidity and which bind non-competitively to all distinct antigenic sites on the antigen of interest.

Further applications of knowledge gained from the use of monoclonal antibodies are suggested for prevention and control of viral infections.

ACKNOWLEDGEMENTS

This work was supported, in part, by grants AT-13989 from the National Institutes of Health and RG-851C6 from the Multiple Sclerosis Society.

REFERENCES

Atassi, M. Z. and Smith, J. A. (1978). *Immunochemistry* **15**, 609–610.
Breschkin, A. M., Ahern, J. and White, D. O. (1981). *Virology* **113**, 130–140.
Croce, M. C., Linnenbach, A., Hall, W., Steplewski, Z. and Koprowski, H. (1980). *Nature* **288**, 488–489.
Fazekas de St. Groth, S. (1978). *Topics Infect. Dis.* **3**, 25–48.
Flamand, A., Wiktor, T. J. and Koprowski, H. (1980a). *J. Gen. Virol.* **48**, 97–104.
Flamand, A., Wiktor, T. J. and Koprowski, H. (1980b). *J. Gen. Virol.* **48**, 105–109.
Gerhard, W. and Webster, R. G. (1978). *J. exp. Med.* **148**, 383–392.
Gerhard, W., Yewdell, J. W., Frankel, M. and Webster, R. G. (1981). *Nature* **290**, 713–717.
Jerne, N. K. (1974). *Annls. Immunol. Inst. Pasteur, Paris* **1250**, 373–389.
Kendal, A. P., Cox, N., Nakjima, S., Webster, R. G., Bean, W. and Beare, P. (1981). *In* "Genetic Variation Among Influenza Viruses" ICN-UCLA Symposia on Molecular and Cellular Biology (D. Nayah and C. F. Fox, Eds), Vol. XXII. Academic Press, London and New York.
Kilbourne, E. D. (1978). *Proc. natn. Acad. Sci. U.S.A.* **75**, 6258–6262.
Laver, W. G., Gerhard, W., Webster, R. G., Frankel, M. E. and Air, G. M. (1979a). *Proc. natn. Acad. Sci. U.S.A.* **76**, 1425–1429.
Laver, W. G., Air, G. M., Webster, Z. G., Gerhard, W., Ward, C. W. and Dopheide, T. A. A. (1979b). *Virology* **98**, 226–237.
Laver, W. G., Air, G. M., Dopheide, T. A. and Ward, C. W. (1980). *Nature* **283**, 454–457.
Lubeck, M. D. and Gerhard, W. (1981). *Virology* **113**, 64–72.
Lubeck, M., Schulman, J. L. and Palese, P. (1980). *Virology* **102**, 458–462.
Moss, B., Underwood, P. A., Bender, V. J. and Whittaker, R. G. (1980). *In* "Structure and Variation in Influenza Virus" (W. G. Laver and G. Air, Eds), pp. 329–338. Elsevier, North Holland.
Nakajima, S. and Kendal, A. P. (1981). *Virology* (in press).
Nakajima, S., Cox, N. J. and Kendal, A. P. (1981). *Inf. Immunol.* **32**, 287–294.
Portner, A., Webster, R. G. and Bean, W. G. (1980). *Virology* **104**, 235–238.

Richman, D., Cleveland, P., Oxman, M., Van Wyke, K. and Webster, R. G. (1981). *Proc. Fifth Int. Congress Virol.* p. 170.

Russ, G., Gerhard, W. and Laver, W. G. (1981). *In* "Genetic Variation Among Influenza Viruses" ICN-UCLA Symposia on Molecular and Cellular Biology (D. Nayak and C. F. Fox, Eds). Vol. XXII. Academic Press, London and New York.

Schild, G. C., Oxford, J. S. and Newman, R. W. (1979). *Virology* **93**, 569–573.

Sleigh, M. J., Both, G. W., Underwood, P. A. and Bender, V. J. (1981). *J. Virol.* **38**, 845–853.

Van Wyke, K. L., Hinshaw, V. S., Bean, W. J. and Webster, R. G. (1980). *J. Virol.* **35**, 24–30.

Wands, J. R., Carlson, R. I., Shoemaker, H., Isselbacher, K. J. and Zurawski, V. Z. (1981). *Proc. natn. Acad. Sci. U.S.A.* **78**, 1214–1218.

Webster, R. G. and Berton, M. T. (1981). *J. Gen. Virol.* (in press).

Webster, R. G. and Laver, W. G. (1980). *Virology.* **104**, 139–148.

Webster, R. G., Kendal, A. P. and Gerhard, W. (1979). *Virology* **96**, 258–264.

Wiktor, T. J. and Koprowski, H. (1978). *Proc. natn. Acad. Sci. U.S.A.* **75**, 3938–3942.

Wiktor, T. J. and Koprowski, H. (1980). *J. exp. Med.* **152**, 99–112.

Wiktor, T. J., Flamand, A. and Koprowski, H. (1980). *J. Virol. Meth.* **1**, 33–46.

Wiley, D. C., Wilson, I. A. and Skehel, J. J. (1981). *Nature* **289**, 373–378.

Wilson, I. A., Skehel, J. J. and Wiley, D. C. (1981). *Nature* **289**, 366–373.

Yewdell, J. W., Webster, R. G. and Gerhard, W. (1979). *Nature* **279**, 246–247.

Yewdell, J. W. and Gerhard, W. (1981a). *Ann. Rev. Microbiol.* **35**, 185–206.

Yewdell, J. W. and Gerhard, W. (1981b). *In* "The Replication of Negative Strand Viruses" (D. H. L. Bishop and R. W. Compans, Eds), pp. 603–608. Elsevier, North Holland.

# 11    Characterization of Epstein-Barr Virus Antigens: Towards a vaccine for malignancies associated with the virus

M. A. Epstein and J. R. North

*Department of Pathology, University of Bristol Medical School, University Walk, Bristol. BS8 1TD*

# I  INTRODUCTION

Epstein-Barr (EB) virus (Epstein *et al.*, 1964), one of the five human herpesviruses, is a lymphotropic agent whose target cells are usually restricted to the B lymphocyte lineage. Thus, only human and certain subhuman primate B cells have receptors for the virus (Pattengale *et al.*, 1973; Jondal and Klein, 1973) and can be infected by conventional methods; however, if the virus DNA is microinjected or receptors are provided artificially, then a variety of other cell types can support some stages of virus replication (Graessmann *et al.*, 1980; Volsky *et al.*, 1980).

The virus has proved difficult to work with in the laboratory since the replicative functions of its genome are not readily expressed *in vitro*, and in the absence of a fully permissive cell system, techniques which are taken as a matter of course with banal "lytic" herpesviruses cannot be employed. Instead, EB virus has to be quantified and its biological activity assessed on the basis of transforming functions which confer on normal target B cells the ability to grow into continuous lines in culture (Pope, 1979). Nevertheless, since some EB virus-carrying lines contain a small number of cells which spontaneously enter the virus productive cycle (producer lines) it has been possible to determine the sequence of antigen expression and other events during virus replication (Epstein and Achong, 1977a), and conversely to elucidate the range and pattern of antibody responses to the various antigens in different EB virus-related conditions (W. Henle and G. Henle, 1979).

# II  EPIDEMIOLOGY OF EB VIRUS INFECTION

EB virus is ubiquitous in all human populations and is spread by horizontal infection. Natural primary infection usually takes place in childhood without clinical manifestations and is always accompanied by seroconversion with development of specific antibodies to virus-determined antigens, by the establishment of permanent immunity to reinfection, and by a harbouring of the virus which persists for the rest of the individual's life. This harbouring takes two forms:– (*i*) a small number of circulating B lymphocytes from any seropositive individual can be shown to carry the virus genome; (*ii*) there is a productive infection such that virus is shed into the buccal fluid. This shedding of the virus is responsible for the horizontal transmission which causes natural primary infections. In developed countries about 75 to 80% of the population ultimately becomes infected, in contrast to developing countries where 99·9% of children are already infected by the age of about 3. These findings have recently been documented elsewhere (Epstein and Achong, 1979a; W. Henle and G. Henle, 1979; G. Henle and W. Henle, 1979).

The immunologically privileged site from which EB virus genome-containing B lymphocytes are released into the blood throughout life despite specific humoral and cellular immunological controls, is not known. Nor is it understood what relationship, if any, this site may have to the source of virus replication which gives rise to the shedding of infectious particles into the buccal fluid. However, it is well known that the incidence of individuals shedding EB virus from the mouth varies in different populations and under different conditions. In developed countries about 20% of healthy seropositive individuals are shedders at any one time and the dependence of this on a delicate immunological balance is evident from the fact that the rate rises significantly to more than 50% of seropositives subjected to immunosuppressive therapy. A similarly raised incidence of shedders has been observed in the general population of developing countries perhaps as a result of the immuno-suppressive effects of malarial and other parasitic infections. During acute infectious mononucleosis (IM), shedding of EB virus into the oropharynx occurs in almost all patients. The various aspects of virus shedding have been discussed by Epstein and Achong (1979a) and G. Henle and W. Henle (1979).

It has usually been assumed that the productive infection in the oropharynx was restricted to B lymphocytes within Waldeyer's Ring, since only B cells were known to have receptors for the virus. However, the finding of EB virus at the orifice of Stensen's duct (Niederman *et al.*, 1976) and the observation that cannulated duct fluid contained considerably more virus than the buccal fluid (Morgan *et al.*, 1979) led to the suggestion that salivary gland epithelial cells may also be involved. The concept of EB virus replication in epithelial cells has become more acceptable in recent years following experiments in which virus production by the virus genome-containing squamous epithelial cells of nasopharyngeal carcinomas (NPC) was demonstrated both after grafting in nude mice and *in vitro* (Trumper *et al.*, 1976 and 1977; Crawford *et al.*, 1979) and the possibility remains that the source of buccal fluid virus may ultimately be traced to some special type of oro/nasopharyngeal epithelial cell.

If natural primary infection is delayed to adolescence or young adulthood, there is a 50% chance that it will be accompanied by the clinical manifestations of IM. Such delayed infection is more frequent in the privileged classes of Western societies enjoying high standards of hygiene, than in the lower socio-economic groups, thus explaining the characteristic association of IM with affluence. The uniformly early age of EB virus infection in developing countries, which leaves no adolescents or young adults susceptible, accounts for the virtual absence there of IM. These epidemiological observations concerning EB virus and IM have recently been reviewed in detail (Epstein and Achong, 1977b; G. Henle and W. Henle, 1979).

Why natural primary infection should usually remain clinically silent in childhood yet carry a 50% risk of IM amongst adolescents and young adults, almost certainly relates to the size of viral dose, mode of infection, and host physiological and immunological responses in the two age groups. Young children appear to be readily infected by casual contamination with a small dose of virus shed into the environment whereas, in contrast, adolescents and young adults can only be infected with considerable difficulty. IM has long been recognized for its association with kissing among young people (Hoagland, 1955) and it would appear that the disease is only induced where a healthy seropositive individual shedding virus passes large quantities of the agent in buccal fluid to a seronegative (and therefore susceptible) partner during direct osculatory contact. Indeed, there is very good evidence that infection is not transmitted where susceptible young adults merely share a room and washing facilities with those in the acute stage of IM (Hallee *et al.*, 1974) when the maximum shedding of virus occurs (Niederman *et al.*, 1976). However, although almost all IM is seen in those aged 15–25, it is worth noting that primary infection in very young children and in quite old adults can very occasionally be accompanied by the fully developed disease (Ginsberg *et al.*, 1977; Horwitz *et al.*, 1976). In any event, the ultimate consequences of IM are exactly the same as with a silent primary infection—seroconversion, solid immunity to subsequent reinfection with EB virus, and life-long harbouring of the virus.

## III ASSOCIATION OF EB VIRUS WITH HUMAN TUMOURS

EB virus is associated with two, and only two, human malignancies, namely endemic (sometimes termed African) Burkitt's lymphoma (BL) (Burkitt, 1958) and undifferentiated or poorly differentiated NPC. It is most important that the exact nature of these two cancers should be understood and defined (Burkitt, 1963; Shanmugaratnam, 1971), since the restriction of the association to these tumours alone is of itself highly significant. Apart from BL, other lymphomas are quite unrelated to the virus, and tumours of the post-nasal space other than undifferentiated

NPC or anywhere in the head and neck outside that narrow topographical region, are likewise unrelated to the virus.

Both BL and NPC are monoclonal tumours. BL is always of B lymphocyte origin, and the tumour cells consistently carry a chromosomal abnormality, t(8q−:14q+), characteristic of many B cell malignancies. In contrast NPC, however undifferentiated at the light microscope level, can always be shown to be of squamous epithelial origin since electron microscopy reveals keratin and desmosomes in the tumour cells. NPC epithelial tumour cells thus provide the only example apart from B lymphocytes of cells which are naturally infected with EB virus, although the agent's mode of entry remains obscure. These findings have been discussed elsewhere (Epstein and Achong, 1979b; Klein, 1979a).

## A. BURKITT'S LYMPHOMA

The recognition of an oncogenic role for EB virus in BL rests on the following points:–

1.   An unusually high level of antibodies to virus capsid antigen (VCA) occurs in BL patients, with geometric mean titres 8–10 times greater than those of control sera from African children or patients with other malignancies. In addition, there is a specific pattern of antibody reactivities with uniquely high titres to early antigen (EA) of the restricted (R) type, and patients with BL show changes in these antibody levels having a close and peculiar association with clinical events in the disease.

2.   All the tumour cells of almost all properly authenticated cases of endemic BL carry the EB virus genome. It is this virus genome which causes the expression in the tumour cells *in vivo* of the EB virus nuclear antigen (EBNA) and the EB virus-determined membrane antigen (MA), and nucleic acid hybridization studies have demonstrated that there are, in fact, multiple copies of EB virus DNA in each BL cell. In many instances, placing tumour cells in culture is sufficient to activate in some cells the resident EB virus DNA, to give a productive infection with release of infectious virus particles—indeed the virus was first discovered in such circumstances.

3.   A World Health Organisation prospective seroepidemiological survey has followed 42,000 Ugandan children for 7 years and found 12 cases of BL; studies of the pre-disease serum samples have shown remarkably raised titres of antibodies to VCA for many months or years

before onset of the tumour, and from these data the risk factor attached to such high serological responses has been calculated. The risk of developing endemic BL was thirty times higher for individuals with VCA antibody titres of two doubling dilutions or more above those of the control population, a risk almost twice that long accepted as establishing an aetiological relationship between heavy cigarette smoking and bronchogenic carcinoma.

4.   EB virus is capable of transforming normal human B lymphocytes into continuously proliferating cell lines carrying the EB virus genome and showing many of the characteristics of malignant transformation.

5.   EB virus has been shown to be experimentally oncogenic in South American sub-human primates; the virus causes malignant lymphoproliferative disease in cotton top marmosets and owl monkeys, and confirmation of a dose response has been obtained.

6.   Animal herpesviruses known to produce malignant tumours either naturally or experimentally provide striking parallels with EB virus in BL and NPC.

Each of these points has been fully documented in recent reviews (Epstein, 1978a; Epstein and Achong, 1979b).

### B. Nasopharyngeal Carcinoma

Although the evidence is so far less extensive, many of the features of the relationship of EB virus to BL have likewise been found in the association of the virus with NPC. Thus, patients have high titre antibodies to the virus with a characteristic pattern of reactivities; in this case the high titre antibodies to EA are directed against the diffuse (D) type of antigen and there is also production of IgA to VCA. Antibody levels usually change in response to clinical events. The virus DNA is present in all the malignant epithelial cells of NPC tumours, causes the expression in them of EBNA, and can be detected by nucleic acid hybridization. References in support of these observations can be found in Epstein (1978b) and Klein (1979a).

### C. Co-Factors

If, as now seems virtually certain, EB virus plays some sort of causative role in endemic BL, it clearly cannot do so alone since the virus is widespread throughout the world (W. Henle and G. Henle, 1979) whereas the high incidence endemic areas of the tumour are restricted to certain parts of tropical Africa and New Guinea showing specific features of temperature and rainfall (Burkitt, 1962a and 1962b; Booth *et al.*, 1967). It has long been clear that the spread of the virus was in no way climate-dependent, and it seems likely now that a co-factor affected by temperature and rainfall is responsible for determining the geographical distribution of the tumour; Burkitt has made a persuasive case for hyperendemic malaria as such a co-factor (Burkitt, 1969) and a considerable body of evidence supports this view (Burkitt, 1969; Williams, 1966; Pike *et al.*, 1970). Even so, other influences must also play a significant part in causation for, where BL is endemic almost the whole population is infected by EB virus at an early age (Henle and Henle, 1969) and hyperendemic malaria, by definition, affects over 50% of young children, yet only small numbers of these doubly infected individuals develop BL. The possible additional co-factors which have been suggested include a specific genetic predisposition, unusually early infection by the virus, or some special temporal relationship between first infection with the virus and infection with malaria. The ways in which the various co-factors might interact have been considered elsewhere (Epstein and Achong, 1979b; De-Thé, 1979; Klein, 1979b).

In the case of NPC, the long-recognized racial predisposition, shown by the high incidence of the tumour amongst Southern Chinese and related races of South East Asia (Clifford, 1970; Shanmugaratnam, 1971) and the moderately high incidence in parts of North and East Africa (Clifford, 1970; Cammoun *et al.*, 1974), has been put on a firm basis by the demonstration of a genetic co-factor. Among Southern Chinese, those having an HLA profile with an HLA-A2 and BW46 haplotype have a three times higher incidence of NPC than the rest of the population (Simons *et al.*, 1976). In addition, environmental co-factors are also involved; Southern Chinese immigrants living in California have the same high incidence of NPC as do the Chinese in Southern China, but their local born descendants have a lower incidence, although this is still strikingly higher than that seen in the surrounding Caucasian population (Henderson, 1974). Furthermore, there is a definite risk factor for members of low incidence racial groups born and raised in high incidence regions (Henderson *et al.*, 1976). However, despite extensive search, the nature of the environmental co-factors responsible has not so far been determined (Clifford, 1970; Shanmugaratnam, 1971).

## IV EB VIRUS-INDUCED ANTIGENS

With the exception of the lymphocyte-detected membrane antigen (LYDMA), all currently known EB virus-associated antigens have been discovered in the course of studies with naturally occurring human antibodies. These serologically defined antigens are discussed below in the order in which they were first reported; full bibliographical details have been provided by Ernberg and Klein (1979).

### A. Virus Capsid Antigen (VCA)

VCA is usually detected by indirect immunofluorescence and occurs in both the nucleus and the cytoplasm. Other detection methods which have been reported include immunoperoxidase and the use of radio-iodinated antibodies. There is some early evidence that seven major proteins are associated with this antigen.

### B. Membrane Antigen (MA)

MA is also demonstrated by indirect immunofluorescence. It has been subtyped into early (EMA) and late (LMA) components; EMA is independent of virus DNA synthesis and is present in fresh BL tumour cells from biopsy samples and in some cells of virus producer lymphoid lines irrespective of their origin. LMA is expressed during the later stages of virus production after virus DNA synthesis has taken place, and is accompanied by VCA. Since MA is carried onto the viral envelope as the virion is released by budding through cellular membranes, it is not surprising that antibodies to MA are also virus neutralizing.

### C. Early Antigen (EA)

The EA complex is seen following indirect immunofluorescence using sera from patients with EB virus-related diseases. Such sera have reactivities, additional to antibodies to VCA, which have permitted the recognition of two components in the EA complex:– the R occurring as clumps in the cytoplasm and destroyed by 95% alcohol; and the D in both the nucleus and cytoplasm, which is alcohol insensitive but rather readily digested by proteases. EA includes a complex of virus-determined inhibitors of cellular nucleic acid and protein synthesis and is not incorporated in the mature virus particle.

## D. EB Virus Nuclear Antigen (EBNA)

EBNA is detected in the nucleus by three-layer anticomplement immunofluorescence and there is good evidence (Reedman *et al.*, 1972; Klein and Vonka, 1974) that it is identical with a heat-stable, complement fixing, soluble (S), EB virus-associated antigen first described by Pope *et al.* (1969), and probably also with a soluble antigen demonstrable by immunodiffusion (Old *et al.*, 1966). EBNA associates with chromosomes during mitosis, binds to double stranded DNA, and shows many similarities to the T antigens of SV40 and other oncogenic papovaviruses. EBNA appears to contain antigenically specific subunits of 48,000 daltons which complex with a non-specific 53,000 molecular weight cellular protein to give a molecule of about 180,000 daltons (Luka *et al.*, 1980); this complex in EBNA is of special interest because the cellular component has also been found complexed with T antigen in SV40 transformed cells and in other malignant cells transformed in various ways (Jay *et al.*, 1979).

## E. Lymphocyte Detected Membrane Antigen (LYDMA)

LYDMA is the only EB virus-induced antigen for which naturally occurring antibodies have not yet been demonstrated. It was originally invoked to explain the apparent specific *in vitro* cytotoxicity for EB virus-carrying B cells, of T cells from IM patients (Svedmyr and Jondal, 1975), and was subsequently thought to be present on all such virus genome-positive cells (Klein *et al.*, 1976). However, there was a disturbing absence of evidence for any restriction by the major histocompatability complex (see chapter 14) of the T cell recognition of LYDMA, and some doubt as to the adequacy of the panel of target cells used in the early experiments to establish the specificity of the phenomenon.

More recently, it has been shown beyond question that all EB virus-infected individuals carry in the peripheral circulation for life, memory T lymphocytes from which cytotoxic cells can be grown up *in vitro*. The cytotoxicity does not require serum or soluble factors but depends absolutely on T cells from seropositive donors, and these T cells are specific for EB virus-carrying target cells (Moss *et al.*, 1978; Rickinson *et al.*, 1979; Moss *et al.*, 1979; Moss *et al.*, 1981a). The cytotoxic T cells show clear-cut HLA restriction on their recognition of EB virus-positive B lymphocytes (Rickinson *et al.*, 1980; Misko *et al.*, 1980; Wallace *et al.*, 1981) and in addition, it has been found that with any given seropositive individual, the "strength" of the memory T cell response remains remarkably constant over months and years (Rickinson *et al.*, 1981). There is no correlation between the expression of MA and LYDMA, and neither the nature of the antigen recognized as LYDMA in association with the HLA determinants, nor its function, are known.

## F. ANTIGEN EXPRESSION IN INFECTED CELLS

Studies on EB virus-carrying producer lines, in which a few cells spontaneously enter the virus productive cycle at any one time, and on normal B lymphocytes to which the virus has been added *in vitro*, have shed light on the cellular events following infection.

Where the virus transforming function is expressed and normal cells are induced to replicate to give a continuously proliferating line, the first antigen to be detected is EBNA which is seen after about 12 hours (Menezes *et al.*, 1978; Einhorn and Ernberg, 1978; Takada and Osato, 1978). EBNA expression is independent of DNA synthesis, is followed by blastogenesis at about 24 hours, and by cellular DNA synthesis at about 36 hours (Takada and Osato, 1978). EMA appears to follow (Ernberg *et al.*, 1974; Sairenji *et al.*, 1977) and recent experiments indicate that LYDMA is also expressed at this time, some 24 hours after EBNA (Moss *et al.*, 1981b); both EMA and LYDMA are independent of DNA synthesis. At an as yet undetermined stage after this the virus DNA is replicated and the transformation event takes place. Transformed cells thus express only EBNA, LYDMA, and EMA, with other viral functions held in abeyance. In these circumstances, EBNA is thought to play a role in initiating or maintaining transformation (Ernberg and Klein, 1979) perhaps in combination with the 53,000 molecular weight protein with which it forms complexes.

When the viral replicative functions predominate it has been considered that infected cells pass through the foregoing stages of antigen expression (Ernberg *et al.*, 1976) but bypass the transformation event; instead, they proceed to the expression of EA which inhibits all cellular RNA, DNA and protein synthesis (Gergely *et al.*, 1971a), to virus DNA synthesis, and finally to the production of VCA and LMA to provide components for the assembly and release of infectious virus particles (Epstein and Achong, 1977a). However, it has recently been suggested that the expression of EBNA may relate exclusively to transformation leaving a different EBNA-negative pathway leading to the virus productive cycle (Volsky *et al.*, 1981). This would fit well with and explain an earlier observation on the presence of EBNA-negative EB virus-containing cells in the blood during IM (Crawford *et al.*, 1978).

## V USE OF MONOCLONAL ANTIBODIES FOR ANTIGEN CHARACTERIZATION

While some progress has been made in assigning EB virus-induced polypeptides to the antigen systems defined by immunofluorescence, the lack of resolution using polyspecific antisera, combined with inevitable uncertainties in molecular weight estimations, has prevented the conclusive identification of the structural and functional roles of most molecules.

### A. MOLECULAR COMPLEXITY OF EB VIRUS-INDUCED ANTIGENS

The double stranded DNA of EB virus has been confirmed as having a molecular weight of $10^8$ daltons (Schulte-Holthausen and Zur Hausen, 1970; Becker and Weinberg, 1972; Pritchett *et al.*, 1975) and if maximum coding potential were realized it should be able to specify more than 100 proteins (Pritchett *et al.*, 1976). Indeed, 33 polypeptides have been resolved in purified virions alone by SDS-PAGE analysis (Dolyniuk *et al.*, 1976a) and 7 of these could be removed by detergent treatment and are likely therefore to be components of the viral envelope (Dolyniuk *et al.*, 1976b). The assignment of polypeptides in the virion, as well as virus-induced non-structural polypeptides, to known antigen systems has, until recently, proceeded slowly owing to the complexity of the antisera available for antigen characterization. As has already been pointed out, human sera with naturally occurring antibodies usually show a spectrum of reactivities to EB virus-induced antigens which varies in different circumstances (W. Henle and G. Henle, 1979), and with one exception (Zajac and Ogburn, 1975) xenogeneic antisera with proven monospecificity have not so far been developed.

Several recent studies have attempted to classify the multitude of EB virus-associated polypeptides synthesized in virus-producing cells or in the EB virus genome-carrying, non-producer cell line, Raji (Pulvertaft, 1964; Epstein *et al.*, 1966) after superinfection, using observations on the time of polypeptide appearance, sensitivity to various metabolic inhibitors, and ability to bind human antisera of known reactivities. These studies have described between 11 and 16 polypeptides in the EA complex, although with discrepancies in molecular weight estimation and the antisera used, it is not yet clear whether each analysis has identified the same set of components (Kallin *et al.*, 1979; Mueller-Lantzsch *et al.*, 1979 and 1980a; Bodemer *et al.*, 1980; Feighny *et al.*, 1981; Bayliss and Wolf, 1981). Two additional polypeptides have also been identified in cells producing virus and these are generally assumed to be the major components of VCA, since molecules of the same size are present in the nucleocapsid; these VCA polypeptides have been estimated to have molecular weights of between 165,000 and 150,000 daltons and 158,000 and 140,000 daltons respectively (Kallin *et al.*, 1979; Mueller-Lantzsch *et al.*, 1979; Kawanishi *et al.*, 1981; Edson and Thorley-Lawson, 1981).

More precise information has been obtained on components of the MA complex despite the limitations of polyvalent antisera, since advantage can be taken of various methods for the identification of molecules originating in the cell membrane (Thorley-Lawson and Edson, 1979; Qualtière and Pearson, 1979 and 1980; Strnad *et al.*, 1979; North *et al.*, 1980; Mueller-Lantzsch *et al.*, 1980b). Such work has demonstrated that some MA polypeptides are glycosylated, and has yielded substantial agreement on the size of three of the molecules; allowing for the variability and imprecision of measurements made on SDS-PAGE, it would appear that the MA on the surface of most EB virus-producing human cell lines includes major glycoproteins having molecular weights of about 320,000, 220,000 and 85,000 daltons (conveniently designated gp 320, gp 220 and gp 85). In contrast, there is disagreement over a further polypeptide of 140,000 molecular weight which may or may not be glycosylated, and over the nature of two other slightly larger molecules.

An interesting feature of MA is that when expressed by EB virus-producing marmoset lines, its two highest molecular weight components are slightly larger than their counterparts on human cells, i.e. 340,000 and 270,000 (designated gp 340 and 270) (North *et al.*, 1980; Qualtière and Pearson, 1980; Edson and Thorley-Lawson, 1981) and it has been suggested that these differences reflect species divergencies in glycosylation pathways. In order to reduce complications arising from these slight species-related differences in molecular weight, the two largest MA glycoproteins will be referred to globally as gp 340/220, irrespective of the particular cells from which they originate.

In addition to differences in MA dependent on species, it has also been found that two commonly used laboratory strains of EB virus (P3HR-1, B95-8) both specify MA complexes which are unusual in the relative amounts of the two highest molecular weight polypeptides, as compared with MA specified by a number of other isolates (Thorley-Lawson and Edson, 1979; North *et al.*, 1980; Qualtière and Pearson, 1980; Mueller-Lantzsch *et al.*, 1980b; Blake *et al.*, 1981). In view of the well known changes in genome undergone by these two aberrant EB virus strains during laboratory passage (Raab-Traub *et al.*, 1978 and 1980; Kieff *et al.*, 1979; Bornkamm *et al.*, 1980), such observations are not surprising.

Since naturally occurring antibodies to MA were found to react with virus particles (Silvestre *et al.*, 1974) it has long been suspected that MA polypeptides would be found on the EB virus. More recent work has shown that xenogeneic antisera to purified virions have anti MA-activity (Thorley-Lawson, 1979a; North *et al.*, 1980), and it has now actually been demonstrated that MA components are present in the viral envelope (North *et al.*, 1980).

## B. Monoclonal Antibodies to EB Virus-Induced Antigens

It is evident from the foregoing that the complexities of EA and VCA have hardly begun to be explored, and although the broad outlines of EBNA and MA are appreciated, many problems remain. The advent of monoclonal antibodies has now provided a new tool for work in this field. Several monoclonal antibodies to EB virus-induced antigens have already been developed, and in all cases so far the procedures used have involved immunization of Balb/c mice with purified EB virus and detection of antibody activity by the ability to bind to EB virus-producing cells. It is not surprising therefore that all the resulting monoclonal antibodies show activity against MA or VCA-like antigens.

Using monoclonal antibodies it has already emerged that gp 340 and gp 220 are structurally related, but antigenically distinct, molecules. Of 25 clones so far described, antibodies from 11 bind both gp 340 and gp 220, while 14 only bind to gp 340 (Hoffman *et al.*, 1980; Thorley-Lawson and Geilinger, 1980; Franklin *et al.*, 1981; Mueller-Lantzsch *et al.*, 1981). This could be explained on the basis that the molecules have identical polypeptide sequences but differ in their sugar side chains, although experiments using tunicamycin, a drug which inhibits glycosylation, imply that similar amounts of carbohydrate are normally present in each molecule (Edson and Thorley-Lawson, 1981). An alternative suggestion, that monoclonal antibodies which precipitate both gp 340 and gp 220 do so through conformational determinants arising from close proximity of the molecules (Mueller-Lantzsch et al., 1981), appears unlikely since such precipitation of the components from lysates of B95-8 and P3HR-1 occurs independently and the components themselves move independently on gel chromatography in deoxycholate (Thorley-Lawson and Geilinger, 1980; Franklin et al., 1981; A. J. Morgan and J. R. North, unpublished). The possibility that carbohydrate antigens are shared or that the molecules are coded for by the same or related genes, cannot yet be evaluated.

An indication of the importance of the role which monoclonal antibodies will play in elucidating the complexities and inter-relationships of all the EB virus-determined antigens is already evident in connection with MA and VCA. Two separate monoclonal antibodies to the gp 340/220 components of MA have shown cytoplasmic staining of acetone fixed cells (Hoffman et al., 1980; Thorley-Lawson and Geilinger, 1980) similar to that seen in the conventional test for VCA (Henle and Henle, 1966), and the close correspondence of the two staining patterns has been demonstrated using double immunofluorescence (Hoffman et al., 1980). In view of the well-known difficulty in discriminating between VCA and EA (R) staining with polyvalent human antisera, the unequivocal demonstration of MA components in the cytoplasm using monoclonal antibodies emphasizes the need for such reagents to disentangle the MA, VCA and EA complexes. It is not surprising that MA should be detectable together with these other antigens in the cytoplasm since like them it is synthesized during virus replication, and as a membrane protein its synthesis must presumably occur on membrane-associated ribosomes. This in turn would explain how MA components are incorporated in the viral envelope (North et al., 1980) during virus release by budding through cytoplasmic membrane, a process known to occur with EB virus in addition to budding at the cell surface (Epstein and Achong, 1979c).

Using conventional antisera, indications have been obtained of antigenic differences between the MA polypeptides induced by different virus isolates (Franklin et al., 1981), and these observations have now been confirmed by the use of a panel of monoclonal antibodies (Mueller-Lantzsch et al., 1981). It seems likely that extension of this type of work will complement comparative DNA sequencing (Bornkamm et al., 1980; Raab-Traub et al., 1980) in the search for disease-related EB virus strain differences which have so far not been identified.

Apart from the clear identification of gp 340/220 as a major component of the MA complex, the roles of the numerous other EB virus-induced molecules of EBNA, VCA, EA, and the smaller components of MA (140,000 and 85,000 daltons) remain to be elucidated. Recently developed monoclonal antibodies to molecules of about the appropriate size (Mueller-Lantzsch *et al.*, 1981) are likely to be of importance in investigations of this type. It is also likely that the true molecular nature of LYDMA will ultimately become clear as soon as serological procedures, based on monoclonal antibodies which recognize this antigen, have been developed. (See note added in proof, p. 300.)

Once all of the EB virus-induced antigens have been defined in molecular terms by investigations based on monoclonal antibodies, it should be possible to dissect the spectrum of naturally occurring antibody responses to EB virus seen in various clinical situations. The precise definition of these various antibodies could well provide the basis for tests of diagnostic and prognostic value in routine clinical practice.

## VI RATIONALE FOR AN EB VIRUS VACCINE

In view of the almost certain contribution of EB virus to the aetiology of BL, and the many similarities in the relationship of the virus to that tumour which are repeated in its relationship to NPC, it would appear that prevention of infection by the virus should reduce the incidence of these two tumours by removing an essential component from the complex of factors responsible for their causation.

Although BL is not a major problem even in the highest incidence areas, a vaccine programme is nevertheless more than justified on the basis of the association of EB virus with NPC. As already pointed out, NPC is the commonest tumour of men and the second commonest tumour of women in populations of Southern Chinese origin (Shanmugaratnam, 1971), and there is a less high but significant incidence of the tumour running in a belt across North Africa, down through the Sudan and into certain upland regions of Kenya (Clifford, 1970; Camoun *et al.*, 1974). Thus, in terms of world health, the tumour is of very considerable importance; Southern Chinese and related races alone constitute about one quarter of the world's population (Shanmugaratnam, 1971).

## A. Ethical Considerations

The possibility of developing an anti-viral vaccine to be used in the control of EB virus-associated malignancies has been urged for some years (Epstein, 1976), but it has been recognized at the same time that any vaccine involving a suspected human tumour virus would only be acceptable for administration to man if it were free from all trace of virus nucleic acid. That such a vaccine could be feasible became clear when it was demonstrated that susceptible chickens can be protected to a very considerable extent against the lymphomas induced by the herpesvirus of Marek's disease, through the use of vaccines free of viral nucleic acid; success was first reported with a vaccine consisting of the purified plasma membranes of Marek's virus-infected tissue culture cells (Kaaden and Dietzschold, 1974), and soluble viral antigens extracted from such cells by non-ionic detergents have also proved efficacious (Lesnick and Ross, 1975). Similarly, solubilized antigens from cells infected with Herpesvirus saimiri have been shown to be antigenic in sub-human primates and to be capable of eliciting virus-neutralizing antibodies (Pearson and Scott, 1977); actual protection against challenge with carcinogenic doses of Herpesvirus saimiri has so far only been induced in cotton-top marmosets by a heat and formaldehyde killed virus vaccine (Laufs and Steinke, 1975).

This type of work has recently been extended to EB virus. It has been known for some time that in man naturally occurring antibodies to EB virus MA are closely related to virus-neutralizing antibodies (Pearson *et al.*, 1970 and 1971; Gergely *et al.*, 1971b; De Schryver *et al.*, 1974), and now an experimentally induced rabbit antiserum which neutralizes EB virus and also binds selectively to MA-positive lymphoid cell lines has been described (Thorley-Lawson, 1979a). Furthermore, antigenic determinants extracted from the membrane of EB virus-infected cells have proved capable of eliciting neutralizing antibodies in experimental animals (Pearson and Qualtière, 1978; Thorley-Lawson, 1979b). Development of a vaccine for human use involving material of this type would meet the principal ethical objections to a more conventional vaccine based on preparations of a virus thought to play a causative role in human carcinogenesis.

## B. Practical Considerations

For the preparation of a purified MA vaccine against EB virus, the large scale production of the necessary cells does not present any special

problems nor is it especially expensive. The most important consideration with regard to such a vaccine concerns verification of the absence of
viral DNA. From the logistic point of view this safety testing is again not
unduly difficult, particularly when compared to the immense efforts
required for the much more complicated problem of safety testing with
killed polio vaccines 25 years ago.

The essential experimental investigation of the antigenicity and protective efficacy of an MA polypeptide vaccine calls for the use of
susceptible animals and here organizational difficulties are likely to be
encountered. As already mentioned, EB virus is capable of causing
malignant lympho-proliferative tumours in cotton-top marmosets and
owl monkeys and both these species are now, unfortunately, becoming
increasingly rare and subject therefore to international restrictions on
their supply. There is thus a special need for the establishment of
breeding colonies of these animals on a large scale.

Once it has been shown that an appropriate nucleic acid-free vaccine
can protect susceptible sub-human primates against tumour induction
on subsequent challenge with infectious EB virus, and that this does not
engender immunopathological complications, the next step must
involve extension of the work to human volunteers. The effectiveness of
the vaccine in man could be investigated in the context of EB virus
seronegative young people at risk for primary infection in Western
countries in the age group where this is accompanied by IM.

Assuming that protection against the development of primary infection accompanied by IM can be successfully achieved, the vaccine
could then be considered for a trial to show that the prevention of EB
virus infection, seemingly a necessary component in the multifactorial
aetiology of BL, significantly reduces the subsequent occurrence of the
tumour in a high incidence trial area. This would parallel the situation
with the herpesvirus of Marek's disease where the agent is widespread
in chicken populations but only exercises its oncogenic potential in
combination with certain individual, environmental, and genetic influences (Payne, 1973), and where vaccine protection against virulent
virus prevents the development of lymphomas.

A field trial involving a vaccine against EB virus in relation to BL has
certain special advantages; firstly, there are well-recognized endemic
areas in which the tumour has a relatively high incidence and where the
effects of a vaccine programme would be readily manifest (Williams *et
al.*, 1978); and secondly, since endemic BL is a disease with a peak
incidence in children around the age of six (Burkitt, 1963), it should be
possible to vaccinate all members of a population between the ages of
three and twelve months in an endemic area and to judge the effect on

tumour development within eight to ten years. Over this period, of course, re-vaccination to maintain immunity is likely to be required, but this should not present any greater logistic difficulties than those encountered in the prospective seroepidemiological survey so success-fully carried out in Uganda during the 1970's under the auspices of the World Health Organisation (De-Thé et al., 1978). And even if actual prevention of infection cannot be achieved, it might well be that a modest boost to immunity against EB virus would be sufficient to provide protection against the induction of BL, merely by some trivial change in the host's immunological balance such as, for example, a reduction in viraemia at a stage after infection critical for the malignant transformation of target cells which must precede the development of the tumour.

## VII ROLE OF MONOCLONAL ANTIBODIES IN VACCINE PRODUCTION

In order to develop an anti-EB virus vaccine based on MA it is neces-sary both to identify which components of the antigen complex elicit virus-neutralizing antibodies, and to elaborate methods for their puri-fication on a large scale.

The first of these tasks has been simplified by the finding that a rabbit antiserum which only reacts with gp 340/220 components of MA, nevertheless possessed considerable EB virus neutralizing activity (North et al., 1980), indicating that immunization with these compo-nents alone would induce neutralizing antibodies. This supposition has been confirmed by the ability of two, independently derived, mono-clonal antibodies to gp 340/220 to neutralize the virus (Hoffman et al., 1980; Thorley-Lawson and Geilinger, 1980). Furthermore, since it is clear that the virus-neutralizing monoclonal antibodies bind to anti-genic determinates shared by both the gp 340 and gp 220 MA glycopro-teins (see above), immunization with either of these molecules should be effective.

For the purification of MA, any efficient method must rely on the distinguishing features of the gp 340/220 polypeptides, and it is fortu-nate that these molecules have a number of useful characteristics which can be exploited. Thus:–

1.   Location on Cellular Membranes. The conventional approach to the preparation of membrane proteins from EB virus-producing cells would involve cell disruption followed by purification of the plasma

membranes by sucrose density gradient centrifugation (Crumpton and Snary, 1974), and indeed such preparations do contain the gp 340/220 components. However, since cytoplasmic membranes of virus-producing cells also bear gp 340/220 (Hoffman *et al.*, 1980; Thorley-Lawson and Geilinger, 1980), greater yields are possible when the whole membrane fraction is retained.

2. Large Size. Because of the unusually large size of the molecules in question, when membranes are solubilized in Triton X100 or de-oxycholate and separated by gel chromatography on Ultrogel Aca-22 (LKB, Bromma, Sweden), gp 340 and gp 220 migrate separately according to their molecular weights as determined on SDS-PAGE, and are thus separated from most other membrane proteins. Incidentally, even better molecular weight separations can be achieved after reduction and blocking of sulphydrile groups, and the use of buffers containing 8M urea and 0·5% deoxycholate on sepharose CL6B (Pharmacia, Uppsala, Sweden). The removal of disulphide links and exposure to 8M urea does not reduce the antigenicity of gp 340/220 (J. R. North and A. J. Morgan—unpublished).

3. Lectin Binding. As regards affinity for lectins, gp 340/220 binds lentil lectin (R. communis agglutinin II) (ricin), and soybean lectin, but not U. europeus or H. pomatia lectins (Thorley-Lawson and Edson, 1979; Strnad *et al.*, 1979). Although lentil and soybean lectins cannot be used in purification procedures owing to difficulties with elution, insolubilized ricin permits 99% of MA activity to be eluted with galactose at approximately 50-fold purification (Thorley-Lawson and Edson, 1979).

4. Ability to Elicit Monoclonal Antibodies. The use of monoclonal antibodies on immunoadsorbent columns (see chapter 22) has been valuable in the purification of various membrane glycoproteins (Sunderland *et al.*, 1979; Brown *et al.*, 1981; Campbell *et al.*, 1981), and the availability of several monoclonal antibodies to gp 340/220 makes it likely that this technique will play an important role in purification. However, since no single monoclonal antibody yet tested is capable of binding all gp 340/220 molecules from a given cell line (J. R. North—unpublished), the use of more than one such antibody on a Sepharose column should considerably increase the efficiency of the process. Lack of binding of all gp 340/220 molecules by individual monoclonal anti-bodies does not necessarily imply low affinity, and preliminary experiments would seem to indicate that this property arises from antigenic heterogeneity within the gp 340/220 population.

In addition to their use on immunoadsorbent columns, monoclonal antibodies provide invaluable methods for the quantification of antigen yields at the various steps of purification in a manner not possible with polyspecific antisera.

REFERENCES

Bayliss, E. J. and Wolf, H. (1981). *J. Gen. Virol.* **56**, 105–118.
Becker, Y. and Weinberg, A. (1972). *In* "Oncogenesis and Herpesviruses" (P. M. Biggs, G. de-Thé and L. N. Payne, Eds), pp. 326–335. IARC, Lyon.
Blake, K., North, J. R., Morgan, A. J. and Epstein, M. A. (1981). (submitted to press).
Bodemer, W. W., Summers, W. C. and Niederman, J. C. (1980). *Virology* **103**, 340–349.
Booth, K., Burkitt, D. P., Bassett, D. J., Cooke, R. A. and Biddulph, J. (1967). *Brit. J. Cancer* **21**, 657–664.
Bornkamm, G. W., Delius, H., Zimber, U., Hudewenz, J. and Epstein, M. A. (1980). *J. Virol.* **35**, 603–618.
Brown, W. R. A., Barclay, A. N., Sunderland, C. A. and Williams, A. F. (1981). *Nature* **289**, 456–460.
Burkitt, D. (1958). *Br. J. Surg.* **46**, 218–223.
Burkitt, D. (1962a). *Nature* **194**, 232–234.
Burkitt, D. (1962b). *Brit. med. J.* **2**, 1019–1023.
Burkitt, D. (1963). *In* "International Review of Experimental Pathology" (G. W. Richter and M. A. Epstein, Eds), 2, pp. 67–138. Academic Press, London and New York.
Burkitt, D. (1969). *J. natn. Cancer Inst.* **42**, 19–28.
Cammoun, M., Hoerner, G. V. and Mourali, N. (1974). *Cancer* **33**, 184–192.
Campbell, D. G., Gagnon, J., Reid, K. B. M. and Williams, A. F. (1981). *Biochem. J.* **195**, 15–30.
Clifford, P. (1970). *Int. J. Cancer* **5**, 287–309.
Crawford, D. H., Rickinson, A. B., Finerty, S. and Epstein, M. A. (1978). *J. Gen. Virol.* **38**, 449–460.
Crawford, D. H., Epstein, M. A., Bornkamm, G. W., Achong, B. G., Finerty, S. and Thompson, J. L. (1979). *Int. J. Cancer* **24**, 294–302.
Crumpton, M. J. and Snary, D. (1974). *Contemp. Topics Molecular Immunol.* **3**, 27–56.
De Schryver, A., Klein, G., Hewetson, J., Rocchi, G., Henle, W., Henle, G., Moss, D. J. and Pope, J. H. (1974). *Int. J. Cancer* **13**, 353–362.
De-Thé, G. (1979). *In* "The Epstein-Barr Virus" (M. A. Epstein and B. G. Achong, Eds), pp. 417–437. Springer—Berlin, Heidelberg and New York.
De-Thé, G., Geser, A., Day, N. E., Tukei, P. M., Williams, E. H., Beri, D. P., Smith, P. G., Dean, A. G., Bornkamm, G. W., Feorino, P., and Henle, W. (1978). *Nature* **274**, 756–761.
Dolyniuk, M., Pritchett, R. and Kieff, E. (1976a). *J. Virology* **17**, 935–949.

Dolyniuk, M., Wolff, E. and Kieff, E. (1976b). *J. Virology* **18**, 289–297.

Edson, C. M. and Thorley-Lawson, D. A. (1981). *J. Virology* **39**, 172–184.

Einhorn, L. and Ernberg, I. (1978). *Int. J. Cancer* **21**, 157–160.

Epstein, M. A. (1976). *J. natn. Cancer Inst.* **56**, 697–700.

Epstein, M. A. (1978a). *In* "Viruses and Human Cancer" (Y. Ito, Ed.), pp. 72–99. S. Karger, Basel.

Epstein, M. A. (1978b). *In* "Nasopharyngeal Carcinoma: Etiology and Control" (G. de-Thé, Y. Ito and W. Davis Eds), pp. 333–345. IARC, Lyon.

Epstein, M. A. and Achong, B. G. (1977a). *Ann. Rev. Microbiol.* **31**, 421–445.

Epstein, M. A. and Achong, B. G. (1977b). *Lancet*, **ii**, 1270–1273.

Epstein, M. A. and Achong, B. G. (1979a). *In* "The Epstein-Barr Virus" (M. A. Epstein and B. G. Achong, Eds), pp. 1–22. Springer—Berlin, Heidelberg and New York.

Epstein, M. A. and Achong, B. G. (1979b). *In* "The Epstein-Barr Virus" (M. A. Epstein and B. G. Achong, Eds), pp. 321–337. Springer—Berlin, Heidelberg and New York.

Epstein, M. A. and Achong, B. G. (1979c). *In* "The Epstein-Barr Virus" (M. A. Epstein and B. G. Achong, Eds), pp. 23–37. Springer—Berlin, Heidelberg and New York.

Epstein, M. A., Achong B. G. and Barr, Y. M. (1964). *Lancet* **i**, 702–703.

Epstein, M. A., Achong, B. G., Barr, Y. M., Zajac, B., Henle, G. and Henle, W. (1966). *J. natn. Cancer Inst.* **37**, 537–559.

Ernberg, I. and Klein, G. (1979). *In* "The Epstein-Barr Virus" (M. A. Epstein and B. G. Achong, Eds), pp. 39–60. Springer—Berlin, Heidelberg and New York.

Ernberg, I., Masucci, G. and Klein, G. (1976). *Int. J. Cancer* **17**, 197–203.

Feighny, R. J., Henry II, B. E., Pagano, J. S. (1981). *J. Virology* **37**, 61–71.

Franklin, S. M., North, J. R., Morgan, A. J. and Epstein, M. A. (1981). *J. Gen. Virol.* **53**, 371–376.

Gergely, L., Klein, G. and Ernberg, I. (1971a). *Virology* **45**, 22–29.

Gergely, L., Klein, G. and Ernberg, I. (1971b). *Virology* **45**, 10–21.

Ginsburg, C. M., Henle, W., Henle, G. and Horwitz, C. A. (1977). *J. Am. med. Ass.* **237**, 781–785.

Graessmann, A., Wolf, H. and Bornkamm, G. W. (1980). *Proc. natn. Acad. Sci. U.S.A.* **77**, 433–436.

Hallee, T. J., Evans, A. S., Niederman, J. C., Brooks, C. M. and Voegtly, J. H. (1974). *Yale J. Biol. Med.* **47**, 182–195.

Henderson, B. E. (1974). *Cancer Res.* **34**, 1187–1188.

Henderson, B. E., Louie, E., Jing, J. S., Buell, P. and Gardner, M. B. (1976). *New Engl. J. Med.* **295**, 1101–1106.

Henle, G. and Henle, W. (1966). *J. Bact.* **91**, 1248–1256.

Henle, G. and Henle, W. (1979). *In* "The Epstein-Barr Virus" (M. A. Epstein and B. G. Achong, Eds), pp. 297–320. Springer—Berlin, Heidelberg and New York.

Henle, W. and Henle, G. (1969). *E. African Med. J.* **46**, 402–406.

Henle, W. and Henle, G. (1979). *In* "The Epstein-Barr Virus" (M. A. Epstein and B. G. Achong, Eds), pp. 61–78. Springer—Berlin, Heidelberg and New York.

Hoagland, R. J. (1955). *Am. J. med. Sci.* **229**, 262–272.

Hoffman, G. J., Lazarowitz, S. G. and Hayward, S. D. (1980). *Proc. natn. Acad. Sci. U.S.A.* **77**, 2979–2983.

Horwitz, C. A., Henle, W., Henle, G., Segal, M., Arnold, T., Lewis, F. B., Zanick, D. and Ward, P. C. J. (1976). *Am. J. Med.* **61**, 333–339.

Jay, G., Deleo, A. B., Appella, E., Dubois, G. C., Law, L. W., Khoury, G., Old, L. J. (1979). Cold Spring *Harb. Symp. quant. Biol.* **XLIV**, 659–664.

Jondal, M. and Klein, G. (1973). *J. exp. Med.* **138**, 1365–1378.

Kaaden, O. R. and Dietzschold, B. (1974). *J. Gen. Virol.* **25**, 1–10.

Kallin, B., Luka, J. and Klein, G. (1979). *J. Virology* **32**, 710–716.

Kawanishi, M., Sugawara, K. and Ito, Y. (1981). *Virology* **109**, 72–81.

Kieff, E., Given, D., Powell, A. L. T., King, W., Dambaugh, T. and Raab-Traub, N. (1979). *Biochim. biophys. Acta Rev.* **560**, 335–373.

Klein, E., Klein, G. and Levine, P. H. (1976). *Cancer Res.* **36**, 724–727.

Klein, G. (1979a). *In* "The Epstein-Barr Virus" (M. A. Epstein and B. G. Achong, Eds), pp. 339–350. Springer—Berlin, Heidelberg and New York.

Klein, G. (1979b). *Proc. natn. Acad. Sci. U.S.A.* **76**, 2442–2446.

Klein, G. and Vonka, V. (1974). *J. natn. Cancer Inst.* **53**, 1645–1646.

Lesnick, F. and Ross, L. J. N. (1975). *Int. J. Cancer* **16**, 153–163.

Laufs, R. and Steinke, H. (1975). *Nature* **253**, 71–72.

Luka, J., Jörnvall, H. and Klein, G. (1980). *J. Virology* **35**, 592–602.

Menezes, J., Patel, P., Dussault, H. and Bourkas, A. E. (1978). *Intervirology* **9**, 86–94.

Misko, I. S., Moss, D. J. and Pope, J. H. (1980). *Proc. natn. Acad. Sci. U.S.A.* **77**, 4247–4250.

Morgan, D. G., Niederman, J. C., Miller, G., Smith, H. W. and Dowaliby, J. M. (1979) *Lancet* **ii**, 1154–1157.

Moss, D. J., Rickinson, A. B. and Pope, J. H. (1978). *Int. J. Cancer* **22**, 662–668.

Moss, D. J., Rickinson, A. B. and Pope, J. H. (1979). *Int. J. Cancer* **23**, 618–625.

Moss, D. J., Rickinson, A. B., Wallace, L. E. and Epstein, M. A. (1981b) *Nature* **291**, 664–666.

Moss, D. J., Wallace, L. E., Rickinson, A. B. and Epstein, M. A. (1981a). *Europ. J. Immunol.* **11**, 686–693.

Mueller-Lantzsch, N., Yamamoto, N. and Zur Hausen, H. (1979). *Virology* **97**, 378–387.

Mueller-Lantzsch, N., Georg, B., Yamamoto, N. and Zur Hausen, H. (1980a). *Virology* **102**, 231–233.

Mueller-Lantzsch, N., Georg, B., Yamamoto, N. and Zur Hausen, H. (1980b). *Virology* **102**, 401–411.

Mueller-Lantzsch, N., Georg-Fries, B., Herbst, H., Zur Hausen, H. and Braun, D. G. (1981). (submitted to press.)

Niederman, J. C., Miller, G., Pearson, H. A., Pagano, J. S. and Dowaliby, J. M. (1976). *New. Engl. J. Med.* **294**, 1355–1359.
North, J. R., Morgan, A. J. and Epstein, M. A. (1980). *Int. J. Cancer* **26**, 231–240.
Old, L. J., Boyse, E. A., Oettgen, H. F., de Harven, E., Geering, G., Williamson, B. and Clifford, P. (1966). *Proc. natn. Acad. Sci. U.S.A.* **56**, 1699–1704.
Pattengale, P. K., Smith, R. W. and Gerber, P. (1973). *Lancet* ii, 93.
Payne, L. N. (1973). *In* "Analytic and Experimental Epidemiology of Cancer" (W. Nakahara, T. Hirayama, K. Nishioka and H. Sugano, Eds), pp. 235–257. University of Tokyo Press.
Pearson, G. R. and Scott, R. E. (1977). *Proc. natn. Acad. Sci. U.S.A.* **74**, 2546–2550.
Pearson, G. R. and Qualtière, L. F. (1978). *J. Virology* **28**, 344–351.
Pearson, G., Dewey, F., Klein, G., Henle, G. and Henle W. (1970). *J. natn. Cancer Inst.* **45**, 989–995.
Pearson, G., Henle, G. and Henle, W. (1971). *J. natn. Cancer Inst.* **46**, 1243–1250.
Pike, M. C., Morrow, R. H., Kisuule, A. and Mafigiri, J. (1970). *Br. J. Prev. Soc. Med.* **24**, 39–41.
Pope, J. H. (1979). *In* "The Epstein-Barr Virus" (M. A. Epstein and B. G. Achong, Eds), pp. 205–223. Springer—Berlin, Heidelberg and New York.
Pope, J. H., Horne, M. K. and Wetters, E. J. (1969). *Nature* **222**, 186–187.
Pritchett, R. F., Hayward, S. D. and Kieff, E. D. (1975). *J. Virology* **15**, 556–584.
Pritchett, R., Pedersen, M. and Kieff, E. (1976). *Virology* **74**, 227–231.
Qualtière, L. F. and Pearson, G. R. (1979). *Int. J. Cancer* **23**, 808–817.
Qualtière, L. F. and Pearson, G. R. (1980). *Virology* **102**, 360–369.
Raab-Traub, N., Pritchett, R. and Kieff, E. (1978). *J. Virology* **27**, 388–398.
Raab-Traub, N., Bambaugh, T. and Kieff, E. (1980). *Cell* **22**, 257–268.
Reedman, B. M., Pope, J. H. and Moss, D. J. (1972). *Int. J. Cancer* **9**, 172–181.
Rickinson, A. B., Moss, D. J. and Pope, J. H. (1979). *Int. J. Cancer* **23**, 610–617.
Rickinson, A. B., Wallace, L. E. and Epstein, M. A. (1980). *Nature* **283**, 865–867.
Rickinson, A. B., Moss, D. J., Wallace, L. E., Misko, I. S., Epstein, M. A. and Pope, J. H. (1981). *Cancer Res.* **41**, 4216–4221.
Sairenji, T., Hinuma, Y., Sekizawa, T. and Yoshida, M. (1977). *J. Gen. Virol.* **38**, 111–120.
Schulte-Holthausen, H. and Zur Hausen, H. (1970). *Virology* **40**, 776–779.
Shanmugaratnam, K. (1971). *In* "International Review of Experimental Pathology" (G. W. Richter and M. A. Epstein, Eds), 10, pp. 361–413. Academic Press, London and New York.
Silvestre, D., Ernberg, I., Neauport-Sautes, C., Kourilsky, F. M. and Klein, G. (1974). *J. natn. Cancer Inst.* **53**, 67–74.

Simons, M. J., Wee, G. B., Goh, E. H., Chan, S. H., Shanmugaratnam, K., Day, N. E. and De Thé, G. (1976). *J. natn. Cancer Inst.* **57**, 977–980.

Strnad, B. C., Neubauer, R. H., Rabin, H. and Mazur, R. A. (1979). *J. Virology* **32**, 885–894.

Sunderland, C. A., McMaster, W. R. and Williams, A. F. (1979). *Eur. J. Immunol.* **9**, 155–159.

Takada, K. and Osato, T. (1978). *Intervirology* **11**, 30–39.

Thorley-Lawson, D. A. (1979a). *Cell* **16**, 33–42.

Thorley-Lawson, D. A. (1979b). *Nature* **281**, 486–488.

Thorley-Lawson, D. A. and Edson, C. M. (1979). *J. Virology* **32**, 458–467.

Thorley-Lawson, D. A. and Geilinger, K. (1980). *Proc. natn. Acad. Sci. U.S.A.* **77**, 5307–5311.

Trumper, P. A., Epstein, M. A. and Giovanella, B. C. (1976). *Int. J. Cancer* **17**, 578–587.

Trumper, P. A., Epstein, M. A., Giovanella, B. C. and Finerty, S. (1977). *Int. J. Cancer* **20**, 655–662.

Volsky, D. J., Shapiro, I. M. and Klein, G. (1980). *Proc. natn. Acad. Sci. U.S.A.* **77**, 5453–5457.

Volsky, D. J., Klein, G., Volsky, B. and Shapiro, I. M. (1981). *Nature* **293**, 399–401.

Wallace, L. E., Moss, D. J., Rickinson, A. B., McMichael, A. J. and Epstein, M. A. (1981). *Eur. J. Immunol.* **11**, 694–699.

Williams, A. O. (1966). *J. Med. Genet.* **3**, 177–179.

Williams, E. H., Smith, P. G., Day, N. E., Geser, A., Ellice, J. and Tukei, P. (1978). *Brit. Cancer* **37**, 109–122.

Zajac, B. A. and Ogburn, C. A. (1975). *In* "Oncogenesis and Herpesviruses" (G. De-Thé, M. A. Epstein and H. zur Hausen, Eds), II, pp. 331–337. IARC, Lyon.

*Note added in proof*

Two groups have recently reported the development of monoclonal antibodies which bind to all EB virus-carrying lymphoblastoid cell lines and most EB virus-positive lymphoma-derived lines; These antibodies react with a 45,000 dalton cell surface polypeptide. Blocking of specific T cell killing of EB virus-carrying target cells has not been achieved, but is it likely that such blocking may require antibody-binding to numerous sites on the target antigen which cannot occur with a single monoclonal antibody. It seems probable, therefore, that these monoclonal antibodies are indeed directed against LYDMA. Kintner, C., and Sugden, B. (1981). *Nature* **294**, 458–460; Rowe, M., Hildreth, J. E. K., Rickinson, A. B. and Epstein, M. A. (1982). *Int. J. Cancer* (in press).

# 12 Monoclonal Antibodies in Bacteriology

D. A. Mitchison and A. R. M. Coates

*MRC Unit for Laboratory Studies of Tuberculosis, Royal Postgraduate Medical School, Ducane Road, London. W12 0HS*

## INTRODUCTION

The purpose of this article is to review the potential value of monoclonal antibodies in clinical bacteriology and to illustrate their use by describing progress made with a set of monoclonal antibodies directed at tubercle bacilli.

## I POTENTIAL VALUE IN CLINICAL BACTERIOLOGY

The ways in which monoclonal antibodies might be of use in the investigation and management of bacterial infections are summarized in Table 12·1. The advantages they might have over polyclonal antisera are often likely to be only matters of convenience and cost, arising from their specificity, reproducibility and unlimited availability. In a few instances their increased specificity could open up a completely new range of possibilities. Serological methods are already used for the definitive classification of certain species within a genus, e.g. salmonella or shigella species, and are of help in other genera, e.g. Lancefield grouping of streptococci. Conventional sera might eventually be replaced by monoclonal antibodies. Subdivision of species by serotyping is of value for epidemiological purposes, particularly when comprehensive bacteriophage or bacteriocin systems are not available. Monoclonal antibodies could be developed for this purpose, e.g. in capsular typing of *Streptococcus pneumoniae* or in Griffith's typing of *S. pyogenes*, but there is increasing evidence from our studies to be described, from unpublished observation with other bacterial genera and from work with viruses that their use leads to the discovery of additional serotypes. In serodiagnosis, monoclonal antibodies might replace currently available polyclonal antisera where it is hoped to detect specific bacterial antigens e.g. in cerebrospinal fluid or sputum. Inhibition assays might be used for the detection of antibody as has been demonstrated in parasitic infections (Mitchell *et al.*, 1979). The use of monoclonal antibodies for purposes of immunization is highly speculative. A human hybridoma cell line would be necessary for passive immunization, e.g. against tetanus toxin, and would avoid the difficulty of obtaining sufficient high titre antibody directly from man. Monoclonal antibodies might also be of value in examining the detailed antigenic structure of different immunizing strains and thereby find differences between them undetectable by conventional serology. Finally, one of the most interesting roles for monoclonal antibodies is as probes to separate and identify antigenic fractions from complex mixtures of bacterial macromolecules. They might also provide means of precisely manipulating the immune response, for instance by acting on components of an idiotypic network (Roitt *et al.*, 1981).

TABLE 12·1
Potential uses of monoclonal antibodies
in bacteriology

1. Classification of bacterial species
2. Serotyping within species
3. Serodiagnosis of bacterial infections
4. Immunization
5. Structural probe

## II MONOCLONAL ANTIBODIES AGAINST TUBERCLE BACILLI

### A. Varieties of Tubercle Bacilli

Although tuberculosis is a diminishing problem in technically advanced countries, little real progress has been made in its control in developing countries. On the world scale it still remains among the most important of the communicable diseases and is caused by tubercle bacilli. The term tubercle bacilli is used by students of human pathology to include *Mycobacterium tuberculosis, M. africanum,* and *M. bovis,* all of which are highly pathogenic in man. These species have been found to be serologically identical using polyclonal antisera (Lind, 1960; Topley and Wilson, 1975). Several characteristics of *M. tuberculosis* vary in strains from different regions of the world. Those from South India are distinguishable from European and American strains by animal virulence, susceptibility to hydrogen peroxide and to certain antibacterial drugs as well as by phage typing (Mitchison *et al.,* 1963; Grange *et al.,* 1978). Those from Hong Kong also show some differences (Mitchison, 1970). *M. africanum* is found in West and Central Africa and has characteristics intermediate between *M. tuberculosis* and *M. bovis.*

### B. Production and Properties of Monoclonal Antibodies

The production of a group of monoclonal antibodies directed at tubercle bacilli has been described by Coates *et al.* (1981). The strains used for their production and screening included *M. tuberculosis,* strains H37Rv and H37Ra (the much studied virulent and avirulent variants of a strain from an American patient), strains S1 and 6067 from British patients and strain 7219 from a South Indian patient, as well as the virulent strain Vallée of *M. bovis* and the attenuated BCG strain (Glaxo).

Hybridomas were produced in BALB/c mice by the method of Kohler and Milstein (1975). In the first of the 2 immunizing schedules, $2 \times 10^7$ colony forming units (cfu) of the avirulent H37Ra strain of *M. tuberculosis* were given intraperitoneally on day 0 and the same dose intravenously on days 28 and 29. The aim in using whole living cells was to preserve antigens intact and to create monoclonal antibodies directed mainly at surface antigens. However avirulent strains could differ antigenically from virulent strains. For the second schedule, bacteria were passed through a press (X-press, LKB), centrifuged and the supernatant filtered through a 0·2 μ membrane filter. A dose containing 100 μg protein of the resultant "pressate", prepared from the virulent H37Rv strain of *M. tuberculosis*, was given intraperitoneally on days 0 and 15; these were followed 7 months later by an intravenous dose of $10^8$ cfu heat-killed bacilli of the virulent S1 strain. The purpose of this schedule was to broaden the number of antigens by exposing those within the bacterial cell and by using 2 different strains of *M. tuberculosis*. The supernatants from hybridomas were initially screened by solid phase radio-immunoassay (RIA) with pressates of *M. tuberculosis* strains H37Rv or S1 and *Escherichia coli*. Most clones reacting with *E. coli* were discarded. Cell lines from 7 hybridomas were selected, cloned, established as stable lines and the monoclonal antibody in ascitic fluid was investigated in detail.

The binding of the monoclonal antibodies to pressates of various species and strains of mycobacteria and of *E. coli* were first studied by solid phase RIA (Table 12·2). The origin of the data in Table 12·2 is shown for a single antibody (TB23) and the 3 pressates with which it bound in Fig 12·1. The asymptotic value of maximum binding (MB%) and the $\log_{10}$ titre yielding 50% of maximum binding (B50) was calculated from a fitted curve for each pressate. TB23 apparently bound with 4 strains of *M. tuberculosis* (H37Rv, H37Ra, 6067 and 7219) but not with strain S1. The specificity with which TB23 distinguished strain S1 and some of the more interesting reactions of the remaining monoclonal antibodies were confirmed by an inhibition assay (Fig. 12·2).

Several of the monoclonal antibodies showed a remarkable specificity which has never been demonstrated by polyclonal serology. We have already seen that TB23 distinguished strains S1 from the other 4 strains of *M. tuberculosis*. TB71 and TB72 separated all strains of *M. tuberculosis* from *M. bovis*. TB23, TB77 and TB78 distinguished *M. bovis* Vallée from *M. bovis* BCG. There were varying patterns of binding with pressates of other mycobacterial species, but the binding range of TB68, TB71 and TB72 included only *M. tuberculosis* and *M. bovis*. TB73 had a very wide range of reactivity, binding with all mycobacteria tested with *E. coli*. Monoclonal antibodies with a similarly wide specificity were frequently encountered.

## C. USES

### 1. CLASSIFICATION

*M. tuberculosis*, *M. africanum* and *M. bovis* are currently distinguished by morphological and biochemical tests and by phage typing. The mono-

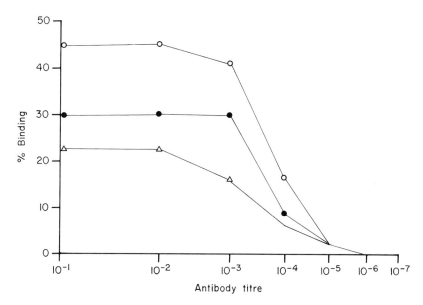

FIG. 12·1 Binding in radioimmune assay of monoclonal antibody TB23 to bacterial pressates. Results against pressates of *M. bovis* Vallée (O), *M. tuberculosis* H37Rv and H37Ra (mean value) (●) and *M. kansasii* (△) are shown.

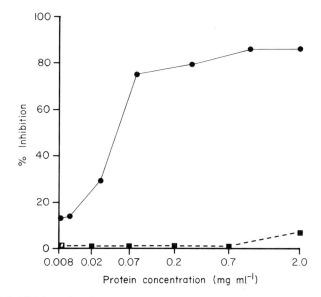

FIG. 12·2 Inhibition of radioimmune assay binding by monoclonal antibody TB23. Results with pressates of *M. tuberculosis* H37Rv (●) and *M. tuberculosis* S1 (■) are shown.

### TABLE 12·2
Binding of monoclonal antibodies by bacterial pressates

| Species | Strain | TB68 MB% | TB68 B50 | TB23 MB% | TB23 B50 | TB71 MB% | TB71 B50 | TB72 MB% | TB72 B50 | TB77 MB% | TB77 B50 | TB78 MB% | TB78 B50 | TB73 MB% | TB73 B50 |
|---|---|---|---|---|---|---|---|---|---|---|---|---|---|---|---|
| *M. tuberculosis* | H37Ra | 3+[a] | 3+[b] | 2+ | 3+ | 1+ | 3+ | 1+ | 2+ | 2+ | 2+ | 2+ | 3+ | 2+ | 2+ |
| | H37Rv | 3+ | 3+ | 2+ | 3+ | 1+ | 3+ | 2+ | 2+ | 1+ | 3+ | 2+ | 3+ | 2+ | 2+ |
| | S1 | 3+ | 3+ | 0 | – | 2+ | 3+ | 1+ | 2+ | 1+ | 3+ | 1+ | 3+ | 2+ | 1+ |
| | 6067 | 3+ | 3+ | 2+ | 3+ | 2+ | 3+ | 2+ | 2+ | 2+ | 2+ | 2+ | 2+ | 2+ | 2+ |
| | 7219 | 3+ | 3+ | 3+ | 3+ | 2+ | 3+ | 2+ | 2+ | 2+ | 2+ | 2+ | 3+ | 2+ | 2+ |
| *M. bovis* | Vallée | 3+ | 3+ | 2+ | 3+ | 0 | – | 0 | – | 2+ | 2+ | 2+ | 3+ | 2+ | 2+ |
| | BCG | 1+ | 1+ | 0 | – | 0 | – | 0 | – | 0 | – | 0 | – | 3+ | 2+ |
| *M. kansasii* | | 0 | – | 2+ | 3+ | 0 | – | 0 | – | 1+ | 3+ | 0 | – | 3+ | 1+ |
| *M. scrofulaceum* | | 0 | – | 0 | – | 0 | – | 0 | – | 1+ | 3+ | 0 | – | 2+ | 1+ |
| *M. avium* | | 0 | – | 0 | – | 0 | – | 0 | – | 0 | – | 0 | – | 2+ | 2+ |
| *M. fortuitum* | | 0 | – | 0 | – | 0 | – | 0 | – | 2+ | 3+ | 1+ | 2+ | 2+ | 1+ |
| *E. coli* | | 0 | – | 0 | – | 0 | – | 0 | – | 1+ | 1+ | 0 | – | 3+ | 2+ |

MB% = maximum binding (%)

[a] MB%

3+ = 50–100
2+ = 20–
1+ = 10–
0 = <10

B50 = log$_{10}$ titre yielding 50% of maximum binding

[b] B50

3+ = 4·0–5·3
2+ = 3·0–
1+ = 2·0–
– = <2·0

clonal antibody could be used to distinguish *M. tuberculosis* and *M. bovis* serologically. However their value cannot be properly assessed until more strains have been tested. No work has been done with *M. africanum*.

## 2. EPIDEMIOLOGY

The usual way of recognising individual strains of *M. tuberculosis* is by their phage typing and pattern of sensitivity to antituberculosis drugs. The utility of phage typing is very limited since there are only 3 common and highly reproducible phage types (A, B and I) (Grange and Redmond, 1978). Furthermore, the occurrence of types I and B only in certain areas of the world limits their use still further (Bates and Mitchison, 1969; Grange *et al.*, 1978). Drug resistance is so rare as to be of only occasional value. Binding of our monoclonal antibodies was not related to the phage type of the strains (Table 12·3). One antibody

TABLE 12·3
Comparison of phage type with serotype

| Species | Strain | Phage type | | | Serotype Monoclonal Antibody | |
|---------|--------|:---:|:---:|:---:|:---:|:---:|
| | | A | B | I | TB23 | TB71 |
| *M. tuberculosis* | H37Rv | − | + | − | + | + |
| | H37Ra | − | + | − | + | + |
| | S1 | + | − | − | − | + |
| | 6067 | + | − | − | + | + |
| | 7219 | − | − | + | + | + |
| *M. bovis* | Vallée | + | − | − | + | − |
| | BCG | + | − | − | − | − |

(TB23) could differentiate *M. tuberculosis* S1 from other strains. Furthermore, several of our antibodies could separate *M. bovis* Vallée from *M. bovis* BCG, though it should be noted that this separation is also possible with phage 33D (Warsaw) (Jones, 1979). Should it be possible to identify further serotypes with appropriate monoclonal antibodies, an important epidemiological tool would emerge. The serotypes could then be used to explore modes of transmission of infection, the epidemiology of small epidemics and the interesting question of whether tuberculosis originates by an infection with one or several bacilli (Bates, 1980).

## 3. SERODIAGNOSIS

There is a great need for an effective serological blood test for active tuberculosis. It would be of particular use in the following groups of patients:

1.   Patients with a differential diagnosis that includes tuberculosis. Since tuberculosis is a protean disease which may affect any of the organs and be inaccessible for bacteriological examination, one could envisage widespread use of the serological test.
2.   Smear-negative, culture-positive tuberculosis, to speed up the diagnosis.
3.   Smear-negative, culture-negative tuberculosis, to establish a diagnosis.
4.   In a case-finding control programme, together with or as an alternative to bacteriological examination.

Although there have been numerous attempts to develop serological tests for active tuberculosis, none has been adopted for clinical use, mainly because their specificity has been unsatisfactory and the proportion of active cases found to have positive results too low (Takahashi, 1962; Parlett, 1964; Nassau *et al.*, 1976; Coates, 1980). The B-cell response of patients with active disease appears to have a mosaic-like pattern, different patients showing wide variation in the range of antigens against which they develop antibodies (Kaplan and Chase, 1980; Reggiardo *et al.*, 1981). Furthermore, the response is often slow with the highest titres and the largest number of antibodies occurring several weeks after the disease is initially diagnosed (Wallace *et al.*, 1967; Reggiardo *et al.*, 1981). Thus a transient infection insufficiently serious to cause clinical disease would produce antibodies against only a few antigens, while active prolonged disease would produce antibodies against numerous antigens. A test with a crude mixture of antigens from tubercle bacilli could not distinguish between these 2 situations. Furthermore there is a possibility of detecting antibodies against nonspecific antigens in such a mixture, as for instance our monoclonal antibody TB73 which reacted not only with all mycobacteria tested but also with *E. coli*. A set of tests against separate pure specific antigens would solve these problems, but the difficulties of the initial calibration and large scale preparation of the pure antigens would be very large. Cross-reactions have been found between our monoclonal antibodies, prepared in the mouse, and sera from human patients with active tuberculosis (unpublished observations). These cross-reactions might make it possible to utilize the specificity of the monoclonal antibodies without actual isolation of the antigens concerned and thereby increase the efficiency of serological testing.

## 4. STRUCTURAL PROBE

Despite the large amount of work that has been carried out during the 100 years since the discovery of the tubercle bacillus by Robert Koch, little is known about which antigens are important in stimulating the bactericidal activity of the host's immune system or those cellular systems which regulate it. Because of the complexity of the cell wall of mycobacteria, the chemical purification and examination of separate fractions has not so far solved the problem. Monoclonal antibodies offer an alternative and simpler approach. They could be used as a source of molecules known to be antigenic and therefore likely to be involved in the immune mechanism. Knowledge of the structure of such a molecule supplemented by an examination of the antiidiotype raised against the monoclonal antibody might allow characterization of specific protective or regulatory antigens. Even if detailed biochemistry were not done, the antigenic molecules that bind to monoclonal antibodies are likely to be valuable probes in examining the physiology of the immune system. The availability of monoclonal antibodies and their corresponding antigens could also allow purification of subsets of T-lymphocytes and the lymphokines that they produce.

## III MONOCLONAL ANTIBODIES AGAINST OTHER BACTERIA

There is little published work on monoclonal antibodies against bacteria. Monoclonal antibodies have been produced to Lancefield Group A streptococci (Herbst and Braun, 1980) and to *S. agalactiae* (Group B), types II and III (Polin and Kennett, 1980). The latter workers have developed a rapid enzyme immunoassay to identify the Group B streptococci, using monoclonal antibodies. Bethseda Research Laboratories (Maryland, USA) have made claims that they have monoclonal antibodies against various serotypes of *S. agalactiae*. We know of several groups currently developing monoclonal antibodies against other bacteria.

REFERENCES

Bates, J. H. (1980). *Clinics in Chest Medicine* 1, 167–174.

Bates, J. H. and Mitchison, D. A. (1969). *Am. Rev. rasp. Dis.* **100**, 189–193.

Coates, A. R. M. (1980). *Eur. J. resp. Dis.* **61**, 307–309.

Coates, A. R. M., Hewitt, J., Allen, B. W., Mitchison, D. A. and Ivanyi, J. (1981). *Lancet* **ii**, 167–169.

Grange, J. M. and Redmond, W. B. (1978). *Tubercle* **59**, 203–228.

Grange, J. M., Aber, V. R., Allen, B. W., Mitchison, D. A. and Goren, M. B. (1978). *J. gen. Microbiol.* **108**, 1–7.

Herbst, H. and Braun, D. G. (1981). Ann. Immunol. (Paris). (in press).

Jones, W. D. (1979). *Tubercle* **60**, 55–58.

Kaplan, M. H. and Chase, M. W. (1980). *J. infect. Dis.* **142**, 835–843.

Lind, A. (1960). *Int. Arch. Allergy* **17**, 300–322.

Mitchell, G. F., Cruise, K. M., Chapman, C. B., Anders, R. F. and Howard, M. C. (1979). *Aust. J. exp. Biol. med. Sci.* **57**, 287–302.

Mitchison, D. A. (1970). *Pneumonologie* **142**, 131–137.

Mitchison, D. A., Selkon, J. B. and Lloyd, J. (1963). *J. Path. Bact.* **86**, 377–386.

Nassau, E., Parsons, E. R. and Johnson, G. D. (1976). *Tubercle* **57**, 67–70.

Parlett, R. C. (1964). *Bull. Int. U. Against Tuberc.* **34**, 9–35.

Polin, R. A. and Kennett, R. (1980). *J. clin. Microbiol.* **11**, 332–36.

Reggiardo, Z., Aber, V. R., Mitchison, D. A. and Devi, S. (1981). *Am. Rev. resp. Dis.* **124**, 21–25.

Roitt, I. M., Cooke, A., Male, D. K., Hay, F. C., Guarnotta, G., Lydyard, P. M., Carvalho, L. P., Thanavala, Y. and Ivanyi, J. (1981). *Lancet* **i**, 1041–1045.

Takahashi, Y. (1962), *Am. Rev. resp. Dis.*, **85**, 708–719.

Topley, W. W. C. and Wilson, G. S. (1975). *In* "Principles of Bacteriology, Virology and Immunity" (G. S. Wilson and A. Miles, Eds), pp. 582–584. Edward Arnold, London.

Wallace, R., Diena, B. B., Jessamine, A. G. and Greenberg, L. (1967). *Canad. med. Ass. J.*, **96**, 585–588.

# 13 Monoclonal Antibodies in Parasitology with Particular Reference to Malaria

Sydney Cohen

Department of Chemical Pathology, Guy's Hospital Medical School, London. SE1 9RT

## I INTRODUCTION

Precise figures concerning the incidence of human parasitic diseases are impossible to obtain, but the overwhelming importance of these infections, especially in developing countries, is indicated by available estimates of annual morbidity attributable to infestation by various protozoa and helminths (Table 13·1). Although clinical manifestations of acquired immunity may be absent or indecisive, all parasites investigated are in fact highly immunogenic and induce specific antibody formation. These responses have provided the basis for a wide range of serodiagnostic tests having practical usefulness. In addition, the

TABLE 13·1
Annual morbidity due to some parasitic diseases
of man
(W.H.O. World Health Statistics report 30,
1977)

| Protozoa | No. cases (millions) |
|---|---|
| Malaria | 150 |
| Chagas disease | 15 |
| Amoebiasis | unknown |
| Leishmaniasis | unknown |
| Helminths | |
| Hookworm | 700 |
| Schistosomiasis | 200 |
| Filariasis | 200 |

demonstration that in some parasite infections, antibodies have a protective role has suggested the feasibility of developing immunoprophylactic measures.

Protozoa and helminths are large organisms and many undergo complicated life cycles within the human host. Their antigenic constitution is correspondingly diverse and it is this complexity which has frequently hindered the development of satisfactory immunodiagnostic tests having appropriate sensititivity and specificity and has complicated the isolation of protective antigens which might comprise useful vaccines. The advent of hybridoma technology has provided an invaluable tool for the analysis and isolation of specific parasite antigens. Monoclonal antibodies are at present, being raised agaist a wide range of protozoal and helminth parasites. The work is at an early stage of development and this chapter will attempt to illustrate some aspects of its potential with particular reference to malaria.

## II MALARIA

Malaria is caused by multiplication of protozoa of the family Plasmodiidae in the blood and other tissues of the host. More than 100 plasmodial species are known causing malaria in a wide range of vertebrates (Garnham, 1966; Coatney et al., 1971). Parasites exhibit narrowly defined host specificity and only 4 species are naturally occurring pathogens of Man; of these the most virulent is *Plasmodium falciparum*, the cause of malignant, tertian malaria. Infection is initiated by the bite of an infected female anopheline mosquito which inoculates motile sporozoites into the bloodstream (Fig. 13·1). In mammalian hosts these are cleared from the circulation within 1–2 hours and localized in hepatic parenchymal cells through mechanisms at present unknown. The extra-erythrocytic (EE) forms become multinucleate, and after a variable period (usually about 10 days) infected liver cells rupture and each discharges several thousand EE merozoites which invade erythrocytes. Erythrocytic (E) schizonts rupture with a periodicity of 24–72 hours, characteristic for individual species and each liberates 10–20 E merozoites which attach to specific receptors on red cell membranes to initiate invasion. The erythrocytic cycle is associated with clinical manifestations of malaria. After a period of purely asexual replication of erythrocytic parasites a proportion of newly invaded merozoites differentiate into male and female gametocytes which mature without under-going cell division over a period of about 10 days. Sexual reproduction follows the ingestion of gametocytes into the gut of the mosquito (Fig. 13·1).

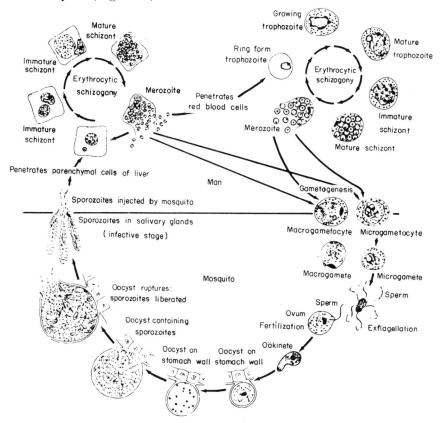

FIG. 13·1 Diagrammatic representation of the mammalian malaria life-cycle.

## A. Immunity to Malaria Sporozoites

Natural sporozite infection in general induces little clinical immunity. Thus, subjects living in hyperendaemic areas and receiving chemotherapy directed against blood-stage parasites are exposed to repeated sporozoite infection and yet remain susceptible to malaria when prophylactic measures are suspended. On the other hand, sporozoites inactivated by irradiation have successfully immunized mice against *P. berghei* (Nussenzweig *et al.*, 1969) and a small number of human volunteers against *P. falciparum* or *P. vivax* (Clyde, 1975). The immunity induced by sporozoite vaccination is strictly stage-specific (Table 13·2). Sporozoites for vaccine preparation are isolated from salivary glands of infected mosquitoes in extremely limited amounts and practical vaccination based on this material cannot be envisaged. The induction of state-specific clinical immunity by inactivated sporozoite vaccines is nevertheless of considerable interest and has stimulated attempts to identify protective sporozoite antigens.

TABLE 13·2
Features of a sporozoite vaccine against malaria

| | |
|---|---|
| Source: | Infected mosquitoes |
| Dose: | $10^5$ Sporozoites (mouse) |
| Inactivation: | Irradiation |
| Requirements: | Fresh preparation |
| | Intravenous route |
| | No adjuvant |
| Effective in: | *P. berghei* (rodent) |
| | *P. falciparum*, *P. vivax* (human) |
| Specificity: | Species specific (some rodent malarias cross protect) |
| | Stage specific (ineffective against bloodstage infection) |
| Duration of Immunity: | 3 months + |

### 1. SPOROZOITE ANTIGENS

Some internal sporozoite antigens cross react with antigens present in erythrocytic parasites of the corresponding species; these antigens common to different stages of parasite development, are revealed by reaction of immune sera with sporozoites whose surface membranes have been partially disrupted for example by air-drying and freezing. Sporozoite surface antigens can be selectively examined in viable, intact organisms, and in all species studied are both species and stage specific which suggests their possible role in protective immunity (Nardin and

Nussenzweig, 1978). Reaction of the surface antigens of viable *P. berghei* sporozoites with serum from sporozoite-vaccinated mice mediates the so-called circumsporozoite precipitin (csp) reaction. This involves a surface antigen with an approximate molecular weight of 41,000 (Gwadz *et al.*, 1978).

2. MONOCLONAL ANTIBODIES AGAINST SPOROZOITES

The first attempt to raise monoclonal antibodies against sporozoites involved the rodent parasite, *P. berghei* (Yoshida *et al.*, 1980). Female Balb/C mice were immunized with *P. berghei* sporozoites by repeated exposure to $\gamma$-irradiated, infected Anopheles stephensi mosquitoes. Four days after the sixth exposure, when the animals were protected against sporozoite challenge and had high titres of anti-sporozoite antibodies, spleen cells from immunized animals were fused with P3U1 plasmacytoma cells (Kohler and Milstein, 1975). Culture supernatants were screened by indirect immunofluorescence using gluteraldehyde fixed sporozoites as antigen. A total of 5 out of 600 cultures were positive for sporozoite antibodies, but only one hybrid cell line was successfully expanded and maintained. The protective effect of antibody produced by this line was shown by the fact that *P. berghei* sporozoites were rendered noninfective by incubation for 45 minutes with culture supernatants or serum from mice bearing the hybridoma. In addition, 10–300 $\mu$g of the monoclonal antibody (isotype IgG1, k), when injected intravenously, protected mice against subsequent challenge with $10^3$–$10^4$ sporozoites. The Fab fragments of the antibody effectively neutralized sporozoite infectivity suggesting a blocking action, for example, on the ability of the parasite to penetrate hepatocytes (Potocnjak *et al.*, 1980). The circumsporozoite precipitin reaction is mediated by the monoclonal antibody, but not by its Fab fragment; however, successive incubation with monoclonal Fab and rabbit antibody to mouse k-chains induces the csp reaction suggesting that this represents a capping phenomenon associated with shedding of immune complexes. Electron microscopy shows that the monoclonal antibody forms an amorphous deposit on the surface of sporozoites (Fig. 13·2). When reacted with sporozoites pre-labelled by lactoperoxidase catalyzed iodination, the monoclonal antibodies bound a component having a molecular weight of 44,000. This antigen is both stage and species specific and is distributed evenly on the surfce of salivary gland sporozoites; the antigen is not detectable on bloodstage parasites or late exoerythrocytic schizonts and has a patchy distribution on occyst sporozoites (Aikawa *et al.*, 1981). Pb 44 antigen has an unusually low

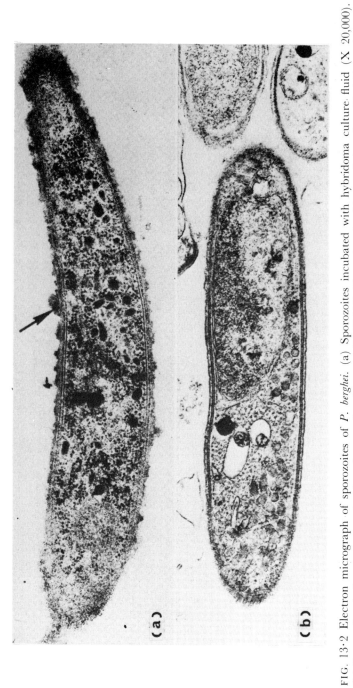

FIG. 13·2 Electron micrograph of sporozoites of *P. berghei*. (a) Sporozoites incubated with hybridoma culture fluid (X 20,000). (b) Sporozoites before treatment showing absence of surface coat (X 26,000) (Reproduced, with permission, from Yoshida *et al.*, 1980. © 1980 American Association for the Advancement of Science.)

isoelectric point which facilitates the separation from contaminants (R. S. Nussenzweig, personal communication).

It is apparent that the application of hybridoma technology has led rapidly to the identification of a protective antigen on the surface of sporozoites from the rodent parasite, *P. berghei*. Parallel work is now in progress using simian and human malaria parasites. Mouse monoclonal antibodies raised against species which are non-infective for rodents, obviously cannot be evaluated for protective activity by direct passive transfer tests. However, mouse monoclonal antibodies of high affinity and appropriate specifity may show protective activity when reacted with sporozoites *in vitro* and then tested *in vivo* for infectivity using an appropriate susceptible host (R. S. Nussenzweig, personal communication).

## B. Immunity to Bloodstage Malaria Parasites

The pattern of acquired immunity to bloodstage infection varies widely in different host-parasite combinations. In some unnatural laboratory infections, for instance *P. knowlesi* in the rhesus monkey, there is no effective immune response and the disease is rapidly fatal. Other forms of experimental malaria, e.g. *P. berghei* in the rat, induce "sterilizing" immunity characterized by complete elimination of the blood parasite and life-long resistance to challenge. In the case of naturally occurring infections, the development of acquired immunity usually controls but does not eliminate the parasite which survives at low density over long periods. This is characteristic of the human malarias which may persist for many years. Such chronicity of infection reflects a complex and subtle balance between the immune reactivity of the host generating responses potentially lethal to the plasmodium, and other mechanisms which promote parasite survival. Specific acquired immunity depends primarily upon antibody which appears to block merozoite invasion of red blood cells. Parasite survival is promoted by the intracellular location of parasites, their antigenic diversity and their capacity to modify host immune responsiveness (Cohen, 1979; 1980). Vaccination against malaria has been attempted with killed or attenuated erythrocytes, and with extracellular bloodstage merozoites (Cohen and Mitchell, 1978); the latter procedure has proved effective against virulent *P. knowlesi* infections in rhesus monkeys and against the human malaria, *P. falciparum*, in douroucouli monkeys (Table 13·3). However, the difficulties which have beset attempts to scale up methods of malaria cultivation, renders a vaccine based upon merozoite produc-

tion an impractical proposition. On the other hand, the success with
experimental vaccination indicates the feasibility of isolating from
bloodstage parasites protective antigens which might prove effective as
vaccines.

TABLE 13·3
Features of a merozoite vaccine against malaria

| | |
|---|---|
| Source: | Cultures of bloodstage parasites |
| Dose: | $10^9$ merozoites (rhesus) |
| Inactivation: | None-merozoites become non-invasive after 30 min at 20°C |
| Storage: | Frozen or freeze dried |
| Route: | Intramuscular |
| Adjuvants: | FCA; Saponin; Stearoyl-MDP |
| Effective in: | *P. knowlesi, P. falciparum, P. fragile* |
| Specificity: | Species specific |
| | Stage specific (ineffective against exo-erythrocytic stage) |
| Duration: | >18 m (*P. knowlesi*) |

## 1. ANTIGENS OF BLOODSTAGE MALARIA PARASITES

During the past decade, analytical techniques giving progressively
higher resolution, have revealed the great complexity of plasmodial
antigens recognized by naturally infected or artifically immunized
hosts. The analysis of *P. knowlesi* by crossed immunoelectrophoresis has
identified more than 20 major parasite antigens and many more minor
components (Schmidt-Ullrich and Wallach, 1978; Deans *et al.*, 1978).
The majority of these antigens appear to be common to several plasmodial species and are therefore unlikely to induce clinical immunity
which characteristically shows species specificity. A comparison of 2
simian parasites which give no clinical cross-protection revealed only
one antigen which was species specific (Deans, 1980). Some antigens
are present throughout the development of bloodstage parasites while
others appear only in more mature forms. More than 40 polypeptide
components, separable by polyacrylamide gel electrophoresis in
sodium dodecyl sulphate and autoradiography, were identified in biosynthetically labelled *P. falciparum* preparations, but relatively few of
these were precipitable by human immune sera (Perrin *et al.*, 1981a).
Aqueous extracts of *P. falciparum* infected blood provide a source of
antigens classified as L (labile) and S (stable) on the basis of their heat
susceptibility. Individual isolates of *P. falciparum* contain a relatively

restricted range of S-antigen specificities which are retained over long periods either *in vivo* or *in vitro*; this observation provides a means of identifying serotypes of *P. falciparum* (Wilson, 1980).

Few plasmodial antigens have been adequately characterized. Among these is an unusual protein containing more than 70% histidine which was isolated from the cytoplasmic granules of the avian parasite, *P. lophurae*. This protein may be concerned in red cell penetration (Kilejian, 1978) and indirect evidence suggests that mammalian parasites contain an analagous histidine-rich protein (Kilejian, 1980).

Several malarial antigens are expressed on the surface of the parasitized erythrocyte and are identifiable by external labelling techniques (Deans and Cohen, 1979; Schmidt-Ullrich *et al.*, 1979) by agglutination (Eaton, 1938; Brown and Brown, 1965) and by electron microscopy (Langreth and Reese, 1979). No blood-stage antigens have been shown to have a protective function, but such identification appears likely with the application of hybridoma technology.

### 2. MONOCLONAL ANTIBODIES AGAINST BLOODSTAGE PARASITES

Hybridomas against bloodstage parasites are being raised in several laboratories and some data concerning rodent, simian and human malarias published or communicated to me are summarized in Table 13·4. Spleen donors have been mice or rats immunized by natural infection or artificial vaccination; the supernatants of fusion products were screened against plasmodial antigen by either indirect immunofluorescence or solid phase radioimmunoassay; the latter procedure was estimated to be $10^4$ times more sensitive than the former and was able to detect 0·5 ng of monoclonal antibody. (Kim *et al.*, 1980).

### (a) *Rodent malaria*
The first study on the rodent parasite, *P. yoelii* demonstrated a protective role for those monoclonal antibodies which were directed against merozoite antigens (Freeman *et al.*, 1980a). Balb/C mice were immunized by infection with *P. yoelii* (17X, mild strain) and challenged on three occasions with *P. yoelii* (YM virulent strain). Spleen cells were fused with P3NS1/1-Ag4-1 myeloma cells using polyethylene glycol. Of 143 culture supernatants screened by indirect immunofluorescence against *P. yoelii* schizonts, 18 reacted with the parasite, and not with normal red cells. On the basis of this initial screening, four specificities were distinguished staining respectively, (*i*) membranes of some infected erythrocytes (*ii*) membranes of all infected erythrocytes (*iii*) all developmental stages of the parasite (*iv*) merozoites. Five clones

TABLE 13·4

Monoclonal antibodies against bloodstage malaria parasites

| Plasmodium | Immunization | Primary screen[a] | No. double cloned | Monoclonal antibodies | | | Reference |
|---|---|---|---|---|---|---|---|
| | | | | Classification | Biological test | Reactive antigens | |
| P. yoelii 17X (mild) YM (lethal) | Natural infection (Balb C mice) | I.F. | 5 | I.F.5 specificities | Passive protection (in vivo) | | Freeman et al. (1980a) |
| P. yoelii 17XL (lethal) | Natural infection | SPRIA | 7 | | | | Kim et al. (1980) |
| P. knowlesi | Merozoite vaccination (AO rats) | SPRIA | 29 | I.F.13 specificities | P. knowlesi growth inhibition (in vitro) | Schizont and merozoite antigen m.w. 66,000 | Deans et al. (1982) |
| P. knowlesi | Merozoite vaccination (Balb C mice) | I.F. | 12 | | Merozoite agglutination Inhibition of merozoite invasion | Merozoite surface antigen m.w. 250,000 (P. knowlesi) | Epstein et al. (1981) |
| P. falciparum | Vaccination with schizonts and merozoites (Balb C mice) | I.F. | 10 | | P. falciparum growth inhibition (in vitro) | m.w. 41,000 m.w. 36,000 91,000 | Perrin et al. (1980, 1981) |
| P. berghei | Natural infection drug-controlled (Balb C mice) | I.F. | 1 | | | m.w. 41,000 | |

[a] I.F. indirect immunofluorescence.
SPRIA solid phase radioimmunoassay.

representative of these specificities were expanded and their isotypes and cross-reactivity with another rodent malaria parasite, *P. vickei petteri*, were determined (Table 13·5). Serum pools containing high titres of anti-*P. yoelii* monoclonal antibodies were obtained from hybridoma tumour-bearing Balb/C mice; the ability of each pool to inhibit parasite growth was tested by passive transfer of 0·5 ml of serum to mice infected with virulent *P. yoelii* (strain YM). Both merozoite specific monoclonal antibodies showed a protective effect (Table 13·5); the other hybridoma products appeared inactive, but may have been tested at significantly lower concentrations as judged by immunofluorescent titres (Table 13·5). The two anti-merozoite monoclonal antibodies bind to merozoites of the lethal (YM) variant of *P. yoelii*, but not to merozoites of the mild 17X strain. Both antibodies protect against only the lethal YM strain and block penetration of parasites into mature red cells but not into reticulocytes. These findings suggest that the two protective monoclonal antibodies recognize merozoite antigen(s) of the lethal YM variant involved in the invasion of mature red cells (Freeman *et al.*, 1980b).

TABLE 13·5
*P. yoelii* monoclonal antibodies secreted by 5 cloned hybridoma lines
(from Freeman *et al.* 1980a)

| Hybridoma | Ig Class | Immunofluorescence | | Passive transfer of immunity | |
| | | *P. yoelii* | *P. vinkei petteri* | Titre of pool | Result |
| --- | --- | --- | --- | --- | --- |
| 25·1 | IgG 2a | Infected erythrocyte membrane | + | 1:30,000 | − |
| 25·54 | IgG 3 | Infected erythrocyte membrane | + | 1:30,000 | − |
| 25·23 | IgG 2a | All parasite stages | + | 1:32,000 | − |
| 25·57 | IgG 1 | Merozoites | − | 1:128,000 | + |
| 25·77 | IgG 2a | Merozoites | + | 1:128,000 | + |

## (b) *Primate malarias*

It is obvious that passive protection tests are not available when rodent monoclonal antibodies are raised against primate malarias which are non-infective for rodents. In these instances, the identification of those monoclonal antibodies which react with putative protective antigens depends upon *in vitro* assays involving measurement of the inhibition of parasite growth or of merozoite invasion of red cells. Such *in vitro* assays for malarial antibodies having a protective function were first elaborated for the simian parasite, *P. knowlesi*, and involved measurement of 3H-leucine incorporation into parasite protein as an index of parasite growth (Cohen, Butcher and Crandall, 1969) or microscopical observation of merozoite invasion of red cells (Butcher and Cohen, 1970). These methods have since been employed for a variety of plasmodial species including the human parasite, *P. falciparum* (Mitchell *et al.*, 1976; Wilson and Phillips, 1976) and various useful modifications have been introduced including the use of red cells labelled with fluorescein isothiocyanate and parasite staining with ethidium bromide as a means of quantifying merozoite invasion (Lamont, Saul and Kidson, 1981).

In the case of *P. knowlesi* where serological variants of the parasite can be identified by a relatively simple agglutination test, the *in vitro* inhibition of growth by antibody was shown to be related to the variant specificity of the parasite being assayed (Butcher, Mitchell and Cohen, 1978). The use of homologous parasites for immunization and subsequent assay is therefore essential for optimum identification of inhibitory antiboides as demonstrated by Wilson and Phillips (1976) for West African isolates of *P. falciparum*. Since both serum and ascitic fluid may contain non-specific inhibitors of parasite growth, it is also essential to assay purified lg preparations before an observed inhibition of parasite development can be regarded as antibody mediated.

In a study of the simian parasite, *P. knowlesi*, Epstein *et al.* (1981) immunized Balb/C mice with erythrocytic merozoites isolated *in vitro* by the polycarbonate seiving method of Dennis *et al.* (1975). Spleen cells of immunized mice were fused with plasmacytoma cells and culture supernatants screened by indirect immunofluorescence against merozoites as antigen. A total of 69 out of 913 wells were positive for anti-merozoite anitbody and 12 were cloned and studied further. Three out of the 12 preparations agglutinated free merozoites and the partially purified Ig from two of these also inhibited merozoite invasion of red cells; the remaining 9 monoclonal antibodies were negative in both tests (Table 13·6). The two active antibodies were shown on electronmicroscopy to react with the entire merozoite surface. Both antibodies precipitated a component of molecular weight 250,000 from biosynthetically labelled schizonts as assessed by SDS-polyacrylamide gel electrophoresis. The inhibitory antibodies reacted with two geographically remote isolates of *P. knowlesi*. These antibodies therefore recognize a protective antigen common to different strains of the organism which has potential as a vaccinating agent against *P. knowlesi* malaria.

Monoclonal antibodies against the human parasite, *P. falciparum*, were produced by fusion of a mouse myeloma cell line (FO) with spleen cells from Balb/C mice immunized by intraperitoeal inoculation of mixed *P. falciparum* schizonts and merozoites (Perrin *et al.*, 1981a; 1981b); in other experiments spleens from Balb/C mice having drug-

TABLE 13·6
Monoclonal antibodies against *P. knowlesi* bloodstage antigens
(from Epstein *et al.*, 1981)

| Monoclonal antibody | Isotype | Merozoite aggln. | Invasion inhibition | Reactive antigen (mol. wt.) |
|---|---|---|---|---|
| 13 C 11 | IgG 2a | +++ | + | 250,000 |
| 16 F 8 | IgG 1 | ++ | + | 250,000 |
| 53 B 3 | IgG 2a | + | − | |
| 9 others | IgG 1 | − | − | |
| | IgA | − | − | |
| | IgM | − | − | |

controlled infections with *P. berghei* were used for fusion. Hybridoma supernatants were screened by indirect immunofluorescence using acetone fixed *P. falciparum* parasitized human erythrocytes as antigen. A total of 47 out of 978 supernatants reacted with *P. faciparum* parasitized red blood cells and two of these were derived from *P. berghei* immunized spleen cells. Fifteen hybridoma lines were double cloned and expanded as ascites tumours; of these 10 samples reacted with trophozoites and schizonts, two with schizonts only and three with all parasite stages. Eleven ascitic fluids were tested at a final concentration of 10% in cultures of *P. falciparum* and 3 inhibited parasite development in 80 hour assays; the Ig fractions isolated from two of these also inhibited parasite growth (Table 13·7). Two of the inhibitory preparations reacted with

TABLE 13·7
Monoclonal antibodies against *P. falciparum* bloodstage antigens
(from Perrin *et al.*, 1981b)

| Hybridoma | Ig Class | I.F. staining[c] | Growth inhibition % 10% Ascitic fluid | Isolated Ig (conc.) | Antigen (mol. wt.) |
|---|---|---|---|---|---|
| Hb 28[a] | IgG 3 | Sz and Tz | 100 | 95 (8 μg ml⁻¹) | 41,000 |
| Hb 26 | IgG 2a | Sz only | 96 | 89 (16 μg ml⁻¹) | 96,000 and 36,000 |
| Hb 31 | IgG 3 | Sz and Tz | 95 | | 41,000 |
| Hb 12[b] | IgG 1 | | 19 | | |
| Hb 9[b] | IgM | | 18 | | |

[a]  Derived from *P. berghei* immunized mouse.
[b]  2 out of 8 non-inhibitory monoclonal preparations tested.
[c]  Immunofluorescent staining of schizonts (Sz) and trophozoites (Tz).

an antigen of molecular weight 41,000 and the other with components of 96,000 and 36,000 (Table 13·7): all were thought to be surface components of merozoite on the basis of immunofluorescent staining patterns. The derivation from a *P. berghei* immunized mouse of a monoclonal antibody which inhibits *P. falciparum in vitro*, is an unexpected finding (Table 13·7) in view of the established species specificity of malarial immunity (Cohen and Mitchell, 1978). The antigens identified by the three inhibitory monoclonal antibodies are clearly of considerable interest as potential materials for use as vaccines against *P. falciparum*.

### C. Monoclonal Antibodies Against Malaria Gametes

The gametes, or sexual stages of malaria parasites, are present only in the midgut of infected mosquitoes and develop from male and female gametocytes ingested with a blood meal (Fig. 13·1). Fertilization follows gamete formation and the zygote develops as an oocyst in the mosquito gut wall; after about 2 weeks sporozoites released from oocysts migrate to the salivary glands. Immunization of chickens with gametes of *P. gallinaceum* does not affect the development of asexual parasites, but the avian host is no longer infectious for mosquitoes. Similar immunity has been induced in rodent and primate models (Carter and Chen, 1976; Mendis and Targett, 1979; Gwadz and Green, 1978). This transmission blocking immunity is mediated by anti-gamete antibodies which prevent fertilization (Gwadz, 1976; Carter *et al.*, 1979).

In work designed to isolate the antigens which induce transmission blocking immunity, Rener *et al.* (1980) produced hybridomas secreting antibodies against surface antigens on male and female gametes. Mouse plasmacytoma cells (P3-X63-Ag8) were fused with spleen cells from Balb/C mice immunized by intraperitoneal and intravenous inoculation of male and female gametes of *P. gallinaceum*. Culture supernatants were screened by indirect immunofluorescence against gametes as antigen. Two of the monoclonal antibodies induced stellate agglutination of male gametes and also reacted with female gametes; when tested for inhibition of infectivity in mosquitoes, each individual antibody was inactive, but in combination these antibodies caused a rope-like agglutination of male gametes and completely inhibited infectivity (Table 13·8).

TABLE 13·8
Monoclonal antibodies against *P. gallinaceum* gametes (from Rener *et al.*, 1980)

| Hybridoma | Isotype | Agglutination of gametes Pattern | Conc. antibody | Inhibition infectivity | Reactive antigen[a] |
|---|---|---|---|---|---|
| 10 G 3 | IgM | Stellate | 0·02–3 mg ml$^{-1}$ | ± | 220,000 |
| 11 C 7 | IgG1 | Stellate | 1·5 –3 mg ml$^{-1}$ | ± | |
| 10 G 3 + 11 C 7 | | Rope-like | 0·02–3 mg ml$^{-1}$ | + + | |

[a] L. H. Miller (personal communication).

## III MONOCLONAL ANTIBODIES IN OTHER PARASITIC INFECTIONS

The production of monoclonal antibodies reacting with protozoal parasites other than malaria, has been initiated in several laboratories (Table 13·9). The overall objectives of such studies which are at an early stage of development, are the isolation and characterization of antigens having a role in immune protection or immunopathology and the production of antigens or antibodies of use in immunodiagnosis and serological typing of parasites. Pearson *et al.* (1980) have described general methods for generating and detecting monoclonal antibodies against protozoal parasites.

*Toxoplasma gondii* is an intracellular protozoan parasite capable of infecting a very wide range of mammalian hosts. Serological studies reveal that 20–90% of human adults have been infected often without clinical symptoms; the disease may be serious in congenitally infected children and in immunosuppressed subjects and is a significant cause of ovine abortion. In a study aiming to characterize membrane antigens of Toxoplasma, Handman *et al.* (1980) hybridized spleen cells from immune mice with myeloma cells and produced 4 monoclonal antibodies which reacted with membrane components radioiodinated with lactoperoxidase and having molecular weights of 35,000 and 14,000, 43,00 and 27,000, respectively.

Monoclonal antibodies have also been raised against a variety of helminths pathogenic for man and domestic or laboratory animals (Table 13·10). The major emphasis of work completed has been upon the development of improved immunodiagnostic tests. The major problem in this regard, relates to the antigenic complexity of preparations conventionally used which leads to inadequate sensitivity and specificity of tests. Hence the improvement of immunodiagnostic methods has centred upon attempts to identify and purify stable anti-

TABLE 13·9

Monoclonal antibodies in protozoal infections other than malaria

| Parasite | Immunization | Screening | Application | Reference |
|---|---|---|---|---|
| *Toxoplasma gondii* | Chronic infection of mice | RIA—intact tachyzoites Indirect I.F. | Identification of membrane antigens | Handman *et al.* (1980) |
| | Infected mice | RIA—sonicated tachyzoites Indirect I.F. | | Sethi *et al.* (1980) |
| *Trypanosoma brucei* | Mice—intraperitoneal variant antigen | RIA—purified variant specific surface antigen | | Pearson *et al.* (1980) |
| | Mice—intraperitoneal variant antigen | RIA—purified variant specific surface antigen | Immunochemistry of surface glycoprotein | Pearson *et al.* (1981) |
| *Trypanosoma rhodesiense* | Mice—intraperitoneal surface coat glycoprotein | I.I.F.—acetone fixed or live trypanosomes | Immunochemistry of surface glycoprotein | Lyon *et al.* (1981) |
| *Theileria parva* | Mice—exposed to bovine lymphoblasts infected with Theileria macro-schizonts | Binding assay to Theileria tranformal cells I.I.F. acetone fixed infected cells | | Pearson *et al.* (1980) |
| | Mice—exposed to bovine lymphoblasts infected with Theileria macro-schizonts | I.I.F. acetone fixed infected cells | Identification of strains of *Theileria parva* | Pinder and Hewett, (1980) |

TABLE 13·10
Monoclonal antibodies in helminth infections

| Parasite | Immunization | Screening | Application | Reference |
|---|---|---|---|---|
| Taenia hydatigena T. ovis T. saginata Echinococcus granulosus | Mice—aqueous sonicates adult worms | ELISA or RIA—sonicated parasites as antigen | Preparation of immuno-diagnostic reagents for use in sheep | Craig et al. (1980) |
| Mesocestoides corti | Chronically infected mice | RIA—acid treated parasites from nude mice | Investigation of model Immunodiagnostic assay in mice | Mitchell et al. (1979) |
| Schistosoma mansoni | Infected rats | I.I.F.—schistosomula | Isolation of reaginic and protective antibodies | Verwaerde et al. (1979) |
| | Infected mice | Circumoval precipitation schistosome eggs RIA—schistosome eggs | Identification of major serological antigen, $MSA_1$ | Hillyer et al. (1980) |
| S. japonicum | Mice—extracts of adult worms | RIA—aqueous extracts of adult worms | Specific immunodiagnosis of S. japonicum | Mitchell et al. (1981) |

gens which may help to detect infection, evaluate its duration, recognize the threat of immunopathology or assess the immune status of the host. It is obvious that monoclonal antibodies are likely to prove invaluable for such specific antigen isolation. The problem of antigenic purification can sometimes be circumvented by the use of monoclonal antibodies. Thus, in a model system involving a larval cestode of mice, *Mesocestoides corti*, a specific and sensitive competitive solid phase radio-immunoassay was elaborated based upon the inhibition of binding of a radiolabelled monoclonal antibody to a crude parasite antigen mixture by sera from *M. corti* infected mice (Mitchell *et al.*, 1979). Such a test is workable only if the animal whose cells are used for fusion and the infected host recognize a similar set of parasite antigens; this may not always be the case with human or vetinary parasitic infections, (Craig *et al.*, 1980); however, a monoclonal antibody with immunodiagnostic potential for the important human pathogen, *Schistosoma japonicum*, has been reported (Mitchell *et al.*, 1981).

## IV CONCLUSION

Animal parasites of man are large organisms with complex life-cycles and a corresponding diversity of antigens. The isolation and characterization of individual parasite antigens is being expedited by the use of monoclonal antibodies. This work is at an early stage of development, but has already been applied to a wide range of protozoa and helminths and shows promise of improving the specificty and sensitivity of immunodiagnostic methods and the efficacy of immunotherapy.

In the case of malaria, experimental vaccination with sporozoites, erythrocytic merozoites and gametes has induced effective immunity against specific stages of the parasite in a variety of experimental hosts. The development of practical vaccines against human malaria based upon these forms of the parasite is however, impractical for several reasons including especially the paucity of available antigenic material. All stages of the differentiating parasite are antigenically complex and the task of identifying protective antigens with potential as immunogens has been greatly facilitated by the advent of hybridoma technology. Work in progress has identified putative protective antigens on the surface of sporozoites, merozoites and gametes and has made feasible attempts to isolate or produce by recombinant DNA technology, specific protective antigens for evaluation as vaccines in experimental and human malaria. Although the major emphasis of current work in malaria is upon vaccine development, there exists the means, as yet unexploited, for developing new forms of passive immunotherapy using human hybridomas, and for elaborating improved immunodiagnostic tests giving greater reproducibility, specificity and sensitivity.

ACKNOWLEDGEMENTS

I am grateful to Drs. G. F. Mitchell, L. H. Miller and R. S. Nussenzweig and their collaborators who kindly made available some of their unpublished data.

REFERENCES

Aikawa, M., Yoshida, N., Nussenzweig, R. S. and Nussenzweig, V. (1981). *J. Immunol.* (in press).
Brown, K. N. and Brown, I. N. (1965). *Nature* **208**, 1286–1288.
Butcher, G. A. and Cohen, S. (1970). *R. Soc. trop. Med. Hyg.* **64**, 470.
Butcher, G. A., Mitchell, G. H. and Cohen, S. (1978). *Immunology* **34**, 77–86.
Carter, R. and Chen, D. H. (1976). *Nature* **263**, 57–60.
Carter, R., Gwadz, R. W. and Green, I. (1979). *Expl. Parasit.* **47**, 194–208.
Clyde, D. F. (1975). *Am. J. trop. Med. Hyg.* **24**, 397–401.
Coatney, R. G., Collins, W. E., Warren, M. and Contacos, P. G. (1971). *In* "The primate malarias". U.S.A. Dept. Health Education & Welfare, Bethesda.
Cohen, S. (1979). *Proc. R. Soc.* B. **203**, 323–345.
Cohen, S. (1980). *In* "Host Invader Interplay". (H. van den Borsche Ed.), p. 191–203. Elsevier, Amsterdam.
Cohen, S., Butcher, G. A. and Crandall, R. B. (1969). *Nature* **223**, 368–371.
Cohen, S. and Mitchell, G. H. (1978). *Curr. Top. Microbiol. Immunol.* **80**, 97–129.
Craig, P. S., Mitchell, G. F., Cruise, K. M. and Rickard, M. D. (1980). *Aust. J. exp. Biol. Med. Sci.* **58**, 339–350.
Deans, J. A. (1980). *Trop. Dis. Res.* Series 4, (in press).
Deans, J. A. and Cohen, S. (1979). *Bull. Wld Hlth Org.* **57**, Suppl 1, 93–100.
Deans, J. A., Dennis, E. D. and Cohen, S. (1978). *Parasitology* **77**, 333–344.
Deans, J. A., Alderson, T., Thomas, A. W., Mitchell, G. H., Lennox, E. S. and Cohen, S. (1982). *Clin. exp. Immunol.* (in press).
Dennis, E. D., Mitchell, G. H., Butcher, G. H. and Cohen, S. (1975). *Parasitology* **71**, 475–481.
Eaton, M. D. (1938). *J. exp. Med.* **67**, 857–869.
Epstein, N., Miller, L. H., Kaushel, D. C., Udeinya, I. J., Rener, J., Howard, R. J., Asofsky, R., Aikawa, M. and Hess, R. L. (1981). Personal Communication.
Freeman, R. R., Trejdosiewicz, A. J. and Cross, G. A. M. (1980a). *Nature* **284**, 366–368.
Freeman, R. R., Trejdosiewicz, A. J., Bushby, L. E. and Cross, G. A. M. (1980b). Fourth International Congress of Immunology (abstracts) 12. 8. 09.

Garnham, P. C. C. (1966). In "Malaria Parasites and other Haemosporidia" Blackwell Scientific Publications, Oxford.

Gward, R. W. (1976). Science 193, 1150–1151.

Gwadz, R. W. and Green, I. (1978). J. exp. Med. 148, 1311–1323.

Gwadz, R. W., Carter, R. and Green, I. (1978). Bull. Wld Hlth Org. 57, (Suppl. 1) 175–180.

Handman, E., Goding, J. W. and Remington, J. S. (1980). J. Immunol. 124, 2578–2583.

Hillyer, G. B. and Pelley, R. P. (1980). Am. J. trop. Med. Hyg. 29, 582–585.

Kilejian, A. (1978). Science 201, 922–924.

Kilejian, A. (1980). J. exp. Med. 151, 1534–1538.

Kim, K. J., Taylor, D. W., Evans, C. B. and Asofsky, R. (1980). J. Immunol. 125, 2565–2569.

Kohler, G. and Milstein, C. (1975). Nature 256, 495–497.

Lamont, G., Saul, A. and Kidson, C. (1981). Exp. Parasitol. (in press).

Langreth, S. G. and Reese, R. T. (1979). J. exp. Med. 150, 1241–1254.

Lyon, J. A., Pratt, J. M., Travis, R. W., Doctor, B. P. and Olenick, J. G. (1981). J. Immunol. 126, 134–137.

Mendis, K. N. and Targett, G. A. T. (1979). Nature 277, 389–391.

Mitchell, G. H., Butcher, G. A., Voller, A. and Cohen, S. (1976). Parasitology 72, 149–162.

Mitchell, G. F., Cruise, K. M., Chapman, C. B., Anders, R. F. and Howard, M. C. (1979). Aust. J. exp. Biol. Med. Sci. 57, 287–302.

Mitchell, G. F., Cruise, K. M., Garcia, E. G. and Anders, R. F. (1981). Proc. natn. Acad. Sci. U.S.A. (in press).

Nardin, E. H. and Nussenzweig, R. S. (1978). Nature 274, 55–57.

Nussenzweig, R. S., Vanderberg, J. and Most, H. (1969). Military Medicine 134, 1176–1182.

Nussenzweig, R. S., Cochrane, A. and Lustig, H. (1978). In "Rodent Malaria" (Peters, W. and Killick-Kendrick, R. Eds) p. 247. Academic Press, London.

Pearson, T. W., Pinder, M., Roelants, G. E., Kar, S. K., Lundin, L. B., Mayor-Withey, K. S. and Hewett, R. S. (1980). J. Immunol. Methods 34, 141–154.

Pearson, T. W., Kar, S. K., McGuire, T. C. and Lundin, L. B. (1981). J. Immunol. 126, 823–828.

Perrin, L. H., Dayal, R. and Rieder, H. (1981a). Trans. R. Soc. trop. Med. Hyg. 75, 163–165.

Perrin, L. H., Ramirez, E., Lambert, P. H. and Miescher, P. A. (1981b). Nature 289, 301–303.

Pinder, M. and Hewett, R. S. (1980). J. Immunol. 124, 1000–1001.

Potocnjak, P., Yoshida, N., Nussenzweig, R. S. and Nussenzweig, V. (1980). J. exp. Med. 151, 1504–1513.

Rener, J., Carter, R., Rosenberg Y. and Miller, L. H. (1980). Proc. natn. Acad, Sci. 77, 6797–6799.

Schmidt-Ullrich, R. and Wallach, D. F. H. (1978). Proc. natn. Acad. Sci. 75, 4949–4953.

Schmidt-Ullrich, R., Wallach, D. F. H. and Lightholder, J. (1979). *J. exp. Med.* **150**, 86–99.

Sethi, K. K., Endo, T. and Brandis, H. (1980). *J. Parasitol.* **66**, 192–196.

Verwaerde, C., Grzych, J. M., Bazin, H., Capron, M. and Capron, A. (1979). *C. R. Acad. Sci. Paris* **289**, 275.

Wilson, R. J. M. (1980). *Nature* **284**, 451–452.

Wilson, R. J. M. and Phillips, R. S. (1976). *Nature* **263**, 132.

Yoshida, N., Nussenzweig, R. S., Potocnjak, P., Nussenzweig, V. and Aikawa, M. (1980). *Science* **207**, 71–73.

# F  GENETICS

# 14 Monoclonal Antibodies to HLA Antigens: new approaches to the study of structure, genetics and function

ANDREW J. McMichael

*Nuffield Department of Medicine, John Radcliffe Hospital, Headington, Oxford. OX3 9DU*

## I INTRODUCTION

Among the first human structures to be recognized by monoclonal antibodies were HLA antigens (Barnstable *et al.*, 1978; Trucco *et al.*, 1978). Since then, many such reagents have been produced, reflecting the abundance and immunogenicity of these cell surface glycoproteins. It has been demonstrated that these antibodies can be used as powerful probes to investigate very basic questions about transplantation anti-gens concerning their structure, genetics and function. This chapter will discuss in detail these aspects, which are of importance in under-standing the immune system and its role in disease processes. Because of the large numbers of antibodies still needed, their use in HLA typing is still in its infancy.

## II  THE HLA SYSTEM: STRUCTURE, GENETICS AND FUNCTION; OUTSTANDING QUESTIONS

The basic features of the HLA system are summarized in Fig. 14·1. There are two types of HLA antigen known as Class 1 (formerly S. D.) and Class 2 (also known as immune associated, Ia) antigens (Klein, 1979). Both are cell surface glycoproteins. Class 1 antigens have a heavy chain of 43,000 daltons, which is noncovalently associated with $\beta_2$ microglobulin, 12,000 daltons. The heavy chain is a transmembrane glycosylated protein with a short lipid soluble hydrophobic region near its carboxy terminal; $\beta_2$ microglobulin is water soluble. There are three series of Class 1 antigens, known as HLA A, B and C in man (H-2 K, D and L in mice) all with the same basic structure. HLA A and B (and almost certainly C) antigens show striking homology in their amino acid sequences with each other (reviewed by Strominger, 1981) and their counterparts in other species (Coligan *et al.*, 1981). The HLA A, B and C heavy chains are controlled by three genetic loci, HLA *A*, *B* and *C*, which map close together on chromosome six in a cluster of genes known as the major histocompatibility complex (MHC). The order of genes is *A*, *C*, *B* with a recombination frequency of about 1% between *A* and *B*. HLA *A*, *B* and *C* loci exhibit genetic polymorphism to an extreme degree. There are respectively at least 20, 30 and 8 alleles defined for each locus (Table 14·1). The individual allelic products are described by a number, preceded by a "w" if it is a provisional work-shop designation, e.g. A3, B7, Cw8. A diploid cell can therefore express six different Class 1 heavy chains, if heterozygous at each locus. The variation between each heavy chain seems to be slight, less than 20% of the amino acid residues, but several of these variations are clustered at particular regions of the molecule, which may be antigenic and involved in function (Strominger, 1981). Analysis of amino acid and DNA sequence data suggests that the HLA *A*, *B* and *C* loci evolved from a common ancestral gene by gene duplication and mutation (Strominger, 1981; Coligan *et al.*, 1981).

Human $\beta_2$ microglobulin ($\beta_2$m) seems to be invariant between indi-

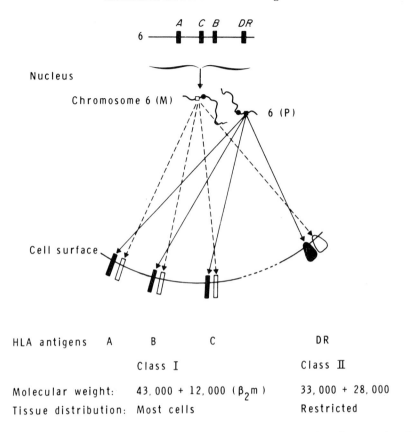

FIG. 14·1 The HLA System. HLA A-B-C-DR antigens are cell surface glycoproteins of two types: Class I and Class II. Each series (A, B, C and DR) is controlled by the major histocompatibility complex (MHC) on the short arm of chromosome 6. Each individual has a maternally (M) and paternally (P) derived chromosome 6. Within the MHC are four loci *A*, *B*, *C* and *DR* which control expression of each series of HLA antigens.

viduals, and is structurally conserved between species (Sanderson, 1977). It is not coded for by the *MHC* and in man is controlled by chromosome 15 (Goodfellow *et al.*, 1975). The structure of $\beta$2m shows striking homology with immunoglobulin domains. These are sequences of about 110 amino acids, held in a loop by a disulphide bridge, each coded for by a separate exon, that make up an immunoglobulin chain: 2 for a light chain, 4 or 5 for a heavy chain. Analysis of the structure of the heavy chain of HLA and H-2 indicates that these are also made up of domains, one of which shows sequence homology with immunoglobulin (Strominger, 1981; Coligan *et al.*, 1981). Three domains are outside the

TABLE 14·1
HLA specificities

| | Locus | | |
| --- | --- | --- | --- |
| A | B | C | DR |
| A1 | B5 | Cw1 | DR1 |
| A2[a] | B7[a] | Cw2 | DR2[a] |
| A3 | B8 | Cw3 | DR3 |
| A9 | B12 | Cw4 | DR4[a] |
| A10 | B13 | Cw5 | DR5 |
| A11 | B14 | Cw6 | DRw6 |
| Aw19 | B15 (w62, w63)[b] | Cw7 | DR7 |
| Aw23 | B16 | Cw8 | DRw8 |
| Aw24 | B17[a] (w57, w58)[b] | | DRw9 |
| A25 | B18 | | DRw10 |
| A26 | Bw21 | | |
| A28[a] | Bw22[a] (w56, w57)[b] | | |
| A29 | B27[a] | | MT1[a] |
| Aw30 | Bw35 | | MT2[a] |
| Aw31 | B37 | | MT3 |
| Aw32 | Bw38 | | MB1[a] |
| Aw33 | Bw39 | | MB2 |
| Aw34 | B40 (w60, w61)[b] | | MB3[a] |
| Aw36 | Bw41 | | |
| Aw43 | Bw42[a] | | |
| | Bw44 | | |
| | Bw45 | | |
| | Bw46[a] | | |
| | Bw47 | | |
| | Bw48 | | |
| | Bw49 | | |
| | Bw50 | | |
| | Bw51 | | |
| | Bw52 | | |
| | Bw53 | | |
| | Bw54 | | |

[a]  Identifiable by monoclonal antibodies, either alone or by combinations.
[b]  Splits defined at the Eighth Histocompatibility Workshop.

membrane, there is a short hydrophobic $\alpha$ helix within the lipid bilayer and the COOH terminal is intracellular. The N terminal domain, unlike the others, is not held by a disulphide bond; it has been suggested that this is held as a loop by $\beta_2$ microglobulin (Strominger, 1981; Coligan et al., 1981).

Class 1 antigens have a widespread tissue distribution, probably being expressed on most nucleated cells. HLA C seems to be a minor component in terms of quantity of antigen expressed on cells (Snary *et al.*, 1977).

Class 2 MHC antigens, HLA DR (H2 Ia in the mouse), have a different structure. There is an $\alpha$ chain of 33,000 daltons and a $\beta$ chain of 28,000 daltons which are non-covalently linked. In the mouse there are two series: I-A and I-E and all four chains are controlled by closely linked genes in the *MHC* (Klein *et al.*, 1981, Uhr *et al.*, 1979). In addition there is serological evidence for at least one other structure, I-J coded for in this region (Murphy, 1978). I-A and I-E antigens have related but distinct amino acid sequences. In the mouse both I-A and I-E are polymorphic but I-A is more so; and most of the variability seems to reside in its $\beta$ chain (Uhr *et al.*, 1979).

HLA DR antigens are much less well characterized. Using conventional antisera, antibodies produced by women in pregnancy, one allelic series has been clearly defined. This *HLA DR* locus maps outside *HLA A, B* and *C* closest to *B* (Fig. 14·1). Like HLA A B and C, HLA DR antigens show marked polymorphism. Table 14·1 lists the HLA A, B, C and DR antigens. It is apparent that the number of possible HLA A-B-C-DR haplotypes is large (75,000) and of diploid genotypes is huge.

HLA DR antigens show sequence homology with I-E antigens (Strominger, 1981; Silver and Ferrone, 1979). A major question, therefore, is whether there is a human equivalent of I-A. While specific allo-antisera to HLA DR antigens 1 through 10 presumably define unique antigenic determinants, three related series of antigens, DC, MT and MB, have been described (Tosi *et al.*, 1978; Park *et al.*, 1980a; Duquesnoy and Marrari, 1980) which could either define "public" antigenic sites which are shared by two or more different HLA DR molecules, or the products of a second locus. This putative second series of antigens would show a smaller degree of polymorphism and allelic association (linkage disequilibrium between particular genes at each locus, e.g. *MT1* with *HLA DR 1, 2* and *6*. The important contributions of monoclonal antibodies to this discussion will be described below.

HLA DR antigens have a restricted tissue distribution. Initially they were demonstrated only on B lymphocytes and monocytes. B lymphocytes prepared from human peripheral blood, are used for HLA DR typing, with alloantisera by complement mediated cytotoxicity, a process which is technically demanding (Park *et al.*, 1980b).

As their synonyms imply, histocompatibility or transplantation antigens are important in graft rejection. Of all cell surface antigens, they provoke the strongest immunological reactions. Furthermore, their extreme polymorphism means that matching between unrelated organ donors and recipients is very difficult to achieve. Although the rejection process, mediated by both antibody and cellular (T cell) immunity, is primarily directed at the Class 1 antigens, the Class II antigens play a crucial role in initiating these immune reactions, as they do *in vitro* by stimulating strong mixed lymphocyte reactions. It is not too surprising, therefore, that recent figures on kidney grafting indicate that HLA DR matching is more important than HLA ABC matching (Ting and Morris, 1978). There is a need, therefore, for improved understanding and techniques in clinical HLA DR matching.

The natural function of the HLA antigens has provoked much interest, partly to explain the extreme degree of polymorphism in functional terms: to demonstrate not only the benefits of heterozygosity but that certain HLA antigens confer particular selective advantages. McDevitt and coworkers (Benacerraf and McDevitt, 1972) showed, ten years ago, that the ability of inbred mouse strains to make immune responses to certain synthetic peptide antigens was controlled by single genes which mapped in the *H-2* complex. These immune response (*Ir*) genes function at the level of the helper T lymphocytes which are essential amplifiers of both B cell (antibody) and T cell (cell mediated immune) responses. When attempts were made to identify the products of *Ir* genes, Ia (Class 2) antigens were discovered (Shreffler *et al.*, 1974). It was then found that helper T lymphocytes recognize foreign antigens in association with Ia antigens on antigen presenting cells, and that particular Ia types affected the immunogenicity of the foreign antigen (Rosenthal *et al.*, 1977). Thus a point mutation in one Ia antigen can qualitatively affect the ability of that mouse to respond to an unrelated foreign protein (Lin *et al.*, 1981). Two alternative explanations have been proposed. T lymphocytes in responding to Ia and foreign antigen (x) on the surface of presenting cells may be affected by different combinations (? complexes) of Ia and x. Alternatively, Ia antigens may control the quality of the T cell receptor for foreign antigen; it is held by some that the T cell receptor repertoire is generated in the thymus by somatic mutation of anti self MHC receptors (Von Boehmer *et al.*, 1978). Whichever explanation is correct, the Class 2 antigens clearly play a role in the regulation of immune responses. This applies not just to antibody responses to synthetic peptides in mice, but to both B and T cell responses to complex antigens in all species tested, including man (Bergholtz *et al.*, 1980).

Class 1 antigens operate in similar ways in the function of another population of T cells, the cytotoxic T lymphocytes (Tc). Zinkernagel and Doherty (1974) showed that Tc, which lyse virus infected cells, recognize virus and Class 1 antigens together, on the cell surface. This has been found to be true in humans where virus specific Tc show specificity for (self) HLA A or B antigens as well as virus (McMichael *et al.*, 1977, Shaw and Biddison, 1979). Furthermore, there is some variability in the response according to HLA type (McMichael, 1978). Whether virus and HLA antigens interact physically on the cell surface is not yet known and explanations of the findings are similar to those postulated for Ir genes.

These studies appear to provide a raison d'etre for the HLA antigens and a potential explanation for the polymorphism, given that the primary role of the immune system is to combat infectious disease. Further support for this comes from studies which show that indiviuals whose cells carry certain HLA antigens are more susceptible to particular diseases (Ryder *et al.*, 1979) (e.g. HLA B27 and ankylosing spondylitis; DR2 and multiple sclerosis; DR4 and rheumatoid arthritis; DR3 and organ specific autoimmune diseases). These clear associations are with disease susceptibility. Associations with resistance to infectious disease must be of greater biological significance but require much more comprehensive surveys to demonstrate (Piazza *et al.*, 1973). The mechanisms that underlie these findings are not understood but the autoimmune nature of many of the diseases for which associations have been discovered strongly supports the notion that the HLA antigen products themselves, rather than products of fortuitously linked genes, are responsible.

The advent of monoclonal antibodies has given immunologists a new tool for analysing further the structure, function and role in disease, of HLA antigens, as well as providing reagents of potential value in tissue typing. In the following discussion their use in analysis of HLA antigen structure, antigenicity, genetic control and function will be illustrated.

## III PRODUCTION OF MONOCLONAL ANTIBODIES TO HLA

The abundance of antibodies that have been made to HLA antigens testifies to the immunogenicity of these structures. To make antibodies to the nonpolymorphic (monomorphic) determinants, no special preparation of antigen is needed for immunization of the mice. HLA bearing lymphocytes or cell lines are sufficient. In fusion experiments from such mice anti HLA antibodies occur, in our experience, at low frequencies (less than 10% of antibody making clones, but provided that these can be identified easily, this is more than adequate. Antibodies specific for Class 1 antigens can be recognized by testing them for binding or cytotoxicity on normal and Daudi cells. The latter is a Burkitt's lymphoma line that lacks HLA A, B and C antigenic determinants due to an inability to make $\beta_2$ microglobulin (Goodfellow *et al.*, 1975). Antibody to Class 2 antigens can be selected by screening culture supernatants on B cell lines and T cell lines. The former are positive for, and the latter negative for, HLA DR antigens. While these tests are sufficient for initial culture selection, further evidence is required to prove that the antibody recognizes HLA antigen. Immunoprecipitation of antigen from radiolabelled cell membranes, tissue distribution studies of antibody binding, competitive binding studies with well defined monoclonal antibodies, and inhibition of binding with purified HLA antigen, have been used (Barnstable *et al.*, 1978, Parham *et al.*, 1979, Trucco *et al.*, 1979).

Purified glycoproteins have been used as immunogens to generate antibodies to Class 1 and Class 2 determinants. They may be prepared by detergent solubilization of plasma membrane, followed by affinity column chromatography on a lentil lectin column with elution by $\alpha$ methylmannoside, or purification with a monoclonal anti HLA antibody coupled to sepharose with elution at high or low pH (Parham *et al.*, 1979; and see chapter 22). Mice can be immunized subcutaneously with the antigen, freed from detergent by precipitation in cold acetone, in complete Freund's adjuvant with a final intravenous boost four days before fusion. These purification steps are not necessary for the production of monoclonal antibodies to monomorphic (i.e. invariant within the species) determinants but are of theoretical advantage in producing antibodies to polymorphic antigenic sites. Because monoclonal antibodies that identify polymorphic determinants are rare, we favour this strategy because it gives a high yield of anti HLA clones compared to hybridoma fusions from mice immunized with whole cells (McMichael *et al.*, 1980, Ellis *et al.*, 1981). This is especially advantageous if screening is by the relatively laborious process of radioimmuno-binding assay to two cell lines, one positive for, and one negative for, the antigen in question. Trucco *et al.* (1979) and Grumet *et al.* (1981) have screened, by complement mediated cytotoxicity, hybridoma colonies prepared from mice immunized whith whole cells and have obtained antibodies to polymorphic determinants. This screening can be carried out on standard tissue typing trays so that large numbers of culture supernatants can be characterized alongside conventional HLA typing reagents. This method does, however, exclude non-cytotoxic (IgG1) antibodies.

# IV MONOCLONAL ANTIBODIES TO CLASS 1 ANTIGENS

Monoclonal antibodies to HLA Class 1 antigens can be divided into two types: those that recognize monomorphic determinants and those that see polymorphic antigenic sites. Both are informative about the nature of the Class 1 antigen in terms of its antigenicity.

## A. MONOMORPHIC ANTIGENIC SITES

Monomorphic antigens are shared between all human HLA A, B and C molecules (Barnstable *et al.*, 1978). No locus specific antigen has yet been described. As the antibodies are made by murine B cells, they reflect differences in the amino acid sequence of Class 1 antigens between the H-$2^d$ antigens of Balb/c mice and HLA. Studies indicate that about 30% of amino acids are different between the two (Strominger, 1981). However, detailed antigenic analysis of proteins whose crystalographic structure is known, such as myoglobin (Crumpton *et al.*, 1970) or influenza haemagglutinin (Wiley *et al.*, 1981, chapter 10), indicates that antigenic sites tend to be relatively few and sited at the corners of the folded molecule. The crystalographic structure of HLA A-B-C is not yet known and not enough sequences are known to define probable antigenic sites precisely. Based on the available data, however, some preliminary observations on HLA antigen structure can be made.

At least three types of monomorphic antibody have been defined, each with different properties (Brodsky *et al.*, 1979a). In these analyses, use is made of the cell line Daudi which cannot make $\beta_2$ microglobulin, yet contains intracellular Class 1 heavy chain, and lines which are hybrids between mouse and human cells. These tend to lose several human chromosomes and it is possible to select lines, which carry chromosome 6 (HLA heavy chain) but not 15 ($\beta_2$ microglobulin). These cells express HLA Class 1 heavy chain associated with mouse $\beta_2$ microglobulin. Cell lines which express human chromosome 15 and not 6 may also be used (Brodsky, 1979). The reaction patterns of the three types of antibody are shown in Table 14·2.

The simplest pattern is that of anti $\beta_2$m which binds only to cells that express human $\beta_2$m (Brodsky *et al.*, 1979a, b; Trucco *et al.*, 1979). An intriguing finding with these antibodies is that they block binding of monoclonal antibodies which are specific for the heavy chain and HLA typing alloantisera. The probable explanation is that $\beta_2$m holds the heavy chain in a stable conformation at the cell surface (Lancet *et al.*,

TABLE 14·2

Reaction patterns of monoclonal antibodies to monomorphic HLA Class 1 antigens

| HLA-H $\beta_2$m Antibody | Daudi (+) − | Target cells[a] | | | Specificity |
|---|---|---|---|---|---|
| | | Lymphocytes + +(h) | m-h-H Chr6 + +(m) | m-h-H Chr15 − +(h) | |
| BBM1 | − | + | − | + | $\beta_2$m |
| BB7·5 | − | + | − | − | H-$\beta_2$m(h) |
| W6/32 | − | + | + | − | H-$\beta_2$m |

[a]   Target cells were: Daudi which synthesizes HLA Class 1 heavy chain (HLA-H) in the absence
     of $\beta_2$ microglobulin ($\beta_2$m); peripheral blood lymphocytes which express HLA Class 1 heavy
     chain in association with human $\beta_2$ microglobulin -$\beta_2$ m(h); mouse-human hybrid cells which
     carry human chromosome 6 but not 15 (m-h-H Chr6) and express HLA Class 1 heavy chain
     associated with mouse (m) $\beta_2$m; and mouse-human hybrids which express human
     chromosome 15 but not 6 (m-h-H Chr15) and so can express H-2 with human $\beta_2$m.
     Data adapted from Brodsky et al., 1979; Parham and Brodsky 1981.

1979, Cepellini et al., 1981). Thus, almost all the antibodies which bind
to the heavy chain do so only when it is associated with $\beta_2$m, or show
only very weak binding to isolated heavy chain (Trucco et al., 1979,
Brodsky et al., 1979b). An interesting observation is that there are some
antibodies that require human $\beta_2$m whereas others bind to heavy chain
associated with either human or mouse $\beta_2$m (Parham and Brodsky,
1981). This may indicate that part of the $\beta_2$m chain which differs in the
two species forms part of the antigenic site or that the heavy chain
conformation is affected by very slight differences in the $\beta_2$m. A fourth
type of antbody binding pattern is binding to isolated heavy chain.
Ploegh et al. (1979) have reported a xeno-antiserum that bound to intracellular HLA heavy chain, but did not lyse intact cells including Daudi
in the presence of complement. Another interesting point in the relationship between heavy chain and $\beta_2$m comes from studies in primates
(Brodsky et al., 1981b; Parham and Ploegh 1980; Parham and Brodsky,
1981). W6/32 binds to Class 1 antigens on old-world but, with one
exception, not new-world monkeys. The exception is the owl monkey
where two strains show a difference with binding to cells in one but not
the other; W6/32 does bind to free heavy chain in the "negative" group
however and Parham and Brodsky (1981) have suggested that the $\beta_2$
microglobulin may differ in the two groups.

   The picture that emerges, therefore, is of a molecule that can
have a variable antigenic form, depending on its interaction with $\beta_2$
microglobulin. The possibility that disturbances of this antigenic conformation might be important in the function of HLA antigens in T
lymphocyte immune responses will be discussed later.

## B. POLYMORPHIC ANTIGENIC SITES

Monoclonal antibodies to polymorphic Class 1 antigenic sites are harder to prepare. Those that have been made can also be used to analyse the antigenic structure of the HLA molecule. In conventional HLA typing, use is made of human antisera donated by recently-pregnant women, who have been immunized to paternal HLA antigens of the foetus. Antisera that are specific for a single HLA antigen, e.g. B7, are selected by a complicated screening process; many antisera contain antibodies to more than one antigen, e.g. B7 and A3. Typing sera have been extensively analyzed in a series of collaborative international workshops (Terasaki, 1980). What is not clear is whether each antigen carries unique antigenic specificities (epitopes) or, whether an antigen merely carries an unique combination of epitopes, each of which is shared by other antigens. Monoclonal antibodies specific for single epitopes can distinguish between these possibilities.

Two antigens have been studied in some detail, HLA A2 and B7. Both have been sequenced (reviewed by Strominger, 1981) so that it should, ultimately, be possible to locate each antigenic site precisely. Both antigens show crossreactivity with others (Joysey and Wolf, 1978) and these are shown in Fig 14·2.

The monoclonal antibodies relevant to this discussion are listed in Table 14·3. HLA A2 has been described by antibodies of the types

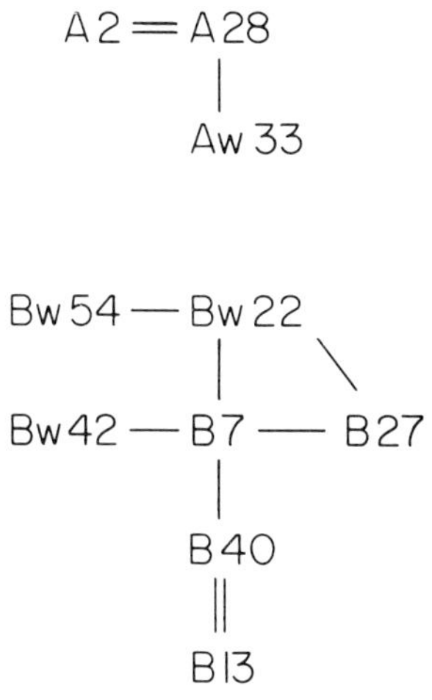

$$A2 = A28$$
$$|$$
$$Aw33$$

$$Bw54 - Bw22$$

$$Bw42 - B7 - B27$$
$$|$$
$$B40$$
$$\|$$
$$B13$$

FIG. 14·2 The HLA A2 and HLA B7 crossreacting groups. (adapted from Joysey and Wolf, 1978) = strong crossreaction; − crossreactions.

TABLE 14·3

Reaction patterns of antibodies to polymorphic HLA Class 1 antigenic determinants

The A2 group:

| Antibody:[a] | A2 | A28 | Target cells carrying A28* | B17 | Others | | |
|---|---|---|---|---|---|---|---|
| PA2·1 | + | − | + | − | − | | |
| MA2·1 | + | − | − | + | − | | |
| MA28·1 | + | + | + | − | − | | |
| FMC5 | +[b] | − | n.t. | − | − | | |

The B7 group:

| Antibody:[a] | B7 | B27 | B40 | B22 | B42 | Others |
|---|---|---|---|---|---|---|
| BB7·1 | + | − | − | − | − | − |
| MB40·3 | + | − | + | − | − | − |
| MB40·2 | + | − | +[b] | − | − | − |
| ME1 | + | + | − | + | n.t. | − |
| anti B27m | + | + | − | + | + | − |

[a] See text for references.
[b] Antibody does not bind to all HLA antigens of this type and therefore identifies subgroups.

indicated (Parham and Bodmer, 1978; Brodsky *et al.*, 1979; McMichael *et al.*, 1980; Beckman *et al.*, 1981). Each shows a different reactivity pattern and therefore is likely to see a different epitope. All except one react with all HLA A2 antigens tested, including two shown to be variants by cytotoxic T cells (Biddison *et al.*, 1980; Pfeffer and Thorsby, 1981). One, FMC5, does identify HLA A2 subgroups but has not yet been tested on those defined by cytotoxic T cells (Beckman *et al.*, 1981). One antibody, MA28·1 (Parham and Brodsky, 1981) reacted with HLA A2 and A28. Others react with HLA A2 and an A28 variant found initially on only one cell line IDF (and on normal lymphocytes from the original IDF blood donor) (Brodsky *et al.*, 1981) but more recently also on cells from other donors (J. Bodmer personal communication); the antigen is called here A28*. MA2·1 shows an unexpected cross-reactivity with HLA B17 (McMichal *et al.*, 1980); this was not previously recognized as a crossreaction by alloantisera but Morton *et al.*, (1971) had some evidence for its existence. Interestingly, our measurements of the binding avidity of MA2·1 for A2 and B17 give the same result $(2 \times 10^{-9})$ suggesting identity of the antigenic determinants and hence of a stretch of amino acid sequence. The anti A2 antibodies, therefore, clearly define at least three antigenic determinants. Furthermore, they provide evidence for heterogeneity of both the A2 and A28 molecules, a feature which had not been suspected from conventional HLA serology.

There are four antibodies that describe the B7 family. BB7·1 binds to an unique epitope, (Brodsky *et al.*, 1979), MB40·2 (Parham, 1981) recognizes a determinant shared by B7 and B40, and ME1 (Ellis *et al.*, 1981) sees an epitope shared by B7, B27 and B22. These antibodies almost certainly see different antigenic sites. Parham (1981) has identified a variant of HLA B40 seen only by MB40·2.

HLA B27 is an antigen of special interest because of its association with ankylosing spondylitis (Brewerton *et al.*, 1973). 95% of patients carry this antigen which is found in about 7% of controls. The association is maintained in different ethnic groups, strongly favouring the hypothesis that B27 itself is involved in the disease process. Yet more than 80% of B27 individuals do not develop this disease or the related Reiter's disease, even when exposed to known triggering agents (Calin and Fries, 1975). It is possible, therefore, that the HLA B27 antigen associated with the disease is different from that in healthy individuals. Two anti HLA B27 antibodies have been described (Grumet *et al.*, 1981; Ellis *et al.*, 1982), both of which recognize the same crossreacting group of antigens B7–B27–B22. With both antibodies there was preliminary evidence, in indirect binding assays, that the reagents bind best to B27 and only weakly to B22. No differences in binding, however, were found for either antibody when cells from patients with ankylosing spondylitis were compared to normal controls so that for this epitope at least the disease associated B27 is the same as the normal. ME1, which is not a complement fixing antibody, blocks lysis by alloantisera specific for B27 and by those specific for B7. This could mean that the eipitope seen by ME1 is close to the unique B27 and B7 specificities in their respective molecules. This epitope which is shared by B7 and B27 may be distinguishable by alloantisera, which are mixtures of antibodies, by their reactions with other antigenic sites. While B7 has a "private" epitope (Brodsky *et al.*, 1979) it is possible that HLA B27 could have no single unique antigenic determinant.

Besides these antibodies, that identify single or related groups of antigens, some have been found that show broad crossreactivity (Parham and McLean, 1980).

The picture that emerges, therefore, is that Class 1 molecules do have several antigenic epitopes, at least four monomorphic and up to four polymorphic. In addition the B locus antigens have the public allelic antigens B4/B6 defined by alloantisera and now by a monoclonal antibody (P. Parham and F. M. Brodsky personal communication).

Monoclonal antibodies specific for HLA Class 1 alloantigens will ultimately be used for HLA typing. Those described in Table 14·3 could be used to type for the antigens shown. An important methodological issue arises, however, because many are not cytotoxic and therefore cannot be used with existing typing methods. It will probably transpire that the cytotoxic antibodies will be used on existing HLA typing trays as they are made. The other reagents would require a change in technique, perhaps to automated ELISA testing but this will only occur when a panel of reagents is available that can distinguish all, or nearly all, sixty Class 1 antigens.

## V MONOCLONAL ANTIBODIES TO HLA DR (CLASS 2) ANTIGENS

The Class 2 antigens are as yet rather poorly understood and mono clonal antibodies should help considerably in their analysis. There are some fundamental questions to answer. Is there a second major locus, equivalent to I-A of the mouse and are there other related loci such as I-J? If so, do the presently defined specifiities all map at one locus or do the polyclonal antibodies react with antigenic specificities which are present on products of more than one locus and appear as single antigens because of strong linkage disequilibrium? Is this kind of pauci-locus hypothesis too naive in view of recent information about immuno-globulin gene structure; could there be multiple exons some of which could contribute to more than one polypeptide chain? (Bodmer, 1981).

### A.    MONOMORPHIC ANTIGENIC SITES

There are monoclonal antibodies that are specific for HLA DR which recognize both monomorphic and polymorphic determinants. The monomorphic antibodies are normally defined by their characteristic binding pattern to B cells and monocytes, patchy distribution on organs such as kidney (Hart et al., 1981) and absence from unstimulated T cells. They precipitate two chains from radiolabelled cells: p33 and p28 of 33,000 and 28,000 daltons respectively. Competitive binding studies may indicate that they bind to determinants which are similar, or closely-related, to those seen by previously characterized reagents.

Attempts have been made to determine whether monomorphic anti-bodies identify more than one type of HLA DR antigen. Charron and McDevitt (1979, 1980) followed up the pioneering work of Jones (1977) and used two dimensional gels to analyse HLA DR antigens. In this technique cells are radiolabelled by culture in $^{35}$S methionine, their membranes are solubilized with detergent and HLA DR antigen is precipitated by the monoclonal antibody. The precipitate is applied to a tube gel system which separates by charge (non-equilibrium pH gradient electrophoresis—NEPHGE) and after a fixed time this gel is loaded lengthwise on the top of a SDS-polyacrylamide gel, which separates proteins by molecular weight. The resulting two dimensional separation of the components of the precipitate is visualized by exposing the gel to x-ray film to give a pattern such as that shown in Fig. 14·3. The most prominent spots are actin (an artefact) and a protein at the basic end of the gel with a molecular weight of approximately 31,000 daltons, known as invariant (i) spot. These two spots, because of their

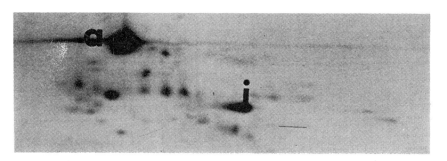

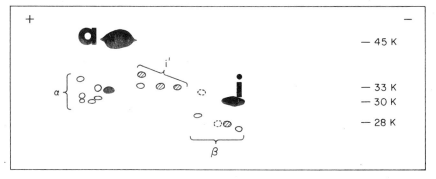

FIG. 14·3 2D gel analysis of HLA DR antigens precipitated from radio-labelled cells by an anti HLA DR monoclonal antibody specific for a monomorphic determinant. The precipitate was first run on a non equilibrium pH gradient electrophoresis tube gel (in the horizontal plane) and this was applied to the top of an SDS-polyacrylamide gel (vertical plane). The first dimension separated by charge; the second by molecular weight. The top panel is a photograph of the autoradiograph; the lower panel is a drawing to demonstrate the major groups of spots (separated polypeptides). a is actin; i is invariant spot; i′ are spots which may be related to i; $\alpha$ are the HLA DR $\alpha$ chain spots; $\beta$ are the $\beta$ chain spots. 45K, 33K, 30K and 28K show the molecular weights in kilo-daltons of the separated polypeptides. I am grateful to Dr. W. Makgoba for allowing me to show this autoradiograph.

constant positions, are useful as reference markers. All monoclonal antibodies to HLA DR, except one (Lloyd *et al.*, 1981), have precipitated the i-polypeptide from internally labelled proteins. A similar structure has been found in analysis of mouse Ia (Jones, 1977). Trypsin digestion of invariant spot, cut out of gels, has revealed a structure dissimilar to p33 and p28, which discounts the hypothesis that it is a precursor molecule (McMillan *et al.*, 1981). Its nature, function and genetic control remain unknown.

Charron and McDevitt (1979), Shackleford and Strominger (1980) and de Kretser *et al.* (1982) have analyzed the p33 and p28 HLA DR antigens, precipitated from several HLA DR homozygous cell lines with a number of monoclonal anti DR antibodies. The spot patterns are complex, although much of the heterogeneity is due to post synthetic glycosylation with addition of charged sialic acid residues. Thus, when glycosylation was blocked by incubation of the cells with tunicamycin, or pulse chase experiments were performed to observe precursor-product relationships, the patterns were much simpler (Charron and McDevitt 1980, de Kretser *et al.*, 1982). Similarly, simpler patterns were obtained from neuraminidase treated HLA DR positive melanoma cell membranes (Lloyd *et al.*, 1981). As predicted from preliminary peptide mapping (Silver and Ferrone, 1979), all of the heterogeneity between precipitates from different cell lines appears in the p28 region (beta chain). Charron and McDevitt (1979, 1980) showed that the position of at least two p28 spots in precipitates from tunicamycin treated cells, varied in position but they were not certain how many gene products these represented. De Kretser *et al.* (1982) have analyzed the 2 D spot patterns obtained by immunoprecipitation from several HLA DR homozygous cell lines, derived from donors who were the offspring of consanguinious marriages. They showed that there were two p28 polypeptide clusters of spots, $\beta1$ and $\beta2$; both varied in position between different DR types but whereas one group was constant within one DR type, the other could vary. They suggested, therefore, that the constant $\beta$ spots correspond to the HLA DR locus product and that the variable $\beta$ spots were derived from a separate gene. These results do not contradict those of Charron and McDevitt (1979, 1980); they add to data from groups of HLA matched consanguinious cell lines. It is not clear yet whether $\beta1$ and $\beta2$ correspond to the I-A and I-E $\beta$ chains of the mouse.

Further evidence for more than one HLA DR product comes from studies with monomorphic monoclonal antibodies that appear to identify distinct antigens. Lampson and Levy (1980) described two, each of which precipitated two polypeptide chains of 33,000 and 28,000 daltons but neither would clear the antigen seen by the other. There appears to be disagreement as to whether 2-D gel analysis of the products reveals significant differences (McDevitt 1980, Strominger 1981). Both could block cytotoxicity by the same complement fixing monomorphic monoclonal antibodies (Grumet *et al.*, 1980). It is hard to reconcile all these observations at present unless the two antibodies identify different glycosylated forms of the same gene products (Shackleford *et al.*, 1981).

Nadler *et al.* (1981a, b) and Pesando *et al.* (1982) have described three monoclonal anti DR antibodies which seem to identify distinct HLA DR antigens. One of these identified a polymorphism which did not correspond to any known HLA DR type (Nadler 1981a). Accolla *et al.* (1981) have found two monoclonal antibodies which define two sets of HLA DR antigens which are clearly different when their $\beta$ and $\alpha$ chain peptide maps are analyzed by 2-D gels.

Taken together, all these data imply that there are at least two sets of HLA DR antigens. Apparent lack of linkage disequilibrium between the two has been hinted at in two studies (Nadler *et al.*, 1981b; de Kretser *et al.*, 1982) so that the second locus may map well away from the first. This might correspond to the SB antigen defined as a mixed lymphocyte reaction stimulating antigen by Shaw *et al.* (1981) which maps between HLA DR and *GLO* (the *GLO* gene locus codes for glyoxylase, is polymorphic and maps outside HLA on chromosome 6). It would be interesting to determine which, if any, of these antibodies will inhibit T cell recognition of SB antigens.

Another approach has been to use monoclonal antibodies raised against rodent Ia antigens to detect crossreactive human DR molecules. MRCOX3, a mouse anti rat Ia reagent crossreacts with a murine Ia specificity which maps at the I-A locus and with a determinant shared by cells positive for HLA DR1, 2 and 6 (McMaster and Williams, 1979; Brodsky *et al.*, 1979). This does not necessarily mean that DR1, 2 and 6, or an antigen in linkage disequilibrium with these three, is the equivalent of the mouse I-A Ia molecule, because the beta chains of both I-A Ia and I-E Ia map in the *I-A* region (Jones *et al.*, 1978). Pierres *et al.* (1981) have shown that mouse monoclonal alloantibodies specific for I-E/C$^k$ or I-A$^k$ antigens crossreact with human DR. Again, these antibodies appear to identify distinct gene products.

## B. Polymorphic Antigenic Sites

Monoclonal antibodies that detect polymorphic HLA DR determinants have also been described and are listed in Table 14·4. The

TABLE 14·4

HLA DR antigens defined by alloantisera and monoclonal antibodies

| | | Alloantisera defined private specificities | | | | | | | | | | |
|---|---|---|---|---|---|---|---|---|---|---|---|---|
| | | DR1 | DR2 | DR3 | DR4 | DR5 | DR6 | DR7 | DR8 | DR9 | DR10 | |
| Alloantisera | MT1(MB1) | + | + | − | − | − | + | − | − | − | − | |
| | MT2 | − | − | + | − | + | + | − | + | − | − | |
| | MT3 | − | − | − | + | − | − | + | − | − | − | |
| | MB2 | − | − | + | − | − | − | + | − | − | − | |
| | MB3 | − | − | − | + | + | − | − | − | − | − | |
| Monoclonal antibodies[a] | DA2 | + | + | + | + | + | + | + | + | + | + | monomorphic |
| | Genox 3·32 | + | + | + | + | + | + | − | + | + | + | |
| | 1·1 | + | + | + | ± | + | + | + | + | + | + | |
| | MRCOX3 | + | + | − | − | − | + | − | − | − | − | MT1, MB1 |
| | Genox 3·53 | + | + | − | − | − | + | − | − | − | − | MT1, MB1 |
| | 8w1247 | − | − | + | − | − | + | − | − | − | − | MT2 |
| | 17·5 | − | − | − | + | + | − | ± | − | − | − | MB3 ± MT3 |
| | NFK3 | − | + | − | − | − | − | − | − | − | − | DR2 |
| | FMC2 | − | − | − | + | − | − | − | − | − | − | DR4 |

[a] See text for references.

specificities detected by alloantisera fall into two groups, the probable private specificities DR1-10 and the related crossreactive determinants MT1-3 and MB1-3. The latter may be public antigens shared by some but not all of the DR antigens, or they could be antigenic variants of the products of a second locus (Park *et al.*, 1980), each of which is in linkage disequilibrium with one or more first locus antigens. The MT1 (Brodsky *et al.*, 1979) and 2 (Trucco *et al.*, 1979, Garotta *et al.*, 1980) specificities have been defined by monoclonal antibodies. MT1 is also picked up by MRCOX3 and may therefore be an I-A locus equivalent. MB3 and "part of" MT3 is identified by another monoclonal antibody (Hansen *et al.*, 1981). Another type of crossreactive antibody reacts with most, but not all HLA DR antigens. Examples are Genox 3·32 which fails to bind to DR7 (Brodsky *et al.*, 1979) and I·1 which fails to bind to one HLA DR4 homozygous cell line (Nadler *et al.*, 1981). Antibodies of this type are hard to distinguish from antibodies which detect monomorphic specificities unless several homozygous cell lines are tested; they may therefore be commoner than is generally realized.

Very few monoclonal antibodies have been described which are specific for single HLA DR antigens. Antibodies specific for DR2 (Fuggle *et al.*, 1981) and 4 (Zola *et al.*, 1980) have been found but have been subjected so far to only preliminary analysis. One problem that has arisen is that some of these antibodies, which detect polymorphisms, such as NFK3 and MRCOX3 only detect DR antigens on lymphoblastoid cell lines and not on normal B cells. This must indicate some difference in antigen expression or exposure in transformed or dividing cells and requires further investigation.

In conclusion, monoclonal antibodies to HLA DR antigens are undoubtedly capable of unravelling the complexity of the HLA DR system. The present data are compatible with the economical hypothesis that there are a minimum of two pairs ($\alpha$ and $\beta$) of D region loci, one *I-A*-like which may code for the MT (and related MB and DC) determinants and one *I-E*-like coding for the DR with perhaps a third coding for SB specificities. Many other interpretations are possible at this stage and it remains to be seen whether more loci will be revealed.

## VI ANALYSIS OF HLA ANTIGEN FUNCTION USING MONOCLONAL ANTIBODIES

As described in the introduction to this chapter, HLA molecules, Class 1 and Class 2, play important roles in antigen recognition by T lymphocytes. Cytotoxic T cells (Tc) see HLA Class 1 antigens and virus antigens together on the surface of infected cells (McMichael, 1978;

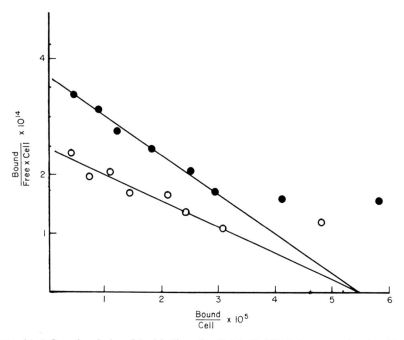

FIG. 14·4 Scatchard plot of the binding of radiolabelled PA2·6, a monoclonal antibody that binds to a monomorphic determinant on HLA Class I antigens, to untreated (O———O) and influenza A virus infected (●———●) peripheral blood lympho-cytes, under equilibrium conditions. The slope of the line measures the affinity (associa-tion constant) which increases from $4·4 \times 10^{-8}$ to $6·5 \times 10^{-8}$ litres $mol^{-1}$. The point where the lines cross the x axis gives the number of antigenic sites: $5·5 \times 10^5$ per cell. (Data from Hildreth, Makris and McMichael, unpublished; see also Hildreth and McMichael, 1981; Liberti *et al.*, 1979 and Trucco *et al.*, 1980.)

Shaw and Biddison, 1979). Helper T cells ($T_H$) are triggered by foreign antigen and Ia antigen on macrophage-like cells (Bergholtz *et al.*, 1980). Tc also respond primarily to foreign Class 1 antigen and $T_H$ cells to Classs 2 antigens in transplantation reactions *in vitro*. These conclusions are based on experiments where HLA matched or mismatched cells are mixed together. Thus, influenza specific Tc lyse only target cells that express virus antigen and are HLA A and B matched with self, probably because they were primed, *in vivo*, by that combination (McMichael, 1978; Shaw and Biddison, 1979). Monoclonal antibodies have been used to confirm these findings; antibodies specific for monomorphic and polymorphic HLA Class 1 determinants blocked virus specific Tc killing (McMichael *et al.*, 1980; Wallace *et al.*, 1981). The antibody had to be at a concentration sufficient to block all the HLA antigenic sites to achieve maximal inhibition. Anti HLA DR allo-antibodies blocked antigen specific T helper cell proliferation induced by foreign antigen on macrophages *in vitro* (Bergholtz *et al.*, 1978). Problems have arisen in the use of monoclonal antibodies to block antigen induced proliferation because antibody dependant cell mediated cytotoxicity (ADCC) may occur (Bright and Munro, 1981).

An approach to the question of whether these T cells respond to altered self HLA or whether there is separate recognition of HLA and foreign antigen has been made by Liberti *et al.* (1979) and Hildreth and McMichael (1981). There is an increase in binding affinity of mono-clonal antibodies to MHC Class I and II antigens on influenza virus infected cells (Fig. 14·4). This effect occurs with monoclonal Fab fragments and is therefore not due to an aggregation of antigen after infection, with an increase in bivalent antibody binding. No such increase was observed for binding to Thy-1, on murine T cells (Liberti *et al.*, 1979) or leucocyte common antigen (Hildreth and McMichael, 1981a) on human cells. These results suggest that influenza virus, possibly through its neuraminidase (Liberti *et al.*, 1979), specifically alters HLA A, B, C and DR antigen conformation on the surface of infected cells. This may not be too difficult to understand for HLA Class I molecules which, according to the evidence outlined above, are sub-ject to variable conformational forms. It should be emphasized, how-ever, that no firm evidence for association between influenza virus and MHC antigen has yet been found, using techniques such as co-precipitation or co-capping.

## VII EXPRESSION OF HLA ANTIGENS ON TISSUES

Monoclonal anti HLA antibodies have been used to examine the expression of HLA antigens on both normal and abnormal cells. The number of HLA molecules on the cell surface can be determined by binding under saturating conditions and then measuring the quantity of antibody bound by either a radioimmunoassay for mouse immuno-globulin or by adding a second radiolabelled antibody, rabbit anti mouse Ig, also under saturating conditions (Morris and Williams, 1975). An alternative, and probably more accurate, method is to measure the binding of radiolabelled monoclonal antibody at different concentrations to construct a Scatchard plot (Fig. 14·4). The number of molecules bound can be calculated from the point where the line crosses the abscissa. All these methods come up with a similar answer

TABLE 14·5
Number of HLA antigenic sites defined by Scatchard plots[a]

|  | $\beta_2$m | HLA A-B-C | HLA DR |  |
|---|---|---|---|---|
| Peripheral blood lymphocytes |  | $2 \cdot 5 - 5 \cdot 5 \times 10^5$ |  | Hildreth and McMichael, 1981 |
| Peripheral blood T cells | $1 \cdot 25 \times 10^5$ | $1 \cdot 0 \times 10^5$ |  | Trucco et al., 1980 |
| Peripheral blood B cells | $3 \cdot 7 \times 10^5$ | $2 \cdot 6 \times 10^5$ | $0 \cdot 8 \times 10^5$ | Trucco et al., 1980 |
| B lymphoblastoid cell line |  | $50 \times 10^5$ | $2 \cdot 0 \times 10^5$ | Hildreth and McMichael, 1981 |
| B lymphoblastoid cell line | $14 \cdot 0 \times 10^5$ | $9 \cdot 5 \times 10^5$ | $4 \cdot 6 \times 10^5$ | Hildreth and McMichael, 1981 |
| T cell line | $0 \cdot 8 \times 10^5$ | $0 \cdot 7 \times 10^5$ |  | Trucco et al., 1980 |
| T cell line |  | $12 \times 10^5$ |  | Hildreth and McMichael, 1981 |

[a] Note that different cell lines, and monoclonal antibodies, were used by the two groups which could account for the few discrepancies.

for HLA Class 1 molecules on peripheral blood lymphocytes of between two and five hundred thousand molecules per cell. Trucco et al. (1980) have used this Scatchard method to estimate numbers of molecules on different cell types for both Class 1 and Class 2 molecules (Table 14·5).

Monoclonal antibodies are particularly suitable reagents for staining tissue sections using second antibodies (anti mouse Ig) coupled with fluorescein, rhodamine or peroxidase. The last method (see chapter 24) is possibly the most sensitive and allows characterization of the cells by conventional staining techniques. Studies of the tissue distribution of HLA antigens in various tissues have yielded interesting results.

Class 1 antigens are widely distributed. They are absent from red blood cells, disappearing as the haemoglobin content of the normoblast increases (Brown et al., 1979), and trophoblast (Trowsdale et al., 1980). The latter may explain in part the resistance of the (foetal) trophoblast to attack by maternal T cells. Class 1 antigens are found on most other nucleated cells, in obviously large amounts on epithelial surfaces, endothelium and lymphoreticular cells. In the kidney HLA A-B-C antigens were shown, by immunofluorescence and peroxidase staining, to be present on the glomeruli, tubules and vascular endothelium (Hart et al., 1981). Fleming et al. (1981) using fluorescence found little staining on sections of brain and liver, other than vascular endothelium or epithelium. The study has been repeated using the immunoperoxidase technique and again it was found that most normal hepatocytes did not express detectable HLA Class 1 antigens (Barbatis et al., 1981, and see chapter 18). Negative findings must always be interpreted subject to the sensitivity of detection, which is probably around $5 \times 10^3$ molecules per cell. This may be further influenced by the avidity of the antibody used and possible artefacts such as antigen denaturation on fixing or freezing (unlikely if other tissues stain), antigen accessibility on the cell surface and the possibility that particular epitopes may be masked. In the study of hepatocytes, these objections have been controlled for as far as possible by testing more than one antibody of known high avidity that bind to different sites. Fleming *et al.* (1981) also found that some breast carcinomas were negative when stained with monoclonal antibody specific for HLA Class 1 antigens. Again, such negative results should be interpreted with great caution, but some cell lines derived from malignant tumours are also negative for HLA Class 1 antigens (Brodsky *et al.*, 1979; Bodmer, 1981) and similar observations have been made in the mouse (De Baetselier *et al.*, 1980). Not all breast tumours examined appeared negative and in some, staining was patchy (Fleming, 1981). No correlation with metastatic behaviour of the malignant tissues has yet been made. Although lack of HLA A, B, C antigens would render a malignant cell resistant to T cell attack, it is unlikely that this would be true if HLA antigen expression was only just below the threshold for detection, because complete inhibition of cytotoxic T cell mediated lysis of virus infected cells only occurred when all HLA sites were masked (McMichael *et al.*, 1980).

Monoclonal antibodies to HLA DR antigens have been used to investigate the expression of Class 2 molecules on different cells. B lymphocytes, monocytes and 15% of bone marrow cells are positive. Vascular endothelial cells also express HLA DR antigens. Particularly intriguing was the finding of HLA DR (and HLA A, B, C) positive dendritic cells which were present in the renal parenchyma (Hart *et al.*, 1981). Because these cells were positive for the leucocyte common antigen, they were not capillary endothelial cells and probably represent the human equivalent of the cell type described by Steinman and Cohn (1973) in rodents. A complete survey of the distribution of HLA DR antigens in other organs has yet to be made. Preliminary results (Daar, A. Fuggle, S. and Fabre, J. W. personal communication) indicate that small bowel epithelium is positive but in other organs only endothelial and dendritic cells stain. Melanocytes may also express HLA DR antigens because melanoma cells are positive (Lloyd *et al.*, 1981). Activated T lymphocytes express DR antigens which are of the same structure of those derived from B cells from the same individuals (Charron *et al.*, 1980).

With reference to clinical problems, it is important to determine the role of HLA DR antigens in organ transplantation. The evidence suggests that HLA DR matching is more important than HLA A, B, C matching (Ting and Morris, 1978). If HLA DR antigens are the targets for graft rejection, their patchy distribution might imply that rejection would be patchy; it is much more likely, however, that the HLA DR antigens are involved in triggering immune responses which may then be directed at the relatively ubiquitous HLA A-B-C antigens. It may also be important to consider the relative contribution to these reactions made by the products of different HLA DR loci, especially if it is found that the tissue distribution of each varies.

## VIII CONCLUSIONS AND PROSPECTS

In this chapter the main emphasis has been on ongoing research studies aimed at a deeper understanding of the HLA system and its genetics, structure and function. The field is moving rapidly, especially so since the advent of these reagents. It is likely that many of the issues discussed here will be resolved within a few years. Epitope mapping of HLA A, B, C and DR antigens should become possible as more HLA amino acid or DNA sequences are determined and the crystalline structure is analyzed. The question of how many types of DR antigens there are will be quickly settled as peptide maps and partial amino acid sequences of precipitated antigens are studied. More and more antibodies should be found specific for private antigenic specificities which together with those specific for epitopes of limited polymorphism will make HLA typing by monoclonal antibodies possible. The antibodies that are cytotoxic (in the presence of complement) can be added to typing trays as they arise.

One of the more useful applications of the human-human cell hybridomas described in chapter 2 would be to make monoclonal antibodies to HLA specificities; this should, in theory, be easier provided that the B cells can be boosted adequately *in vitro*. Monoclonal antibodies are desirable for HLA typing from the point of view of standardization and the possibility of automating the procedure would make it more generally accessible. The need for HLA typing in organ transplantation is likely to continue.

The study of HLA association with disease should receive new impetus as HLA antigens are better defined. Already de Kretser *et al.* (1981) have shown that HLA DR3 homozygous cell lines differ in their "second" HLA DR type. HLA DR3 has multiple associations with autoimmune diseases and it will be important to know how these different haplotypes relate to susceptibility to these various diseases.

Much of our interpretation of HLA antigen structure and antigenicity is likely to be influenced by the detailed structural analysis of HLA genes that is now in progress. Already it is known that the Class 1 probes find multiple (15–20) copies in the mouse genome (Cami *et al.*, 1981). The possibility that exons may be shared between products of different loci may lead to some rethinking. Monoclonal antibodies may advance these studies, in the preparation of messenger RNA and identification of cell free translation products.

Such advances in the knowledge of the structure of genes and antigens will still not explain how HLA antigens function. There is clearly a need to study the antigens *in situ* and look for possible interactions with other structures in the membrane. Studies on whole cells and antigens, purified with monoclonal antibodies, in lipid vesicles should be revealing. At the other end of the problem, study of antigen recognition by cloned and fused T cells should determine whether one, two, or more receptors are being sought. Monoclonal antibodies will very likely be the tools that finally answer this question.

Expression of HLA antigen on different tissues may also yield clues to function, as will abnormal expression on infected or maligant cells. It is possible that HLA or HLA-related structures are involved in cell-cell recognition outside the immune system (Dausset and Contu, 1980). Such molecules, and the recognition structures involved, will also be accessible to monoclonal antibodies.

The HLA system still presents us with a host of problems. Monoclonal antibodies are now, and will continue to be, essential tools for the experimentalist who wishes to solve them.

ACKNOWLEDGEMENTS

I am grateful to my colleagues James Hildreth and William Makgoba for many helpful discussions and to Drs. J. Fabre, S. Fuggle, P. Parham, F. Brodsky, C. Grumet, J. Hansen, M. Crumpton, W. F. Bodmer, T. de Kretser, J. Bradley and E. Yunis for kindly allowing me to refer to their work in press.

REFERENCES

Accolla, R. S., Gross, N., Carrel, S. and Corte, G. (1981). *Immunobiology* **159**, 1.
Barbatis, C., Wood, J., Morton, J. A., McMichael, A. J. and McGee, J. O'D. (1982). *Gut* (in press).
Barnstable, C. J., Bodmer, W. F., Brown, G., Galfre, G., Milstein, C., Williams, A. F. and Ziegler, A. (1978). *Cell* **14**, 9–20.

Beckman, I. G. R., Bradley, J., Macardle, P. J., Bashir, H., Wolnizer, C. M. and Zola, H. (1982). *Tissue Antigens* (in press).

Benacerraf, B. and McDevitt, H. O. (1972). *Science* **175**, 273–279.

Bergholtz, B. O., Thorensen, A. B. and Thorsby, E. (1980). *Scand. J. Immunol.* **11**, 541–548.

Biddison, W. E., Krangel, M. S., Strominger, J. L., Ward, F. E., Shearer, G. M. and Shaw, S. (1980). *Human Immunol.* **3**, 225–232.

Bodmer, W. F. (1981). *Tissue Antigens* **17**, 9–20.

Brewerton, D. A., Caffrey, M., Hart, F. D., James, D. C. O., Nicholls, A. and Sturrock, R. D. (1973). *Lancet* **i**, 904–907.

Bright, S. and Munro, A. (1981). *Tissue Antigens* **18**, 217–231.

Brodsky, F. M. (1979). D.Phil. thesis, University of Oxford.

Brodsky, F. M., Bodmer, W. F. and Parham, P. R. (1979a). *Eur. J. Immunol.* **9**. 536–545.

Brodsky, F. M., Parham, P., Barnstable, C. J., Crumpton, M. J. and Bodmer, W. F. (1979b). *Immunol. Rev.* **47**, 3–62.

Brown, G., Biberfeld, P., Christensson, B. and Mason, D. Y. (1979). *Eur. J. Immunol.* **9**, 272–275.

Calin, A. and Fries, J. F. (1975). *New Engl. J. Med.* **293**, 835–839.

Cami, B., Bregegere, F., Abastado, J. P. and Kourilsky, P. (1981). Nature **291**, 673–675.

Cepellini, R., Garotta, G., Malavasi, F. and Trucco, M. (1981). *Tissue Antigens* **17**, 28–36.

Charron, D. J. and McDevitt, H. O. (1979). *Proc. natn. Acad. Sci. U.S.A.* **76**, 6567–6571.

Charron, D. J. and McDevitt, H. O. (1980). *J. exp. Med.* **152**, 18s–36s.

Charron, D. J., Engleman, E. G., Benike, C. J. and McDevitt, H. O. (1980). *J. exp. Med.* **152**, 127s–136s.

Coligan, J. E., Kindt, T. J., Vehara, H., Martinko, J. and Nathenson, S. G. (1981). *Nature* **291**, 35–39.

Crumpton, M. J., Law, H. D. and Strong, R. C. (1970). *Biochem. J.* **116**, 923–925.

Dausset, J. and Contu, L. (1980). *Human Immunol.* **1**, 5–18.

De Baetselier, P., Katsav, S., Gorelik, E., Feldman, M. and Segal, S. (1980). *Nature* **288**, 179–181.

De Krester, T. A., Crumpton, M. J., Bodmer, J. G. and Bodmer, W. F. (1981). *Eur. J. Immunol.* (in press).

Duquesnoy, R. J. and Marrari, M. (1980). *In* "Histocompatibility Testing" (P. Terasuki Ed.) 552–555.

Ellis, S. E., Taylor, C. and McMicheal, A. J. (1982). *Human Immunology.* (in press).

Fleming, K. A., McMicheal, A. J., Morton, J. A., Woods, J. and McGee, J. O'D. (1981). *J. Clin. Path.* **34**, 779.

Fuggle, S. V., Kirkley, J., Ting, A. and Morris, P. J. (1982). In preparation.

Garotta, G., Barbanti, M., Calabi, F., Neri, T. M., Trucco, M. M. and

Cepellini, R. (1980). *In* "Histocompatibility Testing" (P. Terasuki Ed.) 864–865.

Goodfellow, P. N., Jones, E. A., van Heyningen, V., Solomon, E., Bobrow, M., Miggiano, V. and Bodmer, W. F. (1975). *Nature* 254, 267–269.

Grumet, F. C., Charron, D. J., Fendly, B. M., Levy, R. and Ness, D. B. (1980). *J. Immunol.* 125, 2785–2789.

Grumet, F. C., Fendly, B. M. and Engleman, E. G. (1981). *Lancet* ii, 174–176.

Hansen, J. A., Martin, P. J., Kamoun, M., Nisperos, B. and Thomas, E. D. (1981). *Human Immunol.* 2, 103–111.

Hart, D. J., Fuggle, S. V., Williams, K. A., Fabre, J. W., Ting, A. and Morris, P. J. (1981). *Transplantation* 31, 482–433.

Hildreth, J. E. K. and McMichael, A. J. (1981). Mechanisms of Lymphocyte Activation. (Resch, K. and Kircher, H. Eds) pp. 599–602. Elsevier/North Holland, Amsterdam.

Jones, P. P. (1977). *J. exp. Med.* 146, 1261–1279.

Jones, P. P., Murphy, D. B. and McDevitt, H. O. (1978). *J. exp. Med.* 148, 925–939.

Joysey, V. G. and Wolfe, E. (1978). *Br. med. Bull,* 34, 217–222.

Klein, J. (1979). *Science* 203, 516–521.

Klein, J., Juretic, A., Baxevanis, C. N. and Nagy, Z. A. (1981). *Nature* 291, 455–460.

Lampson, L. and Levy, R. (1980). *J. Immunol.* 125, 293–295.

Lancet, D. P., Parham, P. and Strominger, J. C. (1979). *Proc. natn. Acad. Sci. U.S.A.* 76, 3844–3848.

Liberti, P. A., Hackett, C. J. and Askonas, B. A. (1979). *Eur. J. Immunol.* 9, 751–756.

Lin, C. S., Rosenthal, A. S. and Hansen, T. H. (1981). *Immunobiology* 159, 181.

Lloyd, K. O., Ng, S. and Dippold, W. (1981). *J. Immunol.* 126, 2408–2413.

McDevitt, H. O. (1980). *J. exp. Med.* 152, 83s.

McMaster, W. R. and Williams, A. F. (1979). *Immunol. Rev.* 47, 117–137.

McMichael, A. J. (1978). *J. exp. Med.* 148, 1458–1467.

McMichael, A. J., Ting, A., Zweerink, H. J. and Askonas, B. A. (1977). *Nature* 270, 524–526.

McMichael, A. J., Parham, P. R., Rust, N. and Brodsky, F. M. (1980a). *Human Immunol.* 1, 121–130.

McMichael, A. J., Parham, P., Brodsky, F. M. and Pilch, J. R. (1980b). *J. exp. Med.* 152, 195s–203s.

McMillan, M., Frelinger, J. A., Jones, P. P., Murphy, D. B., McDevitt, H. O. and Hood, L. (1981). *J. exp. Med.* 15, 936–950.

Morris, R. J. and Williams, A. F. (1975). *Eur. J. Immunol.* 5, 274–281.

Morton, J. A., Pickles, M. M., Sutton, L. and Skov, F. (1971). *Vox Sang* 21, 141–153.

Murphy, D. B. (1978). *Springer Semin. Immunopath.* 1, 111–131.

Nadler, L. M., Stashenko, P., Hardy, R., Pesando, J. M., Yunis, E. J. and Schlossman, S. F. (1981a). *Human Immunol.* 2, 77–90.

Nadler, L. M., Stashenko, P., Hardy, R., Tomaselli, K. J., Yunis, E. J., Schlossman, S. F. and Pesando, J. M. (1981b) *Nature* **290**, 591–593.

Parham, P. (1981). *Immunogenetics* **13**, 509–528.

Parham, P. R. and Bodmer, W. F. (1978). *Nature* **276**, 397–399.

Parham, P. and McLean, J. (1980a). *Human Immunol.* **1**, 131–140.

Parham, P. and Ploegh, H. L. (1980b). *Immunogenetics* **11**, 131–144.

Parham, P. and Brodsky, F. M. (1982). *In* "Monoclonal Antibodies and T cell hybrids" (E. J. Hammerling, U. Hammerling and J. F. Kearney Eds). Elsevier/North Holland, Amsterdam. (in press).

Parham, P. R., Barnstable, C. J. and Bodmer, W. F. (1979). *J. Immunol.* **123**, 342–349.

Park, M. S., Terasaki, P. I., Nakata, S. and Aoki, D. (1980a). *In* "Histocompatibility Testing" (P. Terasaki Ed.) 854–857.

Park, M. S., Nakata, S. and Omori, K. (1980b). *In* "Histocompatibility Testing" (P. Terasaki Ed.) 161–164.

Pesando, J. M., Nadler, L. M., Lazarus, H., Tomaselli, K. J., Stashenko, P., Ritz, J., Levine, H., Yunis, E. J. and Schlossman, S. F. (1982). *Human Immunol.* (in press).

Pfeffer, P. and Thorsby, E. (1982). *Transplantation* **33**, 52–63.

Piazza, A., Belvedere, M. C., Bernoco, D., Conighi, C., Contu, L., Cutroni, E. S., Mattiuz, P. L., Mayr, W., Richiardi, P., Scudeller, G. and Cepellini, R. (1972). *In* "Histocompatibility Testing" (J. Dausset Ed.) 73–84.

Pierres, M., Rebouch, J. P., Kourilsky, F. M., Dosseto, M., Mercier, P., Mawas, C. and Malissen, B. (1981). *J. Immunol.* **126**, 2424–2429.

Ploegh, H. L., Cannon, L. E. and Strominger, J. L. (1979). *Proc. natn. Acad. Sci. U.S.A.* **76**, 2273–2277.

Rosenthal, A. S., Barcinski, M. A. and Blake, J. T. (1977). *Nature* **267**, 156–158.

Ryder, L. F., Andersen, E. and Svejgaard, A. (1979). HLA and Disease Registry, Third Report (Munksgard, Ed.) Copenhagen.

Sanderson, A. R. (1977). *Nature* **269**, 414–417.

Shackleford, D. A. and Strominger, J. L. (1980). *J. exp. Med.* **151**, 144–165.

Shackleford, D. A., Lampson, L. A. and Strominger, J. L. (1981). *J. Immunol.* **127**, 1403–1410.

Shaw, S. and Biddison, W. (1979). *J. exp. Med.* **149**, 565–571.

Shaw, S., Johnson, A. H. and Shearer, G. M. (1980). *J. exp. Med.* **152**, 565–580.

Shaw, S., Kavathas, P., Pollack, M. S., Charmot, D. and Mawas, C. (1981). *Nature* **293**, 745–747.

Shreffler, D., David, C., Gotze, D., Klein, J., McDevitt, H. O. and Sachs, D. (1974). *Immunogenetics* **1**, 189–199.

Silver, J. and Ferrone, S. (1979). *Nature* **279**, 436–439.

Snary, D., Barnstable, C. J., Bodmer, W. F. and Crumpton, M. J. (1977). *Eur. J. Immunol.* **8**, 580–584.

Steinman, R. M. and Cohn, Z. A. (1973). *J. exp. Med.* **137**, 1142–1162.

Strominger, J. L. (1981). *In* "Progress in Immunology" (J. Dausset Ed.) 541–554.

Terasaki, P. (1980). (Ed.) Histocompatibility Testing.

Ting, A. and Morris, P. J. (1978). *Lancet* i 575–577.

Tosi, R., Tanigaki, N., Centis, D., Ferrar, G. B. and Pressman, D. (1978). *J. exp. Med.* **148**, 1592–1611.

Trowsdale, J., Travers, P., Bodmer, W. F. and Patillo, R. A. (1980). *J. exp. Med.* **152**, 11s–17s.

Trucco, M. M., Stocker, J. W. and Cepellini, R. (1978). *Nature* **273**, 666–668.

Trucco, M. M., Garotta, G., Stocker, J. W. and Cepellini, R. (1979). *Immunol. Rev.* **47**, 219–252.

Trucco, M. M., De Petris, S., Garotta, G. and Cepellini, R. (1980). *Human Immunol.* **1**, 233–245.

Uhr, J. W., Capra, D. J., Vitetta, E. S. and Cook, R. G. (1979). *Science* **206**, 292–297.

Von Boehmer, H., Haas, W. and Jerne, N. K. (1978). *Proc. natn. Acad. Sci. U.S.A.* **75**, 2439–2442.

Wallace, L. E., Moss, D. J., Rickinson, A. B., McMichael, A. J. and Epstein, M. A. (1981). *Eur. J. Immunol.* (in press).

Wiley, D. C., Wilson, I. A. and Skehel, J. J. (1981). *Nature* **289**, 373–378.

Zinkernagel, R. M. and Doherty, P. C. (1974). *Nature* **251**, 547–548.

Zola, H., Bradley, J., McArdle, P., McEvoy, R. and Thomas, M. (1980). *Transplantation* **29**, 72–73.

# 15 Monoclonal Antibodies and Human Gene Mapping by Somatic Cell Genetics

PETER GOODFELLOW AND ELLEN SOLOMON

*Imperial Cancer Research Fund, Lincoln's Inn Fields, London. WC2A 3PX*

## I INTRODUCTION

Mapping of the human genome has made direct contributions to our understanding at the molecular level of several genetic disease states. In the future, further advances in technology combined with a knowledge of linkage relationships may facilitate early prenatal diagnosis of deleterious phenotypes. Genetic mapping studies in man have made widespread use of serologically identified markers, such as the red blood cell antigens of the ABO, Rh, and Xg systems (Race and Sanger, 1975).

Because many of these markers are highly polymorphic, e.g. the histocompatibility antigens HLA-A, B, C, or are comprised of variants which exist at reasonable population frequencies, e.g. ABO, they have been some of the most useful markers for family studies or linkage analysis. Among the first demonstrations of linkage groups including rare genetic disorders were ABO and nail patella syndrome, (Renwick and Lawler, 1955) and Rh and elliptocytosis (Lawler, 1954). Serologically based linkage studies have relied upon human alloantisera. With the development of monoclonal antibody technology (Kohler and Milstein, 1975) many of the reagents for such studies shall undoubtedly become available more widely and in a more standardized form. In addition, monoclonal antibodies can provide new information as to the genetic complexity of these polymorphic systems. However, because of small family sizes, long generation times, and widespread geographical distribution of modern families, data for linkage studies is often difficult to obtain, even with the increasing number of serologically, and biochemically, well-defined polymorphic markers. Another problem is that although linkage groups may be established by family studies, the assignment of these groups to particular chromosomes is dependent upon the finding of chromosomal heteromorphisms or rearrangements. Until 1968 a number of linkage groups had been identified, but, no autosomal assignment had been made.

An enormous expansion in the number of assignments to the human gene map has occurred in the last ten years, due largely to the development of somatic cell genetics. By May 1981, 264 autosomal assignments had been made and of these, 167 were made by somatic cell genetics. In this method human somatic cells are fused with rodent somatic cells under selection conditions which allow only the hybrid cell to grow. The resulting hybrid often retains the full complement of rodent chromosomes, but retains only a random selection of human chromosomes. Gene assignments to human chromosomes depend upon, (i) expression of the gene product of interest in the hybrid cell; (ii) detectable variation between the human and rodent gene product; (iii) identification of the human chromosomes present. Hybrids are scored for the presence or absence of the human gene product and presence or absence of each of the human chromosomes. Concordance between these is taken as evidence for the assignment of a marker to a chromosome. In this area of human genetics the development of monoclonal antibodies has proved enormously helpful. Somatic cell genetics relies upon variation between species rather than variation among individuals, and monoclonal antibodies, especially as produced in mice, have been particularly useful as reagents which easily detect human/rodent differences.

This applies both to situations in which monoclonal antibodies have provided species-specific reagents to recognize previously defined molecules, as well as in cases in which a molecule is originally defined by a species-specific monoclonal antibody.

Once a monoclonal antibody has been used to genetically map a cell surface expressed determinant, it may then be used for the genetic manipulation of somatic cell hybrids, both in the specific elimination of individual human chromosomes and, more rarely, in the positive selection of hybrids containing a specific human chromosome. The serological problems encountered in these experiments in the past, using multi-specific sera, have often been formidable and have limited the general application of the techniques. This has been due to the complex character of the antisera and the often inappropriate assay used in the original definition of the antigen, for example red cell agglutination. Before these antisera can be used with somatic cell hybrids they must frequently be redefined with respect to specificity and exhaustively absorbed to remove so-called heterophile antibodies. The use of monoclonal antibodies avoids many of these problems and greatly simplifies studying the genetics of serological determinants by somatic cell genetics.

In this review we describe several instances of the use of monoclonal antibodies to assign genes to human chromosomes using somatic cell genetics. These are either genes which may have been previously refractory to mapping, and for which purposes monoclonal antibodies have been useful, or genes which have been initially defined by the monoclonal antibody itself. While the principles of gene mapping using these antibodies are the same in each instance, we have chosen examples from our own work which illustrate different biochemical and immunological techniques. Examples are also given to describe the use of monoclonal antibodies for the manipulation of the chromosome constitution of somatic cell hybrids.

## II AN INTRODUCTION TO THE TECHNIQUES OF SOMATIC CELL GENETICS

Somatic cell hybrids are produced by the induced fusion of somatic cells. Two agents are widely used for fusing cells: inactivated sendai virus (Harris and Watkins, 1965; Neff and Enders, 1968) and, more recently, polyethylene glycol (Pontecorvo, 1975). The resultant hybrids are usually isolated by a technique which gives the hybrid cells a selective advantage over the parental cells. The most commonly used system is the HAT (hypoxanthine, aminopterin, thymidine) selective medium (Littlefield, 1964; Szybalski *et al.*, 1962). In the presence of aminopterin cells are prevented from the *de novo* syntheses of nucleotides and are dependent on exogeneously added hypoxanthine and thymidine. In order to utilize the added hypoxanthine and thymidine, cells use the enzymes thymidine kinase (TK E.C. 2.7.1.75) and hypoxanthine guanine phosphoribosyl transferase (HPRT E.C. 2.4.2.8). If an $HPRT^-$ $TK^+$ cell is fused to an $HPRT^+$ $TK^-$ cell, the resultant hybrid will be able to grow in HAT by complementation. The parent cells fail to grow in HAT medium. The fact that the HPRT gene is X-linked makes HAT selection particularly useful for studies on the X-chromosome. Fusion of a human cell with an $HPRT^-$ rodent cell followed by growth in HAT medium selects for the presence of an active human X-chromosome. Clones which have lost the X-chromosome can be obtained by growing the hybrid cells in 8-azaguanine (Littlefield, 1964). Numerous variations on the basic hybrid selection technique exist, including the use of dominant drug resistant markers such as ouabain (Kucherlapati *et al.*, 1975) and the half selective system where one parent is prevented from growing by the HAT medium and the other parent cell does not grow in culture (Nabholz *et al.*, 1969). Once hybrids have been produced it is essential to determine their human chromosome constitution. This can be determined either directly by examination of the chromosomes, or indirectly by assaying enzymes or antigens coded for by each of the chromosomes.

While karyotyping is in many ways the most difficult technically, it also provides the most complete information regarding the human chromosomal contribution of the hybrid cell. The complexity of the karyotype of many mouse cell lines and the difficulty in distinguishing the human acrocentric chromosomes from mouse chromsomes has led to the development of techniques which can be used to distinguish between human and mouse chromosomes. This is most frequently done by the G-11 method whereby chromosome spreads are treated with giemsa at pH 11·3 (Bobrow and Cross, 1974). The mouse chromosomes stain deep magenta, with pale blue staining centromeres; the human chromosomes are pale blue and some of these have a magenta centromere. Fig 15·1 shows an example of G-11 staining of a spread of the hybrid C121 which contains 3 copies of human chromosome 7. The human chromosomes can be seen to stain much more lightly than the mouse chromosomes and the dark staining centromere is apparent. Identification of particular human chromosomes can be achieved with subsequent quinacrine (Q banding) staining (Caspersson *et al.*, 1970) on the same spreads as have been G-11 treated. Trypsin/giemsa G banding (Seabright, 1972) may also be performed as an independent confirmation of the analysis.

The second important technique used for characterizing somatic cell hybrids is isoenzyme analysis. Cell extracts, produced by sonication or freeze/thawing, are subjected to electrophoresis in a variety of buffer systems employing, usually starch or cellulose acetate support media (Harris and Hopkinson, 1977). Using specific staining systems, visualization of bands of enzymic activity can be achieved. Again, the essential requirement of this technique is that it distinguishes the human and

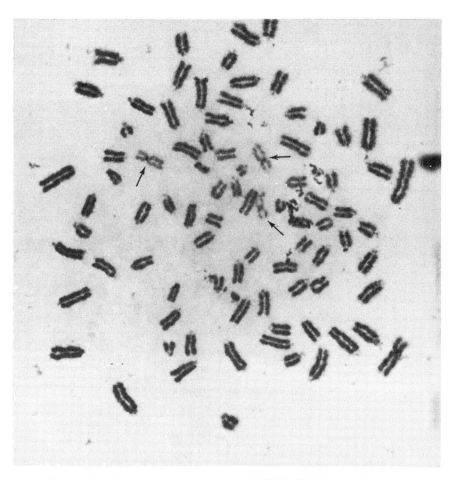

FIG. 15·1  G-11 staining of a metaphase spread of C121. The human chromosomes are indicated by arrows.

rodent enzymes, generally by differences in their electrophoretic mobility. There is at least one enzymic marker specific for each human chromosome which can be used in human-mouse somatic cell hybrids (Evans *et al.*, 1979).

Potentially the most convenient way of characterizing hybrids is the use of cell surface antigenic markers. The ease of performing multiple assays and the small number of target cells needed suggest that, with development of suitable markers, antigenic analysis will play a much larger part in somatic cell genetics. Our initial experiments on cell surface antigenic markers made use of the complement dependent cytotoxicity test (Goodfellow *et al.*, 1975), other workers used immuno-fluorescence (e.g. Buck and Bodmer, 1975) and complement fixation (e.g. Fellous *et al.*, 1974). In recent experiments the cytotoxicity test has been superseded by the indirect radioimmunoassay (IRIA). The details of the radioimmunoassay as performed in our laboratory are outlined in Fig. 15·2. This assay has several advantages over the cytotoxicity assay:

1. The IRIA does not depend upon having a cytotoxic class of antibody.
2. The IRIA result is monitored by a gamma counter and is, therefore, more objective than the cytotoxicity assay which requires microscope observation. The more objective form of the cytotoxicity assay which utilizes $^{51}Cr$ release, suffers from the disadvantage that many cells show a high spontaneous release of chromium.
3. The major disadvantage of the cytotoxicity test is the requirement for a suitable source of complement. The heterophile anti-mouse antibodies found in the rabbit sera used as a complement source cause serious problems of non specific cytotoxicity. These problems can only be avoided by extensive screening of individual rabbits and by careful absorption (Goodfellow, 1975). The IRIA uses a standard second reagent which suffers from none of the disadvantages of complement.

Once hybrids have been produced and their human chromosome composition determined, several other criteria must be met for gene mapping with monoclonal antibodies to be feasible.

First, the monoclonal antibody must show species specificity, that is, it must distinguish between the human antigen and the equivalent rodent antigen. An exception to this rule can only be made if the rodent parent cell is known to lack the antigen under investigation (see, for example, the expression of fibronectin by L cells and hybrids, Eun and Klinger, 1980); however, the possibility of re-expression of the rodent product should always be considered. Second, the antigen must be

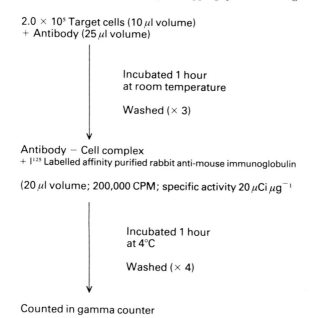

2.0 × 10⁵ Target cells (10 μl volume)
+ Antibody (25 μl volume)

Incubated 1 hour
at room temperature

Washed (× 3)

Antibody — Cell complex
+ I¹²⁵ Labelled affinity purified rabbit anti-mouse immunoglobulin

(20 μl volume; 200,000 CPM; specific activity 20 μCi μg⁻¹

Incubated 1 hour
at 4°C

Washed (× 4)

Counted in gamma counter

FIG. 15·2 The indirect radioimmunoassay (IRIA).

expressed in the set of hybrids under investigation. Differentiated functions are often extinguished if cells at different states of differentiation are fused (Davidson, 1974). This makes it difficult to predict if a differentiated function will be expressed in a hybrid or not. For example, mouse teratocarcinoma stem cell lines lack Thy-1; hybrids made between mouse teratocarcinoma stem cells and Thy-1 positive mouse thymocytes fail to express Thy-1 (Andrews and Goodfellow, 1980). In contrast when EGF (epidermal growth factor) receptor negative L cells were fused with EGF receptor negative human lymphocytes, the hybrids expressed human EGF receptors (see below). By far the best strategy, when possible, is to contstruct hybrids from parental cells which both express the phenotype being studied. The requirement for gene expression in hybrids although essential for using monoclonal antibodies can be overcome if specific DNA probes are available to investigate the genome of hybrids directly. Using this approach we have recently confirmed the assignment of the human immunoglobulin heavy chain genes to chromosome 14 (Hobart *et al.*, 1981). This method was simpler than constructing antibody producing hybrids (Croce *et al.*, 1979) and analyzing the immunoglobulins produced.

## III GENE MAPPING OF CELL SURFACE ANTIGENS

Gene assignment using somatic cell hybrids requires the use of a large number of independent, well characterized, hybrid cell lines. The hybrids we have used in our studies are described in Table 15·1.

Table 15·2 summarizes the gene assignment, or confirmations of previous assignments, which have been made in our laboratory by exploiting the specificity of monoclonal antibodies. As one example of

TABLE 15·1
Hybrids used in gene assignment experiments

| Hybrid series | Human parent | | Mouse parent | | References |
|---|---|---|---|---|---|
| | Name | Type | Name | Type | |
| DUR | DUV | Primary fibroblast | 1R | L cell | Solomon *et al.*, 1976 |
| MOG | H.M. | Primary fibroblast | RAG | Renal adenocarcinoma | Solomon *et al.*, 1979 |
| SIR | S.S. | Primary fibroblast | 1R | L cell | Solomon E. unpublished |
| ThyB | – | Thymocytes | BW5147 | Thymoma | Goodfellow *et al.*, 1980 |
| HORL | H.C. | Peripheral blood lymphocytes | 1R | L cell | van Heyningen *et al.*, 1975 |
| HORP | H.C. | Peripheral blood lymphocytes | 1R | L cell | van Heyningen *et al.*, 1975 |
| FIR | FRIL | Primary fibroblast | 1R | L cell | Solomon E. unpublished |
| C121 | LNSV | SV-40 transformed fibroblast | – | Primary macrophage | Croce *et al.*, 1973 |
| W[a] | M.N. | Peripheral blood lymphocytes | 1R | L cell | Nazholz *et al.*, 1969 |
| CTP | C.K. | Peripheral blood T lymphocytes | PG19 | Melanoma | Jones *et al.*, 1976 |
| POT | – | Peripheral blood lymphocytes | 3T3 | Fibroblastoid | Solomon, E., Sheer, D. and Hiorns L. unpublished |
| MCP-6[b] | G3·32·2 | Burkitt's lymphoma | PCC4 | Teratocarcinoma | Goodfellow P., Banting G. and Solomon E. unpublished |
| P7A | 110 | Primary fibroblast | CL·1D | L cell | Fellous *et al.*, 1973 |

[a]  In the hybrid name the W is preceded and followed by a number. e.g. 3W4.
[b]  Produced by microcell transfer of an X-6 translocation from G1R-6, a hybrid produced between G3·32·2 and 1R.

the general method used for gene assignment we will consider the gene controlling the expression of the antigen defined by the monoclonal antibody 12E7.

The monoclonal antibody 12E7 was raised against the leukaemic T cells of a child with acute lymphocytic leukaemia (Levy *et al.*, 1979). Originally the antibody appeared to react specifically with thymocytes, but using a more sensitive assay the 12E7 antigen was found to be generally expressed on human cells, including all cultured human cells tested (Goodfellow *et al.*, 1980; and unpublished results). Fig. 15·3 demonstrates the reaction of 12E7 in an indirect radioimmunoassay with a human T-cell line (MOLT-4) and a mouse T-cell line (BW5147): 12E7 clearly demonstrates species specificity for the human cell line. A dilution of 12E7 giving maximum binding of antibody to MOLT-4 was taken from Fig. 15·3 and used for subsequent tests on a panel of independent human-rodent somatic cell hybrids (Table 15·3). All the rodent cell lines employed as parents of the somatic cell hybrids were 12E7 antigen negative while several hybrids reacted strongly with

TABLE 15·2

Summary of gene assignments made with monoclonal antibodies

| Antibody | Antigen recognized | Locus name[a] | Locus assignment | Reference to previous | Reference to assignment or confirmation using monoclonal antibody |
|---|---|---|---|---|---|
| OKT-9 | Transferrin receptor | TFR | 3 | — | Goodfellow P., Banting G., Sutherland R., Greaves M., and Solomon E. (in press). |
| W6/32 | HLA-A,B,C | HLA | 6 | Jongsma *et al.*, 1973 | Barnstable *et al.*, 1979 |
| EGFR1 | EGF receptor | EGFR | 7 | Shimizu *et al.*, 1979 | Goodfellow P., Banting G., Waterfield M. and Ozanne B. (in press). |
| W6/34 | — | MIC1 | 11 | — | Barnstable *et al.*, 1979 |
| F10·44·2 | glycoprotein (100,000 daltons) | MIC4 | 11 | — | Goodfellow P., Banting G., Fabre, J. and Solomon E. (in press). |
| 602-29 | — | MIC3 | 12 | — | Andrews P., Knowles, B., Goodfellow P. (in press). |
| BBM1 | $\beta2$ micro-globulin | B2M | 15 | Goodfellow *et al.*, 1975 | Brodsky *et al.*, 1979 |
| R1 | — | MIC5 | X | — | Hope R., Goodfellow P., Solomon E. and Bodmer W.F. (in press) |
| 12E7 | Related to Xg blood group | MIC2 | X | — | Goodfellow *et al.*, 1980 |

[a]   The MIC locus names are local designations of the I.C.R.F. as agreed at Human Gene Mapping 6.

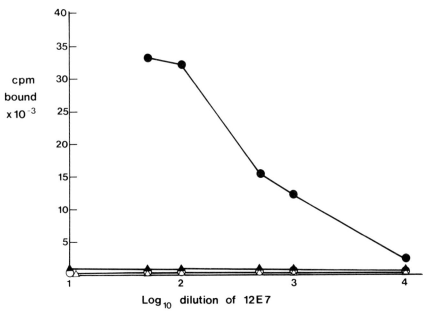

FIG. 15·3 Titration of 12E7 on human (MOLT4) and mouse (BW5147) cell lines. The IRIA was performed as described in Goodfellow *et al.* (1980) and Fig. 15·2. Each point is the average of three determinations. The antibody pool was prepared by ammonium sulphate precipitation from tissue culture supernatant. The undiluted pool of 12E7 contained $1 \cdot 1mg \ ml^{-1}$ antibody as determined by radioimmunoassay. —O— MOLT-4, binding of negative control P3-X63. Ag8; —●— MOLT-4, binding of 12E7; —△— BW5147, binding of negative control P3-X63. Ag8; —▲— BW5147, binding of 12E7.

12E7. Consideration of Table 15·3 suggests that the presence of the human X-chromosome is a necessary condition for 12E7 expression. Confirmation of this hypothesis was obtained from two types of experiment. Firstly, in a set of subclones derived from the positive hybrid ThyB-1 the active human X-chromosome was removed by selection against the HPRT locus using 8-azaguanine (Table 15·4). Concomitant with the loss of the human X-chromosome, 12E7 antigenic activity was lost. Secondly, several human-rodent hybrids which have a human X-chromosome as the only human contribution to the hybrid genome, express the 12E7 antigen (Table 15·5). The X-linked locus controlling 12E7 antigen expression has been named MIC 2. If more than one human gene is required for 12E7 antigen expression in human-rodent somatic cell hybrids all of the genes must be on the human X-chromosome.

Although, the simplest, and most likely explanation, for these results

TABLE 15·3
Reactions of 12E7 with human-mouse hybrids

| Cell | Human chromosome present | CPM bound[a,b] mean (Standard deviation) | |
|------|--------------------------|-------|-------|
| | | 12E7[d] | P3-X63.Ag8[c] |
| SIR·2 | 1,2,3,4,5,6,7,8,10,11,12,13,14, 15,16,17,18,19,20,21,22,X | 14,545 (3165) | 648 (280) |
| SIR7·11 | 1,2,5,7,10,11,12,14,15,16,17,18, 20,21,X | 13,720 (1001) | 717 (42) |
| MOG 7 | 1,3,4,5,7,8,10,11,12,13,15,16, 18,21,X | 28,303 (1147) | 561 (85) |
| MOG 13·17 | 3,21,22,X | 17,363 (1319) | 874 (120) |
| CTP34·B4 | 1,2,3,5,6,7,8,9,12,14,16,17,18,X | 31,198 (3246) | 580 (137) |
| CTP41·2 | 2,4,5,10,13,14,16,20,X | 20,213 (3058) | 637 (194) |
| HORL4·1·1B6 | 1,3,10,11,13,15,18,22,X | 15,599 (118) | 542 (196) |
| HORL4·1·9 | 11,15,X | 22,161 (981) | 1413 (294) |
| ThyB-1·33 | 21,X | 27,236 (2359) | 882 (64) |
| HORP27R | 4,7,11,12,14,15,21,22 | 507 (126) | 413 (51) |
| POT B2·B2 | 12,17,21,22 | 1,186 (137) | 1392 (148) |
| HFL121 | Human primary fibroblasts | 22,335 (115) | 806 (2) |
| JB | Human primary fibroblasts | 18,569 (2,603) | 1135 (30) |
| MOLT-4 | Human T cell ALL line | 35,358 (3,690) | 841 (66) |
| JB | Human peripheral blood lymphocytes | 25,278 (1,740) | 628 (105) |
| 1R | Mouse L cell | 1498 (452) | 1375 (55) |
| PG19 | Mouse melanoma | 1282 (74) | 1102 (190) |
| BW5147 | Mouse thymoma | 540 (53) | 441 (51) |
| 3T3 | Mouse fibroblastoid cell line | 1222 (28) | 1538 (465) |
| RAG | Mouse adenocarcinoma | 2363 (156) | 1757 (135) |

[a]  The conditions for the binding assay are the same as in Goodfellow *et al.*, (1980) and Fig. 15·2.
[b]  Three determination.
[c]  P3-X63.Ag8 (Kohler and Milstein, 1975) was used as the negative control.
[d]  Used as a concentration of approximately 13·0 $\mu$g ml$^{-1}$

is that MIC 2 is the structural gene for the 12E7 antigen it is formally possible that MIC 2 induces the expression of a rodent structural gene for the 12E7 antigen. It would also be necessary to make the unlikely postulate that this gene is not normally expressed in rodents.

Further localization of MIC 2 can be achieved by studying somatic cell hybrids which contain deleted human X chromosomes or X-autosome translocations which have lost part of the human X chromosome. The data presented in Table 15·5 can be used to assign a 12E7 controlling gene to the short arm of the X chromosome. This localiza-

TABLE 15·4
Reactions of 12E7 with subclones and revertant clones of ThyB-1

| | Human chromosomes | CPM Bound $\times 10^{-3}$[a,b] | |
| | | 12E7[d] | CA2·06[c] |
|---|---|---|---|
| ThyB-1 | X,21 | 15·6 | 0·5 |
| ThyB-1RA·1 | 21 | 0·3 | 0·4 |
| ThyB-1·1 | X,21 | 18·6 | 1·0 |
| ThyB-1·1R | 21 | 0·6 | 1·1 |
| ThyB-1·3 | X,21 | 11·4 | 1·2 |
| ThyB-1·3R | 21 | 0·6 | 0·5 |
| ThyB-1·5 | X,21 | 11·6 | 0·7 |
| ThyB-1·5R | 21 | 0·4 | 0·5 |

[a]  See footnote [a] Table 15·3.
[b]  Figures represent the average of two determinants.
[c]  CA2·06 is a monoclonal anti-human DR (Charron and McDevitt, 1979) and was used as the negative control.
[d]  See footnote [d] Table 15·3.

TABLE 15·5
Reactions of 12E7 with "X-only" human-mouse hybrids

| | | CPM Bound $\times 10^{-3}$[a,b] | | |
| | | 12E7[d] | P3-X63.Ag8[c] | Reference/comment |
|---|---|---|---|---|
| Hybrid: | THYB-1·4 | 17·6 | 0·8 | 10% of hybrid cells also |
| Mouse parent: | BW5147 | 1·0 | 0·6 | contain chromosome 21 |
| Hybrid: | MOG13·9 | 20·4 | 1·3 | |
| Mouse parent: | RAG | 1·3 | 0·8 | |
| Hybrid: | HOL9·X | 22·9 | 0·9 | Clone of HORL4.1·9 |
| Mouse parent: | 1R | 0·7 | 0·6 | × 42·2 (Goodfellow, 1975). |
| Hybrid: | 1W1-5 | 0·8 | 0·6 | Xq only |
| Mouse parent: | 1R | 0·7 | 0·6 | |
| Hybrid: | MCP-6 | 0·4 | 0·4 | Contains an X-6 translocation |
| Mouse parent: | PCC4 | 0·5 | 0·4 | Xq13 − 6p21 |

[a]  See footnote [a] Table 15·3.
[b]  Figures represent the average of two or more determinations.
[c]  See footnote [c] Table 15·3.
[d]  See footnote [d] Table 15·3.

tion was an important clue for suggesting the relationship between the 12E7 antigen and the *Xg* locus (Goodfellow and Tippett, 1981).

Eventually it should be possible to find generally expressed antigenic markers specific for each of the human chromosomes, as can be seen from Table 15·2 we have made some progress in this direction. As more antigenic markers become available analysis of human-mouse hybrids and gene assignment will become simpler. An example of this approach can be seen in Fig. 15·4. Previous work had assigned the locus controlling expression of the antigen recognized by the monoclonal antibody

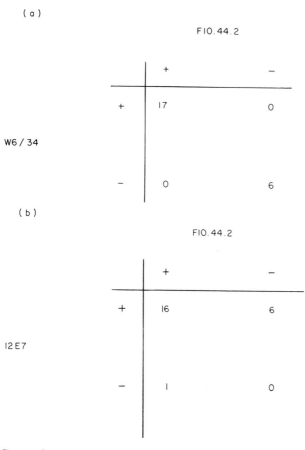

FIG. 15·4 Comparison of reactions of W6/34, F10.44.2 and 12E7 on 23 human-mouse hybrids. (a) Two by two comparison of the reactions of F10.44.2 and W6/34. (b) Two by two comparison of the reactions of F10.44.2 and 12E7. Antigen presence was determined by IRIA; reactions equal to or greater than 3 times background were regarded as positive.

W6/34 to chromosome 11 (Barnstable et al., 1978, this locus has been named MIC 1). The W6/34 antigen is carried on a glycolipid (personal communication W. F. Bodmer) which is generally expressed on human cells. The monoclonal antibody F 10.44.2 was raised against B cell depleted lymph nodes and recognizes an antigenic determinant carried by a human glycoprotein with a molecular weight of approximately 100,000 daltons (Dalchau et al., 1980). A clear correlation is seen between the reactivity of these two monoclonal antibodies on somatic cell hybrids; for comparison the lack of correlation with 12E7 reactivity is also shown (Fig. 15·4). This data suggests the locus, MIC 4, controlling F 10.44.2 antigen expression is on chromosome 11. F 10.44.2 also reacts with somatic cell hybrids which have chromosome 11 as the only human genetic contribution (unpublished results); confirming the assignment to chromosome 11.

## IV GENETIC ANALYSIS OF CELL SURFACE RECEPTORS FOR GROWTH FACTORS

Cell surface receptors are recognized and defined either by functional assays, such as EGF induced mitogenesis or by direct ligand binding (reviewed for EGF, Carpenter and Cohen, 1979). Although differential effects are sometimes seen when the same ligand is bound to cells of different species (for example, diphtheria toxin binding can be used to kill human cells or human-mouse hybrids containing chromosome 5, Creagan et al., 1975; Swallow et al., 1977) often these techniques do not detect species differences. We have exploited the species specificity of monoclonal antibodies to study the genetics of two cell surface receptors which previously could only be studied by ligand binding.

Mouse and human EGF binds with the same affinity to both mouse and human EGF receptors (Carpenter and Cohen, 1975). Previous attempts to study the genetics of the human EGF receptor relied upon the finding that several mouse cell lines, notably including L cells, failed to bind significant amounts of labelled EGF. Two groups demonstrated that in hybrids made between mouse cells lacking EGF receptors, and human cells expressing EGF receptors, binding of labelled EGF to the hybrids correlated with the presence of human chromosome 7 (Shimizu et al., 1980; Davies et al., 1980). Without a direct assay for the human EGF receptor, however, it was not possible to decide if the gene on chromosome 7 was the structural gene for the human receptor or a gene that complemented the mouse defect and permitted expression of the mouse receptor.

In collaboration with our colleagues B. Ozanne and M. Waterfield, we have produced a monoclonal antibody EGFR1 which binds to the human EGF receptor and fails to react with the mouse receptor. Using this antibody we have confirmed the assignment of a structural gene, EGFR, for the EGF receptor to chromosome 7.

EGFR1 was shown to recognize the EGF receptor by 3 types of experiment:

1.   EGFR1 and the EGF receptor give an identical pattern of reactivity when tested on a variety of different human cells.
2.   In immunoprecipitation experiments EGFR1 recognizes a phosphorylated 150,000 dalton polypeptide.
3.   EGFR1 can precipitate labelled EGF which is cross-linked to the EGF receptor.

EGFR1 shows no reaction with mouse cells, even those like 3T3-K which can be shown to bind to EGF. This species specificity implies that EGFR1 does not bind to the presumably conserved EGF binding site; this was confirmed by the finding that EGFR1 does not inhibit the binding of labelled EGF to its receptor. Consideration of a panel of human-rodent somatic cell hybrids suggested that a gene controlling EGFR1 antigen expression was present on chromosome 7. Particularly relevant was the finding that EGFR1 bound to the human-mouse hybrid C121 (Fig. 15·5) which has chromosome 7 as its only human genetic contribution (Fig. 15·1). Also of interest is the reactivity of the chromosome 7 containing hybrid 2W1-R70 (Nabholz *et al.*, 1969); this hybrid was produced from the fusion of the EGF receptor negative L cell 1R with receptor negative human lymphocytes. Although the possibility of a rare EGF receptor positive cell contaminating the parent lymphocyte population can not be excluded, this result suggests induction of expression of the human EGF receptor gene in the hybrid. Further experiments are in progress to study this regulatory phenomenum.

The second ligand receptor we have studied is the transferrin receptor. M. Greaves and colleagues denmonstrated that the monoclonal antibody OKT-9 recognizes the human transferrin receptor (Sutherland *et al.*, 1981). The antibody shows species specificity for the human receptor and does not react with mouse cells. This specificity is demonstrated in Fig. 15·6 which shows binding of OKT-9 to the human-mouse hybrid MOG13/10 but failure to bind to the mouse parent RAG. On a panel of independent hybrids OKT-9 reactivity segregated with human chromosome 3. Similar segregation of OKT-9 antigen expression and chromosome 3 occured in the subclones of MOG13 (Table

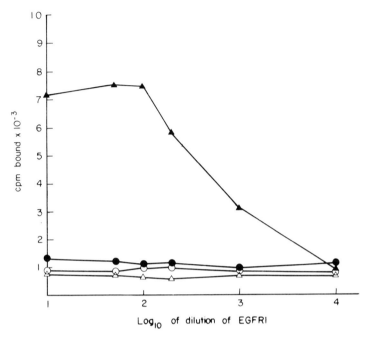

FIG. 15·5 Titration of EGFR1 on the human-mouse hybrid C121. —▲— C121, binding of EGFR1; —△— C121, binding of 12E7 (used as the negative control); —●— 3T3 (mouse cells) binding of EGFR1; —O— 3T3 (mouse cells) binding of 12E7. The IRIA was performed as described in the legend to Fig. 15·3. The EGFR1 antibody pool used was a concentrate of tissue culture supernatant containing 2 mg ml$^{-1}$ antibody. The 12E7 antibody was the same pool as described in Fig. 15·3.

15·6). The OKT-9 antigen and transferrin receptor have a biochemical structure of two disulphide bond linked, 90,000 dalton glycopeptide chains. Similar structures have been described on a variety of actively growing cells and transformed cells (Omary *et al.*, 1980; Judd *et al.*, 1980; Dippold *et al.*, 1980; Woodbury *et al.*, 1980). The structure is also reminiscent of the malignancy associated proteins of Bramwell and Harris (1978, 1979) and the cell surface glucose regulated proteins described by several groups (see, for example, Shiu *et al.*, 1977). Somatic cell genetics can be used to resolve the relationships between these apparently similar molecules.

## V MAPPING OF A SOLUBLE PROTEIN

Mapping of the C3 structural gene is a good example of the use of a monoclonal antibody to map the gene controlling the expression of a

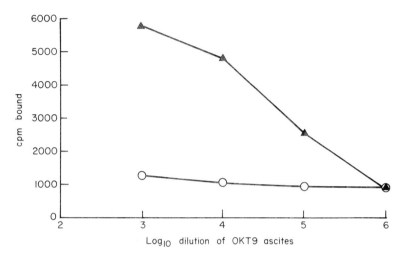

FIG. 15·6 Binding of OKT-9 to the human chromosome 3 positive hybrid MOG13. 10. —▲— MOG13.10 binding of OKT-9; —O— RAG (mouse adenocarcinoma) binding of OKT-9. The IRIA was performed as described in the legend to Fig. 15·3. The human chromosome constitution of hybrid MOG13. 10 is given in Table 15·6. The OKT-9 pool used was ascites containing 20 mg ml$^{-1}$ antibody as determined by radio-immunoassay.

TABLE 15·6
Reactions of OKT-9 with subclones of MOG13

| Cell | Human chromosomes present | CPM Bound mean [a,b] (Standard deviation) | |
| --- | --- | --- | --- |
| | | OKT-9[d] | P3-X63·Ag8[c] |
| MOG 13·9 | X | 852 (96) | 702 (184) |
| MOG 13·10 | 1,3,21,22,X,Y.[5] | 7,100 (749) | 418 (43) |
| MOG 13·17 | 3,21,22,X.[5] | 8,500 (680) | 580 (77) |
| MOG 13·2 | 1,21,22,X | 789 (86) | 472 (40) |
| RAG | Mouse adenocarcinoma | 1,218 (172) | 831 (21) |
| HFL 121 | Human fibroblast | 13,140 (933) | 1,133 (17) |

[a]  See footnote [a] Table 15·3.
[b]  3 determinations.
[c]  See footnote [c] Table 15·3.
[d]  Used at a concentration of approximately 10 μg ml$^{-1}$.
[e]  MOG 13 clones contain marker chromosomes which are described in detail in Solomon et al., 1979.

purified, soluble, serum protein, rather than a cell surface component.

The third component of complement (C3) is a glycoprotein of molecular weight 184,000, comprised of two disulphide bonded chains, $\alpha$ and $\beta$, of molecular weights 112,000 and 72,000 respectively (Tack and Prahl, 1976). Two other complement components, C4 and C5, are very similar to C3 in terms of chain size and structure, mode of activation, mode of inactivation, and the fragments generated by proteolysis. Furthermore, each is derived from a single chain precursor from which a small portion is excised posttranslationally to give rise to separate disulphide linked chains. It has been suggested that all three are descended from a common ancestral component (see review, Porter and Reid, 1979). However, although C4 (O'Neill *et al.*, 1978) has been mapped close to the B locus of HLA in man, along with C2 (Amason *et al.*, 1977) and factor B, (Meo *et al.*, 1976); efforts to map C3 and C5 by linkage studies involving families with deficiencies or polymorphic variants have been unsuccessful. Using a monoclonal antibody to C3 (Whitehead *et al.*, 1981) and somatic cell hybrids, we have succeeded in mapping this complement component to human chromosome 19.

The monoclonal antibody (WM1) was produced by immunizing with purified human C3. Its specificity was established by demonstrating that it inhibits a standard C3 hemolytic assay and is able to immunoprecipitate C3 from human serum in the presence of Staph A (Whitehead *et al.*, 1981).

To use this antibody for purposes of mapping it was necessary first, to demonstrate that cultured cells produce C3, and second, that the human and rodent forms can be distinguished. C3 is produced *in vivo* principally in the liver. Using WM1, Whitehead *et al.*, (1981) have shown that, in culture, human fibroblasts also produce C3. Previous work of Senger and Hynes (1978) had shown that rodent fibroblasts produce C3 in culture. The monoclonal antibody WM1 however, does not react with rodent fibroblast C3, and this species specificity has allowed us to use it to examine C3 as produced by human fibroblast/ mouse hybrids.

S. Whitehead tested a series of hybrids for C3 production by immunoprecipitation of labelled culture medium using WM1 and Staph A, followed by SDS-PAGE and autoradiography. Production of C3 was evident by the presence of $\alpha$ and $\beta$ chain bands. Three strongly positive hybrids were selected and subcloned to produce segregants. From one of these hybrids, MOG2, (see Table 15·7), several subclones were selected. Of these, six were positive for C3 production, and two were negative. Fig. 15·7 shows that autoradiograph of a gel of the immunoprecipitates from these eight subclones. Tracks A5 and E5 are clearly negative while the others are positive. Chromosome analysis of these MOG2 subclones is shown in Table 15·7. Hybrids which either have a particular chromosome and produce C3 (+,+), or do not have the chromosome and do not produce C3 (−,−) are considered "concordant". Those which have the chromosome and do not produce C3 (+,−) or do not have the chromosome and do produce C3 (−,+) are considered "discordant". Every chromosome except 19 has at least two discordancies with C3, with the exception of chromosome 11 which had one discordancy. Chromosome 19 shows concordant segregation in all cases. Results from the two other hybrids which were subcloned were similar, giving conclusive evidence that C3 production segregates with chromosome 19.

TABLE 15·7
Segregation of C3 in 8 subclones of MOG 2

| Chromosome | Concordant | | Discordant | | Total | |
| --- | --- | --- | --- | --- | --- | --- |
| | + | − | + | − | Concordant | Discordant |
| 1 | 5 | 0 | 1 | 2 | 5 | 3 |
| 2 | 2 | 2 | 4 | 0 | 4 | 4 |
| 3 | 6 | 0 | 0 | 2 | 6 | 2 |
| 4 | 5 | 0 | 1 | 2 | 5 | 3 |
| 5 | 6 | 0 | 0 | 2 | 6 | 2 |
| 6 | 5 | 0 | 1 | 2 | 5 | 3 |
| 7 | 5 | 0 | 1 | 2 | 5 | 3 |
| 8 | 4 | 0 | 2 | 2 | 4 | 4 |
| 9 | 4 | 0 | 2 | 2 | 4 | 4 |
| 10 | 6 | 0 | 0 | 2 | 6 | 2 |
| 11 | 5 | 2 | 1 | 0 | 7 | 1 |
| 12 | 6 | 0 | 0 | 2 | 6 | 2 |
| 13 | 6 | 0 | 0 | 2 | 6 | 2 |
| 14 | 6 | 0 | 0 | 2 | 6 | 2 |
| 15 | 6 | 0 | 0 | 2 | 6 | 2 |
| 16 | 5 | 0 | 1 | 2 | 5 | 3 |
| 17 | 6 | 0 | 0 | 2 | 6 | 2 |
| 18 | 5 | 0 | 1 | 2 | 5 | 3 |
| 19 | 6 | 2 | 0 | 0 | 8 | 0 |
| 20 | 3 | 2 | 3 | 0 | 5 | 3 |
| 21 | 5 | 0 | 1 | 2 | 5 | 3 |
| 22 | 5 | 0 | 1 | 2 | 5 | 3 |
| X | 6 | 0 | 0 | 2 | 6 | 2 |

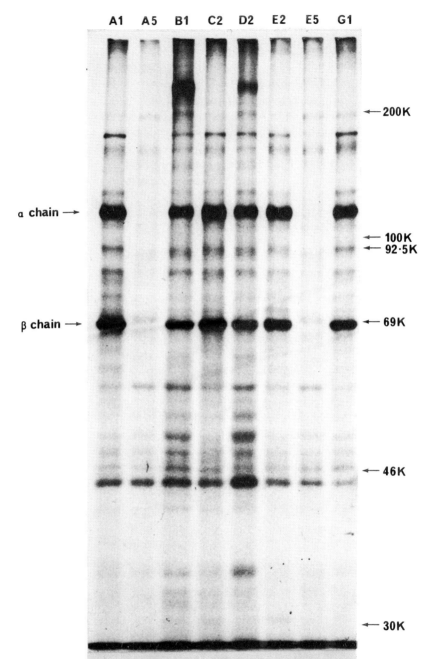

FIG. 15·7 Immunoprecipitation of C3 from MOG 2 subclones, using monoclonal antibody WM1. Cells confluent in 25 cm² flasks were labelled with 0·5 mCi (= 18·5 MBq) ³⁵S-methionine in 2 ml serum and methionine free medium for 48 hours. Culture supernatants were precleared by overnight incubation with 30 μl normal mouse serum

C3 has a small glycosylated portion. In theory, if WM1 were directed against this determinant, we could be mapping a human glycosyl transferase which modified mouse C3. To eliminate this possibility, poly A$^+$ mRNA was prepared from human hepatocytes translated *in vitro* and the produce immunoprecipitated. Polyacrylamide gel analysis of the precipitate revelead an unglycosylated nascent C3 precursor. This was taken as evidence that WM1 recognizes the unglycosylated C3 and that we have mapped the gene coding for the C3 polypeptide.

## VI SOMATIC CELL HYBRIDS AS TOOLS FOR PRODUCING MONOCLONAL ANTIBODIES

Although somatic cell hybrids are mostly used for genetic analysis they can also be used as reagents for the production of monoclonal antibodies and for screening monoclonal antibody fusions for particular antibodies.

Buck and Bodmer (1975) introduced a powerful method for the production of antisera specific for products of defined human chromosomes. Human-mouse hybrids containing a restricted human chromosomal content were used to immunize mice which were syngeneic with the mouse parent cell of the hybrid. After absorption with mouse cells to remove antibodies specific for mouse tumour antigens, antisera were produced specific for products of the human X chromosome (Buck and Bodmer, 1976) and chromosome 11 (Buck and Bodmer, 1975). In collaboration with R. Hope and W. F. Bodmer we have used the same scheme to produce monoclonal antibodies specific for antigens controlled by the human X-chromosome. The hybrid 1W1-5 contains the long arm of the human X-chromosome as its only human genetic contribution on a C3H mouse L cell background. C3H mice were immunized with 1W1-5 and the resultant monoclonal antibody producing colonies were screened on 1W1-5 and L cells. Several colonies were found to produce antibody which discriminated between 1W1-5 and L cells; one of these colonies was cloned and the resultant clone named R1. When tested on a panel of human-mouse hybrids containing only the X chromosome R1 was shown to recognize an

and Staph A precipitation. Each track derives from material precipitated with Staph A from 150 $\mu$l supernatant after a one hour incubation at 4°C with 3 $\mu$l WM1 ascites fluid. Control immunoprecipitations using AAP1 ascites fluid (not shown) failed to reveal C3 $\alpha$ and $\beta$ chain bands. The polyacrylamide gel analysis was using 7·5% polyacrylamide SDS Laemli gels.

antigen controlled by the X-chromosome (Table 15·8). Preliminary gene localization experiments suggest that the R1 antigen controlling gene, MIC5, may map very close to, or is identical with, the gene S5 previously defined by an antiserum raised against 1W1-5 (Buck and Bodmer, 1976). This approach will become more important as markers are required for particular human chromosomes.

If a human product is known to be controlled by a structural gene on a particular human chromosome, judicious use of somatic cell hybrids can be used to screen for specific monoclonal antibodies. The antibody to human epidermal growth factor receptor EGFR1 was derived from an immunization with the epidermoid carcinoma A431. The initial screening was by IRIA on the immunizing cell followed by immuno-precipitation analysis of $^{32}$P phosphate labelled membrane extracts (see previous section). In a reconstruction experiment using the original supernatants we found that screening on the "7 only" human-mouse hybrid C121 also identified the anti-EGF receptor monoclonal antibodies from the fusion (Table 15·9).

## VII SELECTION EXPERIMENTS

Antisera have been used to manipulate the human genetic content of somatic cell hybrids by selecting segregants. Most previous work has used the negative selection technique of complement dependent cytotoxicity in which cells with the unwanted phenotype are removed by cell killing (Puck *et al.*, 1971; Goodfellow, 1975; Jones *et al.*, 1976). Recently, the introduction of the fluorescence activated cell sorter (FACS) (see Herzenberg and Herzenberg, 1978) has facilitated both the isolation of cells with a particular antigen (positive selection) and the isolation of cells lacking a particular antigen (negative selection). Theoretically, using two colour fluorescence, it should even be possible to isolate cells with different combinations of cell surface markers. Monoclonal antibodies which are easily purified and can be directly labelled are particularly suited for these types of experiment.

As part of a series of experiments to evaluate the FACS as a tool in somatic cell genetics we have isolated segregants from the human-mouse hybrid HORL9. The only human chromosomes present in HORL9 are X, 11 and 15 (Goodfellow *et al.*, 1975); previously we had used complement dependent cytotoxicity to isolate segregants which had lost chromosome 11, using anti-S4 (Buck and Bodmer, 1975) and had lost chromosome 15, using anti-$\beta$2 microglobulin (Goodfellow, 1975). We have repeated these experiments using positive and negative

## TABLE 15·8
### Reaction of R1 with "X-only" human-mouse hybrids

| | | CPM Bound X10$^{-3}$[a,b] | | |
| | | R1[d] | CA2·06[c] | Comment |
|---|---|---|---|---|
| Hybrid: | HORL9·X | 10·0 | 2·0 | "X-only" hybrid |
| Mouse parent: | 1R | 2·6 | 2·5 | |
| Hybrid: | 1W1-5 | 13·6 | 1·7 | "Xq only" hybrid |
| Mouse parent: | 1R | 2·6 | 2·5 | |
| Hybrid: | GEOC-5[e] | 4·7 | 0·6 | "X only" hybrid |
| Mouse parent: | PCC4 | 1·4 | 1·4 | |

[a] See footnote [a] Table 15·3.
[b] Figures represent average of two determinations.
[c] See footnote [c] Table 15·4.
[d] Used at a concentration of approximately 20 $\mu$g ml$^{-1}$.
[e] Hybrid produced by fusing ThyB-1 to PCC4 (G. Banting and P. Goodfellow unpublished). This hybrid contains an X-chromosome as its only human contribution.

## TABLE 15·9
### Use of somatic cell hybrid C121 to screen for monoclonal anti-EGF receptor antibodies

| | CPM bound × 10$^{-3}$[a,b,c] | | | |
| Clone | A431 | 1R | MOLT-4 | C121 |
|---|---|---|---|---|
| B12 | 7·0 | 2·2 | 1·8 | 9·9 |
| F11 | 12·2 | 2·6 | 3·3 | 6·9 |
| H12 | 9·1 | 8·1 | 8·0 | 10·8 |
| H9 | 12·0 | 2·9 | 2·3 | 5·8 |
| B10 | 18·1 | 1·8 | 1·3 | 3·0 |
| A11 | 15·9 | 1·8 | 3·6 | 5·9 |
| F12 | 3·1 | 11·2 | 3·4 | 6·8 |
| C11 | 8·4 | 1·9 | 1·2 | 4·8 |
| C9 | 21·9 | 1·3 | 2·2 | 15·0 |
| P3-X63·Ag8 | 0·4 | 1·8 | 0·8 | 1·1 |

[a] See footnote [a] Table 15·3.
[b] Single determination using supernatants.
[c] All the clones except H12 and F12 were shown to be anti-EGF receptor antibodies by immunoprecipitation analysis.

selection on the FACS in an attempt to produce hybrids containing single human chromosomes. As an example, the overall scheme for producing a "15-only" hybrid is presented in Fig. 15·8. HORL9 was backselected in 8 azaguanine to remove the human X chromosome and then a chromosome 11 negative population was isolated by selecting cells which failed to stain with the monoclonal antibody W6/34 (Fig. 15·9). A very clear separation between W6/34 positive and negative cells was achieved. After plating at low dilution a clone, HORLI, was isolated which karyotypically contained only chromosome 15. Unfortunately this clone also contained a subchromosomal fragment of the X-chromosome which was karyotypically undetectable but could be detected by antigenic analysis.

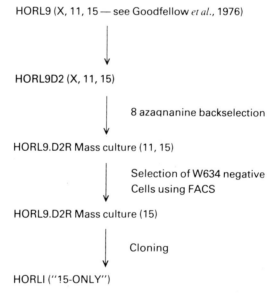

FIG. 15·8 Production of "15-only" derivative of HORL9.

In the future we hope to be able to exploit the FACS for somatic cell genetic analysis in two additional ways. Firstly, it should be possible to sort mixed populations of hybrid cells and directly test the sorted populations for isoenzyme markers. Secondly, two colour fluorescence, where different antibodies are labelled with rhodamine or fluorescine, should enable direct testing of linkage at the single cell level.

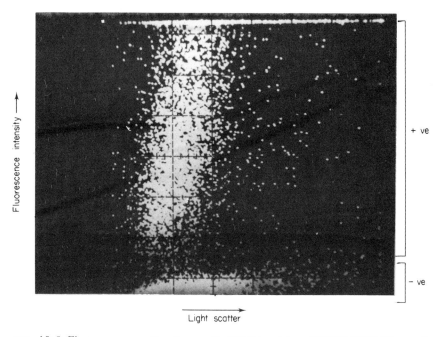

FIG. 15·9 Fluorescence-scatter diagram for W6/34 staining of HORL9D2R. The vertical axis (fluorescence) is a measure of fluorescence intensity; the horizontal axis (scatter) is a measure of cell size. Each spot represents a single cell; 10,000 cells are depicted in the diagram. $5 \times 10^5$ HORL9D2R cells were stained with 50 $\mu$l of W6/34 concentrated tissue culture supernatant containing 200 $\mu$g ml$^{-1}$ antibody. After 1 hr on ice the cells were washed and stained with 1:10 dilution of a fluorescein labelled rabbit anti-mouse Ig preparation (Cappel Laboratories; batch No. 14335). The fluorescence negative population was sorted and cloned.

## VII CONCLUSION

We have presented examples of the ways in which monoclonal antibodies can be utilized for human gene mapping when combined with the techniques of somatic cell genetics. The advantages of monoclonal antibodies for this type of work are their species-specificity, high titre, and monospecificity. Monoclonal antibodies have been particularly useful as reagents to detect human gene products which previously were difficult to distinguish from their rodent counterparts. In addition, monoclonal antibodies have been used to define new cell surface antigens which in turn have been mapped and used in hybrids as markers for specific chromosomes. The increase in chromosome specific antigenic markers will lead to further possibilities for manipulating the chromosome content of somatic cell hybrids and eventually to a more precise map of the human genome.

As more genetic markers become available and the genes controlling their expression are mapped, it should be possible to draw conclusions about the relationship between chromosomal gene order and genome function. Already, some generalizations can be made; the genes coding for dissimilar subunits of multimeric enzymes are usually unlinked, whereas closely related genes often form clusters (for example, immunoglobulins, Croce *et al.*, 1979). A more practical benefit which can be expected from gene mapping studies is related to genetic disease. Some diseases of genetic origin may not be expressed in the cells which can be obtained by amniocentises. For these diseases the only possibility for pre-natal diagnosis is to use polymorphic markers which show linkage to the disease locus in the afflicted families (Solomon and Bodmer, 1979). Technical advances especially in recombinant DNA studies and also in the production of monoclonal antibodies will increase the number of genetically mapped polymorphic markers available and will undoubtedly contribute to advances in prenatal diagnosis.

ACKNOWLEDGEMENTS

We are grateful to all our colleagues who have provided monoclonal antibodies and collaborated with us on the experiments presented in this report. In addition we would like to acknowledge the continuing and very productive collaboration with Dr. S. Povey, Dr. D. Swallow and Mr. Mohamed Parker (isozyme analysis); Dr. D. Sheer and Mrs. S. Chambers (karyotypic analysis) and Mr. G. Banting, Mr. M. V. Wiles and Miss L. Hiorns (serological analysis and cell culture). We would also like to thank Dr. W. F. Bodmer, Dr. F. Benham, Mr. A. Tunneciiffe and Mr. G. Banting for reading and commenting on the manuscript and Miss C. Furse for typing.

REFERENCES

Andrews, P. W. and Goodfellow, P. (1980). *Somatic Cell Genetics* **6**, 271–284.
Amason, A., Larsen, B., Marshall, W. H., Edwards, J. H., Mackintosh, P., Olaisen, B. and Teisberg, P. (1977). *Nature* **268**, 527–528.
Barnstable, C. J., Bodmer, W. F., Brown, G., Galfre, G., Milstein, C., Williams, A. F. and Zeigler, A. (1978). *Cell* **14**, 9–20.
Bobrow, M. and Cross, J. (1974). *Nature* **251**, 77–79.
Bramwell, M. E. and Harris, H. (1978). *Proc. R. Soc. Lond. B.* **201**, 87–106.

Bramwell, M. E. and Harris, H. (1979). *Proc. R. Soc. Lond. B.* **203**, 93–99.

Brodsky, F. M., Bodmer, W. F. and Parham, P. (1979). *Eur. J. Immunol* **9**, 536–545.

Buck, D. W. and Bodmer, W. F. (1975). *In* "Human Gene Mapping 2". Birth Defects: Original Article Series 11, 3, pp. 87–89.

Buck, D. W. and Bodmer, W. F. (1976) *In* "Human Gene Mapping 3". Birth Defects: Original Article Series 12, 7, 376–377.

Caspersson, T., Zech, L. and Johansson, C. (1971). *Hereditas* **67**, 89–102.

Carpenter, G. and Cohen, S. (1975). *Proc. natn. Acad. Sci. U.S.A.* **72**, 1317–1321.

Carpenter, G. and Cohen, S. (1979). *Ann. Rev. Biochem.* **48**, 193–216.

Charron, D. J. and McDevitt, H. O. (1979). *Proc. natn. Acad. Sci. U.S.A.* **76**, 6567–6571.

Creagan, R. P., Chen, S. and Ruddle, F. H. (1975). *Proc. natn. Acad. Sci. U.S.A.* **72**, 2237–2241.

Croce, C. M., Girardi, A. J. and Koprowski, H. (1973). *Proc. natn. Acad. Sci. U.S.A.* **70**, 3617–3620.

Croce, C. M., Thander, M., Martinis, J., Cicurel, L., D'Ancona, G. G., Dolby, T. W. and Koprowski, H. (1979). *Proc. natn. Acad. Sci. U.S.A.* **76**, 3416–3420.

Dalchau, R., Kirkley, J., and Fabre, J. W. (1980). *Eur. J. Immunol* **10**, 745–750.

Davidson, R. L. (1974). *Ann. Rev. Genet.* **8**, 195–218.

Davies, R. L., Grosse, V. A., Kucherlapati, R., Bothwell, M. (1980). *Proc. natn. Acad. Sci. U.S.A.* **77**, 4188–4192.

Dippold, W. G., Lloyd, K. O., Li, C. T. C., Ikeda, H., Oettgen, H. F. and Old, L. J. (1980). *Proc. natn. Acad. Sci. U.S.A.* **77**, 6114–6118.

Eun, C. K. and Klinger, H. P. (1980). *Cytogenet. Cell Genet.* **27**, 57–64.

Evans, H. J., Hamerton, J. L., Klinger, H. P. and McKusick, V. A. (1979). Eds. "Human Gene Mapping 5". *Cytogenet. Cell Genet.* **25**, 1–221.

Fellous, M., Couillin, P., Neuport-Sautes, C., Frezal, J., Billardon, C. and Dausset, J. (1973). *Eur. J. Immunol.* **3**, 543–548.

Fellous, M., Bengtsson, B., Finnegan, D. and Bodmer, W. F. (1974). *Ann. Human Genet.* **37**, 421–429.

Goodfellow, P. N. (1975). D. Phil. Thesis, Oxford University.

Goodfellow, P. N. and Tippett, P. (1981). *Nature* **289**, 404–405.

Goodfellow, P. N., Jones, E. A., van Heyningen, V., Solomon, E., Bobrow, M., Miggiano, V. and Bodmer, W. F. (1975). *Nature* **254**, 267–269.

Goodfellow, P. N., Banting, G., Levy, R., Povey, S. and McMichael, A. (1980). *Somat. Cell Genet.* **6**, 777–787.

Harris, H. and Watkins, J. (1965). *Nature*, **205**, 640–642.

Harris, H. and Hopkinson, D. A. (1977). *In* "Handbook of enzyme electrophoresis in human genetics". North Holland, Amsterdam.

Herzenberg, C. A. and Herzenberg, L. A. (1978). *In* "Handbook of Experimental Immunology". (Weir, D. M. Ed.) 3rd edition. pp. 12·1–12·20. Blackwell, Oxford.

Hobart, M. J., Rabbitts, T. H., Goodfellow, P. N., Solomon, E., Chambers, S., Spurr, N. and Povey, S. (1981). *Ann. Hum. Genet.* **45**, 331–335.

Jones, E. A., Goodfellow, P. N., Kennett, R. H. and Bodmer, W. F. (1976). *Somat. Cell Genet.* **2**, 483–486.

Judd, W., Poodry, C. A. and Strominger, J. L. (1980). *J. exp. Med.* **152**, 1430–1435.

Kohler, G. and Milstein, C. (1975). *Nature* **256**, 495–497.

Kucherlapati, R. S., Baker, R. and Ruddle, F. H. (1975). *Cytogenet. Cell Genet.* **14**, 192–193.

Lawler, S. D. (1954) *Carylogica* **6** (suppl.) 26.

Levy, R., Dilley, J., Fox, R. I. and Warnke, R. (1979). *Proc. natn. Acad. Sci. U.S.A.* **76**, 6552–6556.

Littlefield, J. (1964). *Science* **145**, 709–710.

Meo, T., Atkinson, J., Bernoco, M., Bernoco, D. and Cepellini, R. (1976). *Eur. J. Immunol.* **6**, 916–919.

Nabholz, M., Miggiano, V. and Bodmer, W. F. (1969). *Nature* **223**, 358–363.

Neff, J. M. and Enders, J. F. (1968). *Proc. Soc. exp. Biol. Med.* **127**, 260–267.

Omary, M. B., Trowbridge, I. S. and Minowada, J. (1980). *Nature* **286**, 888–890.

O'Neill, G. J., Yang, S. Y., Tegoli, J., Berger, R. and Dupont, B. (1978). *Nature* **273**, 668–670.

Pontecorvo, G. (1975). *Somat. Cell Genet.* **1**, 397–400.

Porter, R. R., and Reid, K. B. M. (1979). *Adv. Protein Chem.* **33**, 1–71.

Puck, T. T., Wuthier, P., Jones, C. and Kao, F. (1971). *Proc. natn. Acad. Sci. U.S.A.* **68**, 3102–3106.

Race, R. R. and Sanger, R. (1975). *In* "Blood Groups in Man". 6th edition. Blackwell Scientific, Oxford.

Renwick, J. H. and Lawler, S. D. (1955). *Ann. Hum. Genet.* **19**, 312–315.

Seabright, M. (1972). *Chromosoma* **36**, 204–210.

Senger, D. R. and Hynes, R. O. (1978). *Cell* **15**, 375–384.

Shiu, R. P. C., Ponyssegur, J. and Pastan, I. (1977). *Proc. natn. Acad. Sci. U.S.A.* **74**, 3840–3844.

Shimizu, N., Behzadian, M. A. and Shimizu, V. (1979). *Cytogenet. Cell Genet.* **25**, 201–202.

Solomon, E. and Bodmer, W. F. (1979). *Lancet* **i**, 923.

Solomon, E., Bobrow, M., Goodfellow, P. N., Bodmer, W. F., Swallow, D. M., Povey, S. and Noel, R. (1976). *Somat. Cell Genet.* **2**, 125–140.

Solomon, E., Swallow, D., Burgess, S. and Evans, L. (1979). *Ann. Hum. Genet.* **42**, 273–281.

Sutherland, R., Delia, D., Schneider, C., Newman, R., Kemshead, J. and Greaves, M. (1981). *Proc. natn. Acad. Sci. U.S.A.* **78**, 4515–4579.

Swallow, D. M., Solomon, E. and Pajunen, L. (1977). *Cytogenet. Cell Genet.* **18**, 136–148.

Szybalski, W., Szybalski, E. and Rayni, G. (1962). *Natn. Cancer Inst. Monogr.* **7**, 75–89.

Tack, B. F. and Prahl, J. W. (1976). *Biochemistry* **15**, 4513—4521.

van Heyningen, V., Bobrow, M., Bodmer, W. F., Gardner, S. E., Povey, S. and Hopkinson, D. A. (1975). *Ann. Hum. Genet.* **38**, 295–302.

Whitehead, A. S., Sim, R. B. and Bodmer, W. F. (1981). *Eur. J. Immunol.* **11**, 140–146.

Woodbury, R. G., Brown, J. P., Yeh, M. Y., Hellstrom, I. and Hellstrom, K. R. (1980). *Proc. natn. Acad. Sci. U.S.A.* **77**, 2183–2187.

# G  NEUROLOGY

# 16 Differentiation Antigens of the Human Central Nervous System: identification with monoclonal antibodies and potential clinical value

JOHN W. FABRE

*Nuffield Department of Surgery, University of Oxford,*
*John Radcliffe Hospital, Oxford. OX3 9DU*

*Current address: Blond McIndoe Centre, Queen Victoria Hospital,*
*East Grinstead, Sussex. RH19 3D2*

I  Introduction .............................................. 397
II  Problems with Monoclonal Antibody Production to
    CNS Antigens ............................................ 399
    A.  Access to a Frozen Bank of CNS Subregions ............... 399
    B.  Choice of Immunogen ................................. 399
    C.  Assay Systems ........................................ 401
III  Examples of Monoclonal Antibodies to CNS Differentiation
    Antigens ................................................ 402
    A.  Introduction .......................................... 402
    B.  Distribution in Brain .................................. 403
    C.  Biochemical Characterization ........................... 405
IV  Potential Clinical Applications ............................. 405
    A.  Correlations with Disease .............................. 405
    B.  CNS Tumours .......................................... 409
    C.  Treatment of Neuroblastoma ........................... 410
    D.  Other Possibilities .................................... 411

## I INTRODUCTION

The complexity of the human central nervous system (CNS) is daunting, but one should remember that it is at the cell membrane, both in general and at the synaptic points, that the neurons and glial cells communicate with one another both to form and to operate this most complex and intriguing of the body's organs. Any understanding of differentiation and function at the molecular level will therefore rest to an important degree on the identification and characterization of these membrane molecules. Those molecules found largely or exclusively in the CNS are those with which the secrets of function must lie, and the advent of monoclonal antibodies (Kohler and Milstein, 1975) offers an unprecedented opportunity to identify and to characterize these 'differentiation antigens".

It is inherent in the technology of monoclonal antibody production that the reagents one produces recognize individual componnents of complex biological systems and it is this unique resolving power of monoclonal antibodies that is the basis for the revolution they have brought to biology. Nowhere can this capacity to recognize a single component in a complex system be of greater advantage than in an organ like the CNS, where vast numbers of cells with a bewildering complexity of morphology and function are inextricably interlinked in one structure.

Of particular importance are the relatively enormous concentrations of specific antibody routinely available with monoclonal antibodies. This means that one has reagents of the highest quality which can readily be used for precise tissue localization (see chapter 25), which is an important asset in studies of the CNS. Moreover, one is able routinely to construct high capacity immunoadsorbents for the biochemical characterization and purification of molecules for functional and other studies (see chapter 22). This is a far cry from the use of heavily absorbed anti brain xenosera for the identification of CNS differentiation antigens where, quite apart from the usual difficulties as to reproducibility and uncertainties as regards monospecificity, little further than simple identification is usually possible.

At the present time, there are very few reports in the literature of monoclonal antibodies to CNS differentiation antigens, in contrast to the vast amount of published work on monoclonal antibodies to lymphocytes and other leucocytes. Our own interest in the CNS stems in fact from the frequent sharing of antigens between leucocytes and the CNS. The paucity of work on the CNS is a reflection perhaps of the greater practical difficulties inherent in the raising of monoclonal antibodies to the CNS, but is probably also the result of a somewhat delayed response by workers in the field, certainly in comparison to their immunologist colleagues for whom the raising of monoclonal antibodies to the lymphocyte surface would represent a more familiar development. In any case, this review has been written with 3 major aims: to discuss the problems peculiar to monoclonal antibody production to the CNS, so that our experience might be of benefit to others; to demonstrate the scope and power of monoclonal antibodies in this field; and finally to speculate on potential clinical applications.

## II PROBLEMS WITH MONOCLONAL ANTIBODY PRODUCTION TO CNS ANTIGENS

Being a solid, inaccessible organ, every $mm^3$ cube of which contains a great number of different cell types which cannot be dissociated from one another, creates a number of problems that do not arise with studies on, e.g., blood lymphocytes.

### A. ACCESS TO A FROZEN BANK OF CNS SUBREGIONS

Whatever one's primary interest, it is clearly of fundamental importance to know the distribution within the CNS of any antigens to which one raises monoclonal antibodies. It is therefore virtually indispensible to have access to different brain subregions, obtained as soon as possible after death. This requires patience and the help of a considerate pathologist, but one brain can supply almost unlimited amounts of tissue, so that waiting for a fresh specimen is well worthwhile. We have found it useful to very carefully dissect subregions and to use them from one half of the brain for homogenization and storage at $-40°C$, and to store those from the other half of the brain in liquid nitrogen for frozen sections (McKenzie and Fabre, 1981a, 1982; Lakin and Fabre, 1981; McKenzie *et al.*, 1982).

### B. CHOICE OF IMMUNOGEN

The immunogen used will depend on one's interests, but the range of possibilities extends from crude homogenates of whole brain through to purified brain molecules.

If one has a specific goal in mind, the aim is to reduce the heterogeneity of the immunogen as much as possible. One can for example, use homogenates of carefully dissected brain subregions. One can try to overcome the problem of the cellular complexity of the immunogen by using neuronal or glial cell lines, or, to a lesser extent, homogenates of tumours, but all of these last possibilities have the disadvantage that the cells involved are unlikely to be representative of the mature neurons and glia present in the adult CNS. One can also, of course, use foetal brains at various stages of maturation.

In an organ like the CNS, where there is little knowledge of the biochemical make-up of the cell membranes, it is usually a question of immunizing, doing the fusions, and waiting to see what the resultant monoclonal antibodies reveal about the cell membranes. There are, however, exceptions to this. For example, the Thy-1 glycoprotein is a well characterized glycoprotein of rodent brains (Barclay *et al.*, 1975, 1976) for which the complete amino acid sequence is known (Campbell *et al.*, 1981). We therefore initially characterized human Thy-1 using conventional serological techniques (Dalchau and Fabre., 1979), purified human brain Thy-1 and then immunized mice with the pure molecule to obtain a monoclonal anti-human Thy-1 antibody (McKenzie and Fabre, 1981b). If one knows the target molecule to which one wishes to raise monoclonal antibodies, even partial purification of the immunogen will increase the probability of obtaining antibodies of the desired specificity.

One approach which we have used (Lakin and Fabre, 1981) is to immunize with detergent solubilized brain glycoproteins, obtained by affinity chromatography on lentil lectin columns. This approach has 2 potentially important advantages. Firstly, glycoslated molecules are preferentially expressed on the outer surface of the cell membranes and these molecules are therefore the ones that will be of most interest, and will be selected from the homogenate by a lectin affinity step. Secondly, detergent solubilization of the membrane results in the dispersion of the glycolipids into monomeric form in detergent micelles and in this state they are unlikely to be immunogenic. If one wishes to produce antibodies to membrane proteins, rather than glycolipids, this is obviously an advantage. Indeed, if detergents with a small micelle size are used, (e.g. deoxycholate as discussed in chapter 22) the glycolipids can be completely removed from the glycoproteins by a simple gel filtration step, but this is probably not necessary to prevent antibody production to glycolipids.

Once antibodies have been produced to one component of a mixture, the mixture can be depleted of that component using monoclonal antibody affinity columns, as discussed in chapter 22. The glycoproteins used to produce the F3-87-8 antibody (Lakin and Fabre, 1981) were in fact depleted of Thy-1 in this way before being used to immunize mice.

## C. ASSAY SYSTEMS

Once the fusion has been done, one needs a quick method for screening the wells to select those producing antibodies of interest. With a complex, solid organ like the CNS this can present problems, but there are two simple solutions as will be discussed below. In general, a good principle is to use a two-stage screening process. The first asks simply whether or not a particular well is responding with antibodies to the immunogen. This will frequently (but not always) very substantially reduce the number of wells to study. One can then concentrate more attention on these wells in the second stage to ask if the antibodies produced are of interest to the experimenter.

The screening system of choice will depend on the immunogen used and the broad area of interest of the experimenter, but these are 2 main approaches. These are the use of radioactive binding assays and the use of frozen sections.

### 1. FROZEN SECTIONS

There is little doubt that, in most instances, the ideal system for both primary and secondary screening of fusions is the use of frozen sections in combination with immunoperoxidase techniques (see chapter 24). In some cases, where the antibody is seen on the primary screen to detect a subpopulation of cells in the section, the well would usually be selected for further study without secondary screening. If one is attempting to produce antibodies to an unusual cell type in the CNS (e.g. the Purkinje cell) screening on frozen sections is the only possible approach.

### 2. RADIOACTIVE BINDING ASSAYS

(a) *For primary screening*

If one has immunized with a cell line, the best initial screen is to use binding assays with $^{125}$I labelled anti mouse immunoglobulin (Morris and Williams, 1975) to ask if antibodies are being produced to the surface of the cell used as immunogen. One can also use tissue homogenates in this sort of binding assay (Fabre and Williams, 1977; Barclay, 1977) and detailed protocols for this have been published (Hart and Fabre, 1980). The disadvantage of using homogenate of a complex tissue like brain as targets in binding assays for screening fusions is that one is likely to detect only major components shared among many of the different cell types present in the homogenate. This is the system we have used to date, and the antibodies we have detected have in fact been major components of CNS tissue (e.g. Lakin and Fabre, 1981).

(b) *For secondary screening*

Once antibody producing wells have been identified, one must select those producing interesting antibodies. An excellent, although time-consuming, approach is to perform quantitative absorption analyses using a selection of homogenates such as liver, spleen, kidney and brain. Broadly distributed antigens can then be disregarded. One can also screen positive wells at the secondary screen by direct binding to cell lines of different origins, but this is probably best restricted to fusions where cell lines were used as immunogens in the first instance (e.g. Liao *et al.*, 1981).

## III EXAMPLES OF MONOCLONAL ANTIBODIES TO CNS DIFFERENTIATION ANTIGENS

### A. INTRODUCTION

There must be dozens, and perhaps hundreds, of differentiation antigens on the various neuronal and glial cell types of the CNS awaiting identification with monoclonal antibodies. The most interesting, distinguishing different neuronal and glial cell types, remain to be discovered, but a suggestion of what is ahead comes from data just published, where monoclonal antibodies have been used to distinguish peripheral (dorsal root ganglion) neurons from CNS (cerebellar) neurons (Vulliamy *et al.*, 1981; Cohen and Selvendran, 1981) in the rat.

An interesting and unexplained finding has been the frequency with which antigens have been shared between the CNS and leucocytes, both in the rat (Acton *et al.*, 1974, Williams *et al.*, 1978) and man (Dalchau *et al.*, 1980; McKenzie and Fabre, 1981a, b; McKenzie *et al.*, 1982). At least 2 monoclonal antibodies detecting antigens shared between the CNS and myeloid cells have been prepared (J. Kemshead, ICRF Laboratories, London, personal communication). Both of the brain-leucocyte antigens found in man in this laboratory also react with fibroblasts, and what precisely is the connection between these tissues is unknown.

Our own efforts to date in looking for CNS antigens have been biased to screening methods which select for major components. This is because such molecules, being present in large quantities, can be purified and used in biochemical and other studies. Monoclonal antibodies directed at unusual cell types in the CNS (e.g. Purkinje cells) will be useful primarily for screening purposes, as purification of target molecules in these cases is unlikely to be a realistic possibility, unless the antibody also reacts with cell lines.

## B. DISTRIBUTION IN BRAIN

### 1. ABSORPTION ANALYSES

We have characterized 4 monoclonal antibodies reactive against different human CNS differentiation antigens, two of these being quite specific to the nervous system, and two showing a wider but restricted tissue distribution. The reaction of these antibodies with various parts of the CNS is interesting, and a comparison of these 4 antibodies is given in Fig. 16·1, which shows the results of quantitative absorption analyses with homogenates of cuadate, putamen, thalamus, corpus callosum, cerebral white matter, cerebral cortex and cerebellar folia. Each antibody gives a distinctive and interesting pattern. The F10-44-2 antigen (Fig. 16·1(a)) (Dalchau *et al.*, 1980; McKenzie *et al.*, 1982) is absent wherever areas of pure grey matter are used for absorption (cerebral cortex, cuadate and putamen), suggesting that the antigen is restricted to white matter. This restriction within the CNS is interesting, as this antigen is found on a number of extra-neural tissues including mature T lymphocytes and granulocytes (Dalchau *et al.*, 1980), breast epithelial cells (Daar and Fabre, 1981) and colonic epithelium and fibroblasts, but not on many other tissues, including adrenal medulla (Daar and Fabre, 1982). In contrast, the Thy-l antigen (Fig. 16·1(b)) (Dalchau and Fabre, 1979; McKenzie and Fabre, 1981a, b) is found in large quantities throughout the CNS, although areas of grey matter have 5-20 times as much Thy-l as white matter. The F15-135-1 antigen (Fig. 16·1(c)) (McKenzie and Fabre, 1982) gives an interesting picture, because the cerebral nuclei (putamen, caudate and thalamus) have larger amounts of antigen when compared to other areas of brain, including the cerebral and cerebellar cortices. The F3-87-8 antigen (Fig. 16·1(d)) (Lakin and Fabre, 1981) is found in large and roughly equal amounts throughout the CNS.

### 2. STUDIES ON FROZEN SECTIONS

The value of localizing antigens within the CNS is illustrated by the immunofluorescence pictures given in Fig. 16·2. As expected from the

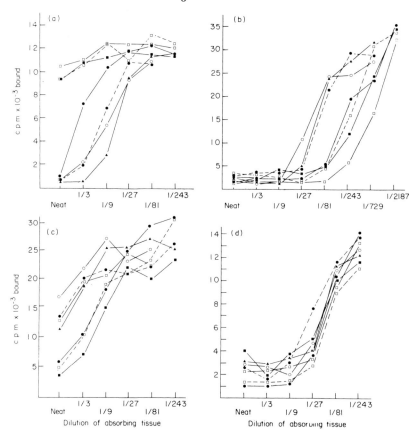

FIG. 16·1 Distribution of 4 brain differentiation antigens within the CNS. Quantitative absorption analysis were performed with the following monoclonal antibodies at limiting dilutions: (a) F10-44-2 (Dalchau *et al.*, 1980; McKenzie *et al.*, 1982); (b) F15-42-1 (anti Thy-l) (McKenzie and Fabre, 1981a,b); (c) F15-135-1 (McKenzie and Fabre, 1982); and (d), F3-87-8 (Lakin and Fabre, 1981). Tripling dilutions of the following homogenates were used for absorption: head of caudate nucleus, ■; putamen; □— — —□; thalamus, ●— — —●; cerebral cortex, □————□; cerebral white matter, △; corpus callosum, O; cerebellar folia, ●————●. Brain homogenate targets were used in the indirect binding assays to detect residual antibody after absorption, and c.p.m. bound refers to [125]I labelled rabbit anti mouse immunoglobulin bound per assay.

absorption analyses (Fig. 16·1(a)), the F10-44-2 antigen did not stain areas of grey matter, the staining in the region of the dentate nucleus (Fig. 16·2(a)) being typical. What was unexpected was that in addition to this general staining of white matter, there was a remarkable concentration of staining around blood vessels (McKenzie *et al.*, 1982) illustrated in Fig. 16·2(b)). The precise significance of this will require ultra-structural studies, but it might represent staining of specialized astrocytes.

The Thy-1 antigen gave granular staining in areas of grey matter, with intense staining of the neuropil and no obvious staining of neuronal cell bodies. This is illustrated with the picture of the cerebellar cortex in Fig. 16·2(d), where one can see intense staining in the molecular layer and in between the neurons of the granular layer, together with an interrupted outline of the body and dendritic processes of a Purkinje cell. The more intense staining of grey matter when compared to white matter is illustrated by the picture of the dentate nucleus, shown in Fig. 16·2(c).

Among other unexpected findings was the demonstration with the F3-87-8 antibody of what appeared to be fibre tracts in the cerebral nuclei. These stained more intensely than the surrounding grey matter, as illustrated for the caudate nucleus in Fig. 16·2(e). Interestingly, these fibre tracts stained less brightly than the surrounding grey matter with the F15-135-1 antibody, occasionally with a bright halo (Fig. 16·2(f)).

### C. BIOCHEMICAL CHARACTERIZATION

As well as precise tissue localization, monoclonal antibodies offer the possibility of biochemical characterization and purification of antigens (see chapter 23). For example, we have used monoclonal antibody affinity chromatography as the main purification step for human brain Thy-1, and have determined the amino acid and carbohydrate composition of this molcule (McKenzie *et al.*, 1981). Using small monoclonal antibody affinity columns, we have demonstrated that the F3-87-8 antigen and the brain form of the F10-44-2 antigen are both glycoproteins, and have molecular weights of 130,000 and 95,000 respectively (Lakin and Fabre, 1981; McKenzie *et al.*, 1982). The determination of the molecular weight of the F3-87-8 antigen is shown in Fig. 16·3, and we present it particularly because it shows how brain homogenate can be radio-labelled for biochemical studies.

## IV POTENTIAL CLINICAL APPLICATIONS

### A. CORRELATIONS WITH DISEASE

Probably the most exciting and, in the long-term, the most useful

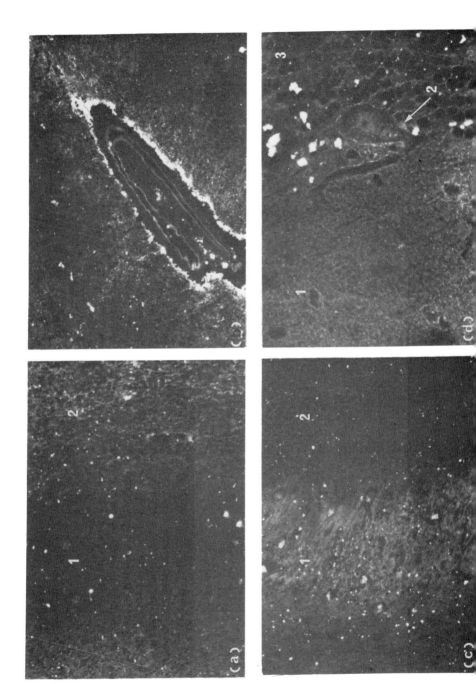

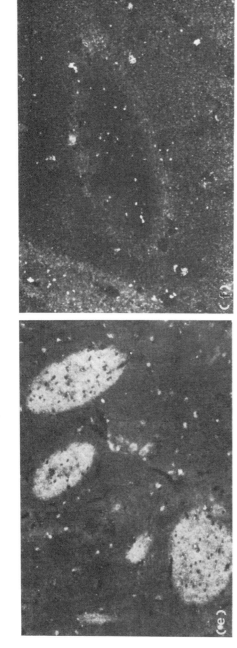

FIG. 16·2 Localization by immunofluorescence on frozen sections of 4 brain differentiation antigens within the CNS. Frozen sections of various brain subregions were incubated with saturating concentrations of monoclonal antibodies and then fluorescein labelled, affinity purified rabbit F(ab')₂ anti mouse F(ab')₂. (a) Region of dentate nucleus (1, grey matter; 2, white matter). (b) Arteriole near thalamus, stained with F10-44-2 antibody (Dalchau *et al.*, 1980; McKenzie *et al.*, 1982). (c) Region of dentate nucleus (1, grey matter; 2, white matter). (d) Cerebellar cortex (1, molecular layer; 2, Purkinje cell; 3, granular layer) stained with F15-42-1 (anti-Thy-1) antibody (McKenzie and Fabre, 1981a,b). (e) and (f) Caudate nucleus stained with F3-87-8 (Lakin and Fabre, 1981) and F15-135-1 (McKenzie and Fabre, 1982) antibody. Magnifications for (a) to (f) were 100, 400, 100, 400, 250, and 400 times respectively.

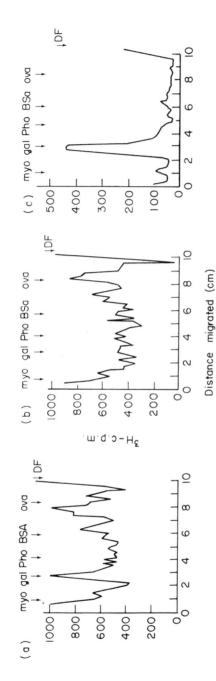

FIG. 16·3  Biochemical characterization of the molecule carrying the F3-87-8 determinant. Homogenate of cerebral cortex was labelled with ³H at the sialic acid residues using periodate and NaB³H₄. It was then solubilized in sodium deoxycholate and analyzed by polyacrylamide gel electrophoresis in sodium dodecyl sulphate, using 5% acrylamide gels. (a) Soluble brain before passage through F3-87-8 affinity column. (b) Soluble brain after passage through the column. (c) Material eluted from the column. The gels were cut into 2 mm slices, and ³H c.p.m. indicates the radioactivity per slice. The number of c.p.m. added to the gels for (a), (b) and (c) was 20,000, 20,000 and 5,000 respectively. Marker proteins with molecular weights in parentheses were myo, myosin (200,000); gal, β galactosidase (130,000); Pho, phosphorylase B (94,000); BSA, bovine serum albumin (68,000); ova, ovalbumin (43,000); and DF, dye front. (From Lakin and Fabre (1981)).

application of monoclonal antibodies will be the correlation of abnormalities in distribution or amount of particular CNS antigens with disease. These correlations should help not only in understanding neurological abnormalities at the molecular level, but will in turn help to unravel the function of particular CNS molecules. Since this is an area where knowledge is virtually non-existent (the CNS molecules themselves, apart from a few, have yet to be identified!) it will be a question of "shot-gun" science, i.e., testing as many abnormal tissues with as many antibodies as one can muster, and waiting for correlations. The only useful guide in attempting to study particular antigens in particular diseases will be knowledge of the neuropathology on the one hand and of the distribution of the antigens in question in the CNS on the other.

It is interesting that outside the CNS complete absence of particular membrane molecules has been found and correlated with disease. For example, in the rare bleeding disorder of Bernard-Soulier disease, where platelet adhesiveness is abnormal, it has been demonstrated that the platelets of these patients are completely lacking in one glycoprotein, called lb, (Nurden and Caen, 1975 and see chapter 8).

## B. CNS TUMOURS

The exciting diagnostic and therapeutic potential of monoclonal antibodies in the field of malignancy (see chapters 5 and 7) will in many instances be complicated as regards CNS neoplasms on account of the blood-brain barrier. The adequacy of delivery from the circulation of tumour-specific monoclonal antibody/toxin conjugates for therapy, and of radio-labelled tumour-specific monoclonal antibodies for localizing and delineating the extent of tumours, will be limited by the extent of breakdown of the blood-brain barrier in the region of the neoplasm. Whether or not this breakdown will be complete enough in all areas infiltrated by tumour to be clinically useful remains to be seen. On the other hand, the detection of tumour-specific or indeed normal CNS antigens in the blood (or the cerebrospinal fluid), if it proves possible, might be useful in the diagnosis and differential diagnosis of CNS tumours.

One potentially interesting and useful area of study involves monoclonal antibodies to normal CNS differentiation antigens. It has been possible to subdivide histologically indistinguishable breast (Daar and Fabre, 1981) and large bowel (Daar and Fabre, 1982) tumours on the basis of whether or not they express differentiation antigens normally found on the epithelial cells of origin. It might therefore be possible to type cerebral tumours according to the membrane antigens they express on their cell surface, and this could be of particular value for a number of reasons. Firstly, in an organ of such cellular complexity as the CNS, the surface antigen phenotype will probably help in defining the precise cell lineage from which the tumour arose, and this could be of prognostic value (as, for example, the subdivision of lymphocytic leukaemias into those of B and T cell lineage has distinguished different prognostic groups). Secondly, the presence or absence of normal differentiation antigens is likely to be a more subtle indicator of cellular maturation and differentiation than the usual cytological criteria, and this might therefore also be of prognostic significance. Finally, the absence of a particular molecule from the cell membrane of the tumour cells is likely to have metabolic or other functional implications and these might influence the biology of the tumour and its response to particular treatments.

Typing of infiltrating cerebral tumours is technically more difficult than with discrete bowel and breast tumours, but studies in this direction might be of value. Ideally, long-term studies correlating presence or absence of differentiation antigens with overall prognosis, response to therapy and other aspects of tumour biology should be performed. Such studies are currently underway for breast and bowel tumours.


## C. Treatment of Nueroblastoma

Where myelotoxicity of cytotoxic drugs or other therapy is an important limiting factor in the curing of tumours (as is almost certainly the case, e.g. with leukaemias and neuroblastomas) an attractive concept is to withdraw marrow from the patient, treat the patient with otherwise toxic therapeutic regimens, and then reconstitute with the autologous marrow (Kemshead and Black, 1980; Gale, 1981). A variation on this theme is to treat the patient and then reconstitute with foreign marrow, but this latter approach is largely limited to those with HLA identical siblings as bone-marrow donors, and has all the complications of graft-versus-host disease.

The autologous marrow approach is of value only if the patient's marrow is completely tumour-free, and this creates problems with leukaemias and neuroblastmas. The difficulty with this approach has always been the removal of tumour cells from the marrow prior to reconstitution. The advent of monoclonal antibodies, however, together with the technology and knowledge accumulated as regards various highly potent cell toxins and their coupling to antibodies (see chapter 7), offers a particularly attractive and sophisticated solution to the problem. If an antibody reacts with the tumour cells but not the haematopoietic stem cells, then the potential exists for incubating the marrow *in vitro* with the monoclonal antibody/toxin conjugate prior to re-infusion into the patient.

Our monoclonal antibody to Thy/1 (McKenzie and Fabre, 1981b) is very likely to be of value in this regard, as it has been shown to react with most neuroblastomas (J. Kemshead, ICRF Laboratories, London, personal communication) but it spares at least the myeloid progenitor cell (Morstyn *et al.*, 1981). There is unfortunately no assay as yet for the human haemopoietic stem cell, so that exclusion of stem cell toxicity is difficult. A variety of tests can be done with human marrow in vitro, and, if the antibody cross-reacts with other primates additional *in vivo* tests can be done with non-human primates. However formal exclusion of toxicity can be done only in the initial clinical evaluation of the therapy, with a batch of untreated marrow stored in case of stem cell toxicity. As regards the anti Thy-l antibody, however, the fact that the picture in human bone marrow resembles very closely that of Thy-l in the bone marrow of the mouse, where stem cells definitely lack Thy-l (Thierfelder, 1977), is very encouraging. Collaborative studies with Dr. P. Thorpe (see chapter 7) and other colleagues are currently underway to evaluate our anti Thy-l antibody for treatment of neuroblastoma.

The major theoretical problem with this approach is antigen heterogeneity among the tumour population, with the possibility that some tumour cells will lack the target antigen of the monoclonal antibody/toxin conjugate. Although one cannot be certain on this point, it is likely that this potential problem will be overcome by using 2 or more antibodies reactive with the particular tumour being treated.

## D. OTHER POSSIBILITIES

There are obviously many areas in neurology where pathological processes might give rise to the presence in the blood and cerebrospinal fluid of CNS antigens (in some cases, possibly specific to particular cell types). It is too early to know how generally useful this aspect of clinical application will be but it is likely that in certain situations it will provide simple but powerful diagnostic aids.

REFERENCES

Acton, R., Morris, R. J. and Williams, A. F. (1974). *Eur. J. Immunol.* **4**, 598–602.

Barclay, A. N. (1977). *Brain Res.* **133**, 139–143.

Barclay, A. N., Letarte-Muirhead, M., Williams, A. F. (1975). *Biochem. J.* **151**, 699–706.

Barclay, A. N., Letarte-Muirhead, M., Williams, A. F. and Faulkes, R. A. (1976). *Nature* **263**, 563–567.

Campbell, D. G., Gagnon, J., Reid, K. B. M. and Williams, A. F. (1981). *Biochem. J.* **195**, 15–30.

Cohen, J. and Selvendran, S. Y. (1981). *Nature* **291**, 421–423.

Daar, A. S. and Fabre, J. W. (1981). *Lancet* ii, 434–438.

Daar, A. S. and Fabre, J. W. (1982). (in preparation).

Dalchau, R. and Fabre, J. W. (1979). *J. exp. Med.* **149**, 576–591.

Dalchau, R., Kirkley, J., Fabre, J. W. (1980). *Eur. J. Immunol.* **10**, 745–749.

Fabre, J. W. and Williams, A. F. (1977). *Transplantation* **23**, 345–359.

Gael, R. P. (1981). *JAMA* **243**, 540–542.

Hart, D. N. J. and Fabre, J. W. (1980). *Clin. exp. Immunol.* **40**, 111–119.

Kemshead, J. and Black, J. (1980). *Der. Med. Child Neurol.* **22**, 816–829.

Kohler, G. and Milstein, C. (1975). *Nature* **256**, 495–497.

Lakin, K. H., and Fabre, J. W. (1981). *J. Neurochemistry.* **37**, 1170–1178.

Liao, S. K., Clarke, B. J., Kirong, P. C., Brickenden, A. B., Gallic, B. L., Dent, P. B. (1981). *Eur. J. Immunol.* **11**, 450–454.

McKenzie, J. L. and Fabre, J. W. (1981a). *Brain Res.* **230**, 307–316.

McKenzie, J. L. and Fabre, J. W. (1981b). *J. Immunol.* **126**, 843–850.

McKenzie, J. L. and Fabre, J. W. (1982). (in preparation).

McKenzie, J. L., Allen, A. R. and Fabre, J. W. (1981). *Biochem. J.* **197**, 629–636.

McKenzie, J. L., Dalchau, R. and Fabre, J. W. (1982). *J. Neurochemistry.* (submitted).

Morris, R. J. and Williams, A. F. (1975). *Eur. J. Immunol.* **5**, 274–281.

Morstyn, G., Metcalf, D., Burgess, A. and Fabre, J. W. (1981). *Scand. J. Haematol.* **26**, 19–30.

Nurden, A. and Caen, J. P. (1975). *Nature* **255**, 720–722.

Ruan, C., Tobelem, G., McMichael, A., Drouet, L., Legrand, Y., Degos, L., Kieffer, N., Lee, H. and Caen, J. P. (1982). *Brit. J. Haematol.* (in press).

Thierfelder, S. (1977). *Nature* **269**, 691–693.

Vulluamy, T., Rathray, S., Mirsky, R. (1981). *Nature* **291**, 418–420.

Williams, A. F., Galfré, G. and Milstein, C. (1978). *Cell* **12**, 663–673.

17　Monoclonal Antibodies to
　　Neurotransmitters: potential value in
　　the understanding of normal and
　　abnormal neurological function

A. Claudio Cuello

*Departments of Pharmacology and Human Anatomy
(Neuroanatomy/Neuropharmacology Group), Oxford
University, Oxford.*

## I INTRODUCTION

In the past decades advances in neurochemistry have opened new frontiers of our understanding of brain function in health and disease. The discovery by Hornykiewicz (1966) that the Parkinsonian condition is accompanied by a specific deficiency in the dopamine content in the striatum is an excellent example of the type of accomplishment in neurological research. There is no doubt that this was the crucial step which allowed the development of compensatory therapy with L-

DOPA in these patients. Abnormalities in brain neurotransmitters have been found in other diseases such as Huntington's chorea (Bird, 1976). Nevertheless, this condition cannot be tied up to changes in one single transmitter. The fact that antidepressant drugs and anti-psychotic drugs act on aminergic mechanisms has contributed to the promotion of a "biogenic amine hypothesis of affective disorders". The discovery and identification of new neuroactive peptides in the mammalian nervous system, such as the endogenous opiate enkephalines (Hughes *et al.*, 1975) and substance P (Chang and Leeman, 1970) provided additional interest in neurochemical studies. All these, and related observations, have prompted a large number of neurologists to search for specific changes in neurotransmitter content, turnover, or their receptors in defined anatomical areas of the human nervous system. This gigantic task is being carried out in several laboratories with a great deal of international co-operation.

The neurotransmitter content in human post-mortem material can be measured by a variety of techniques, such as fluorometric, radio-enzymatic and radioimmunoassay. This type of study provides information on how much transmitter is present in a given nuclear area following homogenization of tissue and extraction of the neuroactive substance, but it does not provide information on its location in neurones or neuronal pathways. This, in turn, can be accomplished by immunocytochemistry. Immunocytochemical studies in post-mortem human brain have just started. Here we comment on the development and application of monoclonal antibodies (Kohler and Milstein, 1975) against neurotransmitter substances and their potential application in neurological research with special emphasis on immunocytochemistry.


## II ANTI-SUBSTANCE P MONOCLONAL ANTIBODY (NC1/34 HL)

Monoclonal antibodies against this peptide have been obtained by the fusion of spleen cells of hyperimmunized Wistar rats against a substance P-bovine seroalbumin conjugate and the mouse myeloma cell line NS1/1. The selected clones produce a complete rat IgG (Cuello *et al.*, 1980a) and performed well in radioimmunoassay and immuno-cytochemistry (Cuello *et al.*, 1979). These antibodies are directed against the C-terminal portion of the peptide and do not cross react with other known mammalian neuropeptides. A 5% intrinsic cross-reactivity was found for the non-mammalian peptide eleidoisin which shares with substance P aminoacids in position 2, 7 and the three

C-terminal aminoacids. In radioimmunoassay the antibody detects down to fentomole amounts of the peptide in liquid phase. In tissue preparations (Cuello *et al.*, 1979) substance P immunoreactive sites were revealed with NC1/34 in CNS areas as described with polyclonal antibodies (Hokfelt *et al.*, 1975; Ljungdahl *et al.*, 1978; Cuello and Kanazawa, 1978).

In experimental animals the use of this antibody demonstrated the peripheral origin of most of the substance P immunoreactive fibres in the trigeminal system (Del Fiacco and Cuello, 1980), the axonal transport of this peptide (Gamse *et al.*, 1979) and its presence in striato-nigral fibres (Cuello, 1980; Cuello *et al.*, 1981b).

The use of NC1/34 in experimental animals has shown that a specific population of substance P containing amacrine cells is present in the retina of non-mammalian species (Karten and Brecha, 1980). This observation has not been confirmed in the human retina. NC1/34 detects immunoreactive elements in areas of the human nervous system which have not yet been reported in experimental animals. That is the case of the neural lobe. A conspicuous substance P immunoreactive fibre system has been found in this extension of the diencephalon (Stoeckel and Cuello, in preparation). Fig. 17·1 illustrates this observation in an immunofluorescent preparation. The role of the peptide in this neural structure and its relationship to oxytocin or vasopressin containing neurones have yet to be established.

In pharmacological investigations NC1/34 revealed permanent loss of substance P immunoreactivity after capsaicin treatment in newborn animals (Cuello *et al.*, 1981a). This is an observation which could bear some neurological interest as this compound stimulates chemosensitive pain receptors (Jancsó *et al.*, 1967). The administration of this active compound from paprika is accompanied by a temporary (Jessell *et al.*, 1978) or permanent loss of the peptide (Gamse *et al.*, 1980; Nagy *et al.*, 1980; Cuello *et al.*, 1981a). The loss of immunoreactive substance as revealed with NC1/34 is also accompanied by some behavioural changes in pain perception (Paxinos *et al.*, 1980).

Substance P is suspected to be a neurotransmitter utilized by neurones providing primary nociceptive information (Henry, 1976). This peptide is also present in the human spinal cord with similar disposition on the superficial layers of the dorsal horn (Cuello *et al.*, 1976). It is therefore tempting to speculate on the possible diminution of this and similar peptides in conditions in which pain perception is abnormal. Recently with Drs. John Pearson and Leslie Brandeis at New York University we found that by using NC1/34 in immunocyto-chemistry, there was a complete loss of substance P immunoreactivity

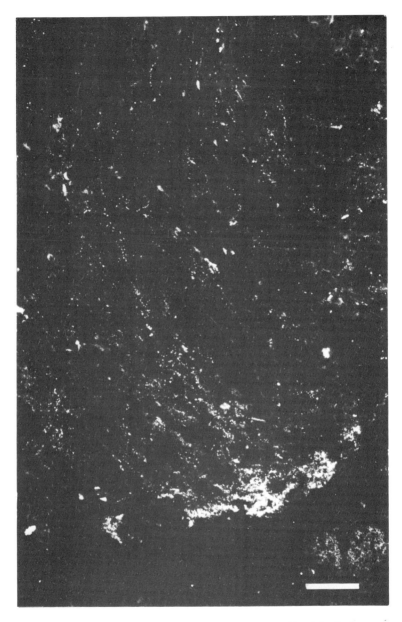

FIG. 17·1 Substance P immunoreactivity (white dots and fibres) in the human neural lobe, as revealed with the monoclonal antibody NC1/34 and developed as an indirect immunofluorescent preparation. Scale bar = 100 µm.

in cases of familial dysautonomia (Pearson *et al.*, 1982). Fig. 17·2 illustrates preparations taken from normal post-mortem material (a) and patients suffering this disease (b) John Pearson (1979) has previously found that this disease is accompanied by a loss of a great number of somatic sensory elements. Research on the distribution of neurotransmitter specific sensory neurones in this condition is awaited.

Most of our preliminary observations with NC1/34 in human post-mortem material confirms the distribution of this peptide in specific neuronal pathways as described with NC1/34 and with polyclonal antibodies in experimental animals. The monoclonal antibody NC1/34 has been used for neuropathological investigations with radioimmunoassay and interesting findings in changes of this peptide in Parkinson and related conditions have been found by Dr. Rinne and collaborators at the University of Turku (personal communication). The fact that this monoclonal antibody is currently available commercially will facilitate further research in the involvement of substance P in various neurological diseases.

## III ANTI-SEROTONIN MONOCLONAL ANTIBODY (YC5/45)

Monoclonal antibodies against a serotonin-bovine serum albumin conjugate were obtained by the fusion of spleen cells of hyperimmune Wistar rats and rat myeloma cell line Y3.Ag 1.2.3. The selected clones produced a complete rat IgG plus a light kappa chain from the parental myeloma (Consolazione *et al.*, 1981). Other clones subsequently lost the parental myeloma kappa chain (Cuello and Milstein, 1981). These were respectively coded YC5/45 HLK and YC5/45 HL. The cells were also grown as in the peritoneal cavity (ascitic fluid) and as solid tumour in the back of the animal (plasma). All these preparations and ammonium sulphate precipitates from supernatants recognized the serotonin-bovine sero-albumin in hemagglutination tests and serotonin immunoreactive sites in formaldehyde fixed preparations. In haemagglutination tests dopamine displaced the binding of the antibody equally as well as serotonin. The serotonin-bovine serum albumin was several thousand-fold more potent in displacing the antibody than the amines. No dopamine immunoreactive sites were found in the central nervous system in areas such as the substantia nigra and other dopamine-rich regions of the brain. Conversely, the monoclonal antibody YC5/45 recognized the classical serotonin containing neurones of the so-called raphe nuclei system of the B-classification of Dahlstrom

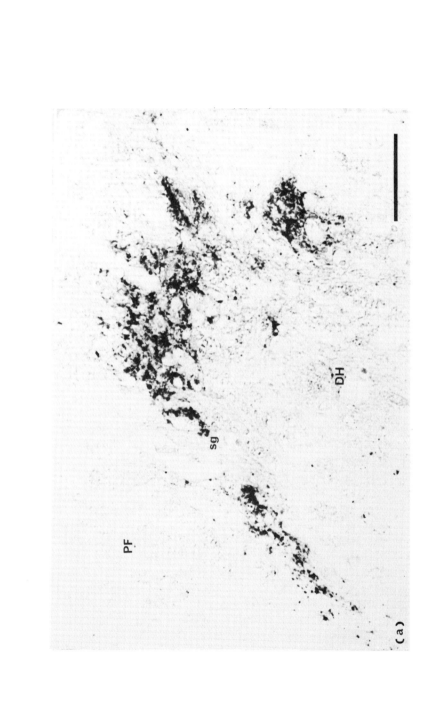

(a)

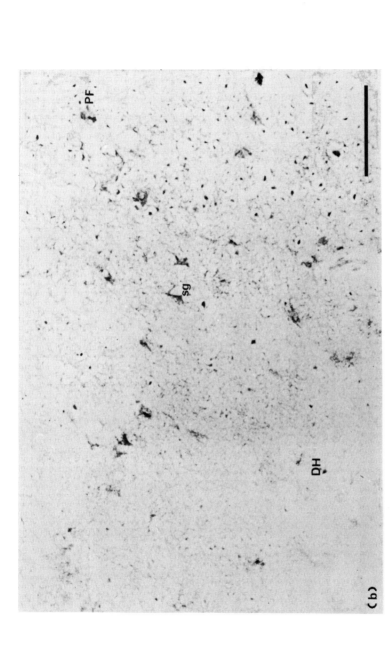

FIG. 17·2 Peroxidase-antiperoxidase preparation using the monoclonal antibody NC1/34 to detect substance P sites (dark deposits) in the human spinal cord. (a) Normal individual. (b) Familial dysautonomia. Note the total absence of peptide in the substantia gelatinosa in familial dysautonomia as compared with a normal control case. PF, posterior funiculus; Sg, substantia gelatinosa; DH, dorsal horn. Scale bar = 50 μm. (from Pearson, Brandeis and ACC, unpublished).

and Fuxe (1964). Fig. 17·3 illustrates the presence of serotonin immunoreactivity in neurones of the nucleus raphe pallidus of the rat. This immunoreactivity disappeared after the administration of parachlorphenylalanine (an inhibitor of the indolamine biosynthetic enzyme, tryptophan hydroxylase) but was not affected by α-methyl-p-tyrosine (an inhibitor of the catecholamine biosynthetic enzyme, tyrosine hydroxylase) (Consolazione et al., 1981). Aspects of fine specificity of this antibody will be dealt with in a separate publication (Milstein, Wright and Cuello, in preparation).

YC5/45 allowed the study of the distribution of 5HT containing neurones in the rat (Consolazione and Cuello, 1981) and also the use of peroxidase-anti-peroxidase (PAP) immunohistochemistry in combination with horse radish peroxidase (HRP) retrograde transport towards the identification of transmitter specific projection neurones (Priestley et al., 1981). The procedure reveals in single sections 5HT-immunoreactive cells by the PAP technique and HRP cytochemistry to identify cells which retrogradely transported the enzyme. The same substrate diaminobenzidene (DAB) is used for both HRP enzymatic reactions. YC5/45 has allowed the identification of a 5HT population of amacrine cells in the frog retina (Osborne et al., 1981). This observation is in line with the presence of this indolamine in the retina of this species as demonstrated by high performance liquid chromatography. Recently Costa and collaborators (1982) completed a systematic anatomical-pharmacological study of the serotonergic enteric nervous system using this monoclonal antibody and compared the results with those of other polyclonal antibodies against serotonin.

No studies have as yet been performed in human brain material using this monoclonal antibody. Nevertheless it has been used to study carcinoid tumours presumably producing serotonin. An example of this is illustrated in Fig. 17·4 from a preparation done in collaboration with Drs. Wells and Milstein.

## IV OTHER MONOCLONAL ANTIBODIES AGAINST NEUROTRANSMITTER SUBSTANCES AND MARKERS

Ideally, neuroscientists in general and neuropathologists in particular would like to have at their disposal, a complete list of monoclonal antibodies to the various neurotransmitter substances and other useful markers such as the neurotransmitter biosynthetic enzymes. This would allow the bridging of the gap between recent discoveries in basic neurosciences and neuropathology.

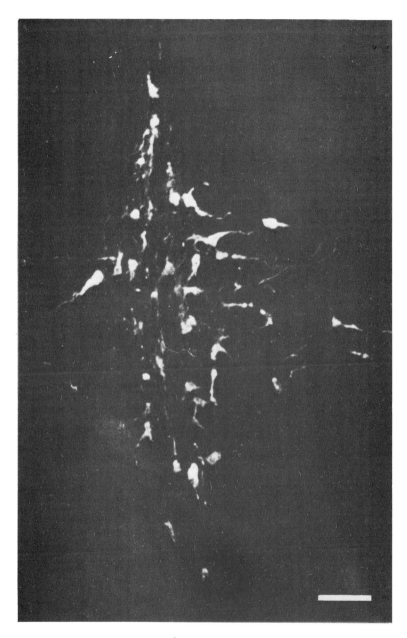

FIG. 17·3 Nucleus raphe pallidus of the rat showing intensely fluorescent serotonin containing neurones as revealed by the monoclonal antibody YC5/45. Scale bar = 100 μm.

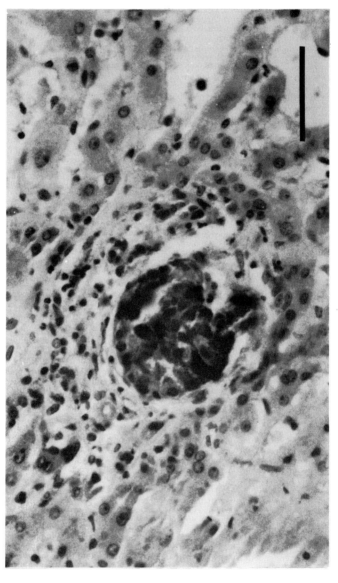

FIG. 17·4 Serotonin immunoreactivity detected in metastatic carcinoid cells in the liver using the monoclonal antibody YC5/45 and developed as immunoenzyme preparation. Reactive cells appear darkly stained in the centre of the field, surrounded by reactional tissue and liver parenchima. Scale bar = 100 $\mu$m.

In collaboration with César Milstein, we recently succeeded in obtaining monoclonal antibodies against Leu- and Met-enkephalin. These monoclonal antibodies have been coded NOC$_1$ and NOC$_2$. The full characterization of these monoclonal antibodies is now in progress. It is hoped that the availability of these antibodies will contribute to our understanding of the role of these natural opiates in neurological functions. Fig. 17·5 illustrates the demonstration of enkephalin immunoreactive fibres in the substantia gelatinosa of the spinal nucleus of the trigeminal nerve in the human brain stem. The disposition of this immunoreactivity was found to be analogous to that described previously using polyclonal antibodies (Cuello, 1978).

Recently Ross and collaborators (1981) developed a monoclonal antibody against tyrosine hydroxylase (the catecholamine rate limiting enzyme). They have demonstrated very elegantly monoamine containing neurones using this monoclonal antibody as primary immunochemical reagent.

Of the biosynthetic enzymes as neurotransmitter markers, choline acetyltransferase is of great importance since very little is known of the cholinergic system in the central nervous system of experimental animals and much less in the human species. Some successful attempts to produce antibodies against this enzyme have been reported recently by various groups (Kimura *et al.*, 1980; Cozzari and Hartman, 1981; Eckenstein *et al.*, 1981; Eder-Colli *et al.*, 1981). The interest of obtaining these antibodies monoclonally restricting their immunological definition, has been stressed by Rossier (1981) in an interesting commentary.

## V "RADIOIMMUNOCYTOCHEMISTRY" WITH INTERNALLY LABELLED MONOCLONAL ANTIBODIES

Monoclonal antibodies can be labelled *in vitro* during their biosynthesis at high specific activity with radioactive amino acid precursors. These radioactive immunological probes can be effectively used in radioautography of immunoreactive sites (Cuello *et al.*, 1980b; Cuello and Milstein, 1981), offering an interesting alternative towards the cellular and subcellular localization of immunoreactive substances. Besides these applications, internally labelled monoclonal antibodies can be used for antibody characterization and binding techniques (Cuello and Milstein, 1981).

"Radioimmunocytochemistry" with monoclonal antibodies does not require the use of developing antibodies which are chemically con-

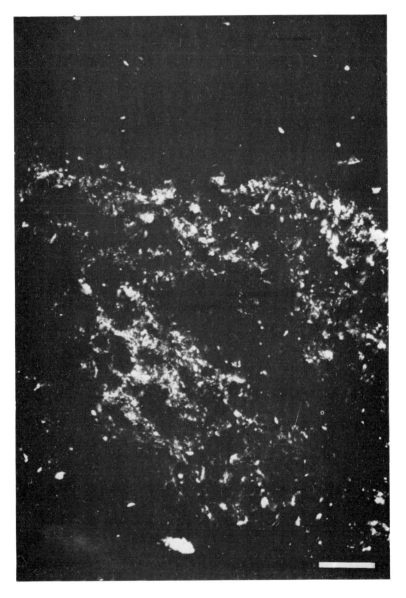

FIG. 17·5 Met-enkephalin immunoreactivity in the substantia gelatinosa of the spinal trigeminal nucleus in the human brain as detected by the monoclonal antibody NOC₂. Fluorescent micrography. Scale bar = 100 μm. (From A.C.C. and Milstein, unpublished).

jugated to suitable markers (FiTC, HRP) or unconjugated, such as in the peroxidase-antiperoxidase technique. The high specificity obtained with these antibodies considerably shortens the time of exposure of the radioautographs. Detailed methodological description of radioimmuno-cytochemistry with internally labelled antibodies can be found else-where (Cuello *et al.*, 1982).

## VI PROSPECTIVE USE OF MONOCLONAL ANTIBODIES IN NEUROLOGICAL STUDIES

Neurotransmitter substances are usually poor immunogens. It is there-fore of great value to immortalize antibodies which recognize these molecules. Monoclonal antibodies will be of great value not only for the small molecular weight neurotransmitter but also for neurotransmitter markers which are difficult to purify as immunogens. This is the case of some neurotransmitter enzymes. Monoclonal antibodies could over-come some of the difficulties such as eliminating unwanted antibodies against substances that are being co-purified with the enzyme. Further-more, the elimination of carrier immunoglobulin always results in clearer immunocytochemistry.

The use of monoclonal antibodies in neurological studies will facili-tate the exchange of information on the fate of neurotransmitter specific neurones in defined neurological states. An example of this is illustrated in the case of loss of substance P immunoreactivity in the spinal cord of patients with familial dysautonomia as revealed with the monoclonal antibody NC1/34 (Pearson *et al.*, 1981). This type of study will be more accessible not only to basic research laboratories, but also in laboratories dealing with post-mortem neuropathological material in hospitals and medical schools. Both of the antibodies here described, NC1/34 and YC5/45, are commercially available (SeraLab Limited, Crawley Down, Sussex, U.K.). It is likely that other monoclonal anti-bodies from different laboratories will be distributed equally widely. This will allow a direct comparison of experimental results and standardization of techniques and criteria of identification of immuno-reactive sites.

Some of the antibodies against neurotransmitter substances such as the case of YC5/45 could exceed the pure neurobiological-neuro-pathological interest. The fact that they can recognize serotonin-containing tumour cells makes this antibody of potential diagnostic interest. Further results are awaited for the generalization of this statement.

Other developments are expected in immunocytochemistry of neurotransmitter substances with the aid of the monoclonal antibodies. It is likely that a number of primary antibodies against these substances will be directly conjugated with tracer substances (HRP, Gold, FiTC., etc), while developmental monoclonal antibodies will probably replace the present polyclonal antibodies.

Radioimmunocytochemistry with internally labelled monoclonal antibodies has proved to be feasible for neurotransmitter substances both at light and electron microscopical levels (Cuello *et al.*, 1980). Radioactive aminoacids are "built-in" in the immunoglobulin secreted by the hybridomas. As a large number of these radioactive aminoacids can be incorporated in a single immunoglobulin molecule a high specific activity is obtained.

It is possible to combine "radioimmunocytochemistry" with conventional immunoenzyme techniques, demonstrating two antigenic sites simultaneously. Examples of these applications are currently being explored in our laboratory. Thus, in collaboration with Priestley and Milstein, we have been able to confirm the co-existence of substance P and serotonin in some raphe nuclei neurones. Similarly, we have gained information on the relationship between enkephalin and substance P-immunoreactive synapses in the substantia gelatinosa of the spinal nucleus of the rat trigeminal nerve at ultrastructural level. In neurological studies the main potential use of this technique will be the quantification of the immunoreaction by densitometry of silver grains or direct measurement of binding by scintillation counting of the radioactivity of microdissected preparations. This could provide information on relative amounts of immunoreactive substances in specific, discrete areas of the human brain in health and disorder.

It is stimulating to think that, in due time, a number of monoclonal antibodies to neurotransmitter substances performing adequately in conventional or newly developed radioimmunoassays and immunocytochemical techniques will contribute meaningfully to neurology-neuropathology. Of particular interest will be neurochemical studies on the neurotransmitters in regional areas of the human brain in conditions such as schizophrenia, other types of dementia, Parkinsonism, Huntington's chorea and other genetic or acquired disorders.

ACKNOWLEDGEMENTS

I would like to thank my collaborators of the Neuroanatomy/Neuropharmacology Group at Oxford and very specially, Dr. César Milstein (MRC Molecular Biology, Cambridge) for a very fruitful

collaboration and critical discussions. The clerical assistance of Mrs
Ella Iles has been invaluable all along this work. These studies were
supported by grants from the Medical Research Council (U.K.), The
Wellcome Trust and The Royal Society. Additional support from the
E.P. Abraham Cephalosporin Fund is also acknowledged.

REFERENCES

Bird, E. D. (1976). *In* "Biochemistry and Neurology" (H. Bradford and D. C.
  Marsden, Eds), pp. 83–92. Academic Press, London and New York.
Chang, M. M. and Leeman, S. E. (1970). *J. biol. Chem.* **245**, 4784–4790.
Consolazione, A. and Cuello, A. C. (1981). *In* "Biology of serotonergic trans-
  mission. (N. N. Osborne, Ed.), pp. 29–61. Wiley, Sussex.
Consolazione, A., Milstein, C., Wright, B. and Cuello, A. C. (1981). *J.
  Histochem. Cytochem.* **29**, 1425–1430.
Cozzari, C. and Hartman, B. K. (1981). *Proc. natn. Acad. Sci. U.S.A.* **77**,
  7453–7457.
Costa, M., Furness, J. B., Cuello, A. C., Verhofstad, A. A. J., Steinbusch,
  H. W. J. and Elde, R. P. (1982). *Neuroscience* **7**, 351–363.
Cuello, A. C. (1978). *Lancet* ii, 291–293.
Cuello, A. C. (1980). *In* "Regulatory Functions of the CNS." (J. Szentagothai,
  J. Hámori and M. Palkovits, Eds), pp. 211–226. Akadémiai Kiadó/
  Pergamon Press.
Cuello, A. C. and Kanazawa, I. (1978). *J. Comp. Neurol.* **178**, 129–159.
Cuello, A. C. and Milstein, C. (1981). *In* "Radioimmunology" (Ch. A.
  Bizollon Ed), pp. 293–305. Elsevier-North Holland, Amsterdam.
Cuello, A. C., Polak, J. M. and Pearse, A. G. E. (1976). *Lancet* ii, 1054–1056.
Cuello, A. C. Galfré, G. and Milstein, C. (1979). *Proc. natn. Acad. Sci. U.S.A.*
  **76**, 3532–3536.
Cuello, A. C., Galfré, G. and Milstein, C. (1980a). *In* "Receptors for
  neurotransmitters and peptide hormones" (G. Pepeu, M. J. Kuhar and S. J.
  Enna, Eds), pp. 349–363. Raven Press.
Cuello, A. C., Milstein, C. and Priestley, J. V. (1980b). *Brain Res. Bull.* **5**,
  575–587.
Cuello, A. C., Gamse, R., Holzer, P. and Lembeck, F. (1981a). *Naunyn-
  Schmiedeberg's Arch. Pharmacol.* **315**, 185–194.
Cuello, A. C., Del Fiacco, M., Paxinos, G., Somogyi, P. and Priestley, J. V.
  (1981b). *J. Neural Transm.* **51**, 83–96.
Cuello, A. C., Milstein, C. and Galfré, G. (1982). *In* "Immunohistochemistry"
  IBRO Handbook Series Methods in the Neurosciences. (A. C. Cuello, Ed.
  Wiley, Sussex. (in press).
Dahlström, A. and Fuxe, K. (1964). *Acta phys. Scand.* **62**, (Suppl. 232). 1–80.
Del Fiacco, M. and Cuello, A. C. (1980). *Neuroscience* **5**, 803–815.
Eckenstein, F. (1981). *Neuroscience* **6**, 993–1000.

Eder-Colli, L., Powell, J., Cuello, A. C. and Smith, A. D. (1981). (submitted).

Gamse, R., Lembeck, F. and Cuello, A. C. (1979). *Naunyn-Schmiedeberg's Arch. Pharmacol.* **306**, 37–44.

Gamse, R., Holzer, P. and Lembeck, F. (1980). *Brit. J. Pharmacol.* **68**, 207–213.

Henry, J. L. (1976). *Brain Res.* **114**, 439–451.

Hökfelt, T., Kellerth, J. O., Nilsson, G. and Pernow, B. (1975). *Science* **190**, 889–890.

Hornykiewicz, O. (1966). *Pharmacol. Rev.* **18**, 925–962.

Hughes, J., Smith, T. W., Kosterlitz, H. W., Fothergill, L. A., Morgan, B. A. and Morris, H. R. (1975). *Nature* **258**, 577–579.

Jancsó, G., Jancsó-Gabor, A. and Szolcsanyi, J. (1967). *Brit. J. Pharmacol.* **31**, 138–151.

Jessell, T. M., Iversen, L. L. and Cuello, A. C. (1970). *Brain Res.* **152**, 183–188.

Karten, H. J. and Brecha, N. (1980). *Nature* **283**, 87–88.

Kimura, H., McGeer, P. L., Peng, J. H. and McGeer, E. G. (1980). *Science* **208**, 1057–1059.

Kohler, G. and Milstein C. (1975). *Nature* **256**, 495–497.

Lungdahl, A., Hökfelt, T. and Nilsson, G. (1978). *Neuroscience* **3**, 861–880.

Osborne, N. N., Nesselhut, T., Nicholas, D. A. and Cuello, A. C. (1981). *Neurochem. Int.* **3**, 171–176.

Paxinos, G., O'Brien, M., Cuello, A. C. and Del Fiacco, M. (1980). *In* "Problems in Pain" (C. Peck and M. Wallace, Eds), pp. 61–72. Pergamon Press, Oxford.

Pearson, J., Brandeis, L. and Cuello, A. C. (1982). *Nature* **275**, 61–63.

Pearson, J. (1979). *J. Autonom. Nerv. System* **1**, 119–123.

Priestley, J. V., Somogyi, P. and Cuello, A. C. *Brain Res.* **220**, 231–240.

Ross, M. E., Reis, D. J. and Joh, T. H. (1981). *Brain Res.* **208**, 493–498.

Rossier, J. (1981). *Neuroscience* **6**, 989–991.

# H   OTHER AREAS

# 18 Monoclonal Antibodies to Mallory Bodies/Intermediate Filaments, and HLA (Class 1) Antigens in Human Liver Disease

J. O'D. McGee, J. A. Morton, C. Barbatis,
J. F. Bradley, K. A. Fleming, A. M. Goate
and J. Burns.

*University of Oxford, Nuffield Department of Pathology, John
Radcliffe Hospital, Oxford. OX3 9DU*

## I MONCLONAL ANTIBODIES TO ALCOHOLIC HYALINE (MALLORY BODIES) AND INTERMEDIATE FILAMENTS

### A. Introduction

One of the histological hallmarks of both acute and chronic alcoholic liver disease is the appearance of hyaline eosinophilic inclusions in hepatocytes. These inclusions have been designated alcoholic hyaline or Mallory bodies (MB); the inclusions were first described in alcoholic cirrhotics by Mallory (1911). They have been documented in fatal cases of Wilson's disease (66–100%), primary biliary cirrhosis (17–46%), Indian childhood cirrhosis (14–82%), large bile duct obstruction (7%) chronic active hepatitis (3%), non-alcoholic cirrhosis (1·5%) and occasionally in other liver diseases. (Gerber *et al.*, 1973; Bhagwat and Pandit, 1979). By comparison they occur in 94–100% of alcoholic cirrhotics (Gerber *et al.*, 1973) but the number of hepatocytes containing MBs in alcoholic cirrhotics is generally much higher than in those disorders listed above. It is evident, therefore, that MB formation is a non-specific response to hepatocellular injury. It should be noted that MBs do not occur in cells of other organs except in pneumocytes in some cases of asbestosis (Kuhn and Tseng-Tong Kuo, 1973).

Alcohol induced cirrhosis is the commonest form of chronic liver disease in the U.K. and in North America. It is estimated, however, that only 10–30% of heavy drinkers develop cirrhosis (Popper, 1977). A major problem in hepatology, therefore, is to understand what mechanisms underlie the progression of acute to chronic alcoholic liver disease. It has been claimed that MBs are chemotactic for polymorphs (Kanagasundarum, 1973) that lymphocytes from patients with alcoholic liver disease on exposure to isolated MBs release a fibrogenic factor (Chen and Leevy, 1973), and that lymphocytes from chronic alcoholics stimulated with MBs are cytotoxic for hepatocytes (Zetterman *et al.*, 1976). These observations have led to the hypothesis that the development of cell mediated immunity to MBs is responsible for the progression of acute to chronic alcoholic liver disease. It has also been reported that MB antigens occur in the serum of patients with acute alcoholic hepatitis and that in those who progress to cirrhosis, antibodies to MBs also develop. MB antigen and antibody were not found in non-alcoholic liver disorders (Zetterman *et al.*, 1976). The implication of these findings is that humoral immunity to MBs is also important in the development of alcoholic cirrhosis. A numbe· of laboratories have been unable to confirm these reports on cell and humoral immunity to MBs. It is likely that the discrepant results of different laboratories is due to the fact that neither the antigen or polyclonal antibodies used in the experiments were pure or specific, respectively, for MBs.

Ultrastructurally MBs are composed of filaments 14–20 nm in diameter (Franke *et al.*, 1979) and sometimes also contain an electron dense amorphous component. Because of their filamentous appearance it has been tempting to assume that MBs are derived from one of the cytoskeletal elements of normal hepatocytes. The cytoskeleton of most cells, including hepatocytes, consist of 3 components *viz.* microfilaments, microtubules and intermediate filaments (Franke *et al.*, 1979). Microfilaments have a diameter of 4–6 nm and contain actin. It has been reported that MBs react with human serum containing anti-actin antibodies (Nenci, 1975) suggesting that they derive from microfilaments. However, MBs do not bind heavy meromyosin (French *et al.*, 1977) and others have not confirmed their reaction with anti-actin (Franke *et al.*, 1979). In view of the latter and the large difference in diameter of microfilaments and MB filaments (4–6 nm versus 14–20 nm) it would appear unlikely that MBs derive from this filament class. Microtubules have a mean diameter of 22 nm and their main polypeptide subunit is tubulin. Since MBs can be induced in mice with griseofulvin (an anti-microtubular reagent) it was surmized that MB formation may be related to a defect in microtubular function. Disruption of microtubular function may be significant in MB formation but it is unlikely that MB filaments are actually composed of microtubule components since the physical diameter of both are widely different and furthermore MBs do not contain tubulin. Evidence that MBs are formed from intermediate filaments (Franke *et al.*, 1979) is accumulating but the details of this hypothesis have not been fully defined (see next section). Intermediate filaments, although physically homogenous in all cell types (mean diameter 10 nm) are biochemically and immunologically heterogeneous (see later). The major subunits of epithelial cell intermediate filaments are thought to be prekeratins (Franke *et al.*, 1981). MBs react with antisera to prekeratins but it is not possible to demonstrate the presence of epidermal prekeratin containing intermediate filaments in normal hepatocytes with antisera raised against epidermal keratins (Franke *et al.*, 1981). In addition MBs contain antigens identified by polyclonal antibodies to MBs which do not react with epidermal prekeratin (Morton *et al.*, 1980).

In view of the possible significance of MBs in the perpetuation of acute to chronic alcoholic liver disease and the debate over the origin of these structures this laboratory has produced monoclonal antibodies to purified MBs and used them to examine some of the hypotheses outlined above.

## B. Production of Monoclonal Antibodies to MBs

MBs were purified (to about 95% homogeneity) from a number of alcoholic cirrhotic livers obtained at autopsy by techniques described elsewhere (Morton *et al.*, 1980). Briefly these techniques depend on the high density of MBs and their marked insolubility in non-denaturing reagents. Purified MBs are poor immunogens in rabbits and goats (Morton et al., 1980). However, a protein designated Mallory body protein (MBP) derived by denaturation, reduction and alkylation of MBs is highly immunogenic in all species examined including mice (Morton et al., 1981). MBP is a protein of approximate Mr 53,000 daltons.

Monoclonal antibodies were produced by the technique of Kohler and Milstein (1975). Balb/c mice were injected subcutaneously with 40 $\mu$g of MBP with complete Freunds adjuvant in a final volume of 0·4 ml. Two booster injections were given at two-weekly intervals. Blood was taken from the tail vein 10 days after the last injection and tested for antibody to MBs by immunofluorescence on sections from an alcoholic liver containing MBs. One of the animals which had developed antibodies was boosted again; the spleen was aseptically removed, made into a single cell suspension, and these cells fused with NS1 cells (see Chapter 21 for fusion techniques). This fusion resulted in 3 clones which produced monoclonal antibodies of different specificities to MBs (Morton et al., 1981). The 3 antibody producing clones were grown in large quantities in 25cm² Falcon flasks and the medium from these flasks stored at −20°C. Ascitic fluid from positive clones was produced by standard procedures. The Ig concentrations in medium and ascitic fluid were determined by radioimmunoassay.

It should be noted that the screening procedure used here for the detection of monoclonal antibody production is highly sensitive and rapid but suffers from one disadvantage in that only about 50 wells can be assayed in any one experiment.

The three monoclonal antibodies produced which react with MBs or MB derived material have been called anti-JMB1, anti-JMB2 and anti-JMB3 and the determinants with which they react JMB1, JMB2 and JMB3 respectively (Morton et al., 1981).

## C. REACTIONS OF MONOCLONAL ANTIBODIES TO MBs/INTERMEDIATE FILAMENTS

### 1. ANTI-JMB1

Culture fluid from this clone (concentration of 6$\mu$g Ig ml⁻¹) labelled MBs in alcoholic cirrhotics intensely (Fig. 18·1) It did not react with liver or other cells in alcoholic cirrhotics or in normal liver tissue. Negative reactions were also obtained by this method on a variety of

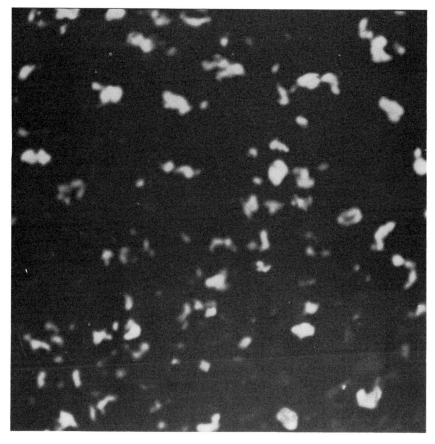

FIG. 18·1 Immunofluorescent labelling of MBs in an alcoholic cirrhotic liver with anti-JMB1 culture fluid.

other human organs. From these observations it was assumed that JMB1 is a determinant unique to MBs. However, it is now clear that JMB1 can be detected at apparently low concentration in normal hepatocytes and bile ducts and in other organs using high titre ascitic fluid diluted 1 : 100 (i.e. 60 $\mu$g Ig ml$^{-1}$) in the more sensitive immuno-peroxidase procedure. Using the latter on sections from alcoholic cirrhotics not only are classic MBs labelled but also much smaller structures (Fig. 18·2) which may be early forms of MBs or possibly MBs undergoing regression. Denk *et al.* (1979), have made similar observations using anti-prekeratin antibodies in alcoholic cirrhotics and in the livers of griseofulvin fed mice. Of much more interest, however, is the fact that ascitic fluid reveals a cytoplasmic filament

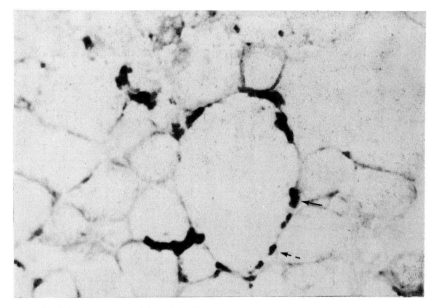

FIG. 18·2 Immunoperoxidase labelling of small granular structures in hepatocytes (arrows) with anti-JMB1 culture fluid.

system in hepatocytes and bile ducts of normal liver. The ascitic fluid antibody gives a weak reaction with these cell types in normal liver but a very much stronger reaction with hepatocytes in alcoholic cirrhotics even when these hypatocytes do not contain MBs (Fig. 18·3). It would appear, therefore, that the concentration of JMB1 either increases generally in all hepatocytes or alternatively the antigen becomes more accessible to antibody following alcohol injury (Morton *et al.*, 1980). Anti-JMB1 (ascitic fluid) also labels cells in other normal tissue similar to that described for anti-JMB2 (see Table 18·1). The nature of the JMB1 determinant and its relationship to JMB2 is discussed below.

2. ANTI-JMB2

This monoclonal antibody (either in the form of culture or ascitic fluid) not only labels MBs in alcoholic cirrhotic livers but also reacts with a cytoplasmic filament system (see below) in non-Mallory body containing hepatocytes and also with bile ducts in the same livers (Figs 18·4(a) and 18·4(b) ).

More surprisingly, this antibody also decorates a cytoplasmic filament system in hepatocytes and bile ducts in normal liver. In hepato-

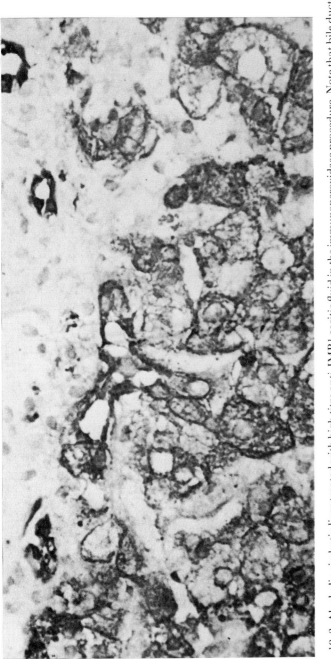

FIG. 18·3 Alcoholic cirrhotic liver treated with high titre anti-JMB1 ascitic fluid in the immunoperoxidase procedure. Note that bile ducts stain and that a filament system can be detected in hepatocytes which do not contain MBs. High titre anti-JMB1 does not react with hepatocytes in normal liver.

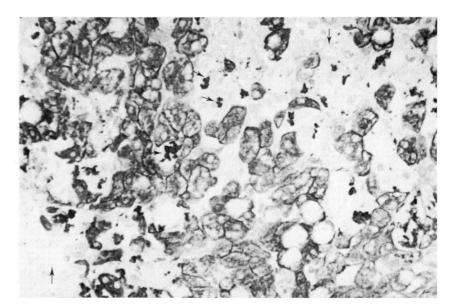

FIG. 18·4(a) Alcoholic cirrhotic liver treated with anti-JMB2 as in Fig. 18·3 MBs (small arrows) and a filament system in some hepatocytes react with antibody. Note, however, that those cells which contain MBs do not have a detectable cytoplasmic filament system and in addition many cells which do not contain MBs (large arrows) also lack these filaments. Compare with Fig. 18·4(b).

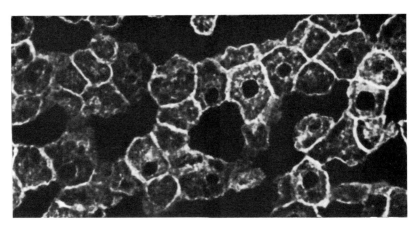

FIG. 18·4(b) Immunofluorescent labelling of normal liver with anti-JMB2. A cytoplasmic filament system is demonstrated in all hepatocytes. This is present in highest concentration under the plasma membrane. This antibody also stains bile ducts (not shown) in normal liver.

TABLE 18·1

Location of JMB2 in normal organs determined by immunoflorescence

| Organ | Cell type |
|---|---|
| Small intestine and colon | Crypt cells |
| Kidney | Cells of proximal convoluted tubules |
| Sweat and mammary gland | Duct lining cells |
| Pancreas and salivary gland | Duct and acinar cells |
| Liver | Hepatocytes and bile duct epithelium |
| Lung | Bronchial epithelium |
| Choroid plexus | Ependymal cells |
| Pituitary | ACTH and GH producing cells |
| Adrenal | Zona reticularis cells |
| Thyroid | Follicular epithelium |
| Testis | Epididymal lining and sertoli cells |

cytes this filament system extends throughout the cytoplasm but is apparently present in highest concentration at the plasma and nuclear membranes (Fig. 18·4(b) ). Ultrastructural studies of normal hepatocytes indicate that intermediate filaments are present throughout the cytoplasm but are present in highest concentration at the same sites as JMB2 (Franke *et al.*, 1979). This suggests that the JMB2 determinant may be associated with intermediate filaments.

Four separate types of experimental evidence support the conclusion that JMB2 is associated with intermediate filaments. The first line of evidence derives from experiments on Chang liver cells. These cells when grown in culture, washed, and fixed in acetone at $-20°C$ for 15 mins react with anti-JMB2 (Fig. 18·5(a) ). The component labelled with anti-JMB2 is clearly a cytoplasmic filamentous system which has a distribution similar to that found in other epithelial cells in culture. Furthermore, these cytoplasmic filaments contract into a perinuclear whorl (which is also anti-JMB2 positive) when the cells are grown in colchicine or vinblastine (Fig. 18·5(b) ). One operational definition of some intermediate filaments is that they contract into a perinuclear position after treatment with these compounds. Ultrastructural immunohistochemistry also shows that anti-JMB2 reacts with 10 nm filaments in chimp liver cells (see Fig. 18·6 for details). The third line of evidence leading to the conclusion that MBs are derived from intermediate filament components is that there is some homology between the amino acid analysis of isolated MBs from alcoholic livers and intermediate filaments (Goate *et al.*) isolated from normal livers (Table 18·2). Clearly, there is not complete homology between MBs and hepatic intermediate filaments. This is to be expected since inter-

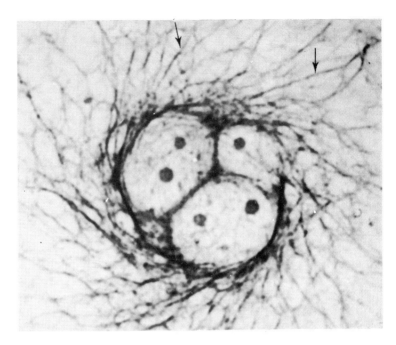

FIG. 18·5(a)

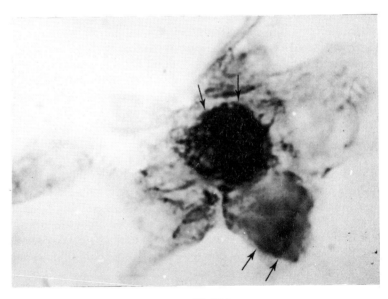

FIG. 18·5(b)

TABLE 18·2

Amino acid analysis of human liver intermediate filaments and isolated
Mallory Bodies (MBs)[a]

| Amino Acid | Intermediate filaments | MBs | Amino Acid | Intermediate filaments | MBs |
|---|---|---|---|---|---|
| Asp | 1·25 | 6·3[b] | Met | 0 | 0 |
| Thr | 3·7 | 4·1 | Ile | 3·7 | 3·3 |
| Ser | 7·4 | 7·4 | Leu | 6·9 | 6·0 |
| Glu | 9·0 | 8·4 | Tyr | 2·9 | 1·9 |
| Pro | 0 | 6·3[b] | Phe | 1·3 | 2·9 |
| Gly | 13·3 | 16·5 | His | 3·0 | 0·9[b] |
| | === | === | Lys | 8·1 | 3·4[b] |
| Ala | 6·6 | 8·9 | NH3 | 22·3 | 12·3 |
| Val | 4 | 6·7[b] | Arg | 6·2 | 4·4[b] |

[a]  MBs from an alcoholic cirrhotic liver and intermediate filaments from a normal liver were
isolated by methods described elsewhere (Morton *et al.*, 1980; Lazarides, 1980).
Note the high concentration of glycine in both; hydroxyproline was not detected in MBs or
intermediate filaments.
[b]  Indicate significant differences in amino acid content of MBs and intermediate filaments.

mediate filaments isolated from whole liver tissue will consist not only of
hepatocyte filaments but also filaments from other cell types such as
endothelial cells etc. which are known to be composed of different
polypeptide subunits from those constitutive to epithelial cells. An
additional more cogent reason, for the lack of complete homology is that
MBs have a larger diameter (14–20 nm) than intermediate filaments
(7–11 nm) indicating that MBs contain components in addition to
those derived from intermediate filaments. Finally, it has been shown
that isolated intermediate filaments from normal liver obtained at
autopsy (Goate *et al.*) contain a 45,000 dalton polypeptide and two
polypeptides with approximate Mr 18–23000 daltons. The latter 2
bands which may be breakdown products of the first, have been shown
to react with anti-JMB2 on immunoblots (Fig 18·7). It is clear from the
above experiments that JMB2 is a constitutive or associated component
of intermediate filaments. The distinction between the constitutive or
associated nature of JMB2 has not yet been determined.

FIG. 18·5(a)  Immunoperoxidase labelling of intermediate filament (arrows) in Chang
liver cells with anti-JMB2.

FIG. 18·5(b)  Immunoperoxidase labelling of Chang cells with anti-JMB2 after the
cells had been treated with colchicine. Note that all of the intermediate filaments have
contracted into a perinuclear whorl (large arrows). The nucleus (small arrows) has
almost been extruded from the cell.

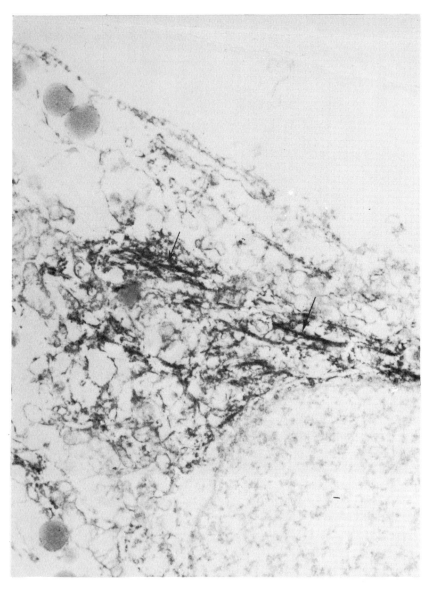

FIG. 18·6 Immunoperoxidase, ultrastructural localization of JMB2 antigen in chimp liver cells grown in culture. The electron dense reaction product is localized to intermediate filaments (arrows) which radiate from the nucleus. This cell was not stained with lead or uranyl acetate.

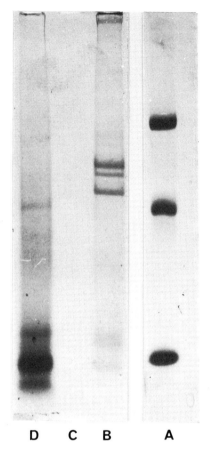

FIG. 18·7 7·5% SDS PAGE of intermediate filaments isolated from normal liver obtained at autopsy and cultured chimp liver cells. Track A contains standards (bovine serum albumin, ovalbumin, myoglobin). Track B contains purified intermediate filament from cultivated chimp liver cells. Track C is blank. Track D contains purified intermediate filament from normal human liver.

As mentioned earlier intermediate filaments are biochemically and immunologically heterogeneous (Lazarides, 1980). Five classes of intermediate filaments have been distinguished on the basis of their polypeptide subunit constitution. The supposed major polypeptides of epithelial cell (including hepatocytes) intermediate filaments are prekeratins, those of mesenchymal cells and muscle cells being vimentin and desmin respectively, while the subunits of neuronal and glial cells are different from each other and also from the other polypeptides mentioned. The question obviously arises, therefore, whether JMB2 identifies a further intermediate filament class or not. A survey of all organs in the body shows that anti-JMB2 reacts with almost all epithelial cells except epidermis and also with cells presumably of nonepithelial derivation such as pleural and peritoneal mesothelial cells and the ependymal lining of the cerebral ventricles (Table 18·1). By comparing the tissue distribution of JMB2 with the other known intermediate filament classes it is clear that anti-JMB2 defines a sixth type of intermediate filament class (Table 18·3).

TABLE 18·3
Intermediate filament subunits in different cell types[a]

| Cell type | JMB2 | Vimentin | Desmin | Keratin | GF | NF |
|---|---|---|---|---|---|---|
| Muscle | − | ± | + | − | − | − |
| Epidermis | − | − | − | + | − | − |
| Pancreatic acini | + | − | − | − | − | − |
| Kidney (PT) | + | − | − | − | − | − |
| Hepatocytes | + | − | − | − | − | − |
| Salivary acini | + | − | − | − | − | − |

[a]  JMB2 was detected by immunofluorescence. The distribution of vimentin etc., in the various cell types has been reported elsewhere (Lazarides, 1980).

The finding that anti-JMB1 (from ascitic fluid) and anti-JMB2 react with cytoplasmic filaments in the same cell types raises the possibility that both antibodies react with the same polypeptide subunits of intermediate filaments and that the antibodies only differ in their binding constant for the determinant on these polypeptides. This may indeed be so because anti-JMB1 reacts with the same intermediate filament subunits as anti-JMB2 (Goate et al.) shown in Fig. 18·7 (but see below).

In alcoholic liver disease associated with marked fibrosis (e.g. cirrhosis) anti-JMB2 reacts not only with MBs but also with non-MB containing hepatocytes (Fig. 18·4(a) ). Two further reactions, however, were also noted in these livers. Those hepatocytes which contain MBs do not contain a discernable intermediate filament system and in addition many hepatocytes which do not contain MBs are completely devoid of detectable intermediate filaments (Fig. 18·4(a) ). This suggests that in alcoholic liver disease there is a widespread disruption in the organization and presumably metabolism of filaments of the inter-mediate class. How this disruption of intermediate filaments results in hepatocellular dysfunction is not clear since even in cells in culture, the exact function(s) of these filaments has not been defined. It is proposed that they are integrators of cytoplasmic space (Lazarides, 1980).

As mentioned earlier, in contrast to JMB2, JMB1 appears to increase in non-Mallory body containing hepatocytes in alcoholic liver disease. This is against the concept that both determinants are similar. Further experiments are necessary to resolve the complete similarity or otherwise of JMB1 and JMB2 determinants.

Anti-JMB1 and anti-JMB2 also label the MBs of hepatocytes in primary biliary cirrhosis indicating that these inclusions in this disease and alcoholic hepatitis are antigenically similar. The likelihood, there-fore, is that MB formation in both alcoholic liver disease and primary biliary cirrhosis result from a similar disruption in intermediate fila-ment metabolism (Barbatis *et al.*, 1981). Those other liver disorders (see above) in which MBs are formed have not yet been studied with either of these monoclonal antibodies.

3. ANTI-JMB3

This is the least well characterized of the 3 monoclonal antibodies to MBs (Morton *et al.*, 1981). Anti-JMB3 reacts only with mesenchymal cells in sinusoids and fibrous septa of alcoholic cirrhotic livers (Fig. 18·8). In our experience to date this reaction has only been documented in 4 out of 18 alcoholic cirrhotic livers and in no other type of liver disease. Furthermore, this antibody does not react with any of the organs listed in Table 18·1. As anti-JMB3 does not react with MBs it could be argued that this monoclonal antibody is not directed against MBP but against some undetected contaminant in MBP. This explana-tion seems unlikely because the reactivity of anti-JMB3 for mesenchymal cells is completely abolished by absorption with MBP and normal liver but not by MBs themselves (Morton *et al.*, 1981). The most likely interpretation of these observations is that the extraction of MBP from MBs, reveals a determinant which is occluded in intact MBs but is revealed in mesenchymal cells which have "processed" MBs after digestion. Finally, the nature of the mesenchymal cells which contain JMB3 has not yet been determined and the characterization of this antigen and its significance in alcoholic liver disease remain to be clarified.

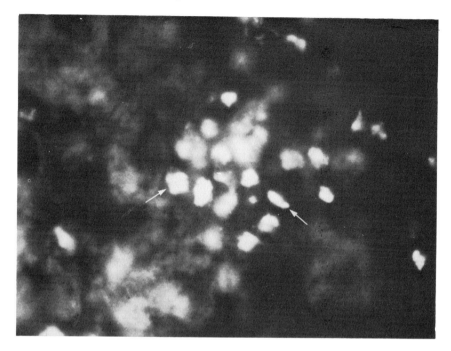

FIG. 18·8  Immunofluorescence labelling of mesenchymal cells (arrows) in an alcoholic cirrhotic liver with anti-JMB3.

## D. MALLORY BODY ANTIGENS IN SERUM

Leevy and his co-workers (Kanagasundaram *et al.*, 1977) have claimed that MB antigens and antibodies are present in the serum of patients with alcoholic liver disease and that the presence of antibody is of value in predicting which patients will progress from acute (reversible) to chronic (irreversible) end stage liver disease. Although numerous laboratories including that of the authors have been unable to confirm these findings with polyclonal antibodies to MBs, this may be due to differences in the purity and specificity of the isolated MBs and the antiserum respectively. Using monoclonal antibodies to MBs which can be produced in abundance it should be possible to determine whether MB antigens and antibodies do occur in alcoholic sera when appropriate assays have been developed.

In summary, monoclonal antibodies to MBs have revealed that MBs in alcoholic liver disease are composed at least in part of intermediate filament polypeptides; that intermediate filament organization in many hepatocytes (including those which do not contain MBs) is grossly disrupted in alcoholic cirrhosis; that MBs are probably processed by mesenchymal cells in the liver; and that the use of one monoclonal antibody to MBs (anti-JMB1) may be used to measure MB antigens in human serum and may result in a test of prognostic value in patients with alcoholic liver disease.


## II MONOCLONAL ANTIBODIES TO HLA (CLASS 1) ANTIGENS IN LIVER DISEASE


### A. INTRODUCTION

HLA antigens are glycoproteins which are thought to be largely restricted in distribution to cell surfaces. There are 2 main groups of HLA antigens *viz*. HLA-Class 1 and HLA-DR.

HLA (Class 1) antigens act as binding sites for cytotoxic T cells and appear to regulate immune responses including those involved in discrimination between self or non-self (Paul and Benacerraf, 1977; Munro and Waldmann, 1978). Cytotoxic T cells appear to exert their cytolytic action on virus infected (McMichael, 1980), hapten or chemically altered cells (Shearer and Schmitt-Verhulst, 1977; Dickmeiss *et al.*, 1977) only when T and target cells share the same Class 1 antigens. Cells infected with virus but which lack the appropriate Class 1 antigens resist cytolysis when exposed to appropriately sensitized T cells (see chapter 14 for a review of HLA structure and function).

Until a few years ago it was surmized that HLA (Class 1) antigens were present on the plasma membrane of all nucleated cells except trophoblast (Amos and Kostyu, 1980). This was based mainly on absorption studies using polyclonal antibodies to these antigens and on immunocytotoxicity assays (Berah *et al.*, 1970; Mattiuz *et al.*, 1973; Seigler and Metzgar, 1970). More recent studies, however, on tissue sections using monoclonal antibodies to HLA Class 1 antigens (Fleming *et al.*, 1981., Barbatis *et al.*, 1981) have shown that in addition to quantitative differences among tissues, certain cells in many tissues do not show detectable amounts of these antigens when examined by immunohistochemical techniques.

In this section the distribution of HLA (A,B,C) antigens in normal and diseased human liver as determined by immunohistochemistry will be described.

## B. HLA Class 1 Distribution in Normal and Diseased Liver

The monoclonal antibody used in the studies to be described below has been designated PA 2·6. It is secreted by a mouse hybridoma line generated by Parham and Brodsky and cloned by McMichael (Brodsky *et al.*, 1979). Briefly, it was produced by fusing spleen cells with a mouse myeloma cell line NS1. One of the clones resulting from this fusion (PA 2·6) secretes an antibody which binds to HLA A,B and C chains and precipitates a polypeptide from lymphocyte membranes which is composed of 2 subunits of Mr 43,000 and 12,000 daltons. Mouse ascitic fluid from this hybridoma was diluted 1:1000 in 0·01M phosphate buffer (pH 7·4) containing 0·15 M NaCl for all immunohistochemical testing for HLA Class 1 antigens in liver; the second antibody was a rabbit anti-mouse IgG conjugated with horseradish peroxidase. All liver biopsies studied were frozen onto metal chucks in liquid nitrogen immediately the biopsy was taken from the patient. Cryostat sections were cut at 6 $\mu$m and fixed in acetone at $-20°C$ for 15 minutes before processing through the immunohistochemical procedure.

### 1. NORMAL LIVER

In normal liver, hepatocytes do not exhibit detectable HLA Class 1 antigens as defined by PA 2·6 either on the cell membrane or in the cytoplasm (Fleming *et al.*, 1981; Barbatis *et al.*, 1981). Bile duct epithelium, sinusoidal lining cells, all blood vessel endothelium and the fibroblasts showed strongly positive membrane staining (Fig. 18·9(a) ). HLA A,B,C antigens were also demonstrable in the cytoplasm of sinusoidal lining cells (Fig. 18·9(b) ).

An immunofluorescent study of other normal human tissues has also shown that HLA Class 1 antigens cannot be detected on many other cells. Those cells, which were consistently positive in this assay, were lymphocytes, endothelial lining cells of small vessels and all epithelium examined (Table 18·4). This latter finding implies that normal hepatocytes are not unique in lacking detectable HLA Class 1 antigens on their cell membranes although other epithelial cells, namely bile duct lining cells, in the same liver stain strongly for HLA Class 1 (Fig. 18·9(a) ). Two other monoclonal antibodies, one of which (W6/32) reacts with all known HLA-A,B and C heavy chains and the other (PA 2·12) which is specific for $\beta_2$ microglobulin gave the same distribution of immunofluorescence in liver as the monoclonal antibody PA 2·6; $\beta_2$ microglobulin and HLA Class 1 antigens are molecularly associated on cell surfaces. The inability of monoclonal antibody PA 2·6 (and W6/32) to detect Class 1 antigens in normal hepatocytes could be due to the fact that these molecules assume a different conformation on hepatocyte plasma membranes, or that these membranes are inaccessible to monoclonal antibodies. The first of these possibilities cannot be excluded on present data; the second possibility seems unlikely since monoclonal antibodies to antigens unrelated to HLA react with hepatocyte membranes in frozen sections (unpublished observations). It is also possible that the procedures used here are not sensitive enough to detect small amounts of Class 1 antigens. It should be noted, however, that the monoclonal antibody to Class 1 antigens used here readily detects the small amount of Class 1 molecules on cortical thymocytes. Direct comparison of immunofluorescence and immunoperoxidase staining with the same antibody has shown that the latter method is more sensitive (Barbatis *et al.*, 1981). In spite of the increase sensitivity of the

TABLE 18·4
Distribution of HLA Class 1 antigen in normal tissue[a]

| Tissue | Positive cells[a] |
| --- | --- |
| Lymphoreticular system (thymus, spleen, lymph node, tonsil) | All lymphoid cells |
| Gastrointestinal system (tongue, oesophagus, stomach, pancreas, small and large intestine) | All epithelial cells of surface and glands |
| Respiratory system (larynx, trachea, bronchus, lung | |
| Skin | |
| Breast | |
| Cardiovascular system (heart, aorta, common carotid artery) | Endothelial cells of small vessels |
| Urogenital system (kidney, bladder, ovary, testis) | Glomeruli; transitional epithelial cells and cytoplasm of renal tubular cells |
| Liver | Biliary epithelial cells and cytoplasm of sinusoidal lining cells |
| Central nervous system (motor cortex, cerebellum, spinal cord) | None |
| Skeletal system (smooth and voluntary muscle, fibrous, and adipose tissue) | Fibroblasts and cytoplasm of occasional smooth muscle fibres |
| Endocrine system (thyroid, adrenal, islet of Langerhans) | None |

[a] In addition to the positive cells listed, the lining cells of small vessels were positive in all tissues. Unless otherwise stated, the positive staining involved only the cell surface.

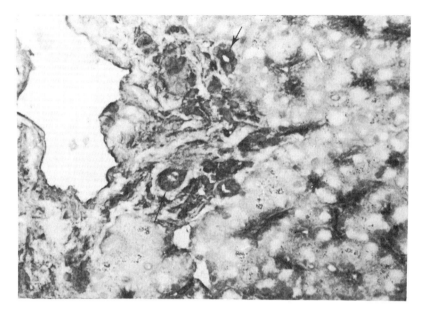

FIG. 18·9(a)

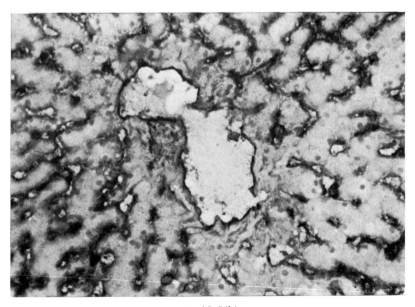

FIG. 18·9(b)

immunoperoxidase procedure it is impossible to exclude the possibility that HLA Class 1 antigens exist in trace amounts on hepatocyte cell membranes.

Allogeneic human liver grafts show a low incidence of rejection compared to renal and heart transplants. Several investigations have shown that HLA compatibility is not of paramount importance in liver transplantation; that hyperacute rejection never occurs in liver; that acute rejection is easily controlled and chronic rejection is rare (Starzl *et al.*, 1976). Morphological observations on rejected liver allografts indicate that when rejection does occur the mononuclear infiltrate in the portal tracts surrounds and involves bile duct epithelium; in the sinusoids foamy histiocytes and mononuclear cells have been described but direct contact of these cells with hepatocytes is not common (Starzl *et al.*, 1976). The latter observations may be explained by the fact that bile duct epithelium and sinusoids contain HLA Class 1 while these antigens cannot be detected on normal hepatocytes. The absence of detectable amounts of HLA Class 1 antigens on hepatocytes could confer resistance to T cell mediated rejection during transplantation, assuming that hepatocyte rejection is HLA Class 1 dependent.

## 2. LIVER DISEASE

In contradistinction to normal hepatocytes, HLA Class 1 antigens were detected on the surface and in the cytoplasm of these cells in several liver disorders. In all cases of acute alcoholic hepatitis (with or without chronic alcoholic liver disease), most cases of primary biliary cirrhosis, and some cases of acute or chronic hepatitis HLA Class 1 antigens were detected on the cell membrane of hepatocytes. HLA distribution was mainly focal; only small groups of hepatocytes showed cell membrane staining and were predominantly located in the periportal zone (Fig. 18·10(a) ). All cases of alcoholic liver disease examined showed variable degrees of fatty change; however, in this series there were no cases of simple fatty change only.

In two cases of acute alcoholic hepatitis superimposed on alcoholic cirrhosis, almost every hepatocyte exhibited cell membrane staining (Fig. 18·10(b) ). 2 cases of non A, non B hepatitis did not show

FIG. 18·9(a) Immunoperoxidase detection of HLA Class 1 antigens in normal liver using monoclonal antibody PA 2·6. These antigens are present on bile ducts (arrows), in sinusoidal lining cells and in mesenchymal cells in portal tracts.

FIG. 18·9(b) Higher power view of liver illustrated in Fig. 18·9(a). This clearly shows the presence of HLA Class 1 antigens in sinusoidal lining cells, and endothelial cells of a central vein. These antigens are not detectable in hepatocytes.

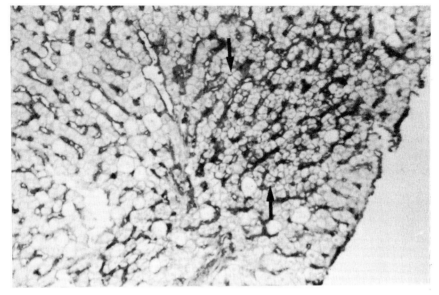

FIG. 18·10(a)

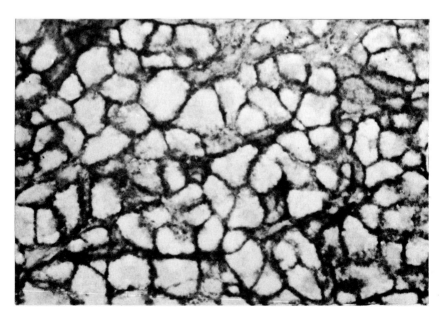

FIG. 18·10(b)

membrane HLA but instead there was a diffuse cytoplasmic granular staining with simultaneous reduction in the intensity of staining of sinusoidal lining cells. Of 9 cases of miscellaneous aetiology only one (due to large duct obstruction) showed HLA Class 1 positivity on hepatocyte cell membranes (Table 18·5).

TABLE 18·5

Detection of HLA Class 1 antigens in hepatocytes in normality and liver disease

| Condition | No. of cases | No. of cases showing hepatocyte HLA Membrane | Cytoplasm |
|---|---|---|---|
| Normality | 8 | 0 | 0 |
| Acute alcoholic hepatitis without cirrhosis | 3 | 3(F)* | 0 |
| Alcoholic hepatitis and cirrhosis | 10 | 8(F) 2(D)† | 0 |
| Alcoholic fibrosis | 6 | 3(F) | 0 |
| Alcoholic cirrhosis | 3 | 0 | 0 |
| PBC | 5 | 4(F) | 0 |
| CAH | 3 | 2(F) | 0 |
| Acute hepatitis | 3 | 0 | 2 |
| Miscellaneous | 9 | 1(F) | 0 |

*F = focal positivity of hepatocytes for HLA Class I (see Fig. 10a)
†D = diffuse membrane staining of hepatocytes throughout the biopsy (see Fig. 10b)

One explanation of the finding that HLA Class 1 antigens can be detected focally or diffusely on hepatocyte cell membranes in acute and chronic liver disease and other liver diseases of diverse aetiology is that certain clones of hepatocytes can express HLA (A,B,C) on the cell surface after exposure to alcohol or other agents. It is conceivable that the detection of HLA (A,B,C) on hepatocyte cell membranes may not necessarily indicate induction of expression of HLA but absorption from plasma; however, the focal distribution of HLA in most cases makes the latter mechanism less probable. In the two cases of non-A, non-B hepatitis diffuse granular cytoplasmic HLA was observed. This also may be due either to induction of HLA expression or diffusion of

FIG. 18·10(a) Focal staining of hepatocytes for HLA Class 1 in acute alcoholic hepatitis (arrows).
FIG. 18·10(b) An alcoholic cirrhotic liver treated with monoclonal antibody to HLA Class 1 antigens. All hepatocyte membranes contain these antigens but sinusoidal lining cells are negative.

HLA (A,B,C) antigens into damaged hepatocytes. The presence of HLA (A,B,C) antigens on the cell membrane or in the cytoplasm of hepatocytes in all of these diseases may render them susceptible to sensitized cytotoxic T cells and so enable the immune system to recognize and eliminate viral infected cells. However, it is also possible that the presence of these antigens on alcohol damaged hepatocytes could lead to perpetuation of immune damage to liver cells even when the patient ceases to drink ethanol.

In summary monoclonal antibodies to HLA Class 1 antigens have revealed that normal hepatocytes lack detectable amounts of these antigens on their cell membranes and this may be of significance in understanding why liver allografts are less frequently rejected than other organs. The monoclonal antibody to this HLA Class has also demonstrated that these antigens are present on alcohol and viral damaged hepatocytes. This finding may be of importance in the mechanisms underlying the progression of acute to chronic alcoholic liver disease and the elimination of hepatocytes infected with virus.

REFERENCES

Amos, D. B. and Kostyu, D. D. (1980). *Adv. human Genet.* **10**, 137.
Barbatis, C., Morton, J. A., Bradley, J., Woods, J. and McGee, J. O'D. (1981). *J. Path.* **134**, 331.
Barbatis, C., Woods, J., Morton, J. A., Fleming, K. A., McMichael, A. and McGee, J. O'D. Immunohistochemical analysis of HLA (A,B,C) antigens in liver disease using a monoclonal antibody. (1982). *Gut* (in press).
Barbatis, C., Morton, J. A. and McGee, J. O'D. (1981). *Gut* (submitted).
Barnstaple, C. J., Bodmer, W. F., Brown, G. *et al.* (1978). *Cell* **14**, 9.
Berah, M., Hors, J. and Dausset, J. (1970). *Transpl.* **9**(3), 185.
Bhagwat, A. G. and Pandit, J. (1979). *Bull. P.G.I.* **13**, 204.
Bradley, J. F., Morton, J. A. and McGee, J. O'D. (unpublished observations).
Brodsky, F. M., Parham, P., Barnstable, C. J., Crumpton, M. J. and Bodmer, W. F. (1979). *Immunol. Rev.* **47**, 3.
Chen, T. and Leevy, C. M. (1973). *Gastroenterology* **64**, 178.
Denk, H., Franke, W. W., Eckerstorfer, R., Schmid, E. and Kerkaschi, D. (1979). *Proc. natn. Acad. Sci. U.S.A.* **76**, 4112.
Dickmeiss, E., Soeberg, B. and Svejgaard, A. (1977). *Nature* **270**, 526.
Fleming, K. A., McMichael, A., Morton, J. A., Woods, J. and McGee, J. O'D. (1981). *J. Clin. Path.* **34**, 779.
Franke, W. W., Schmid, E., Kartenbeck, J., Mayer, D., Hacker, H., Bannash, P. *et al.* (1979). *Biol. Cellulaire* **34**, 99.
Franke, W. W., Denk, H., Kalt, R. and Schmid, E. (1981). *Exp. Cell Res.* **131**, 229.

French, S. W., Sim, J. S., Franks, K. E., Burbridge, E. Z., Denton, T. and Caldwell, M. G. (1977). *In* "Alcohol and the liver". (M. M. Fisher and J. G. Rankin, Eds), p. 261. Plenum Press, New York.

Gerber, M. A., Orr, W., Denk, H., Schaffner, F. and Popper, H. (1973). *Gastroenterology* **64**, 89.

Goate, A., Al-Saigh, K. and McGee, J. O'D. (unpublished observations).

Kanagasundaram, N., Kakumu, S., Chen, T. and Leevy, C. M. (1977). *Gastroenterology* **73**, 1368.

Köhler, G., Milstein, C. (1975). *Nature* **256**, 495.

Kuhn, C. and Tseng-Tong Kuo. (1973). *Cytoplasmic hyaline in asbestosis. Arch. Path.* **95**, 190.

Lazarides, E. (1980). *Nature* **283**, 249.

Mallory, F. B. (1911). *Bull. Johns Hopk. Hospt.* **22**, 69.

Mattiuz, P. L., Massobrio, M., Richiardi, P. (1973). *Minerva ginecologica* **25**, 8.

McMichael, A. J. (1980). *Springer Semin. Immunopathol.* **3**, 3.

Morton, J. A., Fleming, K. A., Trowell, J. M. and McGee, J. O'D. (1980). *Gut* **21**, 727.

Morton, J. A., Bastin, J., Fleming, K. A., McMichael, A., Burns, J. and McGee, J. O'D. (1981). *Gut* **22**, 1.

Munro, A. and Waldmann, H. (1978). *Br. Med. Bull.* **34**, 253.

Nenci, I. (1975). *Lab. Invest.* **32**, 257.

Paul, W. E. and Benacerraf, B. (1977). *Science* **195**, 1293.

Popper, H. The pathogenesis of alcoholic cirrhosis. (1977). *In* "Alcohol and the liver" (M. M. Fisher, J. G. Rankin Eds), p. 289. Plenum Press, New York.

Seigler, H. F. and Metzgar, R. S. (1970). *Transpl.* **9**(5), 478.

Shearer, G. M. and Schmitt-Verhulst, A. M. (1977). *In* "Advances in Immunology" 55. Academic Press, London and New York.

Starzl, T. E., Porter, K. A. Putnam, C. N., Schroter, G. P. S., Halgrimson, C. G., Weil III R., Hoelscher, M. and Reid, H. A. S. (1976). *Surg. Gynec. Obstet.* **142**, 487.

Zetterman, R. K., Luisada-Opper, A., Leevy, C. M. (1976). *Gastroenterology* **70**, 382.

# 19 Monoclonal Antibodies and Human Pregnancy: identification and possible significance of antigens specific to the human placenta

C. A. SUNDERLAND, C. W. G. REDMAN AND
G. M. STIRRAT

*Nuffield Department of Obstetrics and Gynaecology, John
Radcliffe Hospital, Headington, Oxford. OX3 9DU*

## I INTRODUCTION

In the field of human reproduction, as in so many other fields, mono-clonal antibodies are providing new tools with which to examine old problems. Why is the fetus not rejected as any other allograft? What is the biochemical basis and immunological significance of the invasion of trophoblast into the maternal endometrium and how is this controlled? Does pre-eclamptic toxaemia have an immune aetiology? This chapter aims to illustrate how monoclonal antibodies may be used to approach these and other problems rigorously and incisively.

The focus is the human placenta, a fetal tissue with an amazing diversity of functions. Many of these functions are mediated by trophoblast, which represents at all stages of pregnancy the outer placental layer in maternal contact. Thus it is through the trophoblast layer that all metabolites, gases, ions, nutrients, antibodies etc. must pass in the continuous maternofetal exchange. It is trophoblast which as the outer layer of the implanting blastocyst, mediates the invasion of the conceptus into the maternal uterus. It is trophoblast which secretes an array of pregnancy-specific hormones which play an as yet unde-fined role in the maintenance of the pregnancy. Finally, it is the trophoblast layer which stands as the principal fetal tissue in maternal contact and as the potential focus of feto-maternal immunological interactions.

A number of these functions are likely to be mediated by molecules found only on trophoblast and not on other human tissues. Monoclonal antibodies directed to such trophoblast-specific antigens may be valu-able in many different experimental and clinical situations. For exam-ple, specific trophoblast markers can be used directly in histological studies of normal and abnormal placentae, in detection of trophoblast products in neoplastic tissue and particularly in increasing understand-ing of placental biochemistry. This last point derives from the potential for using monoclonal antibodies to purify and so to characterize the molecules they recognize (see chapter 22 of this volume). Particular molecules with defined biochemical roles may therefore be assigned to trophoblast function. The work outlined in the next section describes our progress in the generation of monoclonal antibodies to trophoblast-specific molecules.

## II MONOCLONAL ANTIBODIES TO TROPHOBLAST-SPECIFIC ANTIGENS

### A. Preparation of the Monoclonal Antibodies

Standard techniques (see chapter 21) were followed in the immuniza-tion of mice, the selection of hybrid cells and cloning of hybrids by limiting dilution. The immunogen was trophoblast membrane, derived from term placentae by allowing the syncytiotrophoblast membrane to exfoliate from placental chorionic villi by stirring in saline, isolation of a membrane fraction by differential centrifugation and final purification by sucrose density centrifugation. (Smith *et al.*, 1974: Sunderland *et al.*, 1981a).

Supernatants from hybrid cell cultures were screened in an indirect radioimmunoassay by incubation with glutaraldehyde-fixed trophoblast membrane. The membrane was then washed and bound antibody detected using $^{125}$I-rabbit F (ab')$_2$ anti mouse IgG in a second incubation (Sunderland *et al.*, 1981a). Supernatants were screened immediately to eliminate those of broad tissue specificity. This was done by attempting to absorb the antibodies at limiting dilution with washed tissue homogenates of adult liver and brain at approximately 20 mg protein per ml. Of 31 supernatants tested in this manner, 27 were absorbed by one or other of these tissues. The remaining supernatants were then tested for direct binding to peripheral blood cells and by absorption with homogenates of adult heart, kidney and normal human serum. Two antibodies, which showed no reaction with these cells or tissues have now been cloned. These antibodies have been named NDOG1 and NDOG2.

### B. Properties of the Monoclonal Antibodies

NDOG1 and NDOG2 have now been tested in a number of different systems for cross reaction with other human tissues. The results are summarized in Table 19·1. NDOG2 antibody reacts with no adult cell or tissue so far examined but does bind to the fetal membrane, chorion, and to placental villous syncytiotrophoblast. NDOG1 antibody shows a similar pattern of reactivity except that it does not bind to chorion but does stain specialized regions of connective tissue in adult breast and ureter (to be published).

Discrimination between NDOG1 and NDOG2 antibodies is also achieved by absorption with sera (Table 19·1). Thus, whilst neither antibody is inhibited by normal human serum, NDOG1, but not NDOG2, is blocked by a component of pregnancy serum. There are a large number of pregnancy-specific serum components described in the literature, in various stages of characterization (reviewed by Klopper and Chard, 1979). Work is in progress to discover which, if any, of these components is detected by NDOG1 antibody. Thus, NDOG1 is not inhibited by purified human chorionic gonadotrophin (hCG), human placental lactogen (hPL) (Sunderland *et al.*, 1981a), $\beta_1$ specific glycoprotein (SP1) or PP5 at levels equal to or greater than their maximal concentrations in pregnancy sera. Other experiments (Sunderland *et al.*, 1981a) have demonstrated that NDOG1 antigen is not PAPP-A or placental alkaline phosphatase.

TABLE 19·1
The distribution of NDOG1 and NDOG2 antigens

|  | NDOG1 | NDOG2 |
|---|:---:|:---:|
| (*i*) By absorption assay[a] | | |
| Heart | − | − |
| Liver | − | − |
| Kidney | − | − |
| Brain | − | − |
| Group AB serum | − | − |
| Late pregnancy serum | + | − |
| Placenta | + | + |
| (*ii*) By direct binding[a] | | |
| Erythrocytes | − | − |
| Lymphocytes | − | − |
| Granulocytes | − | − |
| Trophoblast membrane | + | + |
| (*iii*) By immunohistological staining | | |
| Adult endometrium | − | − |
| Adult myometrium | − | − |
| Adult breast | + | − |
| Adult ureter | + | ND |
| Villous syncytiotrophoblast | + | + |
| Villous cytotrophoblast | − | − |
| Chorion | − | + |

[a]  (Sunderland *et al.*, 1981b)
ND  Not determined

The localization of the NDOG1 and NDOG2 antibodies in the placenta has been examined using an indirect immunoperoxidase technique (see Chapter 24). In the term placenta, NDOG1 and NDOG2 antigens show a similar distribution, staining only apical aspects of syncytiotrophoblast (Fig. 19·1). Recent electron micrograph studies have shown that this staining is actually limited to syncytiotrophoblast membrane (K. Gatter—unpublished work). At 6–10 weeks gestation, NDOG1 antibody again stains apical aspects of syncytiotrophoblast, but some staining of stromal areas is also apparent on frozen sections. In contrast NDOG2 antibody does not stain chorionic villi until approximately the sixteenth week, when it appears in its characteristic syncytiotrophoblast location.

## III TROPHOBLAST AND IMMUNOLOGICAL INTERACTIONS BETWEEN MOTHER AND FETUS

The mechanisms by which the fetal allograft is maintained successfully throughout pregnancy are of considerable interest, not only theoretically but also clinically. Thus it is possible that, through the study of such processes, information might be gained relevant to clinical transplantation and attempts to prevent allograft rejection. Also there are abnormal conditions of pregnancy whose aetiology may lie in the breakdown of normal fetal allograft tolerance, for example preeclamptic toxaemia (discussed more fully in Section V) and spontaneous abortion (Stimson *et al.*, 1979). In this section we will show how monoclonal antibodies may now be used to further knowledge in this area.

### A. TROPHOBLAST AND HLA ANTIGENS

In 1962, Simmons and Russell showed that trophoblast cells, obtained from the ectoplacental cone of mouse placenta, survived about 11 days when transplanted under the kidney capsule of mice presensitized to paternal antigens, whereas the associated embryo was rejected in six days. This and several other experiments (Kirby *et al.*, 1966; Simmons *et al.*, 1971) were taken as evidence favouring a lack of transplantation antigens by trophoblast. Siegler and Metzgar (1970) then showed that cultures of human trophoblast did not bind antibody to HLA A and B antigens as measured by absorption in a mixed haemagglutination assay.

More recently the lack of detectable HLA A, B and DR antigens on human chorionic villous trophoblast has been demonstrated by staining of frozen sections with heterologous anti-HLA sera (Faulk and Temple, 1976; Faulk *et al.*, 1977) and biochemically by examining the properties of a partially purified trophoblast membrane preparation in absorption of assays for HLA A, B and DR antibodies (Goodfellow *et al.*, 1976).

These results have, however, been contradicted by others (Loke *et al.*, 1971) and the field has remained in some confusion. Monoclonal antibodies now provide reagents of assured specificity. Using monoclonal antibodies to monomorphic determinants of HLA A, B and C antigens (W6/32—Barnstable *et al.*, 1978) and HLA DR antigens (Cr 3/43—Sunderland *et al.*, 1981b), we have studied the distribution of these

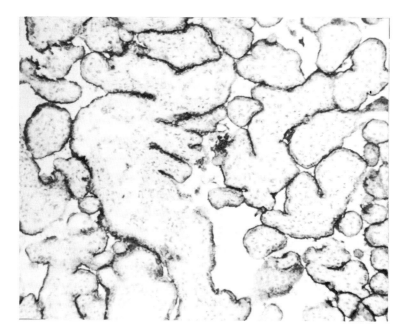

FIG. 19·1(a)

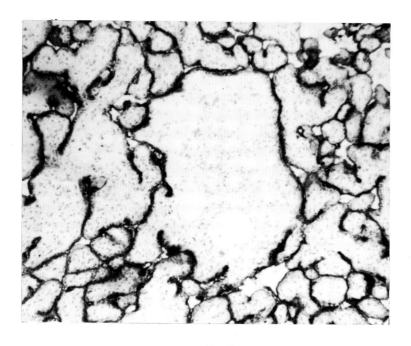

FIG. 19·1(b)

antigens in frozen sections of placentae taken from 6 weeks' gestation until term using the indirect immunoperoxidase technique. The trophoblast cells of the chorionic villi are uniformly negative with both of these antibodies in all placentae examined. An example of this for the eight week placenta is shown in Fig. 19·2. Each chorionic villus is seen to be surrounded by a double layer of nuclei denoting the cytotrophoblast and syncytiotrophoblast layers. On neither of these trophoblastic layers are HLA A, B, C or DR evident whilst NDOG1 provides a control demonstrating the presence of the syncytiotrophoblast membrane in these frozen sections.

HLA A, B, C antigens are, however, evident on elements of the mesenchymal stroma of the villi (Fig. 19·2(a) ). In contrast, HLA DR antigen is almost totally absent from the eight week placenta (Fig. 19·2(b) ) but, at term, is found to stain a few elongated dendritic-like cells of the villous stroma (Fig. 19·3). These cells may be analogous to the Steinman dendritic cell described in mouse lymphoid organs (Steinman and Nussenzweig, 1980) and recently found to be present in the connective tissues of many organs in the rat, except brain. (Hart and Fabre, 1981a). The Steinman cell is considered to be of potential immunological significance and Hart and Fabre (1981b) consider it to be a candidate for the "passenger leucocyte" which may play a major role in stimulating tissue allograft rejection. If these DR-staining cells in term placenta are Steinman cells, then they may therefore be of particular relevance to the problem of fetal allograft immunity.

Purification of syncytiotrophoblast membrane has allowed a more direct examination of its antigenic properties. Absorption studies using monoclonal antibodies have demonstrated that such membrane preparations express very few HLA A, B, C or DR antigens and that this expression is not affected by solubilization of the membrane proteins, thus eliminating the possibility that antibody binding is prevented by steric constraints of the membrane structure (Sunderland *et al.*, 1981b).

The lack of HLA antigens on villous trophoblast has important immunological consequences.

The fetus is an allograft in the sense that it bears a foreign (paternal) genotype. Its successful growth and development during pregnancy demonstrates that it is not subject to immune rejection processes typical of normal tissue transplants. The precise mechanisms by which such

FIG. 19·1 Cryostat sections of term placentae were stained with (a) NDOG1 monoclonal antibody; (b) NDOG2 monoclonal antibody using an indirect immunoperoxidase technique. Nuclei were counterstained with hemotoxylin. (Magnification × 120).

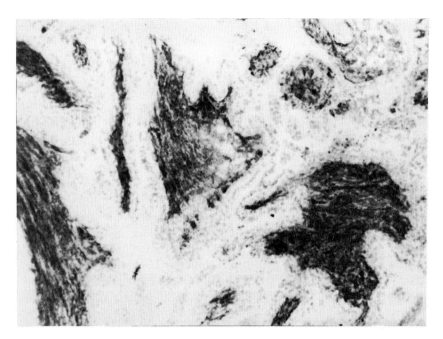

FIG. 19·2(a)

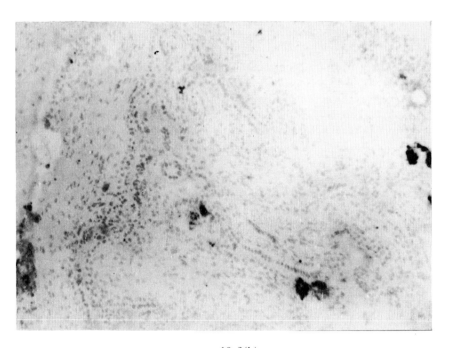

FIG. 19·2(b)

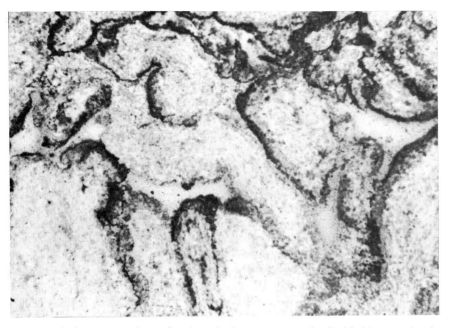

FIG. 19·2 Cryostat sections of an 8 week placenta were stained with (a) monoclonal anti-HLA A, B, C antibody; (b) monoclonal anti-HLA-DR antibody; (c) NDOG1 monoclonal antibody to syncytiotrophoblast. Nuclei were counterstained with hematoxylin. (Magnification × 120).

transplant rejection normally occurs are not yet fully understood, but it is clear that reaction to major histocompatibility antigens is an important component of rejection. Chorionic villous trophoblast is the principal fetal tissue in maternal contact during pregnancy and makes up an area of several square metres in the term placenta. Its lack of HLA antigens therefore considerably limits the potential exposure of the mother to these antigens and may be a vital factor in fetal allograft success.

The fetus differs from normal tissue transplants in bearing the self (maternal) as well as the foreign (paternal) genotype. It is now apparent that cytotoxic T lymphocytes recognize a number of antigens only if they express some shared (i.e. self) HLA antigens (Goulmy *et al.*, 1977; Dickmeiss *et al.*, 1977; McMichael *et al.*, 1977). The lack of any HLA antigens on villous trophoblast may then strictly limit the type of immune attack to which this membrane is susceptible. Indeed it is possible that cellular immune attack to all non-HLA antigens, whether they be viral, polymorphic or trophoblast-specific in nature, may be

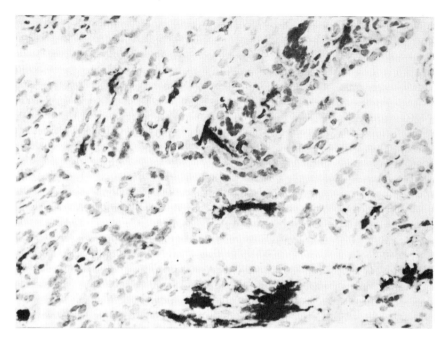

FIG. 19·3 Cryostat section of a term placenta stained with monoclonal anti-HLA-DR antibody. Nuclei were counterstained with hematoxylin. (Magnification × 300).

abrogated by the lack of HLA on this membrane (Barnstable and Bodmer, 1978).

There are, however, other minor trophoblast forms in contact with maternal tissue whose antigenic properties should be considered. In particular, in early pregnancy, the villous cytotrophoblast undergoes a period of rapid proliferation in which it invades the maternal uterus to form the cytotrophoblastic shell. A preliminary study of samples taken from a chorionic sac of six weeks' gestation has shown that this proliferating, non-villous trophoblast carries HLA A, B, C but not DR antigens (Sunderland, Redman and Stirrat, 1981c). Other forms of trophoblast are currently being examined. It may be that it is HLA antigens on such minor trophoblast forms which provoke the formation of antibodies to HLA during pregnancy (Overweg and Engelfriet, 1969) and which have been detected on trophoblast cultured *in vitro* (Loke *et al.*, 1971).

## B. Other Immunological Mechanisms Relevant to Fetal Allograft Survival

Many other contributory mechanisms have been suggested to account for fetal allograft success although the experimental evidence on which they rest is often difficult to evaluate.

Changes in lymphoid anatomy do occur during rodent pregnancy including an increase in size and cellularity of para-aortic lymph nodes which drain the uterus. This increase is greater in allogeneic than syngeneic pregnancies, a difference which is abrogated if rodents are previously made tolerant to the relevant alloantigens (Beer *et al.*, 1975). This work has been interpreted in terms of the generation by these lymph nodes of paternal antigen-specific suppressor T cells or humoral blocking factors.

Maternal humoral immunity is clearly not subject to non-specific suppression during human pregnancy and antibodies to Rhesus factor, blood group antigens A and B, as well as to HLA A, B, C and DR antigens can be generated by pregnancy (Rocklin *et al.*, 1979). It is possible that maternal antibody is produced in pregnancy specifically towards trophoblast antigens. The IgG transporting function of trophoblast makes it impossible to distinguish between specifically and non-specifically bound antibody. Monoclonal antibodies may allow purification of trophoblast membrane components. The testing of such purified components for specific maternal antibody might then be achieved by standard radioimmunoassay techniques. Alternatively, now that it is possible to make human monoclonal antibodies (see chapter 2 of this volume) it may soon be feasible to analyse directly the antibodies produced during pregnancy by fusion using peripheral blood lymphocytes of pregnant women.

The role of cellular immunity in pregnancy must be regarded as an open question despite many years of research (reviewed in Rocklin *et al.*, 1979). This confusion probably results chiefly from the lack of simple, reliable assay systems. Monoclonal antibodies may allow progress in this area in a number of ways. Firstly, with the availability of monoclonal antibodies to functional subsets of peripheral lymphocytes, it is now possible to examine the proportions of these subsets in the blood of pregnant and non-pregnant individuals. Such a study is currently in progress in our laboratory and may serve to indicate both whether a cellular immune response to pregnancy is occurring and whether this response is positive or suppressive in nature (also see section V).

Secondly, cellular responses to placenta are normally examined using crude placental antigen preparations. The raising of monoclonal antibodies to trophoblast molecules opens up the possibility of purifying such molecules (chapter 22). Such purified molecules might then be examined individually for their ability to elicit cellular immune responses.

Finally, there are a number of proposals concerning the possibility of a localized, non-specific immuno-suppression occuring around the chorionic villous trophoblast. Thus Faulk *et al.* (1978) have shown that a trophoblast membrane fraction P1, inhibits allogeneic but not mitogenic transformation of lymphocytes. Assurance of the significance of this finding awaits purification of the molecule involved. This, again might be achieved by monoclonal antibody techniques.


## IV TROPHOBLAST AND NEOPLASIA

Among the distinctive properties which malignant neoplasms have in common, two, namely host invasion and metastasis, are shared to some extent with normal trophoblast. For example, blastocyst implantation proceeds through active phagocytosis of maternal tissue by syncytiotrophoblast (Boyd and Hamilton, 1970) during which plasminogen activator is released (Sherman *et al.*, 1976). This also occurs during *in vitro* assays of tumour cell invasion (Ossowski *et al.*, 1973). Furthermore, blastocyst invasion in the mouse is facilitated by autolytic degeneration of epithelial cells in front of trophoblast (El-Shershaby and Hinchliffe, 1975; Smith and Wilson, 1974). Such degeneration also occurs in tumour invasion and may be mediated by molecules common to trophoblast and tumour. Invasion of maternal tissue continues on into later pregnancy, and reaches into the myometrium and maternal spiral arteries. Unlike tumour invasion, however, the invasion of trophoblast is strictly limited in its extent. Thus, spiral artery invasion ceases abruptly at the distal end of the radial arteries.

Throughout the second and third trimester of human pregnancy syncytiotrophoblast tissue can be detected in the maternal bloodstream (Douglas *et al.*, 1959). This tissue is thought to arise by budding of chorionic villous syncytiotrophoblast and has obvious analogies to tumour cell metastasis. Syncytiotrophoblast deportation is, however, of no apparent consequence to the mother. Trophoblastic elements can be found in the maternal lung which do not grow but appear to lyse without producing any inflammatory response.

These properties of trophoblast are not shared with other normal human tissues and so might be mediated by molecules specific to the trophoblast. It is therefore possible that a series of monoclonal antibodies such as NDOG1 and NDOG2, might detect molecules which include some of those involved in trophoblast invasion and metastasis. It is possible that purification and characterization of these molecules might elucidate their biochemical functions. This in turn may add to our understanding of some aspects of malignant neoplasia.

Such trophoblast-specific molecules are also of considerable interest as possible tumour markers. Monoclonal antibodies to such molecules may therefore be valuable long before we understand the functions of the molecules which they recognize. The theoretical and practical implications of monoclonal antibodies in the diagnosis and therapy of tumours is fully discussed in chapters 5, 6 and 7 but the particular role of trophoblast-specific markers in this field is outlined below.

## A. Gestational Trophoblast Neoplasia

The trophoblast tumours, hydatidiform mole, invasive mole and gestational choriocarcinoma secrete human chorionic gonadotrophin (hCG), a trophoblast-specific product produced by all such tumours and of proven clinical value in tumour detection and the monitoring of metastasis (Bagshawe, 1976). At the present time the success of hCG as a marker for these tumours makes it difficult to see what clinical role other trophoblast-specific markers might play. Human placental lactogen (hPL) may be of some value in that it is secreted in very low, but detectable amounts by these tumours. This contrasts with its high level of production during normal pregnancy and measurement of the hPL:hCG ratio may be useful in discriminating normal pregnancy from trophoblastic neoplasms (Rosen, 1975).

Monoclonal antibodies to hCG and hPL are likely to be of only marginal value in serum detection because the molecules concerned are already available at high purity, allowing the production of heterologous antisera of high specificity. The ability to generate homogeneous monoclonal antibodies, of defined class and affinity may, however, have a significant role to play in tumour localization and therapy (see chapters 5 and 7).

## B. Germ Cell Tumours

Germ cell tumours present in an amazing variety of forms and with variable prognoses despite a multiplicity of treatment regimens. Trophoblastic tissue in these tumours is predictive of a high degree of malignancy and before the advent of chemotherapy, such tumours were usually fatal (Maier and Sulak, 1973). This observation gives weight to the possibility that there are biochemical similarities between trophoblast and neoplastic tissue. Recently, two serum markers alphafetoprotein and hCG, have been used both in the classification of these tumours by direct tissue staining and monitoring of metastasis by serial assay of serum levels after removal of the primary tumour. (Javadpour *et al.*, 1978). Both markers are of considerable value but because about 20% of the tumours do not express hCG or AFP the discovery of additional tumour markers would be beneficial. Attempts to develop monoclonal antibodies to teratoma cell lines have so far not produced reagents of sufficient tumour specificity, probably because the predominant immunogens on the teratoma cell surface are carbohydrate and lipid moieties of broad tissue distribution (McIlhinney, J.—Personal communication). Trophoblast is the first observable differentiated tissue in the development of the conceptus and may therefore share molecules with the totipotential stem cells from which germ cell tumours derive. Monoclonal antibodies might therefore be derived which are trophoblast specific and which cross-react with germ cell tumours. Markers specific for the totipotential stem cells would be ideal reagents in this area, because they would be found in all tumours and would mark the cells from which the tumour originates, rather than its differentiated products.

## C. NON-TROPHOBLASTIC NEOPLASMS

The abnormal phenotype of many tumours includes expression of molecules normally limited to the fetal stage of development and expressed either in very low amounts or not at all in the normal adult. Such molecules are potentially useful tumour markers and include carcinoembryonic antigen (CEA) and alphafeto-protein (AFP). The proportion of the total number of malignant tumours expressing CEA or AFP is, however, fairly low. Thus raised serum levels of CEA are found in 73% of patients with colorectal carcinoma, 76% with pulmonary carcinoma and 91% with pancreatic carcinoma (Hansen *et al.*, 1974). Frequencies of positive CEA are markedly lower with other tumour types, although figures are difficult to ascertain due to the acknowledged multispecificity of anti-CEA sera. A similar situation pertains to the incidence of high serum AFP. Another limitation is that both these molecules are present in low amounts in normal serum

(Ruoslahti and Seppala, 1971; Chu *et al.*, 1972) and levels may be raised in non-malignant disease (Smith 1971; Moore *et al.*, 1971).

It is now apparent that trophoblast markers may be found at relatively low, but significant frequencies (less than 40%) in the serum of a large variety of non-trophoblastic malignancies. Such markers include hCG, hPL, SP1 ($\beta_1$ specific glycoprotein) and placental alkaline phosphatase. These markers often do not occur together. Thus in a survey by Rosen (1975) of 295 patients with varied malignant tumours 20 had detectable levels of hPL but only five of these also had elevated hCG.

The principle problem in clinical application of trophoblast/tumour markers is their low frequency of occurrence. In this respect, it should be noted that if larger numbers of markers are generated and these markers are used in concert, then a high proportion of malignant tumours might become detectable. Screening programmes for malignancy using serum may then become a real possibility.

Monoclonal antibodies raised to trophoblast-specific molecules are likely to detect additional, heretofore, uncharacterized trophoblast products which may show tumour cross-reactions. Trophoblast may therefore represent a valuable alternative to the more obvious approaches of using tumour cell lines or solid tumour tissue in the generation of monoclonal antibodies as tumour markers (Chapter 5). It is therefore our intention to screen our monoclonal antibodies, as they are raised, on a variety of tumours.

## V TROPHOBLAST AND PRE-ECLAMPSIA

Pre-eclampsia is a specific disorder of human pregnancy which for many years has been thought to have a possible immune aetiology. The evidence for this is circumstantial and so far the pathogenesis of the disease remains unexplained (Redman, 1980). Pre-eclampsia is particularly, but not exclusively, a disorder of first pregnancy. Even an earlier miscarriage confers some protection against its development in a subsequent full-term pregnancy (MacGillivray, 1958). This well-established fact is difficult to explain without invoking immune mechanisms—in particular by proposing that previous maternal exposure to fetal antigens is in some way protective. This implies a different mechanism from that of Rhesus isoimmunization where maternal sensitization to the fetus is directly damaging. In effect it is postulated that during normal pregnancy there is a beneficial maternal immune reaction to fetal antigens, the absence of which causes pre-eclampsia.

This would be most likely in a first pregnancy with a first-set immune response than in later pregnancies.

Central to this argument is the need to know how the maternal immune system is stimulated by and responds to, the fetal allograft. The absence of histocompatibility antigens on villous trophoblast has already been discussed. Nevertheless, pre-eclampsia tends to occur where there is a large trophoblast mass such as in multiple pregnancy, placental hydrops or hydatidiform mole (Jeffcoate and Scott, 1959), and it has been suggested that the mother is in these circumstances exposed to an abnormally large antigenic burden. There are poorly substantiated reports of maternal immune reactions to other placental components in pre-eclampsia. More convincing is the evidence that human placentae and kidneys share common antigens (Baxter and Goodman, 1956; Okuda and Grollman, 1966) and that experimental immunization with placental extracts can cause nephritis. Thus, it is possible that the renal features of pre-eclampsia stem from cross-reactivity of this sort. These issues will not be resolved until the biochemical and antigenic structure of trophoblast membrane has been defined. As has already been discussed, monoclonal antibodies will play a central role in this task.

The basic pathological lesions of pre-eclampsia are found in the uterine spiral and basal arteries which supply, respectively, the intervillous space and decidua. In normal pregnancy (as has been mentioned) the spiral arteries are retrogradely invaded by trophoblast cells, which form an inner lining to these vessels for much of their course through the myometrium. In pre-eclampsia the trophoblast invasion is restricted to the terminal decidual segment of the spiral artery (Robertson *et al.*, 1975). In addition, the spiral arteries are partially or completely blocked by a mixture of fibrin, platelet thrombi and lipid-filled cells of uncertain origin (possibly macrophages, possibly smooth muscle cells). The peri-arterial tissue exhibits a low grade lymphocytic infiltration (Robertson *et al.*, 1967).

The histology of the placental bed in both normal and pre-eclamptic pregnancies is therefore complex being formed from a mixture of maternal and trophoblast elements. Thus the trophoblast-specific monoclonal antibodies NDOG1 and NDOG2 provide a powerful new tool for evaluating the pathology of this area.

Any immune theory of the aetiology of pre-eclampsia demands the existence of two maternal immune reactions. The first is the response to an immune stimulus provided by the conceptus which is required for the continuation of normal pregnancy. If this response is absent or defective it allows the development of a second aberrant reaction which triggers the onset of the pre-eclamptic disorder. In the absence of even the most rudimentary data speculation about what these reactions might be tends not to be constructive. It is however relevant to enquire if there is evidence for changes in the circulating maternal immune cell population in both normal and pre-eclamptic pregnancies. This approach has been helpful in defining probable disorders of immune function in multiple sclerosis (Reinherz *et al.*, 1980), primary biliary cirrhosis (Routhier *et al.*, 1980) and other disease states previously assumed to have an immune aetiology (see chapter 3). The newly identified monoclonal antibodies to human suppressor and helper T cell subjects provide a new approach which is currently being tested in our department.

In summary, the application of monoclonal antibodies to the study of the antigenic structure of the human placenta, to the histology of the placental bed in pre-eclampsia and to the characterization of maternal lymphocyte subsets provides important new openings for investigating the aetiology of the single most important antenatal disorder of human pregnancy.

## VI CONCLUSION

It is an often repeated truism that the understanding of basic principles in biology is limited by the methods available for their study. This is certainly so for immunobiology.

The potential for a clearer understanding of feto-maternal immune relations using the powerful monoclonal antibody techniques has been highlighted in the preceding sections of this chapter. It is also becoming apparent that from knowledge gained in that field new insight will be gained in others, and it is likely that as a result there will be exciting developments in areas as yet undreamt of. The prospects are exciting not least because it is at last becoming possible to distinguish specific mechanisms from epiphenomena.

ACKNOWLEDGEMENTS

We are grateful to Dr. A. J. McMichael, D. Y. Mason and A. F. Williams for the provision of monoclonal antibodies, and to Mrs. Caroline Midgely for technical assistance with the project. We acknowledge the support of MRC Grant No. G979/136/C.

REFERENCES

Bagshawe, K. D. (1976). *J. Clin. Path.* **29**, Suppl. 140–144.
Barnstable, C. J. and Bodmer, W. F. (1978). *Lancet* i, 326.
Barnstable, C. J., Bodmer, W. F., Brown, G., Galfre, G. Milstein, C., Williams, A. F. and Ziegler, A. (1978). *Cell* **14**, 9–20.
Baxter, J. H. and Goodman, H. C. (1956). *J. exp. Med.* **104**, 467–485.
Beer, A. E., Scott, J. R. and Billingham, R. E. (1975). *J. exp. Med.* **142**, 180–196.
Boyd, J. D. and Hamilton, W. J. (1970). *In* "The Human Placenta". Heffer. Cambridge, England.
Chu, T. M., Reynoso, G. and Hansen, H. J. (1972). *Nature* **238**, 152–153.
Dickmeiss, E., Soeberg, B. and Svegaard, A. (1977). *Nature* **270**, 526–528.
Douglas, G. D., Thomas, L., Carr, M., Cullen, N. M. and Morris, R. (1959). *Am. J. Obstet, Gynecol.* **78**, 960–973.
El-Shershaby, A. M. and Hinchliffe, J. R. (1975). *J. Embryol exp. Morphol.* **33**, 1067–1080.
Faulk, W. P. and Temple, A. (1976). *Nature* **262**, 799–802.
Faulk, W. P., Sanderson, A. R. and Temple, A. (1977). *Transpl. Proc.* **9**, 1379–1384.
Faulk, W. P., Temple, A., Lovins, R. E. and Smith, N. (1978). *Proc. natn. Acad. Sci. U.S.A.* **75**, 1947–1951.
Goodfellow, P. N., Barnstable, C. J., Bodmer, W. F., Snary, D. and Crumpton, M. J. (1976). *Transplantation* **22**, 595–603.
Goulmy, E., Termijtelan, A., Bradley, B. A. and van Rood, J. J. (1977). *Nature* **266**, 544–545.
Hansen, H. J., Snyder, J. J., Miller, E., Vandevoorde, J. P., Miller, O. N., Hines, L. R. and Burns, J. J. (1974). *Human Pathol.* **5**, 139–147.
Hart, D. N. J. and Fabre, J. W. (1981a). *J. exp. Med.* **154**, 347–361.
Hart, D. N. J. and Fabre, J. W. (1981b). *Transpl. Proc.* **13**, 95–99.
Javadpour, N., McIntire, K. R. and Waldmann, T. A. (1978). *Natn. Cancer Inst. Monographs* **49**, 209–213.
Jeffcoate, T. N. A. and Scott, J. S. (1959). *Am. J. Obstet. Gynecol.* **77**, 475–489.
Klopper, A. and Chard, T. (1979). Eds "Placental Proteins". Springer Verlag, Berlin.
Kirby, D. R. S., Billington, W. D. and James, D. A. (1966). *Transplantation* **4**, 713–718.
Loke, Y. W., Joysey, V. C. and Borland, R. (1971). *Nature* **232**, 403–405.
MacGillivray, I. (1958). *J. Obstet, Gynaec. Brit. Comm.* **65**, 536–539.
Maier, J. G. and Sulak, M. H. (1973). *Cancer* **32**, 1217–1226.
McMichael, A. J., Ting, A., Zweerink, H. J. and Askonas, B. A. (1977). *Nature* **270**, 524–525.
Moore, T. L., Kupchik, H. Z., Maron, N. and Zanchek, N. (1971). *Am. J. Dig. Dis.* **16**, 1–7.
Okuda, T. and Grollman, A. (1966). *Arch. Path.* **82**, 246–258.

Ossowski, L., Quigley, J. P., Kellerman, G. M. and Reich, E. (1973). *J. exp. Med.* **138**, 1056–1064.

Overweg, J. and Engelfriet, C. P. (1969). *Vox. Sang.* **16**, 97–104.

Redman, C. W. G. (1980). *In* "Immunological Aspects of Reproduction and Fertility Control" (J. P. Hearn, Ed.), pp. 83–104. MTP, Lancaster.

Reinherz, E. L., Weiner, H. L., Hauser, S. L., Cohen, J. A., Distaso, J. A. and Schlossman, S. F. (1980). *New Engl. J. Med.* **303**, 125–129.

Robertson, W. B., Brosens, I. and Dixon, H. G. (1967). *J. Path. Bact.* **93**, 581–592.

Robertson, W. B., Brosens, I. and Dixon, H. G. (1975). *Eur. J. Obs. Gyn. Reprod. Biol.* **5**, 47–65.

Rocklin, R. E., Kitzmiller, J. L. and Kaye, M. D. (1979). *Ann. Rev. Med.* **30**, 375–404.

Rosen, S. W. (1975). *Ann. Intern. Med.* **82**, 71–83.

Routhier, G., Epstein, O., Janossy, G., Thomas, H. C., Sherlock, S., Kung, P. C. and Goldstein, G. (1980). *Lancet* **ii**, 1223–1226.

Ruoslahti, E. and Seppala, M. (1971). *Int. J. Cancer* **8**, 374–383.

Sherman, M. I., Strickland, S. and Reich, E. (1976). *Cancer Res.* **36**, 4208–4213.

Siegler, H. F. and Metzgar, R. S. (1970). *Transplantation* **9**, 478–486.

Simmons, R. L. and Russell, P. S. (1962). *Ann. N.Y. Acad. Sci.* **99**, 717–732.

Simmons, R. L., Lipschultz, M. L., Rios, A. and Ray, P. K. (1971). *Nature/New Biol.* **231**, 111–112.

Smith, A. F. and Wilson, I. B. (1974). *Cell Tissue Res.* **152**, 525–542.

Smith, J. B. (1971). "Proc. 1st Conf. and W'Shop on Embryonic and Fetal Antigens in Cancer" (N. G. Anderson, J. H. Coggin, Eds), pp. 305–312. Atomic Energy Commission, Tennessee.

Smith, N. C., Brush, M. and Luckett, S. (1974). *Nature* **252**, 302–303.

Steinman, R. M. and Nussenzweig, M. C. (1980). *Immunol. Rev.* **53**, 127–148.

Stimson, W. H., Strachan, A. F. and Shepherd, A. (1979). *Br. J. Obstet. Gynaecol.* **86**, 41–45.

Sunderland, C. A., McMaster, W. R. and Williams, A. F. (1979). *Eur. J. Immunol.* **9**, 155–159.

Sunderland, C. A., Redman, C. W. G. and Stirrat, G. M. (1981a). *Immunology* **43**, 541–546.

Sunderland, C. A., Naiem, M., Mason, D. Y., Redman, C. W. G. and Stirrat, G. M. (1981b). *J. Reprod. Immunol.* **3**, 323–331.

Sunderland, C. A., Redman, C. W. G. and Stirrat, G. M. (1981c). *J. Immunol.* **127**, 2614–2615.

# 20 Monoclonal Antibodies to Drugs: new diagnostic and therapeutic tools

E. HABER

*Cardiac Unit, Department of Medicine, Massachusetts General Hospital, Boston, Mass. 02114. U.S.A.*

## I INTRODUCTION

The measurement of drug concentration by immunoassay has been of immeasurable value to the clinician and pharmacologist over the past decade. The remarkable selectivity of antibodies has allowed the determination of nanomolar concentrations of drugs in the complex mixture of substances that characterized physiologic fluids and has permitted the differentiation between the active form of a drug and its closely related metabolites. The contribution of these studies to an enhanced understanding of pharmacokinetics and drug metabolism has been considerable (Butler *et al.*, 1977a), though the inherent heterogeneity and lack of reproducibility of antibodies has retarded standardization of these methods. Preliminary investigations of antibodies as specific drug antagonists *in vivo* have also shown some promise, but the limited availability of antibodies elicited by conventional immunization has prevented the widespread application of this approach (Butler *et al.*, 1977b). The advent of monoclonal antibodies produced by somatic cell fusion is likely to enhance and extend considerably these applications of antibodies.

I shall first discuss the difference between the elicited and monoclonal antibodies in their application to diagnosis or therapy, and then discuss the use of antibodies in selective immunoassay, reversal of drug effects, and the investigation of drug receptors.

## II CHARACTERISTICS THAT DIFFERENTIATE MONOCLONAL ANTIBODIES FROM CONVENTIONAL ANTIBODIES ELICITED BY IMMUNIZATION

Antibodies represent a set of molecules that exhibit extraordinary specificity and selectivity. This has been appreciated since the work of Landsteiner (1944) who, in the early years of this century, was able to provide examples such as the ability of an antiserum to resolve the d and l stereoisomers of a simple aliphatic molecule, tartaric acid. More complex organic compounds that vary only by a single substituent group (such as the steroids digoxin and digitoxin that differ in one hydroxyl group) may be readily separated (Smith *et al.*, 1970).

The general structure of the antibody molecule is remarkably conserved, so that it is quite difficult for the chemist to tell the difference between two antibodies of varying specificity. There is a small region of the molecule, however, that is highly variable in its structure (the complementarity region) and makes up the surface that binds antigen. It is the amino acid sequence in this region that determines the nature of the antigen recognized. Recent work has uncovered the mechanisms responsible for variation in the amino acid sequence of the complementarity region.

The antibody molecule is comprised of four polypeptide chains, two identical light and heavy chains. The variable region of the light chain is the product of two genes: V, which occurs in several hundred copies, and J, of which four copies have been identified (Brack *et al.*, 1978; Sakano *et al.*, 1981; Seidman *et al.*, 1978; Seidman *et al.*, 1979). V and J of the light chain may occur in any combination. The heavy chain's variable region is the product of three genes: V, in several hundred copies, D, in ten or more copies, and J, in four copies (Early *et al.*, 1980; Wiegert *et al.*, 1978). As in the light chain, any permutation and/or combination of these genes may occur. These mechanisms alone account for $10^7$ different antibodies. In addition, somatic-point mutation has been shown to occur. Thus the number of possible antibodies must actually exceed $10^{10}$.

Clinicians have not neglected the immune system, but its deliberate manipulation has been restricted to a limited number of areas. Of course, immunization has long been a cornerstone of preventative medicine. The passive infusion of pneumococcal-specific antisera had a brief vogue in the pre-antibiotic days, while tetanus and Rh antibodies are still of great value today. By providing a method for measuring substances in biological fluids that would not be possible by any other means, the immunoassay has produced a literal explosion in the use of antibodies as *in vitro* diagnostic agents. Yet this remarkable group of compounds has been largely neglected in its potential utility as a source of pharmaceutical agents with both diagnostic and therapeutic applications.

There may be several explanations for this neglect. Prior to very recent times, antibodies were only available as complex mixtures of proteins, isolated in very limited quantities from animal sera. Standardization of an antibody is not possible since each immunized animal provides an antiserum of different properties. There is even variation among the sera of single animals at different times following immunization. An additional problem is the potential immunogenicity of heterologous antibodies in the recipient. Each of these problems has been overcome by application of a new technology that has only been available in the past several years. Antibodies may now be produced by cell culture methods in infinite quantities with previously unimagined homogeneity and reproducibility.

As indicated in the first chapter of this volume, Milstein and his colleagues (Kohler and Milstein, 1975) showed that antibodies might be produced, not only by the conventional injection of antigens into a recipient host and the subsequent collection of sera, but by utilization of the technique of somatic cell fusion. This method allows for the production of cell lines that represent hybrids of two different precursor lines. If the parental lines of the hybrid are normal lymphocytes and cells from a malignant plasmacytoma, one can incorporate both properties of antibody production and growth *in vitro* into the product (colloquially named "hybridoma"). Cells that grow in culture may be cloned, so that all the progeny are daughters of a single precursor cell. A homogeneous culture of this type produces a single antibody that is uniform in structure and antigen binding properties. Since the cultures may be stored indefinitely at low temperatures, the same antibody may always be recovered, and, in addition, production in industrial quantities is possible. For *in vivo* application, antibody fragments may be created that reside within the body for shorter periods of time and are less likely to provoke an immune response (Smith *et al.*, 1979). Human antibodies have been produced by an analogous method (Croce *et al.*, 1980; Olsson and Kaplan, 1980), thus effectively limiting the problem of immunogenicity *in vivo*.

## III MONOCLONAL ANTIBODIES TO DRUGS: A LOGICAL RATHER THAN EMPIRIC APPROACH TO SELECTIVE IMMUNOASSAY

The conventional approach to the production of an antibody suitable for immunoassay of drug concentration begins with immunization of an animal with a drug-protein conjugate and then testing the antisera at various times after immunization with respect to affinity and specificity. As indicated above, each antiserum (whether obtained from the same animal at different times after immunization or from different animals) has a unique spectrum of affinities and specificities for the mixture of antibodies that it contains. There are, however, specificities that tend to be dominant, and it is very often difficult to find antibodies that effect a desired resolution, such as between a drug and its metabolite or among closely related compounds. For example, even after many years of effort, it has not been possible to find a method that reliably produces antibodies that differentiate between the octapeptide angiotensin II and its heptapeptide metabolite (Oparil *et al.*, 1972; Oparil *et al.*, 1974) although antibodies that differentiate between this hormone and its decapeptide precursor, angiotensin I, are readily produced in most immunizations. Thus, in addition to the problem that most antisera present by being mixtures of antibodies rather than single reagents, the problem of preference in the production of certain sets of antibodies (immunodominance) often defeats the investigator. The incredible power of selection possible with monoclonal antibodies should allow one to overcome these difficulties. An example of this remarkable selectivity is seen in a set of monoclonal antibodies specific for the drug digoxin.

Digoxin, one of a large group of cardiac glycosides, is the drug most frequently prescribed for patients with congestive heart failure. Cardiac

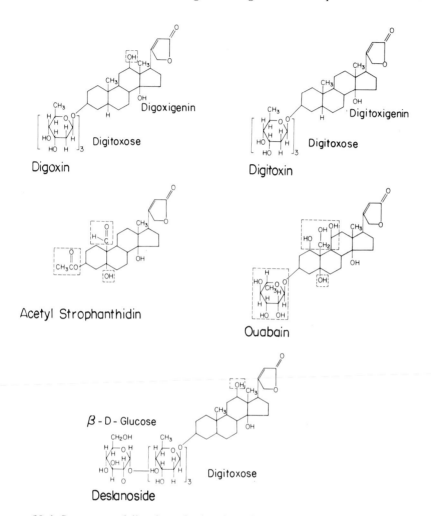

FIG. 20·1 Structures of digoxin and related cardiac glycosides. Differences in steroid ring substitutions are indicated by broken lines. (Reprinted from Margolies *et al.*, (1981), with permission of Elsevier/North-Holland Publishers.)

glycosides are composed of a steroid or aglycone portion and from one to four sugar molecules (Fig. 20·1). The pharmacological activity resides in the aglycone portion of the molecule, and the sugar residues modify water solubility and potency.

Digoxin is an uncharged, chemically well-defined hapten, sufficient in size to occupy most of the antibody combining site. For this reason, cardiac glycosides which include 64 structurally related analogs (Fieser

TABLE 20·1
Hybridoma affinity constants for digoxin

| Hybridoma Clone | H-Chain Isotype | Affinity Constant $K_0(M^{-1})$a | |
| --- | --- | --- | --- |
| | | Culture Media | Antibody Purified from Ascites |
| 26-10 | $\gamma_{2a}$ | $8·5 \times 10^9$ | $4·7 \times 10^9$ |
| | $F_{ab}$ | | $1·2 \times 10^9$ |
| 26-20 | $\gamma_{2a}$ | $1·4 \times 10^9$ | $3·4 \times 10^9$ |
| 26-30 | $\gamma_{2a}$ | $3·9 \times 10^9$ | $5·8 \times 10^9$ |
| 26-40 | $\gamma_{2a}$ | $4·4 \times 10^9$ | $2·6 \times 10^9$ |
| 25-54 | $\gamma_1$ | $2·6 \times 10^8$ | $5·2 \times 10^8$ |
| 35-20 | $\gamma_1$ | $1·9 \times 10^9$ | $1·3 \times 10^9$ |
| Sheep Anti-Digoxin Sera | | | $1·2 \times 10^{10}$ |

Affinity constants (Ko) were determined in an RIA which utilizes [$^3$H-] digoxin and dextran coated charcoal to adsorb free digoxin (Smith, T. W., *J. clin. Invest.* (1972). **51** 1583. Data were plotted according to a modified Sips equation (Nisonoff, A., Pressman, D. *J. Immunol.* (1958). **80** 417. Correlation coefficients varied from r = 0·989 to 0·999.

and Fieser 1959; Fullerton *et al.*, 1979) are suitable for a detailed study of antibody specificity. The rigid four-ring structure common among all cardiac glycosides and other steroids does not allow for major conformational changes as functional groups are substituted at various positions on the rigid steroid backbone. Through an analysis of antibody affinity for related glycosides, the detailed specificity of antibodies may be defined readily. Certain heterogeneous antibodies raised to digoxin have been shown to be very selective in that they discriminate between digoxin and digitoxin, which differ from each other by the presence or absence of a single hydroxyl group at position 12 on the steroid backbone (Fig. 20·1) (Smith *et al.*, 1970). This specificity is very commonly found, however, to the exclusion of others that might be of value or interest in studying cardiac glycosides and their metabolites. Thus we sought to examine a repertoire of monoclonal anti-digoxin antibodies (Margolies *et al.*, 1980; Mudgett-Hunter *et al.*, 1980).

Three high-affinity monoclonal antibodies specific for digoxin have been produced successfully by somatic cell fusion. Each antibody has been analyzed for its affinity and fine specificity for digoxin and related cardiac glycosides. Two of the antibodies, Dig 26-10 (subclass IgG2a) and Dig 35-20 (subclass IgG1), have a high affinity ($10^9$ $M^{-1}$) for digoxin, while the third, Dig 25-54 (subclass IgG1), has an affinity which is an order of magnitude lower affinity ($10^8 M^{-1}$) (Table 20·1).

TABLE 20·2

Monoclonal antibodies tested in a clinical assay for digoxin[a]

| RIA Used: | $^{125}$I-RIA Kit[b] | | $^3$H-Digoxin-RIA[c] | |
|---|---|---|---|---|
| Antidigoxin Ab: | Supplied by Corning | Sheep antisera | Dig 26-10 | Dig 35-20 |
| Digoxin ml$^{-1}$ | ng ml$^{-1}$ | ng ml$^{-1}$ | ng ml$^{-1}$ | ng ml$^{-1}$ |
| *Patient number* | | | | |
| 4601 | 2·6 | 2·8 | 2·6 | n.d. |
| 4605 | 0·9 | 1·2 | 0·8 | n.d. |
| 4614 | 4·4 | 2·8 | 4·0 | n.d. |
| 4615 | 0·4 | 0·8 | 0·8 | n.d. |
| 4616 | 3·5 | 2·8 | 3·0 | n.d. |
| 4617 | 0·8 | 1·0 | 0·7 | n.d. |
| 5875 | 1·3 | 1·4 | 1·6 | n.d. |
| 5876 | 1·3 | 1·1 | 1·2 | n.d. |
| 5884 | 1·2 | 1·6 | 1·6 | n.d. |
| 9708 | 4·4 | 4·8 | 5·4 | 6·0 |
| 9717 | 2·5 | 2·3 | 2·1 | 1·9 |
| 9761 | 2·0 | 1·5 | n.d. | 1·6 |

[a]   Monoclonal antibodies Dig 26-10 and Dig 35-20 were compared to the sheep anti-digoxin sera and to anti-digoxin antibody provided in a commercially available kit for their ability to quantitate digoxin in patient's sera.

[b]   The commercially available $^{125}$I-RIA kit for digoxin was obtained from Corning (New York).

[c]   This [$^3$H-]digoxin RIA is the clinical dextran coated charcoal RIA described in section III.

As demonstrated in Table 20·2, both Dig 26-10 and Dig 35-20 are as capable of quantitating digoxin in human sera as the sheep anti-digoxin antisera raised in this laboratory and commercial heterogeneous anti-digoxin antibodies (Corning, New York). High affinity monoclonal antibodies, which can be obtained in essentially unlimited supply, are particularly attractive as standard reagents in clinical assays for digoxin.

Each of these three antibodies demonstrates a unique specificity pattern (Table 20·3). Based on the results from inhibition of related cardiac glycosides, the following general conclusions can be stated. None of the monoclonal anti-digoxin antibodies are specific for the digitoxose moiety since all of the hybridoma antibodies are reactive towards digoxin and digitoxigenin (Table 20·3). Unlike the sheep antisera, all three monoclonal antibodies are equally reactive to digoxin and to digitoxin (Table 20·3). Hence, none is specific for the hydroxyl at position C12 of the steroid ring. Since the unsaturated lactone ring structure is common to all the cardiac glycosides tested, differences in specificity cannot be attributed to this part of the molecule. Where there are major differences in the functional groups substituted on rings A

484 *E. Haber*

TABLE 20·3
Specificity of hybridoma antibodies for various cardiac glycosides
relative to digoxin[a]

| Hybridoma clone or antisera | Cardiac Glycoside Inhibitors | | | | | |
|---|---|---|---|---|---|---|
| | Digoxin | Digitoxin | Digitox-igenin | Deslanoside | Acetylstro-phanthidin | Ouabain |
| DIG 25-54 | 1·0 | 1·8 | 54·0 | 4·3 | >100 | >100 |
| DIG 35-20 | 1·0 | 4·6 | 2·7 | 3·7 | 110 | 333 |
| DIG 26-10 | 1·0 | 1·3 | 3·7 | 2·6 | 1·50 | 66 |
| DIG 26-20 | 1·0 | 1·0 | 2·2 | 1·5 | 0·70 | 53 |
| DIG 26-30 | 1·0 | 2·6 | 3·6 | 1·6 | 0·85 | 84 |
| DIG 26-40 | 1·0 | 1·4 | 4·0 | 2·0 | 2·30 | 78 |
| Sheep anti-dig serum | 1·0 | 152·0 | 860·0 | N.D. | N.D. | $>10^5$ |

Inhibition of binding to [$^3$H-]digoxin by a series of cardiac glycosides was determined for each hybridoma antibody and for a standard sheep antidigoxin serum. The assay system used was the dextran coated charcoal RIA (Smith, T. W. (1972). *J. Clin. Invest. 51* 1583). The values reported here are amounts of inhibitor required to give 50% inhibition relative to the amount of cold digoxin which gave 50% inhibition.

and B of the steroid structure (Fig. 20·2), major differences in relative affinities for the cardiac glycosides occur. For example, the molecular structures of rings A and B of ouabain and acetyl strophanthidin differ significantly from those of digoxin, digitoxin, and deslanoside (compare Fig. 20·2a and 20·2b and Table 20·3). Thus, the major differences in relative affinities parallel these structural changes (i.e., all three antibodies are less reactive toward ouabain than they are to digoxin, digitoxin, and deslanoside).

In addition to these general trends, each hybridoma antibody may be further analyzed individually with regard to its specific recognition of antigenic determinants of the digoxin molecule. Dig 25-54, for example, has a slightly lower affinity for digitoxigenin because it requires 54 times as much digitoxigenin as digoxin to achieve 50% inhibition (Table 20·3). This reduced affinity for digitoxigenin implies that the digitoxose sugar moiety plays a small role in binding to the Dig 25-54 combining site. Dig 25-54 also bound ouabain and acetyl strophanthidin with affinities reduced by at least two orders of magnitude (Table 20·3). Since the addition of hydroxyl and aldehyde groups at positions 5 and 10, respectively, (Rings A and B; Fig. 20·2) in acetyl strophanthidin would cause steric hindrance to any kind of "contact" with the upper face of rings A and B as the molecule is displayed in Fig. 20·2, it is likely

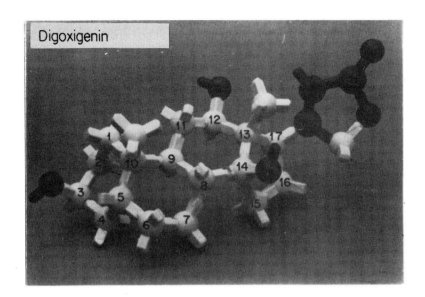

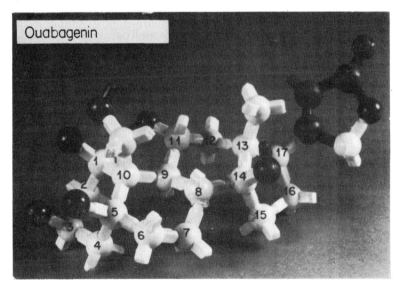

FIG. 20·2 Three-dimensional structures of digoxigenin and ouabagenin. Carbon atoms (white) are numbered as indicated in the steroid backbone illustrated in Fig. 20·1. The -OH functional groups are shown in dark grey. Compare these structural models with the two-dimensional structures depicted for the same molecules in Fig. 20·1.

that Dig 25-54 specifically recognizes the "upper" faces of rings A and B in digoxin. A similar set of steric hindrances are imposed on the upper face of the rings A and B in ouabain with the addition of three hydroxyl groups at positions 1, 5, and 11 (Fig. 20·2b).

The specificity of monoclonal antibody Dig 35-20 is similar to Dig 25-54 since substitutions in rings A and B, which would sterically hinder any bindings to the upper face of these two rings, similarly cause the molecule to bind less tightly to the antibody (Table 20·3). However, since there is essentially no difference in the relative affinity of Dig 35-20 for digoxin and digitoxigenin, the digitoxose sugar groups have no role in binding to this antibody in contrast to Dig 25-54 (see above).

Dig 26-10, as Dig 35-20, does not distinguish between glycosides with or without digitoxose since no significant difference in binding to digoxin and digitoxigenin was observed (Table 20·3). The specificity of Dig 26-10, as that of Dig 35-20 and Dig 25-54, probably resides in rings A and B, but unlike the other two monoclonal antibodies, Dig 26-10 does not discriminate between digoxin and acetyl strophanthidin. Also while the relative affinity of Dig 26-10 for ouabain is reduced, it is not reduced to the extent it is for Dig 35-20 and 25-54 by at least an order of magnitude. Thus, it is possible that Dig 26-10 contacts digoxin at a position from underneath the steroid backbone as it is pictured in Fig. 20·2a, but in such a manner that the addition of hydroxyl groups at positions 1 and 11 (ouabain, Fig. 20·2b) at the far edge of the backbone would interfere in the binding of this antibody.

In many years of study of conventionally obtained digoxin-specific antisera, the kind of molecular discrimination provided by these monoclonal antibodies has not been observed. Such antibodies provide powerful tools for the study of the fine structure of organic molecules. Because of their desirable high affinity, they also offer the possibility of producing a world standard reagent for immunoassay.

## IV ENHANCING SPECIFICITY OF IMMUNOASSAY BY USING TWO MONOCLONAL ANTIBODIES

At times, even careful and extensive screening of antibody-producing clones does not provide the requisite specificity. An example will be given in which two monoclonal antibodies were needed in order to effect the requisite resolution in an immunoassay (Haber et al., in press; Katus et al., 1980).

Monoclonal antibodies recognize a single antigenic determinant which should allow for enhanced specificity of recognition. Thus one could select an antibody specific for the epitope that defines the difference between two very similar molecules. Yet it appears that cross reactivity is often seen. With monoclonal antibodies this is probably a manifestation of the sharing of parts of an epitope by two antigens. A method that entails the combination of two antibodies that recognize different epitopes on the same molecule should enhance specificity markedly. The differentiation between cardiac- and skeletal-muscle myosin appears to offer a good test case. The molecules are different structurally, yet elicited antibodies (mixtures) and most monoclonal antibodies we have tested exhibit varying degrees of cross reactivity. When an assay is constructed so that two different monoclonal antibodies must bind to the same antigen, the resultant cross reactivity observed corresponds, as might be expected from theoretical considerations, to approximately the product of the two fractional cross reactivities.

Cardiac myosin light chains are structurally (Khaw *et al.*, 1979; Khaw *et al.*, 1980) and immunologically (Khaw *et al.*, 1978) different from skeletal- and smooth-muscle myosin light chains and thus may provide a unique cardiac-specific antigen. Unfortunately, there is sufficient immunologic similarity between myosin light chains from various tissues that antibodies that uniquely recognize one and not the others have not been obtained (Khaw *et al.*, 1978; Trahern *et al.*, 1978). The sera of 25 rabbits immunized with human cardiac-myosin light chains were examined by us at varying times after immunization. Cross reactivity between cardiac- and skeletal-muscle light chains varied between 10 and 100%. An antiserum could not be found that would provide the specificity requisite for use in clinical assay. A solution of this problem employs a method that utilizes monoclonal antibodies that recognize two different epitopes on the same antigen and thus markedly enhances the resolution possible in immunoassay. Examples of the varieties of antigenic specificities found are depicted in Fig. 20·3. Antibody 3C7 typifies the most common type. There is complete identity of reactivity between cardiac- and skeletal-myosin light chains, indicating recognition of common antigenic determinants. Antibody 2B2 is representative of a less frequent type. These monoclonal antibodies demonstrate a partial cross reactivity between skeletal- and smooth-muscle light chains. Perhaps only a part of a common antigenic determinant is recognized. The least common monoclonal response is typified by 1E6. This antibody shows no evidence of cross reactivity between skeletal- and smooth-muscle light chains, and thus recognizes the unique determinants of the cardiac light chain, providing the basis

488          *E. Haber*

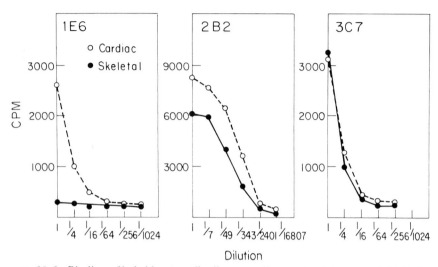

FIG. 20·3. Binding of hybridoma antibodies to cardiac- or skeletal-muscle light chains immobilized on plastic microtiter plates. Dilution of the cell-culture supernatant is plotted against counts per minute of $^{125}$I-labeled goat-(anti-mouse) Fab antibody bound to the plate that recognizes the myosin light chain-specific antibody. (From Haber *et al.* (1981). *In* Monoclonal Antibodies in Endocrine Research". Reprinted with permission of Raven Press).

for development of an entirely specific immunoassay for cardiac cell damage.

Three monoclonal antibodies that exhibited varying degrees of cross reactivity between cardiac- and skeletal-muscle light chains were selected for study. When immobilized on Sepharose, each bound $^{125}$I-cardiac myosin light chains effectively, allowing ready determination of cross reactivity with skeletal-muscle light chains utilizing a solid-phase competitive radioimmunoassay. Increasing concentration of either unlabeled cardiac or skeletal light chains resulted in decreased binding of $^{125}$I cardiac light chains. Antibody 1C5 proved to be fully cross reactive, 2B9 25% cross reactive, and 4F10 17·5% cross reactive. The antibodies appear to possess varying affinities for myosin light chains, the most cross-reactive antibody, 1C5, provided the greatest sensitivity in measurement.

Fig. 20·4 demonstrates the enhanced specificity that is inherent in an assay where two antigenic determinants (epitopes) are independently measured. One monoclonal antibody is immobilized by covalent linkage of Sepharose. When exposed to an antigen mixture, only those molecules recognized by that antibody will adhere. A second antibody, labeled with $^{125}$I, is then added. It will bind only to those antibody

TABLE 20·4
Competitive assay utilizing labeled antigen

| Antibody | Measured fractional cross reactivity |
|---|---|
| 1C5 | 1·00 |
| 2B9 | 0·25 |
| 4F10 | 0·17 |

Bideterminant assay utilizing labeled second antibody

| Antibodies | Calculated cross reactivity | Measured cross reactivity |
|---|---|---|
| 1C5 and 2B9 | 0·25 | 0·25 |
| 1C5 and 4F10 | 0·17 | 0·17 |
| 2B9 and 4F10 | 0·037 | 0·043 |

From Katus, Hurrell, Matsueda *et al.* (1982) *Molecular Immunology*. (Reproduced with permission from Pergamon Press.)

molecules that are both immobilized on the column and possess the epitope for which it is specific. Thus immobilized radioactivity represents the recognition of two different epitopes on the antigen molecule. This form of dual recognition requires that epitopes not be overlapping and be sufficiently distant from one another so that steric hindrance between two antibodies is not encountered.

A logical consequence of the last argument is that the use of the same antibody, both immobilized to Sepharose and labeled, should result in no apparent binding of the label. This is demonstrated in Fig. 20·5. When antibody 2B9 is both immobilized on the support and labeled, no radioactivity remains on the solid support after washing.

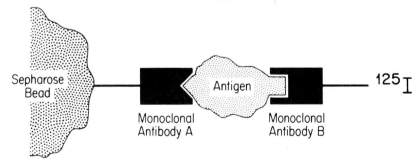

FIG. 20·4 Schematic representation of the bideterminant immunoassay utilizing two monoclonal antibodies. (From Haber *et al.* (1981). *In* "Monoclonal Antibodies in Endocrine Research". Reprinted with permission of Raven Press).

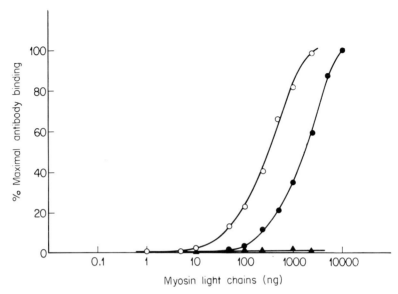

FIG. 20·5 Binding of [125]I-labeled second antibody to antigen that had first been bound to Sepharose-immobilized antibody. Percent maximal labeled antibody binding in antigen excess is plotted against the amount of cardiac- or skeletal-muscle light chain added. Skeletal-muscle light chains (●————●), cardiac-muscle light chains (O————O) measured with antibody 2B9 immobilized on Sepharose and antibody 1C5 labeled. Cardiac-muscle light chains (▲————▲) measured with antibody 2B9 immobilized on Sepharose and antibody 2B9 labeled. (From Katus, Hurrell, Matsveda *et al.* (1982) *Molecular Immunology.* Reproduced with permission from Pergamon Press.)

## V ANTIBODIES IN REVERSAL OF DRUG INTOXICATION

The digitalis glycosides are of great value in the treatment of congestive heart failure and consequently are frequently used in clinical medicine. Unfortunately, they are characterized by a very close toxic-therapeutic ratio. Digitalis intoxication is one of the most frequent adverse drug reactions reported. There is no specific antidote, and the cardiac arrythmias that are a feature of digitalis intoxication are commonly fatal.

We reasoned that if an antibody specific to the digitalis glycosides had a higher affinity for the drug than the physiologic receptor, it should be possible to transfer the ligand from the receptor to the antibody simply by mass action. For optimal effectiveness, diffusion distances should be minimal, the antibody in high concentration in extracellular fluid in proximity to the receptor. It would also be desirable to remove the antibody-drug complex rapidly from the body. Conventional antibody does not allow these goals to be satisfied.

Intact antibody has a number of troublesome properties when used as a drug. When the source is a heterologous species, it is an immunogen. After the first use, an immune response develops that may result in anaphylaxis, serum sickness, or at best accelerated elimination. Antibody is only eliminated by metabolism, with the half-life for endogenous immunoglobulins measured in days or weeks depending on the species and the immunoglobulin isotype. If immune complexes form, elimination is more rapid by the reticuloendothelial system. The presence of immune complexes may adversely affect renal function. The activation of the complement system may likewise be undesirable. The immunoglobulin molecules that bind two moles of antigen per mole be cleaved into smaller fragments by the enzyme papain (Nisonoff, 1964). The resultant Fab bind one mole of antigen each, whereas the Fc contains the complement binding site. Fab has a number of desirable properties when compared with the intact molecule, IgG: equilibrium distribution in extracellular fluid is achieved more rapidly; the volume of distribution is greater; and the fragment is eliminated with a far shorter half-life (Smith *et al.*, 1979). In addition, when injected intravenously, Fab is less immunogenic than IgG (Smith *et al.*, 1979). The immune complexes that may be formed are smaller than those that cause nephrotoxicity (comprising a single antigen molecule with several Fab attached), and complement cannot be fixed because the relevant binding sites on the Fc have been lost.

Digoxin-specific antibody was purified from sheep antiserum utilizing immobilized ouabain. Fab was then isolated after papain cleavage (Curd *et al.*, 1971). After demonstration of safety and effectiveness in animal studies, clinical investigations were initiated. At the time of this writing, 17 patients with life-threatening digitalis intoxication have been studied. The patients ranged in age from infants to septuagenarians, and in each case a dramatic reversal of the signs and symptoms of intoxication occurred (Smith *et al.*, 1976; Aeberhard *et al.*, 1980; Hess *et al.*, 1979).

The history of a recently reported patient is typical of the group (Aeberhard *et al.*, 1980). She is the 34-year-old wife of a physician who, because of marital difficulties, took 20 mg of digitoxin, a massive overdose. She appeared to be well on admission to the hospital except for nausea, but soon lapsed into a series of life-threatening arrhythmias that included multiple episodes of ventricular fibrillation (treated with countershock), as well as asystole (treated with ventricular pacing). At the time the antibody Fab became available to the physicians treating

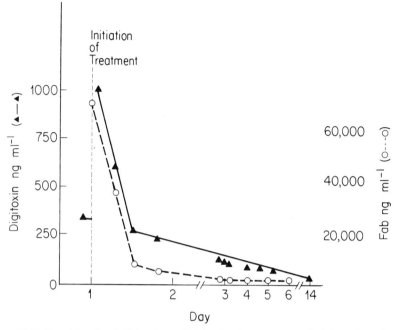

FIG. 20·6  Blood levels of digitoxin and Fab after intravenous administration of antibody Fab to a 34-year-old woman suffering a series of life-threatening arrythmias as a result of a massive overdose (20 mg) of digitoxin. Within an hour of intravenous administration of antibody Fab, atrioventricular conduction had returned. (From Haber (1981). *In* "Contributions of Chemical Biology to the Biomedical Sciences." Reprinted with permission of Academic Press).

her, she was in shock, anuric and exhibited dilated pupils. Her serum potassium was elevated, a grave prognostic sign in digitalis intoxication (Bismuth *et al.*, 1973). Within an hour after the intravenous administration of antibody Fab, her atrioventricular conduction had returned, and she was soon in normal sinus rhythm. No further dysrythmias occurred. The patient was discharged from the hospital without sequellae several days later. Fig. 20·6 demonstrates the initial marked increase of serum digitoxin concentration in this patient as tissue-bound drug equilibrated with the antibody (antibody-bound drug is pharmacologically inactive), followed by rapid clearance of both drug and Fab. It should be noted that the half-life of digitoxin in man is normally 3·5 days with hepatic metabolism of the drug being the major source of removal. It is apparent that excretion has been markedly accelerated by the antibody Fab, the half-life seemingly reduced to about 12 hours. Fig. 20·7 shows that both antibody and Fab appear in the urine largely within the first day after Fab administration.

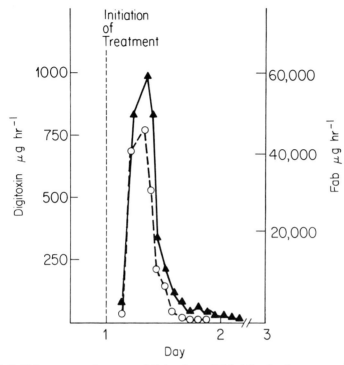

FIG. 20·7 Urinary excretion rates of digitoxin and Fab following intravenous administration of antibody Fab to a 34-year-old woman suffering from digitalis intoxication (20 mg). (From Haber (1981). *In* "Contributions of Chemical Biology to the Biomedical Sciences." (Reprinted with permission of Academic Press).

The digitalis glycosides in most common use are digoxin and digitoxin. They differ from one another very little in their chemical structure, yet most antibodies differentiate between them with differences in affinity of 50- to 100-fold as indicated in section III, above (Smith *et al.*, 1970). It would be desirable to utilize an antibody that bound both digoxin and digitoxin with equal affinity. The monoclonal antibody (26-10) described in section III, above, had an affinity of $5 \times 10^9$ for digoxin and a nearly equal affinity for digitoxin (Margolies *et al.*, 1981). Since a monoclonal antibody is a homogenous protein that recognizes only a single aspect of an antigen molecule, it appears that the hydroxyl group is not a part of the antigenic recognition site of this molecule. This antibody, which can be produced in quantities essentially without limit, has been shown to reverse digoxin intoxication in experimental animals.

It should be apparent that this approach could be applied to many other drugs or toxins. Of particular interest is the acceleration of excretion of a substance that is normally metabolized slowly. Fab is capable of altering the route of disposal from hepatic metabolism to renal excretion (Ochs and Smith, 1977).

## VI ANTIBODIES TO DRUGS AS RECEPTOR PROBES

The hormone receptors of the cell's plasma-cell membrane are present in a very small number of copies (10,000 to 50,000 per cell), which makes their isolation exceedingly difficult. Antibodies to partially purified receptor preparations have been elicited (Wrenn and Haber, 1979), but their utility is limited because these preparations of necessity contain antibodies to other membrane constituents. The ligands for these receptors, however, are usually readily available in quantity. Agonistic substances are often either peptides of modest size or organic compounds, both readily synthesized. For some receptors, a variety of antagonists has been created in the organic chemist's laboratory. Could an antibody for the receptor be obtained by utilizing the ligand (agonist or antagonist) as a template?

The vast diversity of antibody combining sites, as suggested in section II, provides the potential for creating a complementary fit to a molecule of almost any shape. If a figurative plaster mold could be cast upon the surface of the ligand that bound to the receptor, then a second mold made from the first one should have a perfect fit to the receptor. The well-known immunologic principle of raising antibodies specific for another antibody's combining site (anti-idiotypic antibodies) may be utilized as the vehicle for molding the desired shape. The first antibody must bind the ligand generally in the same way as the receptor does, and thus the same atoms and interatomic interactions must be utilized. There are two ways of achieving this short of depending on fortuitous probability. When conventional immunization is employed, many antibodies to the immunogen are formed, each binding to it in a somewhat different manner. The antibodies of this polyclonal response may be fractionated by the use of ligands of different structure. By virtue of being receptor ligands, they are all capable of binding to the receptor and must have some common structures, but if appropriately selected, structures irrelevant to binding are not shared. Those components of the polyclonal antibody mixture that bind to all possible ligands must be most similar to the receptor. The most practical way of achieving fractionation with polyclonal antibodies is sequential affinity chromatography. However, when monoclonal antibody techniques are

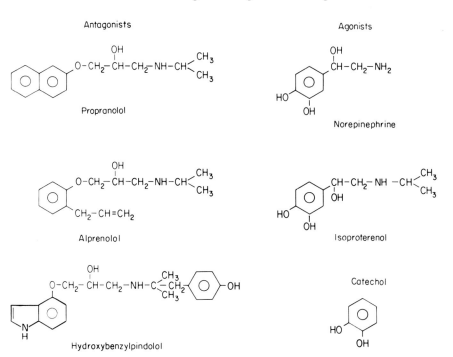

FIG. 20·8 Structures of β-antagonists and agonists. Note the common propanolamine side chain. Catechol, which is neither agonist not antagonist, does not possess this structure. (From Haber (1981). *In* "Contributions of Chemical Biology to the Biomedical Sciences." Reprinted with permission from Academic Press.)

employed, it is simply necessary to use selection techniques that will identify those antibodies that have the property of binding to all possible ligands. This general approach has now been applied to the insulin receptor (Kahn, 1976).

There is a wide variety of structurally different β-antagonists available; all, however, share a common structure, a propanolamine side chain (Fig. 20·8). Rabbits were immunized with an alprenolol-protein conjugate. The resulting antiserum was passed over an acebutolol-affinity column and the fall-through volume discarded. Elution of the affinity column was carried out with 1-propranolol and the eluant antibody characterized after the 1-propranolol had been removed by dialysis. Fig. 20·9 demonstrates the specificity profile of this antibody fraction. Several β-adrenergic antagonists as well as agonists are bound with considerable affinity, in some cases similar to that of the receptor. This fraction also resolved l and d stereoisomers of isoproterenol (not

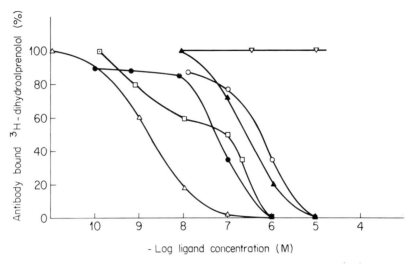

FIG. 20·9 Competitive inhibition of (-)[³H]dihydroalprenolol binding to un-fractionated anti-alprenolol antiserum. Rabbit immune serum (100 μl) was diluted 1:10 in buffer and incubated for 1 hr at 25°C with (-)[³H]dihydroalprenolol and increasing concentrations of (±)-propranolol (△), (±)-alprenolol (□), (±)-hydroxy-benzylpindolol (●), (±)-norepinephrine (O), (±)-isoproterenol (▲), or catechol (▽). Each determination was performed in triplicate and corrected for the non-specific (-)[³H]dihydroalprenolol binding to rabbit preimmune serum. The results are expressed as a percentage of the total antibody-binding capacity for the tritiated antigen. (Reprinted with permission of the American Heart Association; from Rockson *et al.*, Circulation Research, (1980). **45** 808–813.

shown). Thus the antibody fraction could be considered as a qualitative, but not a strictly precise, quantitative model for the β-adrenergic receptor. Antibodies specific for the combining sites of the first antibody set were then raised by immunization of allotypically matched rabbits. The immunogen was identical to the immunoglobulins of the recipient animals except for the variable region of the molecule. Because of tolerance to self-determinants, the immunized animals made antibodies only to unique structures of the immunogen (anti-idiotypes). Table 20·5 shows the inhibition of binding of a labeled β-adrenergic antagonist, [³H]alprenolol, to several kinds of binding sites by the anti-idiotypic antibody. Binding of the ligand, alprenolol, to the idiotype (the first-generation antibody that had been raised in response to alprenolol) is largely inhibited by anti-idiotype (second-generation antibody). Of greater interest is the inhibition of the specific binding of alprenolol to plasma-membrane preparation of several different organs in two different animal species. Scatchard analysis shows the binding of the anti-idiotype to be competitive with β-adrenergic antagonists. The

TABLE 20·5
Inhibition of [³H]alprenolol binding to antibodies and receptors by
anti-idiotypic antibody*

| | Maximal binding with preimmune (dpm) | In presence of anti-idotype (dpm) | Inhibition (%) |
|---|---|---|---|
| Original idiotype (alprenolol) | 10853 ± 250 | 488 ± 250 | 96% |
| Turkey erythrocyte | 19643 ± 540 | 6195 ± 525 | 68% |
| Canine lung | 6385 ± 283 | 4315 ± 190 | 34% |

\* Specific binding at 4-6nM [³H]alprenolol
(From Haber (1982) *Antibodies in vivo*. Reprinted with permission from The American Society for Pharmacology and Experimental Therapeutics).

anti-idiotype also appears to be an inhibitor of adenylate cyclase activation by $\beta$-adrenergic agonists. Increasing concentrations of isoproterenol progressively inhibit adenylate cyclase production in turkey erythrocyte membranes at an isoproterenol concentration of $5 \times 10^{-7}$ M. At a higher concentration of isoproterenol ($10^{-4}$ M), less inhibition is observed, suggesting a competitive nature for this interaction as well. Thus the anti-idiotype behaves as a true $\beta$-adrenergic antagonist, competing with both agonists and antagonists for the receptor site. The obvious potential uses of such receptor-specific antibodies are: the recognition of structural differences among subsets of $\beta$-adrenergic receptors (Burges and Blackburn, 1972); a more rigorous examination of their respective physiologic roles utilizing reagents of greater resolution; and the isolation of receptors with antibody affinity chromatography.

## VII ANTIBODIES AS DRUGS

The development of a new drug is often the result of empiricism, serendipity, or the deliberate modification of an existing natural product. These products of the organic chemist's laboratory are usually characterized by a lack of specificity with a consequent abundance of adverse reactions. If antibodies were the basis of identification of a specific locus of action, one could choose among some $10^{11}$ different combining sites and thus markedly increase the potential for reacting only with the desired site. Specificity would be enhanced and side reactions diminished. The considerably larger size of the antibody combining site in comparison with conventional drugs allows for the establishment of a larger number of interatomic interactions and thus both greater affinity and specificity. While some of the advantages of antibodies are obvious, the disadvantages, discussed in part in previous sections, must also be considered. When binding to a specific site is all that is desired, the activation of the biological effects that are an intrinsic part of an immune reaction is undesirable. The smaller Fab that was discussed above as a possible solution to some of these problems still carries with it an entire domain (one half of its mass) that is of no relevance to antigen binding. Fab from a heterologous species, while of diminished immunogenicity, is likely to cause hypersensitivity when used on a long-term basis.

The solutions to these problems are almost at hand. A much smaller fragment of antibody has been produced that retains all the binding energy and specificity of the intact molecule. Fv comprises a single domain and has a molecular size of 25,000 daltons (Hochman *et al.*, 1976). While the pharmacokinetics of Fv have not as yet been examined, I anticipate that this fragment will be very rapidly cleared and distributed. The advent of the hybridoma method will make possible not only the selection and large-scale production of antibodies of uniform properties, but also the reduction or elimination of the potential problem of hypersensitivity since it will be possible, as indicated above, to produce human antibodies. Will the formation of anti-idiotypic antibodies defeat the long-term utility of antibody therapy? I believe that the well-recognized difficulty in raising anti-idiotypes, even when the effort is undertaken with deliberation, indicates that this problem will rarely manifest itself. The next decade will see a new pharmacology based on the antibody combining site.

REFERENCES

Aeberhard, P., Butler, V. P., Smith, T. W., Haber, E., Tse Eng, D., Brau, J., Chalom, A., Glatt, B., Thebaut, J. F., Delangenhagen, B. and Morin, B. (1980). *Arch. Mal. Coeur.* **73**, 1471–78.
Bismuth, C., Gaultier, M., Conso, F. and Efthymiou, M. L. (1973). *Clin. Toxicol.* **6** 153–162.
Brack, C., Hirama, M., Lenhard-Schuller, R., Tonegawa, S. (1978). *Cell* **15** 1–14.
Burges, R. A., Blackburn, K. J. (1972). *Nature New Biol.* **235** 249–50.
Butler, V. P. Jr., Schmidt, D. H., Smith, T. W., Haber, E., Raynor, B. D. and Demartini, P. (1977a) *J. clin. Invest.* **59**, 345–59.
Butler, V. P. Jr., Smith, T. W., Schmidt, D. H. and Haber, E. (1977b) *Fed. Proc.* **36**, 2235–41.
Croce, C. M., Linnenbach, A., Hall, W., Steplewski, Z. and Koprowski, H. (1980). *Nature* **288**, 488–489.

Curd, J., Smith, T. W., Jaton, J-C., and Haber, E. (1971). *Proc. natn. Acad. Sci. U.S.A.* **68**, 2401–6.

Early, P., Huang, H., Davis, M., Calame, K. and Hood, L. (1980). *Cell* **19**, 981–992.

Fieser, L. F., and Fieser, M. (1959). *In* "Steroids". pp. 727–809. Reinhold Publishing Corp, New York.

Fullerton, D. S., Yoshioka, K., Rohrer, D. C., From, A. H. L., and Ahmed, K. (1979). *Science* **205**, 917–919.

Haber, E., Katus, H. A., Hurrell, J. G., Matsueda, G. R., Ehrlich, P., Zurawski, V. Jr., and Khaw, B. A. *In* "Monoclonal Hybridoma Antibodies: Techniques and Applications." CRC Uniscience (in press).

Hess, T., Stucki, P., Barandun, J., Scholtysik, G. and Riesen, W. (1979). *Am. Heart J.* **98**, 767.

Hochman, J., Inbar, D., and Givol, D. (1976). *Biochemistry* **12** 1130–35.

Kahn, C. R. (1976). *J. Cell Biol.* **70**, 261–286.

Katus, H. A., Hurrell, J., Ehrlich, P., Zurawski, V., Khaw, B. A., Bahar, I. and Haber E. (1980). (Abstract). *Circulation* **62**, (Suppl III) 216.

Khaw, B. A., Gold, H. K., Fallon, J. T., and Haber, E. (1978). *Circulation* **58** 1130–1136.

Khaw, B. A., Fallon, J. T., Katus, H., Elmaleh, D., Strauss, H. W., Locke, E., Pohost, G. M., and Haber, E. (1979). *Circulation* **59–60**, (Suppl II) 135.

Khaw, B. A., Fallon, J. T., Strauss, H. W., and Haber, E. (1980) *Science* **209** 295–297.

Köhler, G. and Milstein, C. (1975). *Nature* **256**, 495.

Landsteiner, K. (1944) "The Specificity of Serological Reactions". (revised edition). Cambridge, MA: Harvard University Press.

Margolies, M. N., Mudgett-Hunter, M., Novotny, J. and Haber, E. 1981 *In* "Monoclonal Antibodies and T Cell Hybridomas". (Hammerling, G., Hammerling, U., Kearney, J. F., Eds) Elsevier/North-Holland, Amsterdam.

Mudgett-Hunter, M., Margolies, M. N., Rosen, E. M. and Haber, E. (1980) (Abstract). *Fed Proc.* **39**, 928.

Nisonoff, A. (1964). *Methods Med. Res.* **10**, 134–141.

Ochs, H. R. and Smith, T. W. (1977). *J. Clin. Invest.* **60** 1303.

Olsson, L. and Kaplan, H. S. (1980). *Proc. natn. Acad. Sci. U.S.A.* **77** 629–631.

Oparil, S., Tregear, G. W., Haber, E. (1972). *In* "Protein and Polypeptide Hormones" (Margolies, M. and Greenwood, F. C. Eds) Proceedings of the 2nd International Symposium. pp. 262–266. Leige, Belgium.

Oparil, S. and Haber, E. (1974). *N. Engl. J. Med.* **291**, 389–401, 446–457.

Sakano, H., Kurosawa, Y., Weigert, M., and Tonegawa, S. (1981). *Nature* **290**, 562–570.

Seidman, J. G., Leder, A., Nau, M., Norman, B. and Leder, P. (1978). *Science* **202**, 11–17.

Seidman, J. G., Max, E. E., and Leder, P. (1979). *Nature* **280**, 370–375.

Smith, T. W., Butler, V. P. Jr., and Haber, E. (1969). *N. Engl. J. Med.* **281**, 1212–16.

Smith, T. W., Butler, V. P. Jr., and Haber, E. (1970). *Biochemistry* **9** 331–337.

Smith, T. W., Haber, E., Yeatman, L. and Butler, V. P. Jr. (1976) *N. Engl. J. Med.* **294**, 797–800.

Smith, T. W., Lloyd, B. L ., Spicer, N, and Haber, E. (1979) *Clin, exp. Immunol.* **36**, 384–96.

Trahern, C. A., Gere, J. B., Krauth, G. and Bigham, D. A. (1978). *Am. J. Cardiol.* **41**, 641–45.

Weigert, M., Gatmaitan, L., Loh, E., Schilling, J. and Hood, L. (1978). *Nature* **276**, 785–790.

Wrenn, S., and Haber, E. (1979). *J. Biol. Chem.* **254**, 6577–82.

# I   PRACTICAL ASPECTS

# 21 Production of Monoclonal Antibodies: a practical guide

Judy M. Bastin,[a] Jean Kirkley[b] and
Andrew J. McMichael[a]

a   *Nuffield Department of Medicine*
b   *Nuffield Department of Surgery, John Radcliffe Hospital, Oxford. OX3 9DU*

## I INTRODUCTION

The aim of this chapter is to describe a method for the production of hybridomas. The approach will be didactic. No two laboratories use exactly the same technique and many of these variations are based on empirical observations. This implies that there is much flexibility possible in the method. There are, however, some common problems and these will be highlighted.

## II PLANNING

Before starting it is necessary to attend to several questions. The first is whether monoclonal antibodies are appropriate for the problem being tackled. Despite our own enthusiasm for the technique, there is still a place for conventional antisera. The rest of this book is a testament to the advantages of monoclonal antibodies and it is appropriate to mention some of the disadvantages. They can be expensive and time consuming to produce; they may be too specific, for instance seeing the "wrong" site on an antigen; they may bind to the epitope with low affinity; they may be of the wrong isotype—IgG1 for instance does not fix complement and is therefore not cytotoxic; mouse antibodies may have disadvantages for therapeutic purposes (see chapter 2).

The cost of the procedure is important to consider. In well equipped laboratories in the John Radcliffe Hospital, Oxford, in 1982, we estimate that one individual working full time on hybrid myelomas will require, in addition to salary, £3,000 per year for consumable expenses, i.e. tissue culture plastics, tissue culture medium, foetal calf serum, $CO_2$ for the incubator, liquid $N_2$ for storage, radioisotopes for immunoassays and mice. These costs apply to laboratories where several workers are involved in hybridoma technology. Working in isolation, the costs might be higher.

The "strike rate" is hard to predict and requires an element of luck as well as expertise and hard work. As a rough guide, we estimate that it takes most people about three months to establish the method to the stage where antibodies are regularly being generated. Some antibodies are relatively easy to produce; in our experience, the most difficult are those specific for rare antigenic determinants on the cell surface such as those that define T lymphocyte subpopulations or the polymorphisms of HLA antigens. In these examples, the strike rate is between one and three per year per full time worker.

The heavy equipment needed is listed in Table 21·1. The $CO_2$ incubator, sterile hood or work station, inverted (phase) microscope and liquid nitrogen storage facility are essential. In addition, access to laboratory mice is needed. These facilities can be shared by more than one worker and in our laboratory we have three hybridoma specialists sharing two hoods, one incubator and one inverted microscope. Attention must be paid to local regulations regarding safety procedures. In the United Kingdom, continuously growing mouse myeloma cell lines and hybridomas are not considered to constitute any special hazard, but it is necessary for users of animals to have the appropriate certificate and licence from the Home Office.

TABLE 21·1
Equipment needed for generation of hybridomas

| | | |
|---|---|---|
| Major items | – $CO_2$—37°C incubator | |
| | Lamina flow hood or work station | |
| | Inverted phase microscope | |
| | Liquid $N_2$ storage tank | |
| | Low speed centrifuge | |
| Access to | – Refrigerator | |
| | −20°C freezer | |
| | −70°C freezer | |
| | Animal facility | |
| Small items | – Micropipettes | |
| | Millipore filters | |
| | 37°C water bath | |
| Consumable items | – Sterile tissue culture plastics: | microtitre 96-well trays (flat bottom) |
| | | 24-well trays |
| | | 25 cm² flasks |
| | | petri dishes |

Before starting, it is essential to devise a suitable assay procedure because rapid efficient screening of culture supernatants is vital. The importance of defining the assay system chosen cannot be over-emphasized.

## III SCREENING ASSAYS

It is beyond the scope of this chapter to give a comprehensive review of antibody screening techniques. The method chosen will obviously depend on the antigen; available techniques range from the measurement of antibody binding to individual target cells in the fluorescence activated cell sorter to virus neutralization. Immunofluorescence and immunoperoxidase techniques, which can both be used for screening, are discussed in chapters 23 and 24 and will not be discussed further here.

Radioimmuno binding assays are particularly useful and can be adapted for use with cells, tissue homogenates, micro organisms or soluble protein antigens. For cells, such as lymphocytes, we use the following procedure which can readily be used to screen over 100 culture supernatants.

Cells, 50 $\mu$l at $10^7$ ml$^{-1}$ suspended in phosphate buffered saline pH 7·4 (PBS) containing 0·5% bovine serum albumin (BSA), are dispensed into 4 cm plastic tubes. An equal volume of culture supernatant (antibody) is added to each tube. After incubation for one hour at 4°C the cells are washed by adding 1·5 ml PBS-0·1% BSA and centrifuged at 1000 × g for five minutes; the supernatant is removed and this process is repeated once. In a volume of 100 $\mu$l in PBS 0·5% BSA, radioiodinated ($^{125}$I) second antibody—anti mouse immunoglobulin (see below) is then added to each tube. After incubation for one hour, the cells are washed as before and then bound antibody is measured in a gamma counter.

For protein antigens, we add 50 $\mu$l antigen at a protein concentration of 0·1–1·0 mg ml$^{-1}$ in protein free PBS to the wells of a flexible plastic microtitre tray. Protein sticks to the negatively charged plastic surface. After overnight incubation at 4°C the solution is harvested (and can be reused) and 100 $\mu$l PBS-0·5% BSA is added to each well to saturate the plastic "sites" and the plate is incubated for a further hour at 4°C. The plate is then washed with PBS-0·1% BSA three times and the monoclonal antibody added, as a culture supernatant, in a volume of 50 $\mu$l. After one hour the plate is washed with PBS-0·1% BSA three times and the radio-labelled anti mouse immunoglobulin (see below) is added in PBS-0·5% BSA. After a further one hour, the wells are washed three times with PBS-0·1% BSA, cut out and counted in a gamma counter.

The quality of the second antibody is critical. The ideal reagent should be made in a rabbit, sheep or goat against mouse IgG F(ab)₂. The antiserum is first passed over an affinity column of mouse IgG F(ab)₂ coupled to sepharose beads. Specific antibody is eluted at low pH and immediately neutralized. The pure antibody can then be digested with pepsin and the F(ab)₂ fragment of antibody separated by a gel filtration on sephadex G200 or sephacryl S200. Aliquots of 25 $\mu$g of antibody are iodinated with 1mCi $^{125}$iodine by the chloramine T method and the reagent is diluted in PBS-0·5% BSA to a final dilution of approximately 3 × $10^6$ cpm per ml (about 0·125 $\mu$g antibody per ml) before use. A detailed description of these steps is given by Jensenius and Williams (1974) and Morris and Williams (1975).

There are preparations of iodinated F(ab)₂ anti mouse F(ab)₂ available commercially (e.g. Amersham International). An alternative is to use affinity column purified IgG without digestion but there is a theoretical disadvantage that some Fc binding may occur with certain types of target cell. Another alternative is to use radio iodinated protein A as the second reagent although antibodies of IgM and IgG1 isotypes may be missed.

## IV IMMUNIZATION

Spleens are normally taken from hyperimmunized mice three or four days after the last injection of antigen. It is advisable to "prime" a few mice as soon as the decision to make hybridomas is taken.

The choice of immunization procedure depends on the antigen. Most laboratories have their own protocols; that shown in Table 21·2 is intended only as a guide. Some laboratories only give one injection of antigen, when the spleen should be taken slightly later, on day 5 or 6. Balb/c mice are normally used so that the hybrid myeloma, derived from a Balb/c plasmacytoma, can be grown in syngeneic animals; ascitic tumours grow particularly well in this strain. Apart from this, there is no reason why other mouse strains should not be used.

For some studies there is a choice to be made between using intact cells or purified antigens as immunogens (e.g. see Chapter 14). A decision has to be taken between spending time purifying the antigen and then obtaining the relevant hybridomas relatively easily, or spending the time looking for the one hybridoma that makes the required antibody out of several hundred. One of the major advances offered by this technique is that the second approach is possible, and given a good screening procedure, often preferable. It is therefore possible to make antibodies to individual antigens on, for instance cell surfaces, which are not even known to exist.

TABLE 21·2
Immunization procedures

---

*Soluble antigen*:
Day   1 – 100 μg subcutaneous (s/c) in Freunds Complete Adjuvant
        28 – 100 μg s/c in Freunds Incomplete Adjuvant
Leave or repeat every three months until mouse required
        4–5 days before fusion:   100 μg IV
*Cell antigens*:
Day   1 – 5 × $10^6$ washed cells in buffered saline i-p
        28 – 1–5 × $10^6$ washed cells in buffered saline i-p
Leave or repeat every three months until mouse required
        4–5 days before fusion:   1–5 × $10^6$ cells IV

---

A problem that we have found more than once is that if the antigen is denatured e.g. by fixing cells with glutaraldehyde, it is possible to make antibody specific for the denatured material. This type of antibody is unlikely to be useful.

A technique that is often discussed when the production of monoclonal antibodies to cell surface antigens is considered, is to coat the cells with antibodies to "unwanted" determinants to mask those antigens and therefore increase the likelihood of making the hybridoma monoclonal antibody specific for the rare antigens. This method has been used successfully in conventional serology. However, if monoclonal antibodies are used to coat the cells, it is theoretically as likely that these will enhance the immune response to the same antigen because not all sites are covered. Our preference, therefore, is to keep immunization procedures simple.


## V CELL CULTURE TECHNIQUE

The meticulous reader is referred to the excellent book by Paul (1975) on general cell culture techniques. The following is meant as a guide for those who prefer to learn as they go, sometimes by their mistakes. Although an advantage, previous experience in cell culture is not necessary and many groups have taught themselves how to grow hybridomas. It is very useful to make contact with a local laboratory with experience, to discuss how to deal with problems, exchange reagents etc.

The principal problem is that of sterility. Most workers add antibiotics to their culture medium so that bacterial contamination with the notable exception of mycoplasma (see below) rarely causes trouble. Yeast and fungi can present problems. Yeast probably comes from fingers and possibly clothing. Other fungi probably come from the air, other contaminated cultures or dirty incubators. Mycoplasma probably most often originates from contaminated cell lines, but may come from the operator.

No-touch technique and clean work cabinets and incubators are essential. Sterile disposable plasticware is normally used in preference to washed glassware. Disposable plastic pipettes and syringes are used to dispense medium and cells. For handling small volumes, micropipettes and multipipettes are invaluable, although their tips must be autoclaved. Millipore filters are useful for sterilizing solutions (e.g. HAT) and "suspect" medium.

Occasional bottles of "sterile" medium from the large suppliers are contaminated and it is advisable to test these by storage at room temperature for 24 hours or at 4° for at least a week before use.

Antibiotics, penicillin and streptomycin, or gentamycin, are added to the culture medium in most laboratories, though some feel that it encourages sloppy technique and the growth of mycoplasma.

## VI GROWTH OF CELL LINES

P3-NS1/1Ag4·1 (NS1) is the myeloma cell line most often used. It is available commercially (Flow Laboratories). The principles involved in growing this line apply not only to the other myeloma cell lines but to the hybridoma lines and will be discussed in detail.

NS1 is grown normally in RPMI-1640 medium (Flow Laboratories or Gibco Biocult) containing 10% foetal calf serum (heat inactivated and virus and mycoplasma screened). The medium is buffered by bicarbonate and, in a 5% $CO_2$-air mixture, maintains a pH of $7 \cdot 2 - 7 \cdot 4$. The medium contains phenol red as an indicator such that the correct colour is orange. Growing cells lower the pH changing the colour to yellow. The medium contains all the essential amino acids and cofactors but as glutamine deteriorates with time, it is usual to add fresh (i.e. from frozen stock) glutamine immediately on opening a bottle (Table 21·3).

NS1 and hybridomas grow in suspension and under optimal conditions divide every 14–20 hours. The optimal cell density is around $2 \times 10^5$ cell $ml^{-1}$ but they do grow happily at densities in the range of $5 \times 10^4$ to $1 \times 10^6$ $ml^{-1}$. If a flask is seeded at $10^5$ $ml^{-1}$, it can be safely left for 48 hours. At higher densities, cells die and the cultured cells look "granular" under the inverted phase microscope. With experience, the colour of the culture becomes an invaluable guide: yellow-orange is all right but daffodil-yellow is too acid. NS1 cultures must be attended to every 2 (possibly 3) days by adding fresh medium to bring the cell concentration down to approximately $5 \times 10^4$ $ml^{-1}$ or by discarding a fraction of the cells and then adding medium back to the original volume. If the medium has been allowed to become too yellow, most of the medium will have to be changed. NS1 cells are normally grown in 25$cm^2$ disposable plastic flasks, kept on their side in a gassed (5% $CO_2$) incubator with the cap loose (or gassed individually with 5% $CO_2$-air and kept with the cap closed tight).

NS1 should be checked periodically for HAT sensitivity by attempting to grow a subculture in HAT medium (see below); if growth occurs, stock culture should be grown in the presence of $10^{-4}M$ 8-azaguanine or discarded.

## TABLE 21·3
## Media and Chemicals

*Media*
Unless otherwise stated reagents may be purchased from Gibco Biocult Ltd. or Flow Laboratories Ltd.

*RPMI 1640*
RPMI 1640 with bicarbonate buffer is supplemented with
   (i)   potassium benzyl penicillin (Glaxo) 100 U ml$^{-1}$
   (ii)  streptomycin sulphate (Glaxo) 100 $\mu$g ml$^{-1}$
   (iii) L-Glutamine 300 mgl$^{-1}$ (300 $\mu$g ml$^{-1}$)
This basic medium is converted to selective HAT medium by addition of
   (i)   Hypoxanthine (Sigma) and Thymidine (Gibco Biocult) (100 × strength).
         To 408 mg hypoxanthine add 100 ml distilled water and then 1M sodium
         hydroxide dropwise until crystals dissolve. Thymidine, 114 mg, dissolves readily
         in 100 ml distilled water. Combine hypoxanthine and thymidine solutions and
         make up to 300 ml with distilled water. Adjust pH to 10·0 with acetic acid,
         millipore filter, aliquot and store at −20°C.
   (ii)  Aminopterin (Methotrexate Sodium, Lederle) (100 × strength).
         To 454 mg Methotrexate add 50 ml distilled water followed by 1M sodium
         hydroxide dropwise until dissolved. Make volume up to 1 litre and adjust pH to
         7·5. Millipore filter, aliquot and store at −20°C.
To make single strength HAT RPMI add 1 ml of 100 × strength hypoxanthine and
thymidine and 1 ml of 100 × concentrated aminopterin stock solutions to 100 ml RPMI
1640. Double these volumes should be added to make double strength HAT RPMI
1640 for addition to fusion plates on Day 1.

*Foetal calf serum*
RPMI 1640 and RPMI 1640/HAT is supplemented with heat inactivated, virus-
mycoplasma screened foetal calf serum (FCS) as necessary.

*Polyethylene glycol* (BDH)
The solid polyethylene glycol 1500 is autoclaved and a 50% solution made with
serum-free RPMI 1640 medium. This is stored at 4°C and will become quite alkaline;
this does not affect the fusion efficiency.

*2 Mercapto Ethanol* (2ME—Sigma)
Prepared at 10$^{-3}$M in RPMI 1640. Use at a final concentration of 10$^{-4}$M in cloning
plates, millipore filtering medium before use.

*Dimethyl Sulphoxide* (Sigma)
Used at a final concentration of 5% DMSO in 95% foetal calf serum, as freezing
mixture.

*8-azaguanine (Koch-Light Ltd.)*
100 × stock solution at 10$^{-2}$M. This may be added to RPMI 1640 in which NS1 is
grown to ensure that HAT sensitivity is maintained.

*Pristane* (Tetramethyl pentadecane) (Pierce and Warriner (UK) Ltd.)
0·5 ml is injected intraperitoneally to each mouse.

Hybridoma cell cultures are initially grown in HAT medium (Table 21·3) and can be weaned off this if desired; in our experience, however, it is easier to maintain them indefinitely in this medium.

## VII FUSION

The mouse is boosted with antigen, intravenously if possible, four or five days before the planned fusion. NS1 cells are grown so that at least $1 \times 10^7$ cells are available.

Table 21·4 gives a check list of the equipment needed for the fusion stage. The procedure itself is described below in stepwise order.

1.  The mouse is killed.
2.  Its spleen is removed using non sterile instruments to cut the skin, which may be washed in ethanol, and sterile scissors and forceps to open the peritoneum and remove the spleen.
3.  The spleen is placed in a petri dish containing 5 ml of RPMI-1640 (no serum added) and cut in half. The cells are then teased out using sterile instruments.
4.  These cells are pipetted into a sterile plastic tube and the clumps allowed to settle over five minutes. The cells are then transferred to a second sterile tube and centrifuged at 300 × g for ten minutes.
5.  In the same centrifuge $10^7$ NS1 cells, which have been washed free of foetal calf serum, are pelleted.
6.  The two pellets are resuspended in 5 ml RPMI-1640 (no serum added), mixed together and recentrifuged at 300 × g for ten minutes.

TABLE 21·4
Fusion check list

| | |
|---|---|
| 1. | Immunized mouse |
| 2. | NS1 cells (at least $10^7$) |
| 3. | One sterile petri dish |
| 4. | 4 24 × 2 ml culture plates or 6 96 × 0·2 ml microtitre plates |
| 5. | 3 15 ml sterile plastic centrifuge tubes |
| 6. | Sterile 1 ml and 10 ml pipettes or<br>    1 ml and 30 ml graduated syringes and needles |
| 7. | Sterile Pasteur pipettes |
| 8. | Sterile instruments: scissors and forceps |
| 9. | Non sterile scissors and forceps |
| 10. | 100–200 ml RPMI 1640 |
| 11. | 10–30 ml FCS |
| 12. | 37°C water bath or beaker of water at 37°C |

(Note that we assume there to be $10^8$ splenic lymphocytes recoverable and aim at a 10:1 ratio of lymphocytes to NS1 cells. Some workers do count the spleen cells after lysing red cells, and adjust the number of NS1 cells accordingly.)

7.    The tube is tapped gently to disrupt the pellets and the tube placed in a 37°C water bath (or beaker of 37°C warm water).

8.    Prewarmed 50% polyethylene glycol (PEG) and RPMI-1640 (no serum) are brought to the culture area.

9.    0·8 of 50% PEG are added dropwise to the cell pellet (approximately $1·1 \times 10^8$ cells) over one minute, keeping all at 37°C.

10.    2 ml prewarmed RPMI-1640 (no serum) are added, starting immediately, dropwise over two minutes; then 8 ml are added over a further three minutes.

11.    The cells are then spun at $300 \times g$ for ten minutes. They are gently resuspended in the required volume of RPMI-1640-20% FCS and plated out.

Various plating out procedures are favoured by different workers. We use either four $24 \times 2$ ml well plates (i.e. $96 \times 1$ ml medium for 96 wells) or $6 \times 96 \times 0·2$ ml well (flat bottomed) microtitre plates (i.e. $576 \times 0·1$ ml $= 57·6$ ml medium for plating out) or a combination of the two. The smaller wells have the advantage that most wells in which cultures grow will contain only one colony (often equalling a clone) of hybrid cells, but the disadvantage that the volume of supernatant available for assay is small.

12.    The plates are placed at 37°C in 5% $CO_2$-air in the incubator, either open, if it is humidified, or in a sealed, gassed, sandwich box.

13.    24 hours later, an equal volume of RPMI-1640-2XHAT-20% FCS is added to each well.

The plates are then left to stand in the incubator until colonies appear.


# VIII EARLY HYBRIDOMA CULTURES

Colonies appear in the culture wells, visible to the naked eye, after 6 to 10 days. They can be seen much earlier using the inverted phase microscope.

No action is required until the colonies are about 2–3 mm in diameter, when the supernatant needs to be screened for antibody activity. In a good fusion in 24-well plates, every culture will need to be tested; in the microtitre plates, about half will carry colonies, but we normally screen only those with single colonies. It is essential to have a good assay procedure already established so that rapid decisions can be taken for each culture well.

Cultures grown in 2 ml or 0·2 ml wells may be fed at this stage, when growth becomes rapid, but there is a danger of disturbing the discrete colonies.

Having identified the culture wells which contain hybridoma cells suitable for further study, we transfer the colony or colonies separately from these wells, using sterile Pasteur pipettes to pick them out, into wells of a new flat bottomed microtitre tray. To each well is added 0·1 ml of normal mouse spleen cells, $2 \times 10^6$/ml in RPMI/10% FCS/2 Mercaptoethanol (2ME) $10^{-4}$M, which act as feeders and encourage growth of the hybridoma cells. These cultures are then observed daily, with the inverted phase microscope, and when they reach confluence over the bottom of the well (24–48 hrs) they are transferred in fresh HAT RPMI-10% FCS to 2 ml wells, again with a vast excess of feeder cells ($2 \times 10^6$ per well). Once growing in this plate the cells may be seeded without feeders, into 25 cm² flasks and the supernatant is assayed to ensure that it is still producing the antibody. The culture may then be cloned by limiting dilution. This can normally be done within one week of first identifying a culture as "interesting".

## IX CLONING

There is no guarantee that a culture which appears as a single colony in the fusion plate is in fact monoclonal. When there are two colonies in the plate, even when far apart and carefully picked out, some mixing of cells must occur. It is therefore essential to clone all cultures. This must be done as early as possible to avoid overgrowth of irrelevant colonies. (A minority of hybridoma colonies actually secrete identifiable antibody). This may happen in the first few days of the life of the culture, but if the colony gets to the stage described above, still secreting antibody, there is an excellent (>95%) chance of recovering the clone and establishing it in long term culture.

Cloning is usually carried out by a limiting dilution method on spleen cell feeders. We use 96 well flat bottomed microtitre plates, seeded with 0·1 ml of mouse spleen feeder cells—$2 \times 10^6$ ml$^{-1}$ in HAT-RPMI 1640-10% FCS-2ME ($10^{-4}$M). The hybridoma cells are diluted to a concentration of 600 cells ml$^-$ and eight doubling dilutions made from this suspension. From each dilution 0·1 ml is added to each of 12 wells of a row in the plate. In this way a range of cell concentrations from 60 to

0·5 cells per well is used. The plate is then observed until colonies appear, normally 7–14 days, and then 6 of the wells that received the fewest hybridoma cells and show single clones are screened for antibody production. Those positive are grown up as described above for the original colony, first on feeders in a new microtitre plate, then to a 2 ml well and then to a 25 cm² flask. They are maintained in HAT RPMI-1640-10% FCS throughout but can be weaned off the 2ME once growing well.

To be rigorous, the process of cloning should be repeated at least two more times, preferably only dispensing one cell per well and calculating the probability of clone being derived from a single cell by the Poisson formula.

In practice, cloning is normally carried out only to ensure that the hybrid myeloma cell line remains stable; we have never observed artefacts in assays arising because of the presence of two antibodies in culture fluid or ascites. Provided uncloned cell stock is stored frozen, so that the line can be cloned again if necessary, and the quality of the antibody is regularly checked, a single cloning procedure is probably adequate.


## X FREEZING HYBRIDOMA CULTURES

At the same time as, or shortly after, cloning it is advisable to freeze down a few (1-5 × 10⁶) cells as an insurance against accidents. The uncloned colony should be grown up in 25 cm² flasks while the cloning plate is incubating and several ampoules of uncloned cells should be frozen (provided they are still producing antibody). When the clone is growing well and in sufficient quantities, freezing again has a high priority.

Freezing mixture is prepared by adding dimethyl sulphoxide (DMSO) dropwise to ice cold foetal calf serum with shaking, to a final concentration of 10% DMSO. The solution is then cooled back to 4°C on ice. The cells are spun down at 300 × g in a cold centrifuge and resuspended at 5 × 10⁶ ml⁻¹ in neat cold foetal calf serum.

An equal volume of the cold freezing mixture is added, with shaking, to the cold cells and 1 ml aliquots pipetted into sterile freezing ampoules. These should be immediately either frozen down in a controlled rate freezer at 1° per minute, or simply placed in a polystyrene box in a −70°C freezer overnight. The following day these ampoules are transferred from the freezer to the gas phase of a liquid nitrogen storage tank.

Controlled rate freezing probably gives higher viability although the simpler method normally gives us cells more than 90% viable. We have also been able to store cells for more than 28 days at $-70°C$ and have still recovered viable hybridomas. (Note that there is some flexibility here because, although not desirable, it is possible to recover clones from frozen stock with very poor viability.)

Frozen cells are thawed by warming at $37°C$ until only a tiny piece of ice remains in the suspension and then 5 ml of ice cold (HAT—RPMI 1640-10% FCS is added dropwise with shaking. The cells are then washed twice by centrifugation and resuspended at $2 \times 10^5$ cells ml$^{-1}$ ready for culture. With valuable clones, it is advisable to thaw and regrow from frozen ampoules a few days after the initial freezing, to check that the stock is safe. It is also advisable to store a few ampoules of precious clones in someone else's liquid $N_2$ storage tank to guard against accidents!

## XI ASCITES

Large amounts of monoclonal antibody (1-10 mg ml$^{-1}$ with titres in excess of $10^{-5}$) can be generated by growing the hybridoma as an ascitic tumour in Balb/c mice.

Repeated intraperitoneal injection of mineral oil, pristane, induces myelomas in Balb/c mice. Single injections of pristane appear to create a favourable environment for the growth of myelomas and hybridomas. Balb/c mice are therefore given a single $0·5$ ml intra-peritoneal injection of pristane at least one week before injection of the hybridoma cells is planned. Although some workers give it only hours before the hybridoma cells with apparent success, it is a good policy to keep a continuous stock of 10-20 pristane primed mice ready in the animal house.

Cloned hybridoma cells do not need to be weaned off HAT before injection and we normally inoculate $1-5 \times 10^6$ cells intraperitoneally as soon as the clone is growing in sufficient numbers. The mice are watched daily for abdominal swelling and when this appears they are tapped by inserting a 19g needle. Ascitic fluid is withdrawn. We normally kill the mice before tapping but it is possible to tap repeatedly from anaesthetized mice for several days and so enhance the yield of fluid.

Ascitic fluid should be centrifuged and stored with sodium azide added to $0·02\%$. Most ascitic fluids store well at $-20°C$ or at $4°C$ but IgM antibodies are better kept unfrozen.

Ascitic tumours may be transferred to pristane treated mice but the antibody titre of the ascitic fluid should be checked carefully at each generation.


## XII TROUBLESHOOTING

Several problems may arise and we list the commoner ones, all of which we have suffered, together with suggested solutions.

1.  *Bacterial infection*: The culture should be discarded and stock bottles such as RPMI 1640 and foetal calf serum cultured to identify the contaminant and its source.

2.  *Yeast infection*: The whole culture should be discarded and stock bottles checked.

3.  *Fungal infection*: This sometimes occurs in isolated wells, in which case the offending wells can be cleaned out with 70% ethanol several times. The plate should be isolated in a sandwich box and observed daily; if repeated infection occurs the plate may have to be discarded.

4.  *Fungal infection in incubator*: This can be avoided if infected cultures are cleared out immediately they are identified. If it does occur it can be very difficult to eradicate. One drastic but effective solution is to clean the incubator with a bleach-detergent mixture which is effective, but as long as a smell of chlorine persists (up to four weeks) cells will not grow!

5.  *Mycoplasma infection*: This is insidious and NS1 cells can be contaminated yet superficially appear to grow normally. In fact, their doubling time is slowed. The infection usually manifests itself as a failure of hybrids to grow after an apparently successful fusion. If this happens, it is advisable to assume mycoplasma infection in the NS1 cells and to arrange for them to be checked. In the meantime it is best to return to frozen NS1 stock, prepare new reagents and to try again. This usually solves the problem. It is fortunately only rarely necessary to clear out all cultures and clean the incubator. The problem can be largely avoided if only clean cell lines are used and particular care is paid to long term cultures such as NS1 and other cell lines such as human lymphoblastoid lines that may be sharing the incubator.

6.  *Hybrids will not grow*: This is strongly suggestive of mycoplasma infection and the procedure outlined above should be followed.

7.  *Hybrids cease to secrete antibody*: This commonly occurs if non secreting clones overgrow and indicates that the culture should have been cloned earlier. Mycoplasma contamination of hybridomas may also cause this problem. If this happens to valuable cell lines it is possible to clean the cells by growing on mouse macrophages (Schimmelpfeng *et al.*, 1980).

8. *Difficulty in cloning*: Some clones seem to grow poorly at low cell density. Addition of extra feeder cells, 2 Mercapto ethanol ($10^{-4}$ Molar) and 20% FCS may help.

## XIII CONCLUSIONS

The method is not as formidable as it might appear at first sight. Many workers with no previous experience in tissue culture have used the technique with great success. The most helpful advice that we were given and can pass on is to clone early and to have a low index of suspicion for mycoplasma infection.

Two outstanding challenges occur to us. One is the successful production of human-human hybridomas, which is discussed in chapter 2. The other is to simplify the technique and equipment required so that it can be used in third world countries where there are limited resources. Recycling of tissue culture plastics and the development of cheap but effective assay procedures would go a long way towards making this feasible. There are many virological laboratories in these countries with experience of cell culture under difficult circumstances and the application of the hybridoma methodology to the study of tropical diseases in tropical countries should not be discounted.

REFERENCES

Jensenius, J. C. and Williams, A. F. (1974). *Eur. J. Immunol.* **4**, 91–97.
Morris, R. J. and Williams, A. F. (1975). *Eur. J. Immunol.* **5**, 274–281.
Paul, J. (1973). *In* "Cell and Tissue Culture". 4th Edition. Churchill Livingstone, Edinburgh and London.
Schimmelpfeng, L., Lagenberg, U. and Peters, J. H. (1980). *Nature* **285**, 661–663.

22　The Purification of Antigens and Other Studies with Monoclonal Antibody Affinity Columns: the complementary new dimension of monoclonal antibodies

ROSEMARIE DALCHAU AND
JOHN W. FABRE

*Nuffield Department of Surgery, University of Oxford, John Radcliffe Hospital, Oxford. OX3 9DV*

*Current address: Blond McIndoe Centre, Queen Victoria Hospital, East Grinstead, Sussex. RH19 3D2.*

# I  INTRODUCTION

The unique resolving power of monoclonal antibodies in detecting individual components of complex biological systems is the basis for the revolution they have brought to biology. This capacity simply to detect individual components is a most powerful experimental tool, as innumerable examples in this volume amply testify. In addition to this, however, monoclonal antibodies make possible another broad and powerful experimental approach, which rests essentially with the ability to construct high capacity and specific immunoadsorbents to almost any antigen one wishes. It becomes a realistic possibility in many situations to obtain pure antigens, complex mixtures specifically depleted of individual components, and other variations on these themes, and therefore to ask questions about structure, function, and molecular interactions in a hitherto unprecedented way.

The techniques involved in monoclonal antibody affinity chromatography are essentially simple, but there are a great many pitfalls in the progression from a cloned antibody-producing hybrid line, through an affinity column, to a pure molecule. To rush at the problem in an unsystematic way and with no awareness of the potential difficulties is to invite failure frequently and unnecessarily. On the other hand, for one reason or another, some monoclonal antibody systems are intrinsically unworkable, and it is important to be able to pin-point these quickly so as not to languish unnecessarily for months on a system that is unlikely ever to be useful.

Our aim in writing this chapter has been to provide the newcomer to this field with a comprehensive set of guide-lines. We present a detailed and systematic approach to the problem, pointing out the pit-falls at every step, and including a large amount of experimental details so that the chapter may be used as a practical as well as a general theoretical guide. We have in addition given examples of the beautiful experiments which are possible with pure molecules, with complex mixtures specifically depleted of individual components, and with related systems.

There are three phases in monoclonal antibody affinity chromatography: preparation of the affinity column, solubilization of the antigen, and the actual chromatography. The rest of this chapter will be devoted almost entirely to a detailed analysis of these steps.

## II PREPARATION OF MONOCLONAL ANTIBODY COLUMNS

### A. Introduction

The essential requirement for a workable affinity column is to have monospecific antibodies of high specific activity. Before monoclonal antibodies such reagents were rare, usually difficult to produce, and available for only a narrow range of antigens. Nowadays of course, monoclonal antibodies can be produced to almost anything one wishes, and when the hybridomas are grown in the form of tumours the resultant antibody preparations have a very high specific activity, containing up to 20 mg ml$^{-1}$ of specific antibody, and accounting for 20% to 90% of the total immunoglobulin present.

The production of affinity columns requires large amounts of antibody. For example, we use on average the antibody from 1 ml of immune ascites per ml of gel. It is clear, therefore, that for even small columns the cost of commercially available monoclonal antibodies is prohibitive. One needs at present to have access to antibody on a non-commercial basis, either by having the hybrid line oneself or via collaborative or other contacts. The sale of antibody coupled to gels is something the commercial distributors of monoclonal antibodies have not yet considered, even though this would fill an important scientific need, and we hope this gap will be filled in the near future.

### B. Producing the Antibody

To produce antibody preparations of the highest specific activity one needs to partially purify the monoclonal antibody from serum or ascites obtained from animals growing properly cloned lines. We have heard of attempts to produce affinity columns from tissue culture supernatants of hybrid lines grown in foetal calf serum but this obviously is unlikely to be successful. The various steps and variables involved in producing appropriate antibody are as follows:

#### 1. NATURE OF THE HYBRID LINE

The proportion of secreted antibody which is specific for the molecule under study will vary with the nature of myeloma used in the fusion. Where the parent myeloma line produces light or heavy immunoglobulin chains, these will scramble with the light and heavy chains produced by the normal lymphocyte, although with some class restrictions on inter-heavy chain scrambling. Thus not all the assembled immunoglobulin molecules will be of the normal lymphocyte type, with antigen specificity. Clearly, non-producer myeloma lines are ideal in this respect and mouse and rat lines of this type are now available. In all of our studies, however, we have used the NS-1 line of Kohler and Milstein (1975), which produces the K light chain but no heavy chain.

## 2. EFFICACY OF CLONING

Proper cloning of the hybrid lines is vital for the production of high titre antibody preparations. In the initial stages this involves removal of contaminating hybrids present in the fusion well selected, and in later stages the removal of non-secreting variants which arise probably because of chromosomal losses. If care is not taken in this respect, the antibody secreting line might be overgrown, and the amount of antibody produced very small.

To avoid any difficulties in this respect we always clone (by limiting dilution, see previous chapter) a line just prior to its injection into mice. Selection of unwanted variants in the mouse may still occur, but we have not found this to be a problem.

## 3. PRODUCTION OF IMMUNE ASCITES OR SERUM

The simplest approach is to inject the hybrid line into histocompatible animals. The NS-1 line is derived from a BALB/c myeloma, so our routine is to immunize only BALB/c mice for fusion experiments, and then to inject the resultant hybrids into BALB/c mice. It is only rarely that it is necessary to immunize mice histoincompatible with the myeloma to be used in the fusion and here the lines can be grown in F1 animals. With interspecies fusions such as between rat and mouse, the hybrid lines have to be injected into immunologically incompetent animals such as nude rats and mice. Whether or not this will work with human hybridomas remains to be seen.

Our routine is to inject a few million hybrid cells intraperitoneally into BALB/c mice which have been injected intraperitoneally with 0·5 ml of Pristane (2, 6, 10, 14 tetramethyl pentadecane, Koch-Light Laboratories, Colnbrook, Bucks, U.K.) anything from 2 weeks to 2 months previously. We are not sure whether or not the importance of pretreating mice with Pristane for the production of ascites has been examined systematically, but it is a custom which has been adopted almost universally following the work of Potter (1972) on mouse myelomas. Somewhere between 10 days to 4 or 5 weeks after injecting hybrid cells, the majority of mice begin to develop visible ascites. Once this is quite prominent the ascites are harvested by inserting a 19 gauge needle into the peritoneal cavity under ether anaesthesia and allowing the ascites to drop out. Seven or eight ml can sometimes be obtained from a single tap, and we average 10 ml or a little more per mouse by serial tapping. If an antibody is at all likely to be interesting it is advisable to inject 15 to 20 mice at the outset to obtain a large pool of ascites, as this saves time in the long run. Once a mouse becomes obviously distressed by the ascites, it is killed, and residual ascites are removed by opening the abdomen. Using this approach, we have had no difficulties in producing large volumes of ascites from any of the 11 hybridoma lines characterized in our laboratory.

Another approach, more suited for the rat, is to grow the hybridoma as a solid tumour subcutaneously. The rat can be serially bled by the tail of 2 ml or so of blood, and a large pool of immune serum thereby accumulated. We have heard that for production of immune ascites in the rat one needs to pretreat with large volumes, of the order of 10 ml, of Pristane intraperitoneally before injecting the hybridoma, although whether or not this will be substantiated remains to be seen.

We pool all the samples obtained on any one day, centrifuge at 1,000g for 10 mins to pellet cells and any debris, and store the supernatant at $-40°C$.

4. PURIFICATION OF THE IMMUNE ASCITES

The immune ascites will contain albumin, immunoglobulin and other serum proteins in addition to the immunoglobulin produced by the myeloma. It might also contain a good deal of fatty material and it is advisable, both on general grounds and also to increase the specific activity of the preparation to perform a simple partial purification of the monoclonal antibody. Two approaches are generally used. The first is to precipitate the immunoglobulins from the immune ascites by adding 16–18% w/v of $Na_2SO_4$ at room temperature (slowly and with constant stirring). The precipitates are then pelleted by centrifuging at 20,000g for 20 min, resuspended in an appropriate buffer and then dialysed to remove any $Na_2SO_4$. It is always advisable to retain an aliquot of the original immune ascites, and to perform a titration of antibody activity of the original ascites and the purified monoclonal antibody, so that yields can be calculated. The supernatant after centrifugation should not be discarded until this has been done, as it is possible although obviously unlikely that a particular monoclonal antibody will behave atypically.

The approach we routinely use is ion-exchange chromatography, which is simple and rapid, and takes advantage of the relatively high pI of immunoglobulins. After thawing and pooling all of the individual aliquots of the immune ascites, it is first centrifuged at 20,000g for 20 mins at 4°C to remove particulate matter and the bulk of the fat, which will be floating at the top. It is then dialysed against 0·025M Tris, 0·1M NaCl, 0·02% Na azide pH 8·4 at 5°C and passed through a column of DEAE CL 6B (Pharmacia, Uppsala, Sweden) equilibrated in the same buffer. The pH is obviously vital in ion-exchange chromatography, and particular care is necessary to ensure that the ascites is at the correct pH after dialysis and that the column is properly equilibrated. One should also be aware of the fairly marked pH changes that occur with temperature in Tris buffers. We generally apply 30–40 ml of ascites to a 100 ml column, but we have applied 200 ml of ascites to a 300 ml column and this has worked well. Fractions are collected from the column and monitored for optical density at 280 nm. We have now treated ascites pools from 12 different hybridomas in this way, and in all cases the antibody activity has come through the column unretarded. Our routine is therefore to slow down or stop the column after the first peak has come through. The fractions in the peak are pooled, and a titration of antibody activity is performed of this pool and of a sample of the dialysed ascites not passed through the column. These are plotted to allow for changes in volume and yield is calculated. Virtually all the antibody activity has to date been found in this peak with about 20% of the protein in the original ascites. In one or two cases, the peak has been a double one, and only one of these contained the antibody. Doubtless, some monoclonal antibodies will be retained by the column under these conditions, in which case pH or salt gradients would be applied to elute them.

Gel filtration (e.g. with G-200 or S300, Pharmacia, Uppsala, Sweden) is another simple purification step that can be used and would be of particular value for IgM monoclonal antibodies. It has the disadvantage that only small volumes can be treated at any one time, e.g. 20ml for a 500 ml. column.

## C. COUPLING OF MONOCLONAL ANTIBODY TO GEL

There are a variety of commercially available gels to which monoclonal antibodies may be covalently coupled without difficulty, these gels differing in the reactive groups used in the linkage. Non-covalently coupled columns are possible, but their use is more restricted, and they will be discussed briefly later. We routinely use cyanogen bromide activated Sepharose 4B (Pharmacia, Uppsala, Sweden), which links the protein via primary amino groups. These columns, if treated with care, can be re-used many times.

The coupling procedure is simple, and consists essentially of mixing the gel and the protein at the correct pH. We usually make about 15–20 ml of gel at any one time. If the protein content of the purified ascites has been measured accurately (e.g. by the method of Lowry *et al.*, 1951) we couple at 10 mg protein ml$^{-1}$ of swollen gel. However, an acceptable way of calculating the approximate protein concentration of the ascites, if a partial purification step has been performed, is to measure the optical density (OD) at 280 nm and to assume that the proteins present have the extinction of pure IgG. The protein concentration will then be $\dfrac{\text{OD at 280 nm}}{1 \cdot 4}$ mg ml$^{-1}$ and our solutions are usually 2–5 mg protein ml$^{-1}$. If this less precise measurement of protein concentration is used, coupling should be done at a ratio of 5 mg of protein per ml of swollen gel, to allow for inaccuracies in the method.

On the day before coupling, the appropriate amount of antibody is thawed and dialysed against $0 \cdot 1$M NaHCO$_3$, $0 \cdot 5$M NaCl, pH $8 \cdot 5$ (the coupling buffer) both to bring the pH up to the range where coupling is efficient and also to remove any Tris present in the antibody solution, since the free amino groups of the Tris will compete with the protein for the reactive groups on the gel beads. On the day of coupling the desired amount of gel powder is weighed out (1g of freeze dried powder gives $3 \cdot 5$ ml of swollen gel) and swollen for 15 min in 100 ml or so of 1mM HCl (pH 3). The gel is then washed on a scintered glass filter (porosity G3) on a Buchner Flask using 200 ml of 1mMHCl per g of dry gel, with the gel being sucked dry on 2 or 3 occasions during the washing. The next step is to wash the gel with 100–200 ml of coupling buffer to bring the pH up to $8 \cdot 5$, and it is vital to check that this has been achieved by measuring the pH of the last few ml of buffer which has passed through the gel. After being sucked dry, the gel is transferred to a suitable tube (e.g. 50 ml screw-cap plastic tube). The pH of the dialysed antibody is checked to be $8 \cdot 5$ and this is added to the gel. The mixture is then mixed continuously by end-over-end rotation for 2 hours at room temperature, during which time the coupling occurs. The mixture is then transferred to the scintered glass filter, sucked dry, and the OD at 280 nm of the fluid is measured to check the efficiency of the coupling. Almost invariably 90% of the protein is bound to the beads. The gel is then washed with a few hundred ml of coupling buffer, and the remaining active groups on the gel are blocked by incubating it for 2 hours at room temperature in 1M ethanolamine at pH 8·0. This can be done on the scintered glass filter by adding 100 to 200 ml of the ethanolamine and allowing it to pass through the gel over the 2 hours, or by transferring the gel to a tube, as for the coupling. At the end of this incubation the gel is sucked dry, and washed with a few hundred ml of coupling buffer. It is then exposed to 3 cycles of alternating low (0·1MNa acetate, 1M NaCl, 0·02% Na azide pH 4·0) and high (0·025 M Tris, 1M Nacl, 0·02% Na azide, pH 8·5) washes to remove any non-covalently adsorbed protein. The pH of the buffer coming through the gel is checked and the buffer changed when the gel has equilibrated. The gel is then washed in Tris buffered saline (0·025 M Tris, 0·15 M NaCl, 0·02% Na azide, pH 7·3 at 5°C) and stored at 4°C in an air-tight container in this buffer. We check the OD at 280 nm against appropriate blanks of all samples that pass through the gel so as to have a good idea of the efficiency of the coupling procedure, and in almost all instances >90% of the initial OD at 280 nm remains bound to the gel.

## III SOLUBILIZATION OF THE ANTIGEN

### A. INTRODUCTION

If the target antigen in which one is interested is available in aqueous solution (e.g. in serum, synovial fluid, etc.) then the most difficult step in affinity chromatography is side-stepped. However, much current work involves integral membrane proteins which, because of the hydrophobic portion inserted into the lipid bilayer of the membrane, are not stable in aqueous solution. A few monoclonal antibodies have been described to membrane glycolipids but almost all currently described monoclonal antibodies directed at membrane constituents interact with membrane proteins, and for this reason we shall concern ourselves solely with the solubilization of membrane proteins.

There are 2 approaches to the solubilization of integral membrane proteins. The first, which is likely to have only limited application, is to use enzymes under carefully controlled conditions to cleave the protein near its point of insertion into the membrane. This approach has been used to solubilize HLA antigens using papain (Springer et al., 1974). However, as the enzymes will cleave proteins at multiple sites, the yield of near-native molecules is likely to be poor even with careful choice of conditions. With few exceptions, therefore, the only viable approach is to use detergents to displace the membrane lipids from the hydrophobic portion of the molecule, resulting in individual membrane proteins stabilized by insertion into a detergent micelle.

## B. GENERAL APPROACHES TO DETERGENT SOLUBILIZATION

Detergents are generally broadly subdivided into ionic and non-ionic varieties. (For reviews see Tanford and Reynolds, 1976; Helenius *et al.*, 1979). Our experience has involved one weakly anionic detergent, sodium deoxycholate, and a variety of non-ionic detergents including Brij 99, Brij 96, Lubrol PX, NP-40, Tween 40 and Triton X-100 (Sigma Chemical Company, London, U.K.). The definition of solubility is an operational one, a molecule being considered soluble in a detergent if it remains in the supernatant after ultracentrifugation (e.g. 80,000 g for 75 min). When this occurs, it is assumed that each molecule is associated with a single detergent micelle, which is probably true if a sufficiently high ratio ($\geqslant 2$ to 1) of detergent micelles to protein molecules is used.

Sodium deoxycholate has proved to be a very valuable detergent. It is extremely efficient at solubilizing membranes and also has the advantage that it has a small micelle size (approximately 1,000 to 10,000 daltons depending on the ionic strength of the medium) so that the size of the molecule plus detergent is usually not much larger than the molecule alone. This latter point is an advantage if one wishes to submit the solubilized membrane to gel filtration, which separates on the basis of molecular size, as differences between molecules are not so blurred as when the detergent micelle has a molecular weight of approximately 50,000 to 100,000 daltons which is usually the case with the non-ionic detergents. Sodium deoxycholate has, however, a number of disadvantages. Firstly, it will lyse the nuclear membrane as well as the external cell membrane, whereas the non-ionic detergents leave the nuclei intact. Secondly, solutions of deoxycholate will become viscous and gel if the pH of the solution falls much below 8 or if the ionic strength of the solution is too high and in particular if it contains divalent cations. Thirdly, being ionic, separation procedures depending on charge (e.g. ion-exchange chromatography, iso-electric focussing) cannot be used on membranes solubilized in deoxycholate. Finally, although antigen denaturation is not a frequent problem, our impression is that deoxycholate is more likely to denature molecules than the non-ionic detergents.

The non-ionic detergents are not such efficient solubilizers as deoxy-cholate, but our experience suggests that the Brij detergents are quite good and are the best of the group in this respect. A 2:1 mixture of Brij 99/Brij 96 is our non-ionic detergent of choice as it remains in solution at 4°C, whereas solutions of Brij 96 tend to come out of solution after several hours at 4°C.

We use the non-ionic detergents directly as supplied, but the deoxy-cholate is used after one crystalization, to remove impurities, particularly any organic impurities and those with absorbance at 280 nm, which vary from batch to batch. This is done as follows (A. F. Williams, personal communication). Approximately 150 g of sodium deoxycholate (Sigma, London, U.K.) is dissolved in 1·2 litres of a 4:1 mixture of acetone and water, in a water bath at 75°C. The acetone/water mixture boils at 63°C, and to avoid inhaling the fumes this should be done in a fume cupboard. The solution is filtered while hot through filter paper using pre-warmed Buchner funnel and flask. It is then allowed to cool slowly and left overnight at 4°C. The crystalline precipitate is removed by filtering through filter paper and washed with some cold acetone/water mixture. The crystals are allowed to dry in a fume cupboard overnight, and the drying process completed by placing them under vacuum with $CaCl_2$ again overnight. The result should be a white crystalline powder.

There are several approaches to the detergent solubilization of a tissue:

## 1. DIRECT SOLUBILIZATION IN DEOXYCHOLATE

This is a very efficient method but it is generally reserved for use with preparations devoid of nuclei. If one adds deoxycholate directly to spleen homogenate, for example, the consequent nuclear disruption and release of DNA results in a solution too viscous to use in affinity chromatography. An exception to this generalization is the direct deoxycholate solubilization of brain homogenate, probably because this tissue contains abundant membranes and relatively few nuclei (Lakin and Fabre, 1981). In these experiments previously washed brain homogenate was pelleted by centrifugation at 20,000 g for 20 min and resuspended to approximately 25% solid tissue (approximately 10 mg homogenate protein $ml^{-1}$) in 0·01M Tris, 0·02% Na azide, pH 8·4 at 4°C. To this was added an equal volume of 4% sodium deoxycholate in the same buffer. The mixture was incubated for 1 hour on ice, with constant stirring after which it was centrifuged at 80,000 g for 75 min. More than 50% of the antigen activity of Thy-1 (unpublished observations) and a brain-specific antigen (Lakin and Fabre, 1981) was in the high speed supernatant.

Where membranes free of nuclei can be readily prepared, for example with erythrocytes and platelets, direct deoxycholate solubilization is a good method to consider in the first instance.

## 2. DIRECT SOLUBILIZATION IN NON-IONIC DETERGENTS

Membrane antigens can be directly solubilized by non-ionic detergents, particularly Brij, but this is entirely unpredictable. Our protocol for solubilization is to take homogenate at 25% solid tissue (approximately 10 mg of homogenate protein $ml^{-1}$) or cells at $5 \times 10^8 \ ml^{-1}$ in 0·01M Tris, 0·15M NaCl, 0·02% Na azide pH 7·3 at 4°C and add an equal volume of 4% w/v of the non-ionic detergent in the same buffer. More recently, we have been using 10% detergent, since with the platelet glycoprotein Ib, 10% Brij gives good solubilization while 4% gives only a poor yield (Ruan *et al.*, 1982). It is probably wiser in fact to use 10% Brij routinely, as rough calculations assuming a Brij micelle molecular weight of 100,000 and average membrane protein size of 20,000 or 30,000 suggest that a 2:1 ratio of micelles/proteins is more likely to be achieved with the higher Brij concentration in our system. The mixture is incubated for 1 hour on ice with constant stirring and then centrifuged for 15 min at 1500 g to remove nuclei. The supernatant is then ultracentrifuged at 80,000 g for 75 minutes.

The choice of appropriate detergent is entirely empirical, and this is best illustrated by studies with 2 human lymphocyte antigens, the leucocyte common antigen (Dalchau *et al.*, 1980a) and an antigen designated F10-44-2 (Dalchau *et al.*, 1980b). Using Lubrol PX and spleen homogenate in the above protocol and following the solubilization of the 2 antigens from the same aliquot of spleen and detergent, it was clear that the leucocyte common antigen was completely solubilized and found only in the ultracentrifuge supernatant, while the F10-44-2 antigen was still in membrane form and was found only in the ultracentrifuge pellet. We do not know the explanation for this, although it is possible that we were seeing selective solubilization from the membrane because of too low a detergent/lipid ratio (Tanford and Reynolds, 1976).

3. SOLUBILIZATION BY USE OF A NON-IONIC DETERGENT
FOLLOWED BY DEOXYCHOLATE

When the antigen is found in the ultracentrifuge pellet following protocol 2. with non-ionic detergents, the detergent appears to act by
disrupting the cell membrane into small fragments which contain the
antigen under study. This was first demonstrated with Tween 40 on
single cell suspensions of thymocytes (Standring and Williams 1978)
and it is a most useful approach to preparing membranes since it is
simple, quick, can be performed on very large samples, and the yields
are excellent (~50%). One should note that the ultra-centrifuge pellet
contains cell organelles in addition to the external cell membranes, and
although this is of no practical importance for the solubilization and
purification of membrane antigens, it is something which one should be
aware of.

The experimental protocol is as for 2., except that the antigen-
containing ultracentrifuge pellet is resuspended in 0·01M Tris, 0·02%
Na azide, pH 8·4 at 4°C, usually to the original volume of cell or
homogenate suspension. However, it could probably be resuspended to
a much smaller volume since the protein concentration of this pellet will
be substantially lower than that of the original cell or homogenate
suspension. After resuspension with a pipette, it is wise to use a ground-
glass homogenizer as the small pellet will frequently be difficult to
disrupt. An equal volume of 4% deoxycholate in the same buffer is then
added, incubated for 1 hour on ice with constant stirring, and then the
mixture ultracentrifuged at 80,000 g for 75 min at 4°C. The antigen
should then be in the supernatant. Because of the small micelle size of
deoxycholate one could probably use a much lower concentration than
4% but we do not routinely do so.

4. VARIATIONS ON PROTOCOLS 1 TO 3

Once it has been established in pilot experiments that a particular
protocol solubilizes the antigen under study, the ultracentrifugation
step may be omitted in some experiments. For example, if direct
solubilization with deoxycholate or a non-ionic detergent is effective,
one may simply add the detergent, incubate, then give a slow spin (e.g.
1,500 g for 15 min) to remove nuclei and any large debris, and take the
supernatant as soluble antigen. With protocol 3 one may add the
non-ionic detergent, incubate, remove the nuclei by centrifuging at
1,500 g for 15 min, add deoxycholate, incubate and then take this as the
soluble preparation. In this case, the non-ionic detergent should be in a

low salt high pH buffer compatible with deoxycholate, e.g. 0·01 M Tris, 0·02% Na azide pH 8·4 at 4°C, (which in our experience does not create problems with tissue homogenates in spite of the low ionic strength). Sometimes after solubilization by a non-ionic detergent as in protocol 2 and if the ultracentrifugation step is omitted, the mixture is made up to 1% deoxycholate (e.g. by adding 1/3 the volume of 4% deoxycholate) to solubilize any membrane fragments present. Again, the non-ionic detergent should be in a buffer compatible with deoxycholate. One should note that the resultant solution contains a mixture of detergents, and that this might complicate matters in certain situations.

## C. ASSAYS IN THE PRESENCE OF DETERGENTS

During solubilization and purification procedures the presence in various fractions of the antigen under study is usually detected by the inhibition of binding of the appropriate monoclonal antibody to a target. If the target is susceptible to detergent lysis, and this will frequently be the case, the target must be protected or a non-lysable system chosen. Possible solutions to this problem are as follows:

### 1. THE USE OF TARGETS "FIXED" BY AGENTS SUCH AS GLUTARALDEHYDE

The simplest procedure is to fix the target cell, homogenate or whatever else one is using with a reagent such as glutaraldehyde (Williams, 1973). The target suspension is washed in protein—free medium three times, and then resuspended to $2 \times 10^8$ ml$^{-1}$ for cells or 2–4 mg of homogenate protein ml$^{-1}$. An equal volume of 0·25% glutaraldehyde in the same buffer is then added, mixed, and incubated for 5 min at room temperature. The reaction is stopped by adding excess protein (e.g. 1/10 volume of 10% bovine serum albumin or undiluted serum) and the targets washed immediately three times by centrifugation in protein containing media. The target suspension frequently turns yellowish in colour and tends to aggregate, so it must be vigorously pipetted and, in the case of cells, preferably filtered through a thin wisp of cotton wool. After fixation, the cells may be stored frozen in aliquots, in protein containing buffers. They are resistant to freezing, non-physiological salt concentrations, detergents, and almost any other insult, but two important things should be noted. Firstly, even after fixation, detergent lysis is occasionally a problem, so appropriate controls must be included even though fixed targets are used (see section

III D. 5). Secondly, even mild fixations as described above will denature some antigenic determinants and 3 of the 12 antibodies we have
studied could not be used with fixed cells for this reason. Therefore,
parallel titrations of the antibody against fixed and fresh targets must be
performed to check for denaturation. Although partial denaturation
usually occurs, this does not preclude the use of the fixed targets.

2. THE USE OF PROTEIN IN THE ASSAY SYSTEM

Living cells or other detergent susceptible targets may be used if one
includes high concentrations of protein in the reaction mixture.
(Springer et al., 1974). How precisely this works is not certain, but even
water soluble proteins have hydrophobic regions which bind detergents, and it appears likely that the protein in the mixture adsorbs the
detergent leaving none free to lyse the targets. In the absence of free
detergent the antigens might aggregate, but this does not appear to
affect their antigenicity. A final concentration of 10% bovine serum
albumin (BSA) in the mixture is what we aim for in the first instance,
but up to 30% may be necessary, depending on the particular detergents in use and their concentrations. Protein may be introduced by
resuspending the target cells in 10% BSA, and diluting the antibody for
titration in 10% BSA. The best way to introduce protein into the
soluble antigen fraction is to add 1/3 volume of 40% BSA (dialysed to
neutral pH) and then make dilutions of the antigen in 10% BSA. This
minimizes dilution of the antigen and keeps the amount of BSA constant at all dilutions. Again, appropriate detergent controls in the assay
system are vital, as protection of the targets by the protein is not always
complete (see section III D.5).

3. THE USE OF PLATE ASSAYS

We have found that some detergent solubilized antigens, but only a few,
will bind to flexible vinyl plates (Flow laboratories, Irvine, Scotland) if
incubated overnight. It is probably not advisable to use this approach
to follow solubilization. However, once the antigen is in soluble form, it
is useful to test its capacity to bind to plates for, if it does, it simplifies
considerably the detection of the antigen during chromatographic procedures. To test binding, $50 \mu l$ of the soluble antigen are added to wells
and incubated overnight at 4°C. The solution is removed from the plate
with a pipette and the wells washed 3 times in 0·5% BSA/PBS. The
washing buffer can be removed by flicking the plate. $200 \mu l$ of 5·0%
BSA are added to each well to saturate protein binding sites. After

incubation for one hour, this is removed and the wells again washed three times. 50 μl of the monoclonal antibody and a control antibody are added at appropriate dilutions to form a titration curve and incubated for 1 hour. The plates are washed 3 times, and 50 μl of $^{125}I$ labelled, affinity purified anti imunoglobulin is added. After a further 1 hour's incubation, the wells are washed 3 times, cut out, and placed into counting tubes to measure radio-activity. Such a titration is illustrated in Fig. 22·1(a) which shows the binding of the F3-87-8 antibody (Lakin and Fabre, 1981) to deoxycholate solubilized brain. Fig. 22·1(b) shows the use of the plate assay to follow the antigen during gel filtration chromatography. It should be noted that non-specific binding of the monoclonal antibodies at high concentrations of immune ascites (e.g. undiluted, 1/10) is frequently seen. One should also note that the system sometimes works better once the antigen has been concentrated by the monoclonal antibody affinity step.

4. OTHER POSSIBILITIES

It is possible to consider other solutions to the problem. For example, we have found that Brij solubilized spleen coupled to cyanogen bromide activated Sepharose 4B (Pharmacia, Uppsala, Sweden) provides an excellent target in binding assays for a number of leucocyte antigens, e.g. the leucocyte common antigen (Dalchau *et al.*, 1980a). With this approach, one should be careful that the detergent used for solubilization does not interact with the reactive groups or the beads chosen for the coupling.

### D. POTENTIAL DIFFICULTIES AND EXPERIMENTAL PROTOCOLS TO DETECT AND AVOID THEM

Once the most suitable approach to solubilization has been considered, and a suitable assay system in the presence of detergents has been devised, one needs to set up pilot experiments with small volumes of tissue to check whether or not solubilization occurs and if any of the potential difficulties will be a problem for the system under study. In the first instance we examine direct solubilization with deoxycholate (if appropriate) or more usually with a 2:1 mixture of Brij 99/Brij 96, as outlined in Fig. 22·2. For example we would thaw a 2·1 ml sample of spleen homogenate (50% solid tissue in phosphate buffered saline), centrifuge it at 20,000 g for 20 min, and resuspend it to 4·2 ml (25% solid tissue) in 0·15M NaCl, 0·01M Tris, 0·02% Na azide pH 7·3 at

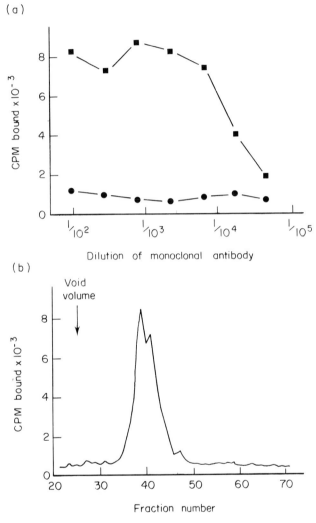

FIG. 22·1 Use of plate assays in the presence of detergents. (a) Deoxycholate solu-bilized brain was incubated in vinyl plates, and binding of F3-87-8 antigen to this plate checked by adding dilutions of F3-87-8 antibody (■) or control (●) monoclonal antibody followed by [125]I rabbit anti mouse immunoglobulin (RAM), as described in text. (b) Monoclonal antibody affinity column purified F3-87-8 antigen was submitted to S-300 gel filtration chromatography and 50 μl of each fraction placed in vinyl plates. Antigen containing fractions were detected by adding F3-87-8 monoclonal antibodies and then [125]I RAM to each well.

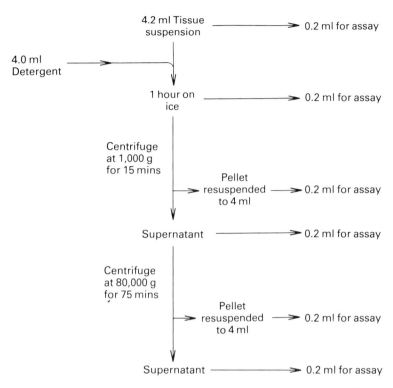

FIG. 22·2 Outline of pilot experiments to test for detergent solubilization of antigen.

4°C. A 0·2 ml sample would be removed and frozen for subsequent assay. We usually add 4 ml of 4% Brij (although 10% Brij is probably better; section IIIB2) and stir the mixture for 1 hour on ice. At the end of the incubation, another sample is taken for assay. The nuclei are then pelleted, the supernatant removed, and a sample of each is taken for assay. The supernatant is then ultra-centrifuged, and again a sample of both pellet and supernatant is taken for assay.

The amount of antigen in each sample must then be assayed by quantitative techniques, and we use quantitative absorptions. Doubling or tripling dilutions of the antigen in 0·5% BSA/PBS 80 $\mu$l of each antigen dilution is placed in microfuge tubes (Beckman RIIC Ltd., Fife, Scotland) and 80 $\mu$l of antibody at a dilution near its titration end-point is added to each tube. After 1 hour on ice the tubes are centrifuged at 23,500 g for 20 min. 25 $\mu$l are transferred in duplicate to LP3 tubes (Luckham Ltd., Sussex, U.K.) and 25 $\mu$l of target suspension is added. After a further 1 hour on ice the targets are washed twice, and 100 $\mu$l of

$^{125}$I labelled, affinity purified anti immunoglobulin antibody (300,000–400,000 cpm per tube) is added to the pellet of the second wash. After resuspension and a further 1 hour on ice, the targets are washed twice and target bound radio-activity is measured. The results of this assay will give a clear indication of whether and in what yield the antigen has been solubilized, and will clearly pin-point any of the potential problems, which are as follows.

### 1. THE ANTIGEN MIGHT BE NOT SOLUBILIZED AT ALL OR ONLY IN LOW YIELD BY THE DETERGENT UNDER STUDY

In a favourable system, the ultracentrifuge supernatant would contain the antigen in good yield, and we would aim at 25%–50% of the antigen activity in the starting tissue. Volume changes in different samples must be considered when calculating yields. A favourable system is illustrated in Fig. 22·3. It is vital to stress that good yields are essential if one is to proceed with studies such as bulk purifications of antigen. It is well worth looking for optimal conditions of solubilization rather than attempt to work with systems giving only 1 or 2% yield of soluble antigen.

### 2. THE CONCENTRATION OF THE ANTIGEN IN THE TISSUE TO BE SOLUBILIZED MIGHT BE TOO LOW FOR DETECTION AFTER THE DILUTIONS INVOLVED IN SOLUBILIZATION

The concentration of antigen in the starting tissue should ideally be detected readily after dilution of at least 1 in 4. This is because of the dilution involved in the addition of an equal volume of detergent and the fact that the yields of soluble antigen that one aims for are in the region of 50%. To counterbalance this, the antigenic activity of the preparation sometimes increases after incubation with detergent, possibly because of release of intracellular or otherwise inaccessible antigen on intact membranes. Sensitivity of assay systems can be increased in absorption analyses by reducing the concentration of antibody, as long as the specific/background ratio remains at least 3 or 4/1. In addition it might be possible to increase by a factor of 2 or 3 the concentration of tissue that we usually use i.e. $5 \times 10^8$ cells ml$^{-1}$ or 10 mg of tissue protein ml$^{-1}$ and increase the concentration of detergent from 4% to 10%. We have not tried this, but it would probably be a reasonable approach. However, if the concentration of antigen or assay sensitivity are too low, clearly one cannot follow the progress of antigen during

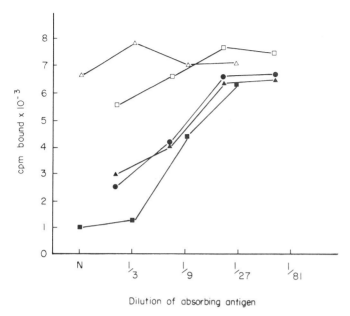

cpm bound x 10⁻³

Dilution of absorbing antigen

FIG. 22·3 Testing a detergent for adequacy of solubilization. Quantitative absorption analysis using F10-44-2 monoclonal antibody (Dalchau *et al.*, 1980b) at 1 in 15,000 dilution and tripling dilutions of spleen homogenate, ■; spleen homogenate plus 4% Brij 99/96 after 1 hour's incubation, ●; ultracentrifuge (80,000 g for 75 min) supernatant, ▲; ultracentrifuge pellet, □; 2% Brij 99/96 control, △. Targets were gluteraldehyde fixed spleen cells at $5 \times 10^7$/ml and cpm bound refer to $^{125}$I labelled rabbit anti mouse immunoglobulin.

solubilization. If this is the case one is working in a very difficult situation and the best one can do is to add the detergents which experience has shown are most likely to solubilize (i.e. deoxycholate or Brij 99/96 plus deoxycholate) and proceed on the assumption the antigen is soluble. If one is attempting bulk purifications from large volumes of tissue, and all the pitfalls are fortuitously avoided, the concentrated antigen eluted from the column might well be detectable.

3. THE ANTIGENIC DETERMINANT UNDER STUDY
MAY BE DENATURED BY THE DETERGENT

4. THE MONOCLONAL ANTIBODY MIGHT BE OF TOO LOW
AFFINITY TO REACT WITH SOLUBLE, MONOMERIC ANTIGEN

If the antigen is denatured by the detergent, or if the affinity of the antibody is too low for interaction with monomeric antigen, little or no

antigen activity will be detected in the assay sample removed at the end
of the 1 hour's incubation in detergent (see Fig. 22·3). This occurred in
our experience only twice with 12 antigen systems studied. One cannot
distinguish readily between these 2 possibilities, and should it occur,
the best thing to do is to proceed with other detergents. If the same thing
happens every time, or at least every time the antigen is in soluble form,
then clearly the system is unworkable either because the antigenic
determinant is readily denatured or masked by detergents, or because
the antibody affinity is too low.

5. THE TARGET CELLS, EVEN IF LIGHTLY FIXED WITH
GLUTARALDEHYDE, MIGHT BE LYSED BY THE DETERGENT

Precise detergent controls must be included. In the experiments outlined in Figs. 22·2 and 22·3 a sample of 2% Brij 99/Brij 96 should be
treated like all the other samples for assay i.e. BSA added, tripling
dilutions made, antibody added etc. This is to check for artefacts
introduced into the system by the detergent(s) in use, principally lysis of
target cells, even of glutaraldehyde fixed target cells. Because the
concentration of detergent diminishes on tripling dilution of the samples, detergent lysis of the targets will also diminish on dilution. The
reduced numbers of targets result in fewer cpm bound in the final
counting of the assay, and the result can be misinterpreted as absorption of antibody activity by antigen.

6. THE MONOCLONAL ANTIBODY MIGHT BE DENATURED
BY THE DETERGENT

This is rarely encountered and we have seen it with only one antibody,
and the denaturation was seen with NP-40 but not other detergents. It
resulted in complete loss of binding of the antibody even at low concentrations of detergent. With conventional sera, such problems would not
be seen because of the broad range of different antibodies contributing
to the antigen binding capacity of the serum, and the inactivation of
some of these would not be detectable. With monoclonal systems one
tends to have all-or-none phenomena in these situations.

## E. INHIBITION OF PROTEOLYSIS

It is vital in many experiments to retain the molecule under study in its
original form. The proteolytic enzymes present in the tissues can cause

considerable problems in this respect and it will usually be necessary to take great care to avoid proteolysis. All 5 of the following precautions should be taken routinely.

1.  Keep all solutions on ice or at 4°C at all times.
2.  Avoid acidic pH's, where acid proteases will be most active.
3.  Avoid the presence of divalent cations, since some proteases require them for activity, and use 5 mM EDTA in all solutions.
4.  Use 2·5 mM iodoacetamide (IAA) in all solutions.
5.  Use 2 mM phenyl methyl sulphonyl fluoride (PMSF) in all solutions.

The PMSF and IAA each inactivate a different class of proteases. IAA is readily soluble in water, and can be used without difficulty. PMSF is poorly soluble in water, but is much more readily soluble in detergents, (it is also very toxic). Problems with proteolysis occur mainly after addition of detergents, so that the PMSF may be dissolved to 4 mM in the detergent prior to addition to the tissue. Both IAA and PMSF must be prepared fresh immediately before use.

## IV AFFINITY CHROMATOGRAPHY WITH MONOCLONAL ANTIBODY COLUMNS

### A. Introduction and Design of Pilot Experiments

Once the antigen has been solubilized in good yield and the affinity column prepared, there are still some obstacles to be negotiated. For this reason it is important to perform pilot experiments to pin-point potential difficulties, and these experiments are best performed with small columns. We routinely use 0·7 ml of gel in disposable plastic columns (econo-columns; Bio Rad, Watford, Herts) or in 2 ml glass syringes with a porous, inert support placed at the bottom. The column is washed with 5 ml of buffer without detergent and then with 5 ml of buffer with 0·5% detergent to equilibrate the column. This is done simply by applying the washing solution to the top of the column with a Pasteur pipette, and takes only a few minutes. Note that it is especially important when using deoxycholate with columns stored in 0·15M NaCl, 0·025M Tris, 0·02% Na azide pH 7·3 at 4°C to wash the column in the low salt, high pH buffer (0·01M Tris, 0·02% Na azide, pH 8·4 at 4°C) before applying deoxycholate, otherwise the detergent will meet with inappropriate condition of pH and ionic strength, as mentioned in section IIIB. The column is then pre-eluted to remove any proteins that can be removed from the column by the eluting procedure in use. One may use either low pH (e.g. 1 M propionic acid, pH 2·6) or high pH (e.g. 0·05M diethylamine, pH 11·5) solutions in 0·5% detergent for elution, although obviously only the high pH solution is appropriate for systems with deoxycholate. 2 or 3 ml of the eluting solution are passed through the column, after which it is brought quickly back to the starting pH by passing through buffer with 0·5% detergent. It is useful to use pH paper to check quickly that the column is back to a reasonable pH. The column is now ready for use.

We apply a few ml, usually 4 ml, of antigen solution to the column at the rate of 2 ml per hr. A useful system which we have devised for use with small volumes of detergent solutions, and in particular for radio-labelled solutions, is given in Fig. 22·4. The solution is forced out of the plastic syringe used as a reservoir by pumping air at a controlled rate into the syringe. This system is doubly useful since, by reversing the flow of air, the sample can be sucked into the syringe to start with.

After 1 or 1·5 ml of sample has passed through the column, a 1 ml sample is collected as the "depleted" fraction. After all the sample has passed through the column, it is washed with 0·5% detergent in the appropriate buffer. The first 1 ml of wash is applied as in Fig. 22·4 at the same rate as sample application, so that the antigen solution in the column will not be wasted by being rapidly washed through. Then 10–20 ml of detergent solution is applied by pipette to wash the column and this can be done quite rapidly. The column is then eluted by low or high pH, or other appropriate solution in 0·5% detergent, by applying 6 × 500 $\mu$l aliquots of the eluting solution and collecting each as a separate fraction. Each fraction should be neutralized immediately if a pH change is used to effect elution. With the 0·05M diethylamine, pH 11·5 buffer, the use of solid glycine in the collecting tube is a useful method, since in saturated glycine the pH is brought rapidly down to approximately 8. If 1M propionic acid is used for elution the sample after collection can be neutralized with 2M Tris, but this can be quite a delicate procedure, and perhaps less concentrated Tris solutions should be used with these small fractions. All else being equal, we routinely use high pH elution in the first instance. Once the eluting solution has been applied, the column should be brought back to more physiological pH by washing with, e.g. 0·15M NaCl, 0·02% N azide, 0·025M Tris, pH 7·4 at 4°C. Note that where deoxycholate is used, it is essential that it be washed out of the column with the low salt, pH 8·4 buffer before the Tris/saline buffer just mentioned is applied.

The starting detergent solution, the depleted samples and the first 4

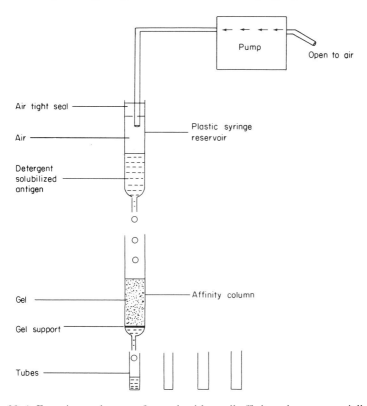

FIG. 22·4 Experimental system for work with small affinity columns, especially when using radio-labelled antigens.

elution fractions are then tested by quantitative techniques for the amount of antigen present. In the majority of cases (in our case 7/12 different affinity columns) the picture seen was similar to that shown in Fig. 22·5 for bulk purification from larger columns, showing complete depletion of antigen from the applied sample, and its recovery in good yield in the eluted fractions. The antigen will usually be concentrated on elution, and the degree of concentration will depend mainly on the ratio of the volume of the applied and eluted samples.

## B. PROBLEMS AND POTENTIAL SOLUTIONS

Our experience has been that if problems arise, attempts to by-pass them are generally unrewarding. However, it is important to be aware

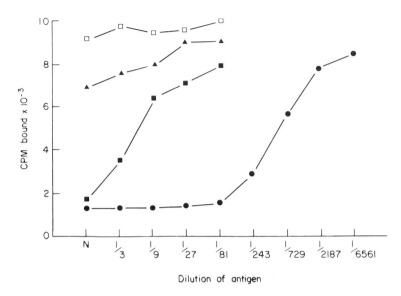

Dilution of antigen

FIG. 22·5 Purification of antigen by monoclonal antibody affinity chromatography. Quantitative absorption analysis using F10-44-2 monoclonal antibody Dalchau *et al.*, 1980b at 1 in 15,000 dilution and tripling dilutions of Brij 99/96 solubilized spleen homogenate before (■) and after (▲) passage through an F10-44-2 monoclonal antibody affinity column; high pH eluate of the column, ●; and 2% Brij 99/96 control, □. 600 hundred ml were passed through the column and the elution volume was 10 ml.

of the potential difficulties particularly as it is sometimes useful to investigate a problem before discarding a system as valueless. The problems that might arise are as follows:

1. THE ANTIGEN PASSES UNRETARDED
THROUGH THE COLUMN

We have seen this with only one of the twelve systems we have studied, and there are two possible causes.

(a) *The antibody is of too low affinity to function effectively*

If all the preliminary work outlined above has been done and no difficulties encountered, this will probably not be a problem. This is because the assays will have involved interactions of antibody with soluble, monomeric antigen, which is what happens on the column. However, this probably was the cause of the problem with the one system with which we had this sort of difficulty.

(b) *The antibody is denatured by the coupling procedure*

The antibody is immobilized usually by multiple points of attachment, and the result could be distortions resulting in loss of antigen binding capacity.

It is important to try to distinguish between these two causes, because too low an affinity of the antibody is an intrinsic and irremediable defect in the system, whereas denaturation on coupling might be circumvented. One can attempt several things. For example, one can construct columns not involving covalent linkage of the monoclonal antibody, using a first step protein A or anti immunoglobulin columns. We have tried the latter, coupling affinity purified rabbit (Fab')₂ anti mouse $F(ab')_2$ at 1 mg ml⁻¹ to CN Br activated sepharose 4B. A 1 ml column was constructed, immune ascites passed through until the column was saturated, and the antigen solution then passed through. This worked well with two antibodies for removal of radio-labelled antigen from a mixture of labelled proteins in solution. Alternatively, one can couple the protein via a different reactive group (e.g. carboxyl groups using AH-Sepharose 4B (Pharmacia Uppsala, Sweden) ) or allow some of the reactive groups on the CN Br activated Sepharose to become inactivated by simply incubating the gel in coupling buffer for a few hours at room temperature before coupling the monoclonal antibody.

## 2. THE ANTIGEN IS RETAINED ON THE COLUMN, BUT ANTIGEN ACTIVITY CANNOT BE ELUTED

We have seen this with two of our 12 columns, and again there are two causes.

(a) *The antigen remains bound to the column in spite of the elution procedure used*

This might sometimes be related to high affinity of the monoclonal antibody, but essentially it means that the distortions in tertiary structure brought about by the elution procedure (e.g. changes in pH or ionic strength) leave the antigen combining site unaltered. With one of our two columns where antigen could not be eluted, the antibody was in fact of unusually high affinity.

(b) *The antigen is eluted from the column, but in a denatured form*

If one is following elution by serological means, denaturation of the antigen will result in no activity being seen in the eluted fractions. We have not come across this problem.

If the column depletes of antigen well, but there is no antigen activity in the eluate, the best thing to do in the first instance is to try other methods of elution. Thus, instead of high pH, one could use low pH, or try elution by changes in ionic strength or with 8M urea. It might be useful in some systems to pass a column volume of eluting solution into the column and allow it to stand for 10–15 minutes before proceeding with the elution. If none of these procedures works, further experiments involve attempts to elute the antigen by techniques which will denature it. For these studies it is obviously necessary to be able to detect the antigen by non-serological methods. For example it might be possible to use radiolabelled antigen which can be identified by polyacrylamide gel electrophoresis in sodium dodecyl sulphate (PAGE in SDS) which is the approach we used with the human leucocyte common (LC) antigen (Dalchau et al., 1980a). Serological analysis of pilot affinity chromatography experiments showed that the columns depleted of the antigen very well, but nothing could be seen on elution. We therefore labelled the sialic acid residues on the surface membrane of human blood lymphocytes (PBL) using $^3$H (Ghamberg and Andersson, 1977) solubilized them and passed the labelled, solubilized membrane molecules through 2 small affinity columns. One was eluted by conventional techniques. The gel from the other colum was removed and boiled for 2 mins in 2% SDS, which will elute any non-covalently linked material from the gel. Control columns were also used. Analysis of the eluted materials by PAGE in SDS showed that the conventional elutions produced nothing, but boiling in SDS gave an excellent peak at the appropriate molecular weight. (Fig. 22·6). Clearly therefore, the antigen was being retained on the column, rather than being denatured on elution in the pilot experiments.

3. ANTIBODY ACTIVITY IS ELUTED FROM THE COLUMN

This can be detected since the amount of antibody activity in the eluted fractions is higher than that used in the assay system. We have seen this twice, in spite of the fact that the antibodies were covalently linked to CN Br activated Sepharose 4B columns, and that we always pre-elute our columns. It might be a result of the monoclonal antibody not having inter-heavy chain disulphide links, resulting in the elution of one half of the antibody molecule by the distortions caused by the elution procedure.

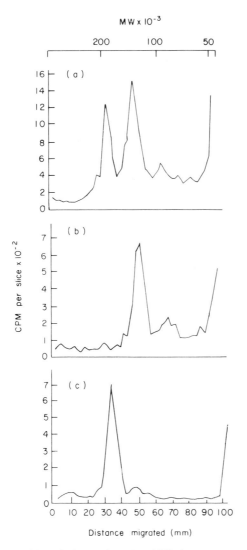

FIG. 22·6 Polyacrylamide gel electrophoresis of ³H thymocyte membrane. Thymocytes labelled at their sialic acid residues with ³H using Na B³H₄ were solubilized with Brij 99/96 and analyzed by PAGE in SDS using 6% gels. (a) sample before application to F10-89-4 (anti leucocyte common antigen) monoclonal antibody affinity column; (b) sample depleted by passage through this affinity column; and (c) eluted material. The gels were cut into 2 mm slices and the radioactivity per slice measured. The cpm added a, b and c were 6,000, 4,500 and 1,200 respectively.

## C. Bulk Purification of Molecules

### 1. INTRODUCTION

A monoclonal antibody affinity column offers the opportunity in one step to purify a membrane molecule one to several hundred fold in relation to total tissue protein. In addition to this high factor of purification, a specific affinity step has theoretical advantages over conventional biochemical techniques, since the purification does not depend on any biological characteristics of the molecule. It can be applied to very large volumes of antigen containing material, and serves as a concentrating as well as a purifying step. An example of bulk purification of a lymphocyte membrane molecule is given in Fig. 22·5.

### 2. PRACTICAL ASPECTS OF CHROMATOGRAPHY

Once the preliminary work has been completed, bulk purification is essentially a scaling up of the procedures outlined in section IVA. We generally use columns containing 8–10 ml of gel, made out of 10 or 20 ml glass syringes with a porous, inert support at the base. We apply 200–500 ml of soluble antigen at 10–20 ml per hour using a pump. The soluble material is passed through a 10 ml column of Sepharose 4B (in series with the affinity column) before passing on to the affinity column to remove any material which might adhere non-specifically to the affinity column. All steps are carried out at 4°C in the presence of proteolytic inhibitors, as outlined in section IIIE.

The solution that has passed through the column is collected into 10 ml fractions and every 5th or 10th fraction is checked for antigen activity, so that one can see when and if the column becomes saturated. After the sample has passed through, the column is washed with at least 100 ml of 0·5% detergent in the appropriate buffer, at 10–20 ml per hour using a pump. Fractions are collected and the optical density at 280 nm is measured. When the optical density is zero, or has stabilized close to zero, the column is eluted as described in section IVA using approximately 5 column volumes of eluting solution. This can be done quite quickly by hand-pipetting, and 5 ml fractions are collected. The fractions are neutralized (if pH change has been used for elution) and the first 5 or 6 fractions, along with the starting and several depleted fractions are analysed for antigen activity. If a plate assay (section IIIC3) is possible for detecting antigen, it can be particularly useful at this and subsequent purification stages. It is vital at this and at all subsequent stages to use disposable plastic or thoroughly cleansed glassware to avoid introducing contaminants into the purified solution.

The antigen containing fractions are pooled, and we routinely apply them to a gel filtration column at this stage, for two reasons. Not only does it serve as an extra purification step, but it effectively "desalts" the antigen containing solutions, removing the eluting and neutralizing substances (e.g. diethylamine, glycine). Concentration of the antigen prior to gel filtration is usually not necessary, as one can load up to 20 ml to a 500 ml column for gel filtration. (We use Sephacryl S-300 (Pharmacia, Uppsala, Sweden) ). The column should of course be equilibrated in 0·5% detergent in the appropriate buffer, and one should take great care to ensure that the antigen concentration in the sample is sufficiently high to be detected after a 5 fold or more dilution as a result of the gel filtration. One should aim to apply 2–4% of the column volume and smaller columns should be used for smaller samples. We collect 100 fractions, each 1% of the column volume, and examine consecutive, or alternate fractions for their content of antigen. Antigen containing fractions are pooled. We find it useful at this stage to concentrate the sample 4 or 5 fold by positive pressure filtration (Amicon, Woking, Surrey) and then, because the detergent will almost certainly be concentrated along with the antigen, to dialyse it against 0·5% detergent in the appropriate buffer. We then divide it into aliquots which are stored at −80°C.

3. CHECKS OF PURITY

At this stage, the purity of the sample should be checked, and SDS gels are now almost universally used for this purpose. It should be stressed that "purity" is a relative and not an absolute term, and, moreover, that it is uncommon for the material eluted from a monoclonal antibody affinity column to give a single band on SDS gels.

One should first determine the concentration of protein in the samples to be analysed, and it is useful to look at the starting detergent solution, the depleted solution, the antigen eluted from the affinity column and the sample after gel filtration. The usual technique for measuring proteins are modifications of the much-quoted paper by Lowry *et al.* (1951). In the context of the present discussion it is vital to note that detergents will frequently form precipitates and interfere with the colour reaction, but this can be overcome by including 1% SDS in the alkaline copper reagent. The standard curve should also contain the same concentration of detergent as that in the sample used to give the protein concentration, and this frequently means that 2 or 3 standard curves are necessary. If these precautions are taken, reproducible and accurate protein measurements will be the result. For the SDS gels we aim to load 10 $\mu$g to 20 $\mu$g of protein for each sample, and perform the electrophoresis on slab gels (which are vastly superior to the cylindrical "disc" gels). If one has no idea of the size of the molecule under study, both high (e.g. 12%) and low (e.g. 6%) percentage acrylamide gels should be used, so that both low and high molecular weight regions can be surveyed. At the termination of electrophoresis, the gels should be stained for both protein (e.g. Coomassie blue) and carbohydrate (periodic acid-Schiff reaction) as we have now 3 examples of membrane proteins which stained very well for carbohydrate but poorly for protein.

We routinely use 3 mm rather than 1·5 mm thick gels, because of the larger sample volume possible with the thicker gels. However, if one has difficulty in obtaining the antigen in a form concentrated enough to load approximately 10 $\mu$g of protein on the gels, one can precipitate the protein by use of acetone or trichloracetic acid. However, we have found it very useful simply to freeze-dry the sample and then resuspend it in loading buffer. If the antigen is in low salt and in 0·5% detergent, 300 to 400 $\mu$l can be freeze-dried and resuspended in 100 $\mu$l of loading buffer without difficulty. Apart from simplicity, freeze-drying does not have the potential problem of selective precipitation, which might occur with the above-mentioned reagents.

It is vital to note that it is not a simple thing to relate a band on a gel to the target molecule of the monoclonal antibody. If one has some previous idea of the expected molecular weight, things are much simpler. But if one has no idea of the size of molecule it is very dangerous to say that a particular band represents the antigen, even if there is only a single band on the gels. We have had the experience of staining a gel for protein and seeing only one major band, with an additional very faint band. On staining for carbohydrate, the weak band gave a very strong reaction, and it was this band that in fact contained the target antigen.

If only one band is seen after staining gels for both protein and carbohydrate, this is good presumptive evidence that the band represents the target antigen of the monoclonal antibody. It is not absolute proof, however. In the absence of other corroborative evidence, one should seek to prove the point by assaying for antigen from the gel itself. In these experiments, the antigen is electrophoresed in low (0·1%) SDS concentrations and without boiling, and immediately the electrophoresis is complete, the gel is cut into 3 mm slices. These are crushed, incubated overnight in a 0·3 ml of buffer and the supernatant assayed for antigen activity. Sometimes the antigen will be denatured by the SDS, but when it is not, this is an excellent way of associating antigen activity with a band on a gel. (e.g. McKenzie *et al.*, 1981). One should in fact run 3 samples of antigen in these experiments: one sample by conventional means, i.e. high SDS and boiling, and 2 samples in low SDS and without boiling. The conventional sample and one of the unboiled samples are then fixed and stained, to check that the electrophoretic mobility of the band under the milder conditions is not altered. A good example of how errors can arise is in relation to antibodies to $\beta_2$ microglobulin (Mol wt 12,000). These will purify HLA ABC antigens from cell membrane, and when run on, e.g. 6% acrylamide gels, the $\beta_2$ microglobulin will migrate with the dye while a major band will be seen at the 45,000 mol wt position. The monoclonal antibody however, is clearly not directed at this band.

If there are several bands on the gel, additional purification procedures might be necessary depending on the use to which the sample will be put. It is frequently useful to pass the sample through gel filtration a second time, and one can use the information obtained from the first run to choose the most appropriate gel for the second run. Thus, if the antigen runs close to the void volume on Sephacryl S300 (Pharmacia, Uppsala, Sweden), one can use Sepharose CL6B (Pharmacia, Uppsala, Sweden) for the second run, to obtain better separation of the antigen from its contaminants. Additional purification procedures can be used. We have used both lectin affinity and ion-exchange chromatography for final purification of Brij solubilized antigen. Preparative iso-electric focusing is also possible, but clearly both ion-exchange and iso-electric focusing techniques can be used only with non-ionic detergents. A number of other approaches are possible (Hoffmann-Ostenhof *et al.*, 1978) but these additional techniques are not as yet widely in use.

Once the antigen is "pure" (i.e. only one band on SDS gels after a reasonable amount, such as 10 $\mu$g, of sample protein is added to the gel) or is as pure as one wishes or is able to obtain it, one should assay this final sample and aliquots from each stage of the purification for antigen activity as well as protein content. After due allowance is made for volume variation during the purification, one can obtain a measure of the yield of antigen and the factor of purification in relation to the total protein in the starting material. For example, a 20% yield of antigen in 0·1% of the initial protein represents a 200 fold purification.

## D. MOLECULAR WEIGHT ESTIMATIONS USING AFFINITY COLUMNS

The usual method for estimating the molecular weights of cell surface proteins is to radio-label the surface molecules, to add a detergent (usually NP-40) to solubilize the membrane, and then to precipitate the target molecule by adding the monoclonal antibody, some normal mouse serum and an anti mouse immunoglobulin serum. The deficiencies of this approach are that one has no idea of the efficiency of the detergent used in the solubilization procedure, or its effect on the antigen or monoclonal antibody, and one has to be careful not to be in antigen or antibody excess in the precipitating step. The use of small affinity columns with systems previously tested as in sections III, IV offers a much more controlled system with which to work. It also means that it is possible to study the sample specifically depleted after passage through the column, and this can give much valuable information. Moreover, questions related to whether or not two antibodies are directed at the same molecule can be answered much more precisely and elegantly than with the current approach of sequential precipitations after "pre-clearing".

One can label cell surface molecules using a number of techniques. In the first instance, because at least the majority of proteins on the outer surface of cell membranes are glycosylated, we prefer to label the terminal sialic acids with $^3$H by use of sodium periodate and NaB$^3$H$_4$ (Ghamberg and Andersson, 1977). This technique is in fact useful only if the molecule under study is heavily glycosylated, but it is an especially attractive system when it works, because of its selectivity. If this fails, we attempt surface iodination with $^{125}$I using the iodogen method (Markwell and Fox, 1978). This is a better technique than lactoperoxidase catalysed iodination, in that the iodination seems to be restricted much more to cell surface proteins. One can also iodinate solubilized proteins in detergent solutions using either the chloramine T or iodogen methods. This results in very high specific activities, but even after careful desalting to remove unreacted $^{125}$I, backgrounds are very high. There is little advantage in the use of this method unless the solubilized material has been substantially purified prior to iodination (e.g. Hart and Fabre, 1981). With cultured cells and lines, one can introduce labelled amino acids or sugars. It should be noted that the surface labelling of cells with $^3$H and $^{125}$I can easily be applied to tissue homogenates (Lakin and Fabre, 1981).

We aim to label a minimum of $2 \times 10^8$ blood lymphocytes by the $^3$H method or $2 \times 10^7$ with $^{125}$I. With blood lymphocytes, generally $10^6$ cpm are incorporated per $10^8$ cells using the $^3$H label, and $5 \times 10^6$ cpm per $10^7$ cells using iodogen for $^{125}$I labelling. Because of the long half-life of $^3$H (12 years) quite large numbers of cells can be labelled, and the soluble, labelled membranes stored frozen. After the cells have been labelled and washed, the volume in which they are solubilized is determined primarily by two considerations: the desirability of having the sample sufficiently concentrated so that it can be run on SDS gels without concentration, and also the desirability of having the sample in a reasonable volume (e.g. 2 ml) for the affinity chromatography step. Detergent/protein ratios are not a problem here because the amount of tissue to be solubilized is relatively small. After $^3$H labelling, we resuspend blood lymphocytes to $1\text{-}2 \times 10^8$ ml$^{-1}$, and after $^{125}$I labelling, to approximately $2 \times 10^7$ ml$^{-1}$ for subsequent solubilization.

After addition of detergents, we proceed as rapidly as possible in the presence of proteolytic inhibitors and being careful to maintain the solutions at 0°C to 4°C at all times, (see section IIIE). We add the appropriate detergent (section II), usually Brij 99/96 with blood lymphocytes, for 30 minutes, and then spin out the nuclei. The supernatant is then quickly frozen at $-80$°C or prepared immediately for affinity chromatography. Although it is not essential, the Brij extract (freshly prepared or just thawed) is usually made up to 1% deoxycholate to ensure complete solubilization of all membranes just before chromatography, even if the antigen system under study does not require deoxycholate for solubilization (see section II). This is done by adding 1/3 the volume of 4% deoxycholate to the Brij extract and incubating for 30 minutes. We have found that over the time period involved in the chromatography (1½ or 2 hours) the deoxycholate does not gel even though the Brij extract is in $0 \cdot 15$M NaCl and at pH $7 \cdot 4$ (see section IIA). It is useful to check the radio-activity of the sample before and after spinning out the nuclei, to see what proportion of the label is lost at this step. The recovery is usually 90% or better with blood lymphocytes, but usually much less with homogenates.

For the chromatography, we use small columns with $0 \cdot 7$ ml of gel and apply the sample precisely as outlined in section IVA. The volume of the sample loaded should be approximately 2 ml, and it can be made up to 2 ml if necessary by addition of the appropriate detergent solution. We aim to load approximately $10^6$ cpm with $^3$H labelled samples and 3 to $5 \times 10^7$ cpm with $^{125}$I, although the amount loaded will vary with the system under study, and the more one loads, probably the better. A depleted sample is collected after 1 column volume of radio-labelled solution has passed through the column. The column is washed as outlined in Section IVA in $0 \cdot 5\%$ of the appropriate detergent, usually with about 10 ml of buffer, checking the radio-activity in the washes. Elution of the antigen may be performed as outlined in section IVA, but for analysis on SDS gels we find that it is better to remove the gel from the column in a small amount of $0 \cdot 5\%$ detergent solution, to sediment the beads by centrifuging at 400 g for 5 minutes in a glass tube, and then to add approximately 0·5 ml of 2% SDS in 0·25M Tris, pH 6·8. This is then placed on a boiling water bath for 2–3 minutes with shaking. For maximum recovery of eluted sample, the gel in 2% SDS is applied in a small column (like that used for chromatography) and the buffer allowed to drain into a tube. A further 0·7 ml of hot 2% SDS is then applied and allowed to pass through the gel to wash out the remaining radio-active material. The amount of radioactivity in the depleted and eluted samples should be measured.

For analysis by PAGE in SDS, we use 3 mm thick slab gels. As outlined in section IV C. 3 both high and low % acrylamide gels should be used if one has no idea of what molecular weight to expect. We aim to analyse the sample before application to the affinity column, the depleted sample and the eluted material. For $^3$H labelled samples we aim to load 50,000 to 100,000 cpm for the starting and depleted samples, and 10,000 to 20,000 cpm for the eluted material. With iodogen labelling of cell surfaces, we tend to load 10,000 to 20,000 cpm for the eluted material. If the samples are too dilute to allow a suitable number of counts to be loaded, one can precipitate protein-bound radioactivity from a larger volume using acetone or trichloracetic acid or, more simply by just freeze-drying a larger volume and resuspending it in loading buffer. A useful piece of advice, when loading samples on slab gels for subsequent slicing (see next paragraph), is to use only every third well, to avoid artefacts caused by diffusion from one track to another. In addition, one should note that with tritiated samples, which will subsequently be analysed by scintillation counting, the gel must be fixed but not stained prior to slicing, because of the quenching effects of the protein stain.

Once the electrophoresis is completed, one can examine the gels either by slicing them and counting the radioactivity per slice (e.g. Dalchau and Fabre, 1981) or by autoradiography. Slicing the gels is time-consuming and requires application and precision, but it is an excellent method and gives a good quantitative idea of the amount of radioactivity in each peak, as shown in Fig. 22·6. The resolution of different bands, however, is not quite as good as with autoradiography and this can sometimes be important. The ideal, of course, is to do both methods.

# V EXAMPLES OF EXPERIMENTS MADE POSSIBLE BY MONOCLONAL ANTIBODY AFFINITY CHROMATOGRAPHY

## A. ANALYSIS OF SPECIFICALLY DEPLETED AND PURIFIED MATERIAL

With only a few ml of solubilized material and with small affinity columns one can make the following reagents available for study:

1.   The original complex solution.
2.   The original solution specifically depleted of one component.
3.   The specific component (depleted in 2) purified several hundred-fold.

These three reagents represent a most powerful approach for the analysis of molecular functions, relatedness between molecules, and similar questions. For example, we were able to show that 2 monoclonal antibodies both specific to leucocytes but showing very different patterns of reactivity amongst leucocytes, were directed at different determinants on the same molecule (Dalchau and Fabre, 1981).

A more common question that arises is whether or not antibodies with similar reactivity patterns are directed at the same molecule. An excellent, and indeed the only certain, way of answering this question is by serological analysis of specifically depleted and purified material. Only one antibody in the group needs to function well in affinity work, and once specifically depleted and purified material is available for this antibody, the remaining members of the group can be checked by inhibition studies.

## B. RECEPTOR LIGAND INTERACTIONS

### 1. USING PURE ANTIGENS

Once a molecule is pure, its interaction with other molecules, particularly on cell surfaces, can be studied. For example, human Thy-1 has been purified in this laboratory (McKenzie *et al.*, 1981) and it has been suggested that Thy-1 might be involved in lymphocyte recirculation by an interaction of Thy-1 on the endothelium of post-capillary venules of lymph node with a Thy-1 receptor on lymphocytes (McKenzie and Fabre, 1981). We therefore incubated rat lymphocytes with pure, detergent-free canine Thy-1 and checked for interaction of Thy-1 with the cell surface by incubating with monoclonal antibody to canine Thy-1 and fluoroscein labelled anti mouse immunoglobulin. This and appropriate controls were then analysed on the fluorescence activated cell sorter. Although the work is still in progress, we have been able to demonstrate very nicely that there is a specific interaction of Thy-1 with the lymphocyte surface (Fig. 22·7). (McKenzie, Dalchau and Fabre in preparation).

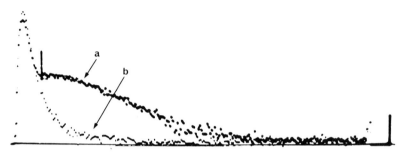

FIG. 22·7 Demonstration of receptor ligand interactions using pure antigen. Purified canine Thy-1 (McKenzie *et al.*, 1981) was incubated with rat lymph node lymphocytes and then (a) anti canine Thy-1 monoclonal antibody (McKenzie *et al.*, 1981b) or (b) with anti human Thy-1 monoclonal antibody (McKenzie *et al.*, 1981a) as a control. They were then incubated with fluorescein labelled anti mouse immunoglobulin and analysed on a fluorescence activated cell sorter.

## 2. USING AFFINITY COLUMNS

After soluble material has been passed through the affinity column and it has been washed, one has a column containing large amounts of the specific antigen on the surface of the beads. Interactions of this molecule with other molecules can be studied in many ways using a variety of indicator systems. We have not yet explored this approach but one possible use would be in relation to the proposed interaction of platelet glycoprotein lb with VIII/von Willebrand factor (Ruan *et al.*, 1981 and see chapter 8). One could take a small anti glycoprotein lb column and pass through Brij solubilized platelet membranes until the column is saturated (Ruan *et al.*, 1982). After washing radio-labelled Factor VIII could be passed through this column, washed, and then eluted. SDS gels could be used to see whether or not the Factor VIII adsorbed to and eluted from the column. Control columns of anti glycoprotein lb without platelet membrane passed through it, and an irrelevant column with platelet membrane passed through, would have to be included.

## C. Antigen Specific Targets

The precise specificity of antibodies is frequently difficult to determine, particularly if the antibodies are of low affinity and if complex sera of multiple specificities are being studied. The use of purified antigens as targets for serological assays offers a particularly attractive solution to this problem, since the specificity of positive reactions is predetermined by the use of single antigens as targets. We are currently using this approach to determine the specificity of autoantibodies in various disease conditions.

## VI CONCLUSION

We hope that this chapter has demonstrated the essential simplicity and wide-ranging potential of monoclonal antibody affinity chromatography, and that it will provide both a stimulus and practical help to the reader interested in the subject.

REFERENCES

Dalchau, R. and Fabre, J. W. (1981). *J. exp. Med.* **153**, 753–765.
Dalchau, R., Kirkley, J. and Fabre, J. W. (1980a). *Eur. J. Immunol.* **10**, 737–744.
Dalchau, R., Kirkley, J. and Fabre, J. W. (1980b). *Eur. J. Immunol.* **10**, 745–749.
Gahmberg, C. S. and Andersson, L. C. (1977). *J. biol. Chem.* **252**, 5888–5894.
Hart, D. N. J. and Fabre, J. W. (1981). *J. Immunol.* **126**, 2109–2113.
Helenius, A., McCoslin, D. R., Fries, E. and Tanford, C. (1979). *Methods in Enzymology* **56**, 734–749.
Hoffman-Ostenhof, O., Breitenbach, M., Koller, F., Kroft, D. and Scheiner, O. (1978). Affinity Chromatography. Pergamon Press, Oxford.
Kohler, G., and Milstein, C. (1975). *Nature* **256**, 495–497.
Lakin, K. H. and Fabre, J. W. (1981). *J. Neurochem.* **37**, 1170–1178.
Lowry, H., Rosebrough, N. J., Farr, A. and Randall, R. J. (1951). *J. biol. Chem.* **193**, 265–275.
Markwell, M. A. K. and Fox, C. F. (1978). *Biochemistry* **17**, 4807–4817.
McKenzie, J. L., Allen, A. K. and Fabre, J. W. (1981). *Biochem. J.* **197**, 629–636.
McKenzie, J. L. and Fabre, J. W. (1981). *J. Immunol.* **126**, 843–850.
Potter, M. (1972). *Physiol. Rev.* **52**, 631–719.
Ruan, C., Dalchau, R., Allen, A. K. and Fabre, J. W. (1982). (in preparation).

Ruan, C., Tobelem, G., McMichael, A., Drouet, L., Legrard, Y., Degos, L., Kieffer, N., Lee, H., Caan, P., (1981). *Brit. J. Haematol.* (in press).

Springer, R. A., Strominger, J. L. and Mann, D. (1974). *Proc. natn. Acad. Sci. U.S.A.* **71**, 1539–1543.

Standring, R. and Williams, A. F. (1978). *Biochem. Biophys. Acta.* **508**, 85–96.

Tanford, C. and Reynolds, J. A. (1976). *Biochem. Biophys. Acta.* **457**, 133–170.

Williams, A. F. (1973). *Eur. J. Immunol.* **3**, 626–632.

# 23 The Use of the Fluorescence Activated Cell Sorter for the Identification and Analysis of Function of Cell Subpopulations

P. C. L. BEVERLEY

*Imperial Cancer Research Fund, Human Tumour Immunology Group, University College Hospital Medical School, University Street, London. WC1E 6JJ*

# I INTRODUCTION

## A. Cell Sorters and Monoclonal Antibodies

It is not the intention of this chapter to attempt a comprehensive review of the application of flow cytometric methods in biological research or even in clinical medicine. Rather I shall attempt to describe the use of monoclonal antibodies with flow cytometry for the identification and enumeration of different cell populations and the separation of these populations for functional analysis.

While cell sorting and analysis has played a role in animal studies for several years because alloantisera with relatively defined specificities have been available, this was not the case for man. The advent of many monoclonal antibodies against human cell surface differentiation antigens however, (see chapters 3, 4, 6, 8, 16 and 19) has provided reagents which in their high degree of specificity match the analytical capabilities of modern flow cytometers. This has led to an increasing use of flow cytometry in human immunology and clinical medicine and it is this area which will be reviewed here.

Comprehensive reviews of the technical aspects of cell sorting are available elsewhere (Melamed *et al.*, 1979) and practical methods for analysis and sorting have also been well reviewed (Herzenberg and Herzenberg, 1978).

## B. How Fluorescence Activated Cell Sorters Work

In present day cell sorters or flow cytometers, cells in suspension are introduced into a stream of liquid which passes through a focused beam of light, usually produced by a laser. Each cell in passing the light beam generates signals by scattering the light or emitting fluorescence and these signals are received by suitably placed photodetectors. In a flow cytometer these signals are amplified, analysed and displayed electronically while cell sorters have the additional capability for separation of cells according to predetermined criteria.

Fig. 23·1 is a simplified block diagram of a fluorescence activated cell sorter (FACS) and illustrates the main features of the instrument. Cells in suspension are introduced into a stream of sheath fluid and pass through a nozzle which vibrates so that the stream breaks up into droplets a short distance below the nozzle. The stream is intersected just below the nozzle by a beam of laser light and signals produced by cells in the stream are detected by photomultiplier (PMT) tubes placed in line and at right angles to the beam of laser light. Amplified signals from the PMT tubes are displayed on a screen in various formats (see below) for analysis.

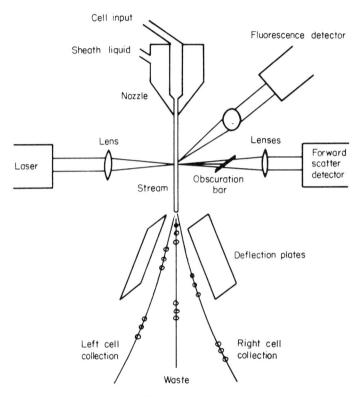

FIG. 23·1 How the cell sorter works.

During sorting, signals generated by each cell are compared to criteria set by the operator which define, for example by fluorescence intensity and light scatter signals, desired populations. If an individual cell meets these criteria a positive or negative charge is applied to the stream so that when the detected cell reaches the stream tip and becomes encased in a droplet, that droplet can be deflected to right or left by charged plates and collected. In practice it is more usual to charge and deflect triplets of droplets to ensure collection of the cell. The limitations and practical problems encountered in this type of sorting will be discussed more fully in section IV.

# II DISPLAY AND ANALYSIS OF DATA

## A. Introduction

Present commercially available cell sorters are capable of measuring several signals simultaneously from each cell passing through the single or dual laser beams. Optical systems to allow this vary, but include the use of beam splitters, dichroic mirrors, selective filters and obscuration bars. With this combination of methods it is usually possible to measure at least two different colours of fluorescence, forward and 90° light scattering, as well as fluorescence polarization. Future machines will probably also incorporate cell volume measurement capability. For work with monoclonal antibodies however the most commonly used analysis involves a single colour of fluorescence and forward angle light scattering as an approximate measure of cell size (see section IID). As an example to illustrate the methods most often used for displaying and analysing data, I shall take the case of human peripheral blood mononuclear cells isolated on ficoll hypaque and stained using indirect immunofluorescence with a mouse monoclonal antibody (UCHT1) against all mature T cells (Beverley and Callard, 1981a). This is not a simple example since the peripheral blood mononuclear fraction is a complex mixture of different mononuclear cell types and is often contaminated by significant numbers of red cells. A common requirement is to obtain estimates of the proportion of different cell types in the mononuclear population so that means for identifying the degree of contamination are required.

## B. Histograms and Gating

The simplest form of data display available is that of the single parameter histogram in which either units of fluorescence intensity or light scattering per cell are plotted on the horizontal axis, which usually consists of 256 channels, and frequency of cells on the vertical axis. Examples of scatter and fluorescence histograms of this type are shown in Figs. 23·2(a) and 23·2(b). The appearance of such a plot may be varied by using a log scale for cell numbers (vertical axis) and it has recently become possible to log transform the fluorescence or scatter signals giving clearer separation of positive and negative peaks.

At first sight such plots, although simple to understand do not appear to allow correlation of different parameters. For example it is impossible to say from inspection of the histograms of Figs. 23·2(a) and 23·2(b) which size of cell is brightly stained by UCHT1. In fact it is possible to extract this information by using a scatter "gate". The gate works as follows. The scatter signal from each cell after amplification and transformation into an electrical pulse whose size is proportional to the original light signal, is compared to values (gates) set by the operator to determine whether that signal is to be included in the data set displayed on the screen. Thus for example it is possible in our example to "gate out" the two left hand peaks of Fig. 23·2(a) which consist of debris, platelets and red cells. Examination of the light scatter of the remaining cells gives a profile with a single peak (Fig. 23·2(c) ). The fluorescence of the scatter gated cells is shown in Fig. 23·2(d) and it can be seen that

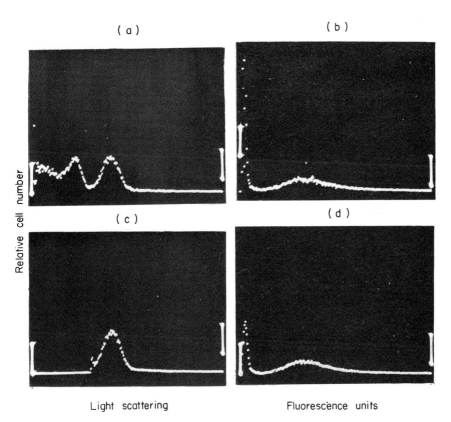

FIG. 23·2 Light scattering and fluorescence histograms. Peripheral blood mononuclear cells were stained for analysis with UCHT1 and FITC sheep anti-mouse immunoglobulin antiserum. Conditions for analysis, laser power 400 mw, photomultiplier 580V, scatter gain 4/1·0 and fluorescence gain 16/0·8. (a) Ungated scatter; (b) Ungated fluorescence; (c) Gated scatter; (d) Scatter gated fluorescence.

the relative size of the two peaks of positive and negative cells differs from that in Fig. 23·2(b). This implies that the small (red) cells which have not been examined in Fig. 23·2(d) were at least largely unstained and must have contributed mainly to the left hand peak in Fig. 23·2(b).

While correlating two parameters using gating and histograms is tedious and similar information can more easily be obtained from dot plots and isometric plots, gating is extremely useful for two main purposes. It is often used in exactly the way illustrated above to exclude from analysis the majority of red cells and dead cells so that subpopulations of nucleated cells can be enumerated (see Fig. 23·4) and it is also possible to set a gate on one parameter, for example light scattering, and then perform analysis of two other parameters, for example red and green fluorescence, on the gated population. The gate therefore effectively allows the analysis of three parameters at once.

## C. DOT AND ISOMETRIC PLOTS

Fig. 23·3(a) shows a dot display of the cell sample illustrated in Fig. 23·2. Each cell appears on the screen as a dot whose x and y axis co-ordinates represent the light scatter and fluorescence signals for the cell. By inspection of such a plot it is easy to gain an impression of which size of cell bears the fluorescent label. In Fig. 23·3(a) for example, it is clear that the majority of fluorescent cells fall in an intermediate size range (small lymphocytes). Both the red cells and larger cells (monocytes) are predominantly unstained as are some small lymphocytes. The dot plot of Fig. 23·3(b) corresponds to the scatter gated fluorescence histogram of Fig. 23·2(d). The stained and unstained populations of small lymphocytes now appear more prominent since with this format a constant number of dots are displayed on the screen and the red cells are no longer shown.

Since each pair of co-ordinates on the screen can only display a single dot the magnitude of homogeneous populations may be underestimated. Isometric plots (Figs. 23·3(c) and 23·3(d) ) overcome this limitation of dot plots by displaying the parameters as a two dimensional histogram. The height of the peaks shows the number of cells in a subpopulation.

All three types of display can be photographed to provide a permanent record of the analysis or alternatively if the instrument is connected to a computer the data can be stored for subsequent plotting in a variety of forms. While visual displays are extremely helpful in the interpretation of data or in sorting populations for subsequent functional analysis, in many cases what is required is a simple numerical division of a population into those which carry a given marker and those which do not. How such figures can be obtained is illustrated in the following sections. Three steps are required: to examine the scatter profile and set a scatter gate, to obtain a fluorescence threshold above which a cell can be considered positive and to determine what percentage of cells fall above this threshold.

## D. SCATTER ANALYSIS

The amount of light scattered at a small forward angle (1–13°) is an approximate measure of cell size. The principle cause of this type of scattering is diffraction but it is also influenced to a lesser extent by other cell properties such as shape, refractive index, number of organelles and size of nucleus. In general however there is a good correlation

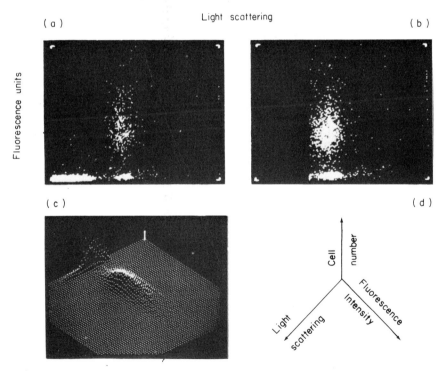

FIG. 23·3 Dot and isometric plots. Peripheral blood mononuclear cells stained and analyzed as for Fig. 23·2. (a) Ungated dot plot; (b) Scatter gated dot plot; (c) Isometric plot, scatter gated; (d) Axes of isometric plot.

between size measured by light scattering or by other methods (Herzenberg and Herzenberg, 1978). Thus by setting a scatter gate as for example in Fig. 23·2(c) it is possible to exclude from analysis the majority of red cells although particularly in some pathological conditions, significant numbers may fall within the nucleated cell size range.

It is also possible using light scattering to exclude from analysis the majority of dead cells since in general these give a smaller scatter signal than a live cell of the same size (Loken and Herzenberg, 1975). In most lymphoid cell populations (blood, spleen, lymph nodes, thymus) dead cells fall in the same scatter range as erythrocytes and can therefore be gated out. Problems may be encountered however, when the size range of the cells is very great or when lymphoid and non-lymphoid cells are analysed simultaneously. Under these conditions the scatter of large dead cells may overlap that of small live cells and make it impossible to set an appropriate scatter gate. This difficulty can sometimes be overcome be labelling viable cells with the dye fluorescein diacetate (Rotman and Papermaster, 1966) though this would obviate the use of fluorescein conjugated antibody for detection of surface markers.

When an appropriate scatter gate has been set an analysis of the fluorescence of the gated population is performed as follows.

## E. Fluorescence Analysis

With monoclonal antibodies there may be readily recognizable separation between positive and negative populations (Figs. 23·2 and 23·3) and it is then straightforward to set a fluorescence threshold (gate) above which a cell is considered positive and below which it is negative. This may not always be so (see for example Fig. 23·5) and it is then usual to set a fluorescence threshold by reference to an appropriate control.

For routine analysis when using indirect immunofluorescence we use as our standard control, cells which have been incubated first with either an irrelevant monoclonal antibody or culture medium and then with the fluorescent anti-immunoglobulin. The scatter gated fluorescence of such a "second layer" control is illustrated in Fig. 23·4(a). A part of the detected fluorescence may be due to non-specific absorption of fluorescent anti-immunoglobulin but with the high amplification of fluorescence signals which is necessary if there are few antigenic sites per cell, even totally unstained cells give detectable signals. It is apparent from a consideration of Figs. 23·4(a) and 23·4(b) that the fluorescence of the brightest control cells is in the same range as that of cells which may be considered positive in the UCHT1 stained sample. Thus the profile in Fig. 23·4(b) consists of two overlapping profiles, of the stained and unstained lymphocytes, which are indicated by the dotted lines. Since the exact shape of the curve produced by the stained cells is not usually known, it is usual to set the fluorescence gate such that only a small number (<5%) of control cells are scored as positive. This is illustrated in Fig. 23·4(b) and gives 3% and 72% positive cells for the control and UCHT1 stained populations respectively.

When working with human peripheral blood mononuclear cells an additional problem remains, that there is often an overlap in size (scatter) between lymphocytes and red cells so that the figures obtained may be underestimates of the true frequencies in the white cell population of positive cells. We have recently developed a simple method to

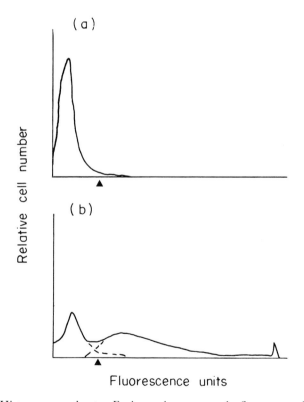

FIG. 23·4 Histograms and gates. Each panel represents the fluorescence histogram of $10^4$ scatter gated mononuclear cells. (a) Second layer control; (b) UCHT1 stained cells. The ▲ shows the positive of the fluorescence gate used to estimate the percentage of antigen positive cells.

estimate the frequency of contaminating red cells (Linch *et al.*, submitted for publication). A sample of the mononuclear cells is stained with a 1:1 mixture of antibodies against a non-polymorphic determinant of HLA and a common leucocyte antigen (Beverley, 1980) and the percentage of positive cells determined. Since the combination of antibodies stains very brightly all nucleated cells, but not red cells, this gives a reliable estimate of red cell contamination and the percentages of positive cells obtained with other antisera can be adjusted accordingly. In the example in Fig. 23·4 the mixture of antibodies stained 95% of the scatter gated cells and the true figures for the control and UCHT1 staining are therefore $(3 \div 95) \times 100$ and $(72 \div 95) \times 100$ expressed as percentages of the white blood cells only.

The type of analysis described above works well if the overlap between positive and negative populations is small. If the overlap is great because each cell has few antigenic sites detected by the antibody in use it is not reliable because it is impossible to set a fluorescence gate which gives a true reflection of the number of (weakly) positive cells. Under such conditions it may be possible to use high electronic amplification to resolve the overlapping populations. This technique has been used to detect low amounts of HLA-DR antigen on human peripheral T cells (Mann and Sharrow, 1981). Other more sophisticated computer based methods of data analysis are also available (Miller *et al.*, 1978) and have been used for example in the analysis of lectin binding to murine thymocytes (Fowlkes *et al.*, 1980).

### F. Preparation of Cells and Reagents

It should be apparent from the foregoing discussion of scatter and fluorescence analysis that interpretation of the data is most simple when clear separation of stained and unstained population is obtained. The best resolution can only be obtained by taking care both with preparation of the cells and the staining reagents.

Since dead cells may cause problems (Section IID), especially if the cell population is very heterogenous in size, it is worth taking pains to ensure maximal viability if necessary by removal of dead cells (Shortman *et al.*, 1971; Von Boehmer and Shortman, 1973; Davidson and Parrish, 1975). Even more important however, is the preparation of good staining reagents and particularly the removal of aggregated immunoglobulin, since this is liable to bind to any cells with Fc receptors. A counsel of perfection is to ultracentrifuge (100,000 × g for 30 minutes) both first and second layer antibodies immediately before use.

This may not always be practicable and we have used the following methods and obtained satisfactory results (Beverley and Callard, 1981a).

For staining with monoclonal antibodies we generally use culture supernatant since this gives low non-specific staining, perhaps because of the low ratio of mouse immunoglobulin to irrelevant serum proteins. The sample is microfuged before use and an additional step which may also be useful is to pass the supernatant through a $0 \cdot 22$ micron filter. Second layer anti-immunoglobulin is carefully absorbed with human immunoglobulin and then immunoabsorbent purified. It is microfuged (and filtered if necessary) before use. Since the concentration of labelled immunoglobulin is usually high we also find it useful to add normal serum (10%) from the species in which the anti immunoglobulin was raised to compete with the labelled material for Fc receptors.

Using these simple measures we have not found it necessary to resort to the use of Fab or F(ab)2 fragments and have been able to stain even cells with readily detectable Fc receptors without undue non-specific background (Callard *et al.*, 1981).

## III ANALYSIS IN CLINICAL MEDICINE

### A. Advantages of FACS Analysis

It is clear that FACS analysis has not as yet become a routine part of clinical investigation. There are a number of obvious reasons for this. The instruments themselves are expensive and for routine use have not been easy to run in such a way as to produce reproducible results on a day to day basis. There have not been suitable reagents (antibodies) available for detection and enumeration of relevant human cells. In addition it has not been obvious to most clinicians, except in the case of a small minority of diseases, that monitoring populations of cells other than by conventional methods is a useful exercise. Finally it is fair to add that in many cases a fluorescence microscope can be used as an alternative to FACS analysis.

Several advances have begun to alter this view. Construction of an analytical flow cytometer is not impossible (Steen and Lindmo, 1979) and commercially available flow cytometers for analysis only are relatively cheap. Monoclonal antibodies to human differentiation antigens are widely available and the functions of populations which they identify are becoming better defined (Reinherz and Schlossman, 1981). Recent results from several laboratories have indicated that in some diseases although total white cell counts´ or lymphocyte counts may remain within normal limits there can be major alterations in leucocyte subpopulations and monitoring such changes may provide diagnostic or prognostic information or be useful in following the effects of treatment (see chapter 3). Finally FACS analysis has the advantages over fluorescence microscopy that it obviates tedious visual counting, is rapid and quantitative and that much larger numbers of cells (tens of thousands compared to a few hundreds) can be enumerated. In the following section, I shall consider some examples of the use of FACS analysis largely taken from our own work.

## B. ANALYSIS OF FOETAL LEUCOCYTES

It is now possible to obtain by foetoscopy samples of foetal blood from about the 14–15th week of gestation onwards (Rodeck, 1980). We have used small amounts of such samples taken for diagnostic purposes to examine in detail the nature of leucocytes in the foetal circulation. Since the amounts of blood available are small (usually less than $400 \mu$ls) and white blood cell counts are low ($2-3 \times 10^9 \, 1^{-1}$) we have developed new methods for the analysis. The foetal blood diluted with an approximately equal volume of heparinized tissue culture medium is mixed 1:1 with hydroxyethyl starch (Plasmasteril, Fresenius, Bad Homburg, Germany) and allowed to stand for 20–30 minutes at room temperature. The leucocyte rich upper layer is collected and washed by centrifugation. No attempt is made to eliminate all red cells as these act as useful carriers during the staining. Aliquots of blood containing as few as $2 \cdot 5 \times 10^4$ nucleated cells are stained in microtitre plates using methods detailed more fully elsewhere (Linch *et al.*, submitted for publication). At the end of the staining by indirect immunofluorescence the cells are resuspended in a small volume (200 microlitres) of medium and the red cells are lysed by addition of 150 microlitres of Zap-oglobin (2 drops in 10 mls Isoton II Coulter Electronics) immediately before the sample is analysed on the FACS. The usual controls are run including one to enumerate all white cells (see section IIE).

Fig. 23·5 shows a series of dot plots from the analysis of a sample from a foetus of gestational age 19 weeks. While the background staining (Fig. 23·5a) is somewhat higher than we are accustomed to with isolated adult cells, the staining with monoclonal antibodies against thymus derived (T) subsets, lymphocytes and granulocytes is clearly distinguishable. We have been able to obtain satisfactory analytical data with up to 6 different sera on as little as 200 microlitres of foetal blood. The high background may be due at least in part to the fact that early lymphocytes are known to possess particularly avid Fc receptors (Seigal, 1976).

While as yet we have not used this method for diagnostic purposes it should be possible to identify at least some forms of severe immunodeficiency. It should also be possible using slightly larger amounts of

( a )              ( b )

( c )              ( d )

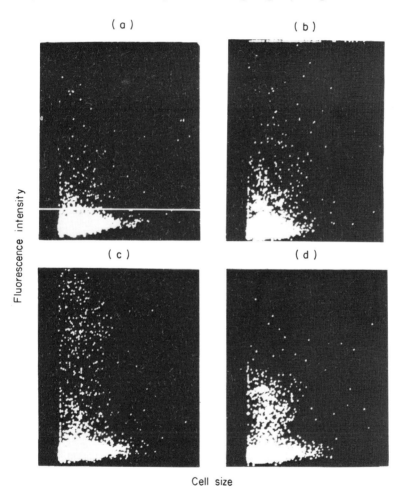

Cell size

FIG. 23·5 FACS analysis of foetal cells. Foetal leucocytes were stained and analyzed on a FACS IV. (a) Second layer control; (b) TG-1 anti polymorph antibody. Many of the cells are very brightly stained at this fluorescence gain and appear at the top of the panel as limiting signals; (c) Leu 2a antibody to cytotoxic/suppressor T subset (d) Leu 3a antibody to helper/inducer T subset.

blood, to isolate subpopulations of foetal leucocytes for further study. Additionally this methodology should be readily applicable to adult blood and may avoid the problem of selective cell loss inherent in ficoll hypaque or other separation methods. It would also decrease the time needed for analysis as well as the amount of blood required.

## C. Analysis of Adult Lymphocyte Subpopulations

As yet there have been few reports of the use of FACS analysis in clinical practice other than in the typing of leukaemias (chapter 6). However, data on the distribution of T cell subsets in multiple sclerosis has been published (Reinherz et al., 1980b). This report is particularly interesting in that there appears to be a correlation between loss of OKT8 positive cells (T suppressor/cytotoxic subset) from the peripheral blood and acute exacerbations or progression of the disease. In this study FACS analysis was not used to obtain data unobtainable by conventional fluorescence microscopy but has the advantage of sampling a much larger number of cells than would be possible by visual counting. It is expected that similar methods will be applied to other diseases in which disturbances in immunoregulation have already been described (Raveche and Steinberg, 1979; Palacios et al., 1981) to obtain more quantitative and reliable data on changes in lymphocyte subpopulations with time and under the influence of therapy.

A different use of FACS analysis is exemplified by our own studies of a group of patients with haemopoietic disturbances, mainly neutropenia and erythroid aplasia. (Callard et al., 1981; Linch et al., 1981). At first sight these patients appear to have an associated disturbance of T cell subsets which is very similar to that seen in the acute stage of infectious mononucleosis (Reinherz et al., 1980a; Crawford et al., 1981) when an excess of suppressor/cytotoxic T cells (OKT3 + OKT8+) is found in the peripheral blood. However, when we used OKT1-like antisera, which had been claimed to be markers for all peripheral T cells (Kung et al., 1979), our initial examination by fluorescence microscopy was difficult to interpret. A few cells stained brightly but the staining of the majority was extremely weak and there was no clear distinction between positive and negative cells. The reason for this is illustrated in the dot plots of Fig. 23·6. While sheep red cell (E) rosette forming cells from the patient stain as well as those from the normal control with UCHT1 (OKT3-like) panels c and d, the patients E+ cells stain poorly with OKT1, panel b. It is also apparent from Fig. 23·6b that there is a continuous distribution of staining ranging from unstained to brightly stained with the majority of cells staining only weakly. In this example therefore the FACS analysis provides convincing confirmation of the reality of the weak staining seen by fluorescence microscopy. Using a fluorescence gate set by reference to a second layer control (see section IIE and Fig. 23·4) it is also possible to obtain a figure for the percentage of positive cells although because of the lack of separation of positive and negative populations this is a rather suspect exercise.

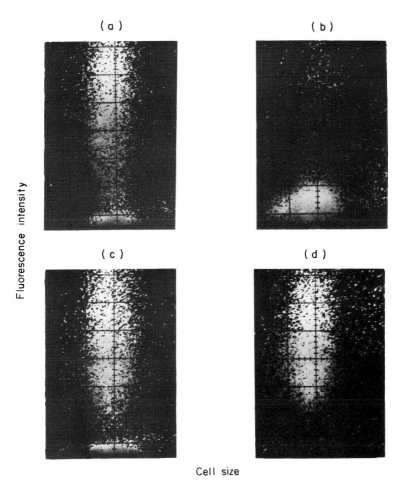

FIG. 23·6 FACS analysis of E rosette forming cells. Isolated E+ cells from a normal individual and a neutropenic patient were stained with either OKT1 or UCHT1 monoclonal antibody. (a) Normal-OKT1; (b) Neutropenic-OKT1; (c) Normal-UCHT1; (d) Neutropenic-UCHT1. (From *Clin. exp. Immunol* **43**, 500. Reprinted with permission from Blackwell Scientific Publications).

In these patients FACS analysis therefore provided clear evidence for the existence of a subset of T cells with the phenotype UCHT1+, OKT1±, OKT8+. We have subsequently confirmed the existence of cells with this phenotype in several more patients and extended our analysis using additional antisera similar to OKT1 (Beverley and Callard, 1981b). Table 23·1 gives data from such an analysis and shows that in addition to the lack of OKT1-like antigen the T cells from these

TABLE 23·1
FACS analysis of E+ cells

| Marker | % +ve cells | |
|---|---|---|
| | Normal | Neutropenia |
| 2nd layer only (control) | 2 | 1 |
| UCHT1 | 96 | 89 |
| OKT1 | 93 | 13 |
| Leu 1 | 94 | 11 |
| UCHT2 | 90 | 5 |
| UCHT3 | 90 | 6 |
| Leu 2a | 32 | 77 |
| Leu 3a | 63 | 11 |
| HLA-DR | 2 | 36 |
| FcγR | 10 | 97 |

UCHT1 recognizes all mature peripheral T cells. OKT1, Leu 1, UCHT2 and 3 recognize closely related surface antigens present on most peripheral T cells. Leu 2a and 3a recognize suppressor/cytotoxic and helper/inducer T subsets respectively.

patients carry FcγR, in contrast to those found in mononucleosis (Haynes *et al.*, 1979), and also show evidence of activation in that they have readily detectable HLA-DR antigen. The intriguing question remains whether these E+, UCHT1+, OKT1±, OKT8+, FcγR+ cells represent a stage in the activation of all cytotoxic/suppressor cells or an expansion of a small subset of normal T cells. We incline to the latter view since we have preliminary evidence for the existence of small numbers of such cells in normal individuals (unpublished data). We, and others, have already presented evidence that neutropenic T cells have distinctive functional properties (Bom-van Noorloos *et al.*, 1980; Callard *et al.*, 1981). A summary of our current idea of the heterogeneity of E rosette forming cells is given in Fig. 23·7.

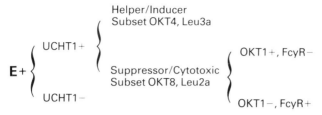

FIG. 23·7 Heterogeneity of E rosette forming cells. The E+ UCHT1+ fraction is about 90% and E+ UCHT1− fraction 10% of AET rosetted mononuclear cells. The E+ UCHT1-cells include a high proportion of FcγR bearing cells (Eγ).

## IV CELL SORTING AND FUNCTIONAL ANALYSIS

### A. LIMITATIONS AND ADVANTAGES

A common requirement in cellular immunology and haematology is to isolate homogeneous subpopulations of cells from a heterogeneous mixture for subsequent functional analysis. There are no ideal methods for doing this. The use of antibodies with complement has the disadvantage of eliminating one population and cells with low density of antigen may be spared. Methods using antibody columns or antibody coated plates have the problem of non-specific adherence and binding of cells by Fc receptors unless Fab or F(ab)₂ fragments are used. Rosette methods share the problem of Fc binding and the necessity for removal of red cells introduces a further difficulty.

In principle at least cell sorting using monoclonal antibodies can overcome some of these problems. Both labelled and unlabelled populations can be recovered simultaneously and the operator can also easily subdivide labelled populations into those with high density and low density antigen. Such a strategy has been used to separate murine T cells into Thy-1 rich and Thy-1 poor subpopulations with different functional properties (Cantor *et al.*, 1975) and to show that cells with high and low OKT1 antigen density function similarly in *in vitro* tests (Reinherz *et al.*, 1979). The ability to utilize two, or with gating (section IIb above) three, parameters can provide additional means of defining and separating populations and with cell sorting, since soluble rather than substrate bound antibodies are generally used, the problem of Fc binding can usually be overcome (see section IIF). With adequate cooling of the input cells non-specific adherence is unimportant.

Cell sorting does however suffer from certain disadvantages. The major problem being the limitations of speed and yield. When adequate purity with a single sort is required it is rarely possible to run the machine at more than $2 \times 10^7$ cells per hour. At higher rates of flow the frequency of discards due to coincidences (undesired cells present in the stream close to the desired cell) is such that yields are not improved. In our experience even at $2 \times 10^7$ cells per hour actual yields of cells after they have been collected, centrifuged and counted are invariably lower than 50% of the input cells. We usually recover 60–80% of the cells recorded as left and right deflections.

Because of the poor recovery and because collecting significant numbers of cells may take a long time if the frequency of the desired cells in the population is low, it is often advantageous to combine other strategies with cell sorting (see sections IV B and C). It may also be more efficient in terms of time saving to perform two sorts, an initial one at high rate with no coincident discards, followed by a slower rate to obtain a pure population. It is also essential to pay attention when sorting to methods for collection of the cells. Siliconized tubes, adequate centrifugation since sorted cells are in dilute suspension, and suitable medium including sheath fluid, to maintain cell viability, are all important.

While the major problem of sorting is the final yield other problems can occur. There may be selective loss of adherent or large cells in the sample input filter and clean separation of populations depends on how well resolved they are by the reagents in use. The efficiency of separation however can readily be estimated by re-analysing samples of the sorted cells. Finally it should not be assumed that the labelling procedure is without effect. While cell sorting itself does not in our experience damage the function of sorted cells in any detectable fashion, some antibodies (and other ligands) can have profound mitogenic or other effects (Van Wauwe *et al.*, 1980). Controls for such effects are simple to perform but not always included in published data.

## B. BONE MARROW PROGENITORS

Human bone marrow is a complex mixture of cell types at all stages of differentiation, from pluripotent stem cells to mature lymphocytes, erythrocytes, granulocytes and monocytes. While there are now *in vitro* assays for erythroid and granulocytic/monocytic colony forming cells and much is known of the regulation of these progenitors, there is still little understanding of how pluripotent cells becomes committed to a particular cell lineage. In part, at least, this has been because it is difficult to isolate pure populations of the earliest progenitor cells. A better understanding of the regulation of this cell pool may be expected to lead to better diagnosis and treatment of leukaemias and other disturbances of haemopoiesis. We have therefore developed a method based on cell sorting to isolate human progenitor cells (Beverley *et al.*, 1980). This method illustrates the strategy discussed above (section IV A) of combining other methods with cell sorting to isolate small subpopulations.

Fig. 23·8a shows a dot plot of ficoll hypaque isolated normal bone marrow cells stained by indirect immunofluorescence with a monoclonal antibody, anti HLe-1, to all leucocytes (Beverley, 1980). The figure illustrates the combined resolving power of light scattering and fluorescence and also that quantititative differences in fluorescence may allow separation of distinct subpopulations. The three populations enclosed by the windows are respectively, cells of the red cell series (1), cells of the granulocytic/monocytic series (2), and lymphocytes (3). Burst forming and colony forming assays showed that all the bone marrow progenitor activity was located in fraction 2, the weakly stained cells. Isolation of this fraction however did not significantly enrich for the progenitors since this fraction contained approximately 50% of the marrow nucleated cells. The use of a second monoclonal antibody TG-1 (anti polymorph) allowed a much greater enrichment. The ficoll hypaque isolated cells were treated with this (IgM) antibody followed by autologous human complement, resulting in lysis of the more mature cells of the granulocytic/monocytic series. Subsequent staining and analysis with anti HLe-1 gave the dot plot shown in Fig. 23·8b. Two fractions differing in size (light scattering) were collected which are highly enriched (up to 100 fold) for burst forming and colony forming activity. The smaller size population is significantly contaminated with small lymphocytes while both may contain up to 50% of undifferentiated blasts some of which contain nuclear terminal transferase (TdT) enzyme.

Thus this protocol utilizing an initial depletion by antibody and complement of irrelevant mature cells followed by cell sorting, can be used to obtain highly purified progenitor cells for functional and cytological analysis. We have so far used cells purified in this manner to examine the cytochemistry and electron microscopical appearance of progenitors and as immunogens in attempts to produce antibodies against stem cells (unpublished data).

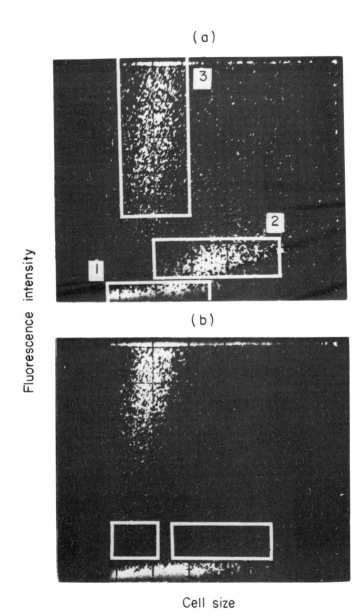

FIG. 23·8 Analysis of normal bone marrow. (a) shows a plot of ficoll hypaque isolated bone marrow cells stained with HLe-1; (b) bone marrow pretreated with anti polymorph antibody (TG-1) and complement prior to staining with HLe-1. (Reprinted by permission from *Nature* **287**, 332. Copyright © 1980. Macmillan Journals Limited.)

## C. Peripheral Blood T Cells

We have used cell sorting in studies of the function of peripheral blood T lymphocytes. The advantages of sorting for this type of study being the recovery of both antigen positive and negative fractions and the relative ease of quantitating contamination of each fraction. The separated cells can either be re-run on the sorter or examined by fluorescence microscopy. The principle disadvantage of cell sorting is the relatively small number of cells which are recovered. For example in the sort illustrated in Fig. 23·9 of 25 × 10⁶ stained E+ cells, only 8 × 10⁶ were recovered in the combined positive and negative fractions.

Nevertheless in spite of the limitation of small numbers we have been able to examine several functions of separated E rosette fractions. In our initial studies we showed that E+ cells which lack the T cell marker defined by the UCHT1 monoclonal antiserum (Fig. 23·7) do not function as classical T cells but have high natural killer (NK) activity. On the other hand E+ UCHT1+ cells have both helper and suppressor activity and respond to mitogens (Beverley and Callard, 1981a). We have followed up these observations by separating E+ cells stained with the antiserum Leu 3a (Ledbetter *et al.*, 1981). When clear separation of

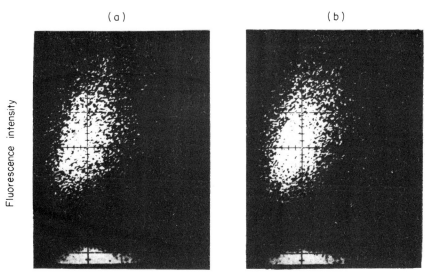

FIG. 23·9 Dot plot of E rosette forming cells stained with Leu 3a antiserum. (a) Scatter gated fluorescence; (b) Windows used for separation of 3a+ and 3a− fractions.

stained and unstained populations is obtained as in this example, there is no problem in setting appropriate windows for sorting (Fig. 23·9b) and the loss of cells which fall in the intermediate area excluded in the sort is small (3%). With other antisera this is not true and the loss must be taken into account in interpreting the data, or different windows set to collect the intermediate cells. Table 23·2 shows some data from such a Leu 3a sort in which separated E+ cells were added to autologous E− cells (null cells, monocytes and B cells) and cultured for six days in a micro variant (Zanders et al., 1981) of the anti influenza culture system described by Callard (1979). The table shows apparently clear separation of helper function in the Leu 3a+ fraction and indeed this is a reproducible finding. This data however is incomplete as it stands for several reasons. It lacks, for example, a control for the effect of coating the cells with antibody. Although in this example coated cells do respond (data not shown), this could be due to a non-specific mitogenic effect of the antiserum. The antigen negative cells may also be heterogeneous and in this example would include E+ T− cells with NK activity (see above and Fig. 23·7). The change in the proportions of helpers and NK cells in the negative fraction might abrogate help. If possible it is therefore useful to perform experiments using an antiserum which stains the negative fraction. We have used the Leu 2a (Ledbetter et al., 1981) antiserum to do this and these experiments confirm the result in Table 23·2 (Callard, Smith and Beverley, in preparation). It is also usual to include a reconstitution control in which the sorted cells are recombined in their original proportions. Such a control is particu-

TABLE 23·2

Function of sorted E+ fractions

| Cells added to 1·5 × 10$^5$ autologous E− cells | Anti influenza response ng ml$^{-1}$ of antibody |
| --- | --- |
| 0 | <1 |
| 0·5 × 10$^5$ E+ | 13·9 ± 4·3 |
| 2 × 10$^5$ E+ | 138·9 ± 24·2 |
| 0·5 × 10$^5$ Leu 3a+ | 2·5 ± 0·9 |
| 2 × 10$^5$ Leu 3a+ | 133·4 ± 22·6 |
| 0·5 × 10$^5$ Leu 3a− | <1 |
| 2 × 10$^5$ Leu 3a− | <1 |

E rosette forming cells were stained and sorted using Leu 3A antibody with the windows illustrated in Fig. 23·9. Sorted fractions were added to E− cells and cultured for six days as described by Callard and Beverley (1981a). Culture supernatants were assayed by enzyme immunoassay.

larly important when the windows for the sort exclude a significant proportion of the cells, in which case the recombination control may indicate selective loss of a subpopulation.

I have sought in this section to illustrate some of the problems and pitfalls of cell sorting in an example where the separation is straightforward and apparently clean (homogeneous) fractions can be obtained. Even in such a model, controls are all important and a minimal requirement would be a control for the effect of coating the cells.

As yet this type of sorting has not been used to any great extent in the analysis of clinical samples. However many diseases show disturbances of lymphocyte subsets and functional analysis of unseparated mononuclear cells often reveals abnormalities. It is the usual practice to assign to the predominant cell type, for example OKT8+ cells in mononucleosis, any functional abnormality revealed in *in vitro* tests but clinical samples are seldom homogeneous and a more reliable analysis will require separation of subpopulations.

### D. Separation of Foetal Cells from the Maternal Circulation

As a last example of the use of cell sorting for functional analysis, I shall return to the subject of antenatal diagnosis (section III B). While amniocentesis and the withdrawal of blood at foetoscopy have important diagnostic uses and can provide samples of foetal blood for identification of many diseases, these procedures are invasive and carry a definite risk to both foetus and mother. Herzenberg and his colleagues (1979) have developed an alternative method of examining foetal cells based on sorting foetal cells from maternal blood.

They used a rabbit antiserum to the HLA-A2 antigen to stain samples of maternal mononuclear cells taken from A2 negative women from 15 weeks of gestation onward. The brightest $0\cdot1-0\cdot8\%$ of cells were collected directly on to microscope slides and stained for Y-chromatin. In every case where an A2 negative female carried an A2 positive male foetus some male cells were detected, though the frequency was low ($\sim7$ per 1,000 cells). Although as yet there have been no reports of the use of this procedure for diagnostic purposes technical developments suggest that this should become possible. Mouse monoclonal antibodies to various HLA alleles are becoming available (Brodsky *et al.*, 1979 and chapter 14, this volume) and these would be ideal reagents for such a procedure (high specificity, low background). It is also now possible to maintain T lymphocytes in culture and expand their number almost indefinitely using T cell growth factor (Gillis and Watson, 1981) so that it might be possible to grow the sorted foetal cells and then re-sort to obtain a purer population for chromosomal or other studies. Our own data (section III B) showing the mature phenotype of foetal lymphocytes as well as other functional data (Rayfield *et al.*, 1980) suggest that this is not an unrealistic proposition.

## V  FUTURE PROSPECTS

### A. DOUBLE LABELS

Techniques for labelling cells with more than one fluorescent labelled antibody have been available for some time and Table 23·3 lists methods applicable when both the antibodies are of the same species (usually mouse). While these methods have been used in experimental studies (see for example Herzenberg and Herzenberg, 1978; Jongkind *et al.*, 1979) they have not as yet played any important role in clinical investigation except in the case of leukaemia and lymphoma (chapters 6 and 24). In part at least, this is because many of the more important normal leucocyte subpopulations can be defined by single labels. In addition the technical problems of two colour analysis when the emission spectra of the fluorochromes used overlap, have limited its routine use. The introduction of dual laser cell sorters and better optical filters however, make the technical problems less formidable and it is to be expected that double labelling methods will find a place in the investigation of clinical samples. It would, for example, be convenient to use two labels to establish that T cells carry HLA-DR antigens in the neutropenic patients illustrated in Fig. 23·6 and Table 23·1.

### B. MIXED LABELLING

Flow cytometers have for some time been used for the analysis of cell cycle after DNA staining with nucleic acid intercalating dyes such as propidium iodide (Krishnan, 1975) or ethidium bromide (Vindelov, 1977). These methods utilize cells usually fixed with ethanol or acetone which may not be optimal for preservation of membrane antigens. However it is possible to combine membrane staining and analysis of cell cycle, either by actual sorting of cells prior to DNA staining or by staining with antibody followed by fixation, DNA staining with propidium iodide and two colour analysis (Roberts *et al.*, 1978).

TABLE 23·3
Methods for double labelling cells

| | Method | Reference |
|---|---|---|
| Direct Labelling | Directly labelled antibodies Antibodies coupled to fluorescent microspheres | Goding (1976) Parks *et al.* (1979) |
| Indirect Labelling | Unconjugated antisera with class specific labelled anti-immunoglobulins Haptenated antibody with labelled antihapten Biotinylated antibody with labelled avidin | Cammisuli and Wofsy (1976) Bayer and Wilchek (1980) |

Recently several dyes have been developed which stain the nucleic acid of viable cells. Hoechst 33342 (Arndt-Jovin and Jovin, 1977) has been used to stain mouse spleen cells and under suboptimal staining conditions allows discrimination between T and B cells (Loken, 1980). Hoechst 33258 has also been used to sort cultured tumour cells on the basis of DNA content (Arndt-Jovin and Jovin, 1978) with little or no toxicity. Nucleic acid staining dyes of this type will be extremely useful in combination with surface labelling by antibodies in the analysis of complicated differentiating tissues such as the bone marrow. Aside from the advantage that the function of the sorted cells can be examined when these DNA vital stains are used, there is the additional advantage that the characteristic scatter properties of the living cell will be preserved and this can be useful both in analysis and sorting (sections II D and IV B).

A number of other fluorescent probes have recently been developed which can measure changes in their environment by alterations in characteristics such as intensity, emission spectrum and polarization. These probes have been used to detect early events in lymphocyte activation. Significant changes can be detected as early as 3 hours after mitogen stimulation (Nairn *et al.*, 1978).

## C. CONCLUSION

I have during the course of this review attempted to suggest some uses of monoclonal antibodies with the cell sorter in clinical medicine. It is clear that the potential of this combination of instrument and reagents has only just begun to be exploited. As antibodies to biochemically defined antigens identifying well characterized leucocyte subsets become widely available, it will become a matter of routine to monitor these subsets. In some cases this may provide diagnostic information, in others be useful in monitoring therapy and in yet others may throw light on the nature of the disease process.

It is to be expected that cell sorting will play a role in isolating cells from patients for further study especially as techniques for immortalizing B cells (Olsson and Kaplan, 1980 and see chapter 2) and growing T cells (Gillis and Watson, 1981) are now available. New techniques for exploring the metabolic state of viable cells with fluorescent probes (section V B) may allow enrichment of cells responding to disease related antigens. Finally new developments in instrumentation will surely also contribute to increasing use of cell sorting in the future.

ACKNOWLEDGMENTS

I should like to acknowledge the collaboration of Drs. R. Callard and D. Linch in the work described in this chapter and the able technical assistance of Mrs. D. Boyle.

OKT antisera were kindly given by Dr. G. Goldstein and Leu antisera by Becton-Dickinson.

I am grateful to Miss S. Chandler for typing the manuscript.

REFERENCES

Arndt-Jovin, D. J. and Jovin, T. M. (1977). *J. Histochem. Cytochem.* **25**, 585–589.
Arndt-Jovin, D. J. and Jovin, T. M. (1978). *Ann. Rev. Biophys. Bioeng.* **7**, 527–558.
Bayer, E. A. and Wilchek, M. (1980). *Methods Biochem. Anal.* **26**, 1–45.
Beverley, P. C. L. (1980). *In* "Transplantation and Clinical Immunology XI" (J. L. Touraine, J. Traeger, H. Betuel, J. Brochier, J. M. Dubernard, J. P. Revillard, R. Triau, Eds), pp. 87–94. Excerpta Medica, Amsterdam.
Beverley, P. C. L. and Callard, R. E. (1981a). *Eur. J. Immunol.* **11**, 329–334.
Beverley, P. C. L. and Callard, R. E. (1981b). *In* "Protides of the Biological Fluids XXIX" (H. Peeters, Ed.), Pergamon Press, Oxford. (in press).
Beverley, P. C. L., Linch, D. and Delia, D. (1980). *Nature* **287**, 332–333.
Bom-van Noorloos, A. A., Pegels, H. G., Van Oers, R. H. J., Silverbusch, J., Feltkamp-Vroom, T. M., Brondsmit, R., Zeijlemaker, W. P., Von dem Borne, A. E. G. K. and Melief, C. J. M. (1980). *New Engl. J. Med.* **302**, 1943–1947.

Brodsky, F. M., Parham, P., Barnstaple, C. J., Crumpton, M. J. and Bodmer, W. F. (1979). *Immunol. Rev.* **47**, 3–28.

Callard, R. E. (1979). *Nature* **282**, 734.

Callard, R. E., Smith, C. M., Worman, C., Linch, D., Cawley, J. C. and Beverley, P. C. L. (1981). *Clin. Exp. Immunol.* **43**, 497–505.

Cammisuli, S. and Wofsy, L. (1976). *J. Immunol.* **117**, 1965–1972.

Cantor, H., Simpson, E., Sato, V., Fathman, C. G. and Herzenberg, L. A. (1975). *Cell. Immunol.* **15**, 180–196.

Crawford, D. H., Brickell, P., Tidmann, N., McConnell, I., Hoffbrand, A. V. and Janossy, G. (1981). *Clin. Exp. Immunol.* **43**, 291–297.

Davidson, W. F. and Parish, C. R. (1975). *J. Immunol. Methods* **7**, 291–296.

Fowlkes, B. J., Waxdal, M. J., Sharrow, S. O., Thomas, C. A., Asofsky, R. and Mathieson, B. J. (1980). *J. Immunol.* **125**, 623–630.

Gillis, S. and Watson, J. (1981). *Immunol. Rev.* **54**, 81–110.

Goding, J. S. (1976). *J. Immunol. Methods* **13**, 215–221.

Haynes, B. F., Schooley, R. T., Grouse, J. E., Payling-Wright, C. R., Dolin, R. and Spruce, A. S. (1979). *J. Immunol.* **122**, 699–708.

Herzenberg, L. A. and Herzenberg, L. A. (1978). *In* "Handbook of Experimental Immunology" (D. M. Weir, Ed.), 3rd Edition. Blackwell Scientific, Oxford.

Herzenberg, L. A., Bianchi, D. W., Schroder, J., Cann, H. M., Iverson, G. (1979). *Proc. natn. Acad. Sci. U.S.A.* **76**, 1453–1455.

Jongkind, J. F., Verkerk, A. and Tanke, H. (1979). *Exp. Cell Res.* **120**, 444–448.

Krishnan, A. (1975). *Cell. Biol.* **66**, 188–193.

Kung, P. C., Goldstein, G., Reinherz, E. L. and Schlossman, S. F. (1979). *Science*, **206**, 347–349.

Linch, D. C., Cawley, J. C., Worman, C. P., Galvin, M. C., Roberts, B. E., Callard, R. E. and Beverley, P. C. L. (1981). *Br. J. Haematol.* **48**, 137–145.

Loken, M. R. (1980). *J. Histochem. and Cytochem.* (1980). **28**, 36–39.

Loken, M. R. and Herzenberg, L. A. (1975). *Ann. N.Y. Acad. Sci.* **254**, 163–171.

Mann, D. L. and Sharrow, S. O. (1981). *J. Immunol.* **125**, 1889–1896.

Melamed, M. R., Mullaney, P. F. and Mendelsohn, M. L. (1979). *In* "Flow Cytometry and Sorting" Wiley, New York.

Miller, M. H., Powell, J. I., Sharrow, S. O. and Schultz, A. R. (1978). *Rev. Sci. Instrum.* **49**, 1137.

Nairn, R. C., Rolland, J. M., Halliday, G. M., Jablonka, I. M. and Ward, H. A. (1978). *In* "Immunofluorescence and related staining techniques" (W. Knapp, K. Holubar, G. Wick, Eds), pp. 57–66. Elsevier/North Holland, Amsterdam.

Olsson, L. and Kaplan, H. S. (1980). *Proc. natn. Acad. Sci. U.S.A.* **77**, 5429–5431.

Palacios, R., Alarcon-Segovia, D., Llorente, L., Ruiz-Argueles, A. and Diaz-Jonanen, E. (1981). *J. Clin. Lab. Immunol.* **5**, 71–79.

Parks, D. R., Bryan, V. M., Oi, V. T. and Herzenberg, L. A. (1979). *Proc. natn. Acad. Sci. U.S.A.* **76**, 1962–1966.

Raveche, E. S. and Steinberg, A. D. (1979). *Seminars in Haematol.* **16**(4), 344–362.

Rayfield, L. S., Brent, C. H. and Rodeck, C. H. (1980). *Clin. exp. Immunol.* **42**, 561–570.

Reinherz, E. L. and Schlossman, S. F. (1981). *Immunology Today* **2**, 69–75.

Reinherz, E. L., Kung, P. C., Goldstein, G. and Schlossman, S. F. (1979). *J. Immunol.* **123**, 1312–1317.

Reinherz, E. L., O'Brien, C., Rosenthal, P. and Schlossman, S. F. (1980a). *J. Immunol.* **125**, 1269–1274.

Reinherz, E. L., Weiner, H. L., Hansen, S. L., Cohen, J. A., Distaso, J. A. and Schlossman, S. F. (1980b). *New Engl. J. Med.* **303**, 125–129.

Rodeck, C. H. (1980). *Br. J. Obstet. Gynaecol.* **87**, 449–456.

Rotman, B. and Papermaster, B. W. (1966). *Proc. natn. Acad. Sci. U.S.A.* **55**, 134–141.

Seigal, F. P. (1976). *Scand. J. Immunol.* **5**, 721–725.

Shortman, K., Williams, N. and Adams, P. (1971). *J. Immunol. Methods* **1**, 273–278.

Steen, H. B. and Lindmo, T. (1979). *Science,* **204**, 403–404.

Van Wauwe, J. P., De Mey, J. R. and Goossens, J. T. (1980). *J. Immunol.* **124**, 2708–2716.

Vindelov, L. L. (1977). *Virchovs. Arch. B. Cell. Path.* **24**, 227–242.

Von Boehmer, H. and Shortman, K. (1973). *J. Immunol. Methods* **2**, 293–299.

Zanders, E. D., Smith, C. M. and Callard, R. E. (1981). *J. Immunol. Methods* **47**, 333–338.

# 24  Immunohistological Applications of Monoclonal Antibodies

D. Y. Mason,[a] M. Naiem,[a]
Z. Abdulaziz,[a] J. R. G. Nash,[a]
K. C. Gatter[a] and H. Stein[b]

[a] *Nuffield Department of Pathology, John Radcliffe Hospital, Oxford. OX3 9DU*
[b] *Institute for Pathology, Christian Albrechts University, Kiel, West Germany.*

## I INTRODUCTION

The preceding chapters in this book have provided ample evidence of the great potential importance of monoclonal antibodies in clinical medicine. Three novel features account for their value. Firstly the fact that the antigen-binding region of a monoclonal antibody lacks the variability inevitably present in polyclonal antibody confers on it a very high degree of specificity. Secondly it is possible to prepare potentially limitless amounts of purified monoclonal antibody, a feature of obvious potential value in a therapeutic context. Finally the production of new monoclonal antibodies represents a very powerful technique for identifying hitherto undiscovered constituents of human tissue. Substances detected in this way, many of which would not be identifiable by any existing technique, may then be isolated (by immunoabsorption techniques, see chapter 22) in substantial amounts for detailed molecular analysis.

Monoclonal antibodies have therefore enormously enlarged the horizons of research in many different medical fields. However it has also become evident that their great potential can only be realized to the full if the techniques by which they are used are optimal. It would, for example, obviously be wasteful of the remarkable capacity of a monoclonal antibody to "home" *in vivo* to a tumour deposit if an inefficient method was used to conjugate the antibody to a toxin or radioisotope. Similarly in the indirect immunofluorescent analysis of a cell population detected by a monoclonal antibody the quality of the fluorescent anti-Ig reagent should match the monoclonal antibody in terms of purity and absence of non-specific binding.

The present chapter is concerned with the use of monoclonal antibodies for methods which have been particularly prone to technical limitations in the past, and have consequently been relatively neglected. Immunohistological procedures are of considerable value in monitoring and characterizing new monoclonal antibodies during their production. Furthermore immunohistological labelling of tissue sections using monoclonal antibodies of known specificity not only offers a means of learning more of the mechanisms underlying human disease, but also of bringing a new objectivity to the process of routine histopathological diagnosis. The field of tissue diagnosis is likely to be one of the first areas in which monoclonal antibodies will come to have a major impact on the everyday practice of clinical medicine.

## II TECHNICAL ASPECTS OF IMMUNOHISTOLOGICAL LABELLING WITH MONOCLONAL ANTIBODIES

Two aspects of this topic should be considered. The results obtained when labelling a tissue section by immunohistological techniques are crucially dependent firstly on the way in which the tissue has been handled before labelling; and secondly on the choice of immuno-histological staining procedure.

## A. PROCESSING OF TISSUE

There are fundamentally two approaches to the processing of tissue samples for immunohistological analysis. Tissues may be frozen with-out prior fixation and cryostat sections prepared. Alternatively tissue may be fixed in one of a variety of fixatives, dehydrated and then embedded in paraffin wax (or less frequently in resin). Sections are then cut, the embedding medium removed and immunohistological label-ling performed.

An intermediate approach, which combines elements of both the techniques above, is to fix a tissue sample before freezing it and cutting cryostat sections. This technique is relatively infrequently used and finds its major application in the field of immunoelectron microscopy where it enables both ultrastructural morphology and antigenic reactivity to be preserved.

### 1. CRYOSTAT SECTIONS

The advantage of using cryostat sections is that the antigenic reactivity of a tissue sample is much more effectively preserved than when the tissue is fixed and embedded. This is particularly true in the case of surface membrane antigens, the majority of which do not survive conventional fixation and embedding.

It should be noted however that there are several exceptions to the rule that membrane antigens do not survive conventional tissue proces-sing procedures. Examples include carcinoembryonic antigen (Isaacson and Judd, 1978) mammary epithelial antigens (Arklie *et al.*, 1981, Sloane *et al.*, 1980) and human syncytiotrophoblast antigens (Sunderland *et al.*, 1981). The important practical implication of find-ing that an antigen survives conventional fixation and embedding is that it may then be studied retrospectively in stored surgical histologi-cal samples. This permits extensive analysis of the antigen's distribu-tion in different disease states, without the necessity for prospectively collecting fresh tissue samples.

### 2. FIXED AND EMBEDDED TISSUES

Sections of tissue processed in this way are most suitable for the demonstration of cytoplasmic antigens, e.g. plasma cell immunoglobulin (Fig. 24·1), neuropeptides etc., presumably because these constituents are present at relatively high local concentrations. However it should be noted that under certain circumstances even cytoplasmic antigens may be undetectable in embedded tissue, due to masking or permanent denaturation (Mason and Biberfeld, 1980).

The effect of fixation and embedding on tissue antigens is relatively poorly understood. It may on occasion be possible to "nurse" a labile antigen through to the final labelling stage by judicious selection of optimal fixation and embedding conditions (Brandtzaeg, 1974; Pearse *et al.*, 1974). This is illustrated by the way in which an antigen common to all human leucocytes could be demonstrated in paraffin embedded sections using a monoclonal antibody provided the tissue had previously been fixed in Carnoy's fixative (Pizzolo *et al.*, 1980). Other fixatives (e.g. formol saline) were not suitable for this purpose.

## B. Choice of Immunohistological Labelling Procedure

By far the most widely used procedures for immunohistological labelling of monoclonal antibodies are those based upon fluorochromes and enzymes (usually horseradish peroxidase) as antibody labels.

### 1. Immunofluorescent labelling

Immunofluorescent staining of tissue sections has much to recommend it. Principal among its advantages are the ease with which it may be performed and the fact that it is relatively simple to label pairs of antigens in contrasting colours using fluorescein and rhodamine as antibody labels.

The major disadvantage of immunofluorescent labelling is that the morphology of the tissue section cannot be visualized simultaneously

FIG. 24·1a and b Immunoperoxidase labelling of human plasma cells with a monoclonal antibody specific for lambda light chains (paraffin embedded tonsil). Strongly labelled cells are seen both within a germinal centre and in extrafollicular tissue (shown at higher magnification in (b) ). This antibody (and a number of other monoclonal antibodies against human Ig) have been found to give staining reactions equal in their intensity to those obtained using conventional antisera. Consequently theoretical objections to the use of monoclonal antibodies for routine immunohistological use (based upon the fact that they usually react with only a single determinant per molecule) are not fulfilled in practice. Haematoxylin counterstain.

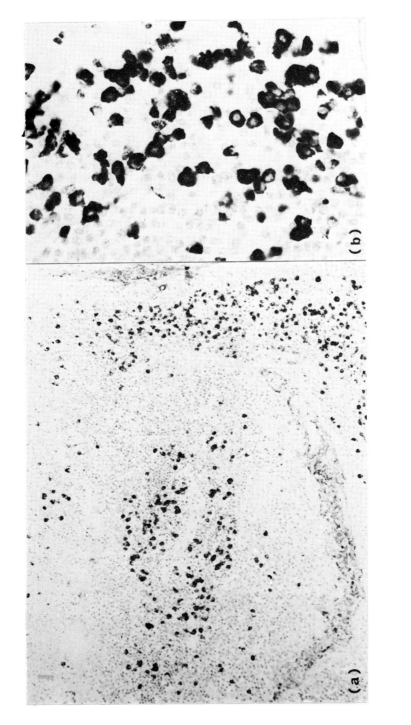

(a)

(b)

with the antibody label so that it is often difficult to be certain of the precise sites to which the antibody binds.[a] Further drawbacks include the fact that fluorescently labelled sections tend to fade on storage and examination, fluorescein suffering more from this than rhodamine. This prevents prolonged examination of sections or their reassessment after an interval, both of which are important practical disadvantages when analysing histologically complex tissue, or when making detailed comparison between the reactivity patterns of different monoclonal antibodies.

It should also be noted that background fluorescence is relatively difficult to exclude completely. Autofluorescence of tissue samples contributes to this problem. However of greater importance is the potential tendency of all fluorescent conjugates to bind non-specifically to tissue sections. Overconjugation of antibodies exacerbates this problem, which may be minimized by absorption of conjugates with liver powder or by ion-exchange chromatography. However, even after these procedures, the removal of the last traces of non-specific reactivity is rarely achieved. It may be added that many fluorescent microscopists consider weak background staining a help rather than a hinderance, since it facilitates the location and orientation of the tissue section under the fluorescent microscope.

## 2. IMMUNOENZYMATIC LABELLING

The most widely used enzyme label is horseradish peroxidase which may be linked to monoclonal antibodies by two different types of procedure (Fig. 24·2).

### (a) *Indirect immunoperoxidase labelling*

In this two-stage technique a covalent conjugate of peroxidase and anti-mouse or anti-rat Ig is used (Fig. 24·2). Technical aspects of the two major conjugation procedures currently used for linking peroxidase to antibody are summarized in Table 24·1. It may be noted that the quality of peroxidase-conjugated antibodies available from commercial sources has greatly improved in recent years and many of them are suitable for immunohistological labelling of monoclonal antibodies (see Appendix).

---

[a]  It may be noted that the localization of antigens by fluorescent microscopy may be improved by the use of a fluorescent label for DNA which strongly labels cell nuclei in tissue sections (Stenman and Vaheri, 1981).

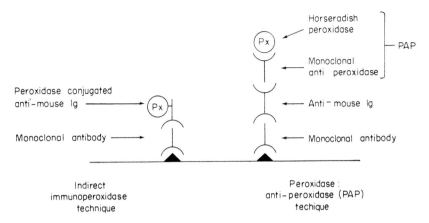

Horseradish
peroxidase

Px

PAP

Monoclonal
anti peroxidase

Peroxidase conjugated
anti-mouse Ig

Px

Anti – mouse Ig

Monoclonal antibody

Monoclonal antibody

Indirect
immunoperoxidase
technique

Peroxidase :
anti-peroxidase (PAP)
techique

FIG. 24·2 Schematic illustration of the two most frequently used immunoperoxidase labelling procedures. The indirect technique (left) resembles other indirect labelling procedures in that the primary antibody is revealed by the use of a labelled second antibody. The peroxidase: anti-peroxidase (PAP) procedure (right)—also referred to as the unlabelled antibody technique—depends upon the ability of the anti-mouse Ig antiserum (second stage) to bind via one antigen-combining site to the primary monoclonal antibody and via the other to soluble PAP complexes (Sternberger, 1979) formed between monoclonal anti-peroxidase and horseradish peroxidase. The anti-mouse Ig antiserum is added in excess to minimize the possibility of both combining sites binding to the primary antibody.

Alkaline phosphatase may be used as an alternative to peroxidase for labelling antibodies (see text and Figs. 24·4–24·8). This may be achieved either by covalently conjugating the enzyme to anti-mouse Ig for use in an indirect technique (Fig. 24·4) or by preparing soluble complexes between monoclonal anti-alkaline phosphatase and alkaline phosphatase (Fig. 24·5–24·8).

Double immunoenzymatic labelling (see Figs. 24·6–24·8) may be achieved by combining peroxidase and alkaline phosphatase labelled sandwiches. At each incubation stage the reagents for each sandwich are mixed before application to the tissue section, and at the completion of the incubation stages the two enzyme substrates are applied in sequence (Mason and Sammons, 1978; Mason *et al.*, 1981a).

## (b) *Peroxidase: anti-peroxidase technique*

An alternative to the indirect immunoperoxidase technique is to use a procedure known as the peroxidase: anti-peroxidase (PAP) technique (Fig. 24·2). The PAP method has been widely used by histopathologists when labelling paraffin embedded surgical biopsies with conventional polyclonal antisera. It is reputed to be of much higher sensitivity than the indirect technique, but this reputation is probably a reflection of the relatively poor quality of the "first generation" commercial peroxidase-conjugated anti-Ig reagents available in the early 1970's rather than of any inherent characteristics of the PAP technique. If optimal covalent

## TABLE 24·1

### Preparation of covalent peroxidase: antibody conjugates

| Technique | Principle | Characteristics of conjugates[b,c] | |
|---|---|---|---|
| | | Advantages | Disadvantages |
| Two stage glutaraldehyde technique[a] | Peroxidase is "activated" by incubation with glutaraldehyde. Owing to the paucity of free amino groups there is minimal cross-linking between peroxidase molecules. Excess glutaraldehyde is then removed (together with any dimeric peroxidase) by gel filtration and the activated enzyme is incubated with antibody. Free aldehyde groups on the glutaraldehyde link with available amino groups on the antibody forming covalent enzyme: antibody conjugates. | Antibody and enzyme activity is well preserved. Conjugates are predominantly of low molecular weight (Ab1 : Px1), facilitating penetration of conjugates into tissues and cells. | The yield is low, approximately 10% of the enzyme being coupled and 40% of the antibody. Free enzyme is easily removed. Free antibody (which competes with conjugated antibody) is difficult to separate however from enzyme: antibody conjugates (because of similarity in molecular weight). |
| Periodate oxidation technique[d] | Incubation with sodium periodate causes oxidation of the carbohydrate moiety of the molecule. The oxidized enzyme is then incubated with antibody and Schiff bases form between the enzyme and free amino groups on the antibody. These complexes are stabilized by sodium borohydride reduction. | The yield of the reaction is high, the majority of the antibody being labelled with enzyme. | The conjugates cover a wide range of molecular weights, often with a predominance of large polymers. Gel chromatography may be used to select optimal smaller complexes. Periodate conjugate may be less stable than glutaraldehyde conjugates. |

The two procedures outlined above are the methods most commonly used to prepare enzyme: antibody conjugates. Potentially superior techniques based upon the use of heterobifunctional coupling agents have been reported (Kitagawa and Aikawa, 1976; Carlsson et al., 1978; Nilsson et al., 1980) but have yet to be widely used for immunohistological labelling.

a  Avrameas and Ternynck, 1971.
b  Boorsma and Streefkerk, 1976, 1979.
c  Nygren and Hansson, 1981.
d  Wilson and Nakane, 1978.

conjugates are used (i.e. those prepared from antibodies purified by elution from Ig immunoabsorbants) it is possible to obtain immuno-histological labelling by the two-stage indirect method which approaches (or may even exceed) the PAP procedure in terms of sensitivity and absence of background staining.

(c)  *Choice of immunoperoxidase technique*

The choice between the indirect conjugate method and the PAP procedure should be based upon the convenience with which the necessary reagents can be prepared or obtained rather than upon considerations of sensitivity. As noted above high quality peroxidase-conjugated anti-mouse Ig reagents are now available commercially (see Appendix). Mouse PAP on the other hand has until now not been widely available from commercial sources, reflecting the difficulty of producing large volumes of polyclonal antibody in the mouse.

One obvious solution is to prepare PAP from monoclonal anti-peroxidase antibody. This has recently been performed in one of the authors' laboratories (Fig. 24·3; Mason *et al.,* 1982) and the PAP complexes prepared in this way have been found to give excellent immunohistological labelling reactions.[b] One theoretical objection to the use of monoclonal PAP is that the antiperoxidase antibody (being of a single sub-class) will not be linked with equal efficiency by the bridging antibody (Fig. 24·2) to all primary monoclonal antibodies (e.g. especially when of different sub-class). However in practice this objection has not proved a major obstacle and the majority of mono-clonal antibodies against human tissue which we have evaluated give good immunohistological labelling by the monoclonal PAP technique.

(d)  *Alkaline phosphatase as antibody label*

Although horseradish peroxidase is by far the most widely used label in immunoenzymatic staining techniques, mention should be made of the use of alkaline phosphatase as an alternative or companion label. Procedures for covalently linking alkaline phosphatase to antibodies are less efficient than those available for coupling horesradish perox-idase, and there are few commercial sources of alkaline phosphatase conjugates. However despite its theoretical inefficiency, the intensity of immunohistological labelling which can be achieved using alka-line phosphatase-conjugated anti-mouse Ig in conjunction with

[b]  Monoclonal PAP was used to perform the immunohistological labelling shown in many of the illustrations to this chapter. Furthermore the reagent has been independently evaluated in two other laboratories and found to give good immunohistological labelling of rat tissues with monoclonal antibodies (Dr. A. N. Barclay and Dr. C. Cuello, personal communication).

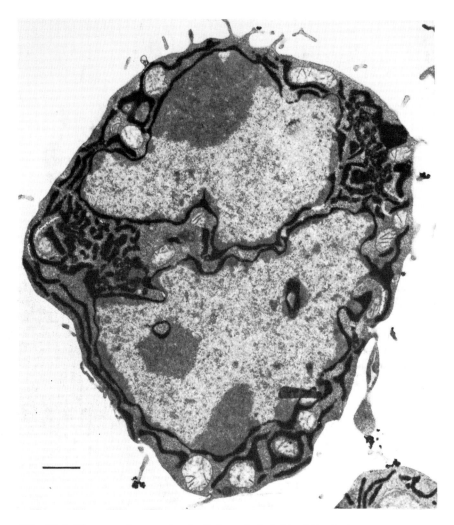

FIG. 24·3 Electron micrographs of cells from the hybrid cell line P6/38 which produces monoclonal antibody against horseradish peroxidase (Mason *et al.*, 1982). This antibody is now routinely used to prepare PAP complexes for immunohistological use (see text and Fig. 24·2). Sites of antibody synthesis within these cells have been

*Immunohistological applications of monoclonal antibodies*

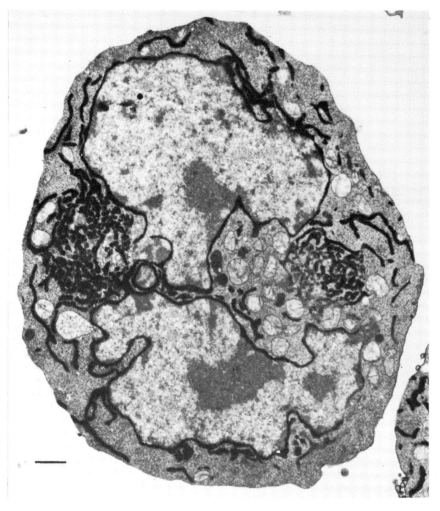

ultrastructurally localized by incubating cells with horseradish peroxidase, followed by washing, fixation and exposure to peroxidase substrate (diaminobenzidine/$H_2O_2$). The black reaction product is present within endoplasmic reticulum, the perinuclear space and the Golgi apparatus. (Bars = $1 \mu$).

monoclonal antibodies compares well with that obtained by immunoperoxidase procedures (Fig. 24·4; Dr. M. G. Ormerod, personal communication).

Just as the PAP system may be used as an alternative to an indirect
peroxidase conjugate method, so alkaline phosphatase may be bound to
the primary monoclonal antibody via an unlabelled bridging antibody
followed by an antibody to alkaline phosphatase (Fig. 24·2). A system
of this sort, based upon rabbit anti-alkaline phosphatase (which may be
called the APAAP procedure as an abbreviation of "alkaline
phosphatase: anti-alkaline phosphatase") has been developed in one of
the authors' laboratories for immunohistological labelling of rabbit
antisera (Mason and Sammons, 1978). More recently we have found
that monoclonal anti-alkaline phosphatase may also be used in the
same type of system for labelling monoclonal antibodies (Fig. 24·5).

One reason for using alkaline phosphatase as an antibody label is
that it may be employed in conjunction with immunoperoxidase staining to give double labelling of pairs of antigens in tissue sections. Figs.
24·6, 24·7 and 24·8 illustrate sections of human lymphoid tissue
stained by a double immunoenzymatic labelling procedure of this sort.
A particular advantage of double immunoenzymatic staining compared to double immunofluorescent labelling is that the two enzyme
products can be visualized simultaneously, whereas fluorescent labels
require sequential visualization using different filter systems. The
important practical consequence is that minor populations of cells
differing in their staining reactions from those of the major population
of labelled cells may be much more rapidly identified using the double
immunoenzymatic procedure. An example is provided by Hodgkin's
disease, in which small numbers of Reed Sternberg cells containing
both kappa and lambda light chains (because of uptake of exogenous
Ig) may be rapidly picked out against a background of single labelled
plasma cells (Fig. 24·8; Mason *et al.*, 1980, Mason *et al.*, 1981a).

A further context in which alkaline phosphatase may be of value is in
avoiding the problems encountered when using immunoperoxidase
staining to study tissues rich in endogenous peroxidase (e.g. bone
marrow). The most frequently used technique for blocking endogenous
peroxidase activity in paraffin sections (exposure to methanol/$H_2O_2$,—
Mason and Taylor, 1975) tends to destroy the reactivity of many
antigens when used on cryostat sections. Endogenous alkaline
phosphatase activity on the other hand can be blocked without the risk
of antigenic destruction by the addition of levamisole to the enzyme
substrate (Ponder and Wilkinson, 1981). This reagent inhibits alkaline
phosphatase activity in most tissues, but does not affect the enzyme

FIG. 24·4 Immunohistological labelling of surface membrane IgD on mantle zone lymphocytes using monoclonal anti-IgD followed by alkaline phosphatase-conjugated anti-mouse Ig (kindly provided by Dr. M. G. Ormerod). Endogenous alkaline phosphatase has been inhibited by the use of levamisole (Ponder and Wilkinson, 1981) although small amounts of enzyme activity persist within vascular endothelium. The enzyme label has been revealed using a substrate containing Fast Red. The distribution pattern of IgD is identical to that obtained using immunoperoxidase techniques (Figs. 24·7, 24·16 and 24·17).

FIG. 24·5 Alkaline phosphatase labelling of lambda light chains in plasma cells (paraffin embedded human tonsil). This staining was achieved using an unlabelled antibody bridge technique (Fig. 24·2) based upon a monoclonal antibody against calf intestine alkaline phosphatase. The enzyme was then revealed using a substrate containing either Fast Red (left) or Fast Blue (right). The Fast Red labelled section was counterstained with haematoxylin.

FIG. 24·6 Double immunoenzymatic labelling of kappa and lambda light chains in human plasma cells (paraffin embedded tonsil) using two unlabelled antibody sandwiches (Fig. 24·2). Kappa light chains stain blue (alkaline phosphatase); lambda light chains stain brown (peroxidase). As noted in the text and in Table 24·6 double staining is of value not only for comparing the relative distribution patterns of pairs of antigens but may also be used to provide information on the specificity of a new monoclonal antibody (by double staining with the antibody in conjunction with an antibody of known specificity).

FIG. 24·7 Double immunoenzymatic labelling of IgD (blue) and T cells (brown) in a cryostat section of human tonsil, using two unlabelled antibody sandwiches (Fig. 24·2). IgD is present on the surface of mantle zone lymphocytes (see Figs. 24·4, 24·16 and 24·17) whilst T cells are plentiful in the extrafollicular areas).

FIG. 24·8 Double immunoenzymatic labelling of kappa and lambda light chains in a lymph node section from a case of Hodgkin's disease. Plasma cells contain only a single class of light chain. A Reed Sternberg cell (arrowed) in contrast is clearly distinguishable since it contains polyclonal Ig (absorbed from its environment) which gives a mixed labelling pattern.

FIG. 24·9 Immunoperoxidase labelling of HLA-DR antigen in a cryostat section of human tonsil. The labelled cells are dendritic cells (interdigitating reticulum cells) in an interfollicular region (compared with Fig. 24·18b). This photomicrograph illustrates the clarity with which cell morphology can be visualized when optimally processed cryostat sections are labelled by the immunoperoxidase technique.

FIG. 24·17 Immunoperoxidase staining of 4 tonsil cryostat sections with monoclonal antibodies against leucocytes (L-C), IgD, T cells and C3b receptor. The sections were mounted on a multi-test slide, carrying four circular areas separated by water-repellant masking (seen in black since the slide was illuminated from behind for photography). Use of multi-test slides facilitates the screening of multiple hybridoma supernatants, since the entire slide can be flooded with reagent (after the primary antibodies have been applied and washed off).

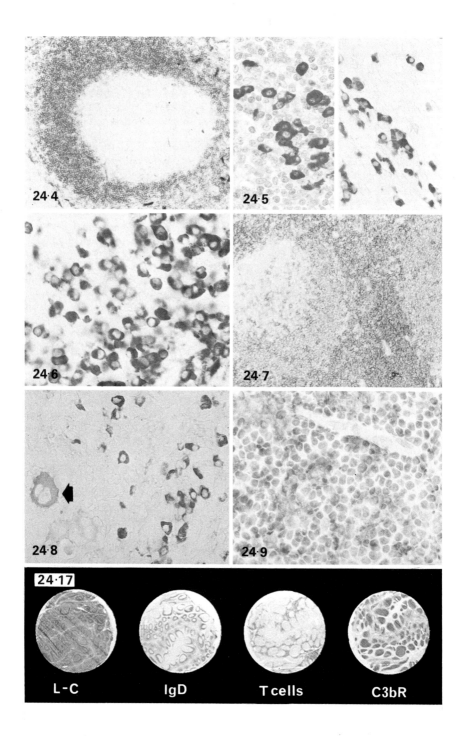

24·4

24·5

24·6

24·7

24·8

24·9

24·17

L-C          IgD          T cells          C3bR

present in intestinal mucosa (the most widely used source of alkaline phosphatase for antibody labelling). In consequence, except when staining samples of intestinal tissue, the endogenous activity in the section is inhibited without affecting the antibody label.

## 3. IMMUNOENZYMATIC VERSUS IMMUNOFLUORESCENT LABELLING

The choice of immunohistological labelling techniques used in any individual laboratory is often based more upon local traditions and availability of reagents than upon more objective criteria. Table 24·2 summarizes the advantages and disadvantages of immunoenzymatic and immunofluorescent techniques, and should help the reader to select the procedure most suited to his need. It may be of value however to make two additional comments.

Firstly it should be recognized that the two techniques are very similar in terms of sensitivity, and that suggestions that immunoperoxidase procedures (and especially the PAP technique) are of much greater sensitivity than immunofluorescent techniques have little foundation in fact. The authors are unaware of any antigen which has been detected using an immunoperoxidase method which has not been demonstrable by immunofluorescent labelling, or *vice versa*. However, one aspect which should be considered when comparing the sensitivity of the two techniques is that in our experience traces of background labelling are much more readily eliminated from immunoperoxidase stained preparations than from immunofluorescently labelled sections (see Immunofluorescent Labelling). The practical relevance of this is that it is generally easier to evaluate labelling (however weak) against a completely negative background, than to assess specific labelling (even when strong) when background staining is present. This is particularly important when using immunohistological procedures to screen numerous culture supernatants for the presence of monoclonal antibodies (see Monitoring of Monoclonal Antibody Production) which may be present at low concentrations. The absence of background staining in the immunoperoxidase procedure greatly facilitates the interpretation of weak positive reactions and thus simplifies the task of screening multiple supernatants.

The second point relating to the choice between immunofluorescent and immunoperoxidase procedures is that it has become traditional, for no very good reason, to use immunofluorescent methods for staining cryostat sections and immunoperoxidase methods for paraffin sections.

TABLE 24·2
Advantages and disadvantages of immunofluorescent and immunoenzymatic labelling techniques

| Technique | Advantages | Disadvantages |
|---|---|---|
| Immunofluorescent labelling | Relatively rapid to perform. When double labelling, each label can be visualized without interference from the other, making it possible to detect small amounts of one antigen even in the presence of large amounts of the other. | Fluorescent labels fade on excitation and storage. Labels cannot be seen simultaneously with a counterstain. When examining double labelled preparations each field must be studied in turn with two different filter systems, making it tedious to pick out small numbers of cells which differ in their labelling pattern from that of the majority of cells. Requires fluorescent microscope. |
| Immunoenzymatic labelling | Label is permanent and can be visualized simultaneously with a counterstain, using a standard microscope. There is no loss of the label intensity when examining sections at low magnifications, and labels may easily be visualized without a microscope (Fig. 24·17). In double stained sections both labels are visualized simultaneously, so that minor cell populations, differing in their reactions from the major population, can rapidly be picked out. | Labelling takes longer to perform than immunofluorescent staining. In double stained preparations one label may mask the presence of trace amounts of the other label. |

The rationale behind the latter tradition is probably the mistaken belief that paraffin embedded formalin fixed tissues give rise to excessive background fluorescence. This is no longer true if modern epi-illuminating microscopes incorporating narrow band interference filters are used.

The use of immunofluorescence as the technique of choice when studying cryostat sections is less readily accounted for, but may stem from poor results (and particularly high levels of background labelling) which have been encountered in the past when using sub-optimal immunoperoxidase techniques based upon poor enzyme-conjugated antibodies. In recent years however a number of laboratories have demonstrated how effectively sections of human tissue can be labelled by immunoperoxidase procedures using both polyclonal and mono-clonal antibodies (Barclay, 1980, Barclay and Meyerhofer, 1981. Hoffman-Fezer *et al.*, 1981, Mason *et al.*, 1982, Naiem *et al.*, 1981a, Poppema *et al.*, 1981, Stein *et al.*, 1980, 1981) and this approach is likely to be used increasingly widely in the future. Of particular value in the context of monoclonal antibodies is the possibility offered by the immunoperoxidase technique of using a counterstain, since this enables labelling patterns to be precisely related to the detailed morphological structure of the section (Fig. 24·9). In contrast, when analysing immunofluorescently labelled cryostat sections, the investigator is (literally) almost completely in the dark as to the morphological relationships of the antigens which are labelled.

The use of immunoperoxidase labelling for cryostat sections has highlighted the importance of using fixation techniques which optimally preserve tissue morphology (Fig. 24·9). Crucial technical aspects include adequate drying of the section and fixation for a sufficiently long period, e.g. for 10 minutes rather than a brief immersion, so that the tissue can survive the subsequent repeated washing and incubation stages.

4. ALTERNATIVE LABELLING PROCEDURES

The immunofluorescent and immunoenzymatic techniques discussed above are those most widely used at the present time for the immunohistological analysis of monoclonal antibodies. However a number of additional procedures, some of which use alternative anti-body labels, have also been investigated with the aim of enhancing sensitivity or offering other practical advantages. Some of these techniques are summarized in Table 24·3.

TABLE 24·3

Alternative immunohistological labelling system

| Technique | Principle | Comments |
|---|---|---|
| Immuno-gold labelling (Gu et al., 1981; Horisberger, 1979) | Colloidal gold is prepared and bound to antibody molecules by electrostatic forces. The label is visible as characteristic electron dense particles in the electron microscope, or by its reddish colour by light microscopy. | The label is more easily identified by electron microscopy than markers such as peroxidase or ferritin. When used in conjunction with double immunoenzymatic labelling techniques it is possible to simultaneously visualize three antigens in a tissue section by light microscopy. By preparing colloidal gold particles of differing sizes it may be possible to perform double labelling at the electron microscopic level. |
| Radiolabelled monoclonal antibodies (Cuello et al., 1980) | Monoclonal antibodies are internally labelled by growing hybridoma cells in the presence of $^3$H-tagged amino acids. Sites of antibody binding are revealed by autoradiography. | Technique is suitable for both optical and electron microscopic use. When used in conjunction with peroxidase staining techniques the double labelling of pairs of antigens at both the optical and electron microscopic technique is possible. |
| Biotin-avidin labelling (Guesdon et al., 1979; Hsu et al., 1981; Warnke and Levy, 1980) | Several systems have been used, but all depend upon the high affinity of avidin (a protein obtained from egg white) for the vitamin biotin. Most commonly the primary antibody is labelled with biotin and then revealed using peroxidase- or fluorochrome-labelled avidin. | May be of higher sensitivity than conventional techniques. Double labelling systems based upon biotin-avidin binding may be used in the future to analyse pairs of monoclonal antibodies (since the use of anti-mouse or rat Ig antibodies is avoided). Endogenous avidin-binding activity is present in many tissues but may be suppressed by prior exposure to free avidin followed by free biotin (Wood and Warnke, 1981). |
| Four stage immuno-peroxidase staining (Poppema et al., 1981) | The primary monoclonal antibody is followed by rabbit anti-mouse Ig, anti-rabbit Ig, and rabbit PAP complexes. | The system has the advantage that widely available reagents (for the PAP system) can be used in conjunction with a monoclonal antibody, and that sensitivity may be enhanced. The major drawback is the necessity for 4 separate antibody incubation steps. |

# III IMMUNOHISTOLOGICAL LABELLING IN PERSPECTIVE

In order to use monoclonal antibodies by immunohistological techniques most effectively it is necessary to appreciate both the advantages and limitations of these techniques.

## A. ADVANTAGES OF IMMUNOHISTOLOGICAL LABELLING

### 1. DEMONSTRATION OF ANTIGEN DISTRIBUTION PATTERNS

When cells are isolated from a tissue sample for immunocytochemical labelling in suspension it is no longer possible to learn anything of the topographical relationships of antigen-positive cells either to each other or to other cell populations or histological features in the tissue. Immunohistological labelling techniques, by analysing cells *in situ*, avoid this limitation. There are two broad contexts in which the ability of immunohistological techniques to visualize the distribution pattern of an antigen is of value. Firstly, when analysing the specificity of a newly produced antibody, its staining reactions on different tissues are often highly informative, and may on occasion make it possible to correctly identify the specificity of a new antibody from its staining reaction on a single tissue section. This aspect of immunohistological labelling is discussed (with illustrations) below under *Monitoring of Monoclonal Antibody Production.* (Section III C. 1).

Secondly, once the specificity of a monoclonal antibody has been established, immunohistological analysis of its reactivity pattern on normal and abnormal tissues may provide valuable information on the nature of disease processes which would not be obtainable by studying the antigen in cell suspensions. This practical application of immunohistological labelling is discussed further in the final section of this chapter.

### 2. DETECTION OF ANTIGENS PRESENT AT LOW FREQUENCY

Provided optimal immunohistological techniques are used, in which non-specific background staining is absent, it is possible to pick out very small numbers of positively labelled cells (or other structures) in a tissue section. Since an average tissue section will usually contain well in excess of $5 \times 10^6$ cells the ability to recognize 5 positively labelled

602         *D. Y. Mason* et al.

cells (which is within the capacity of optimal immunohistological techniques) represents a detection threshold of 0·0001% (Sloane *et al.*, 1980).

This degree of sensitivity (which is beyond the reach of conventional binding assays or immunofluorescent surface labelling) is of value in several different practical contexts. Particular mention may be made of the importance of analysing antibodies which appear to be specific for a single organ or tissue by immunohistological techniques. Antibodies of such restricted reactivity are of obvious potential value. However their specificity should not be considered established until sections from numerous different tissue samples have been screened immunohistologically, since small numbers of antigen-positive cells may be

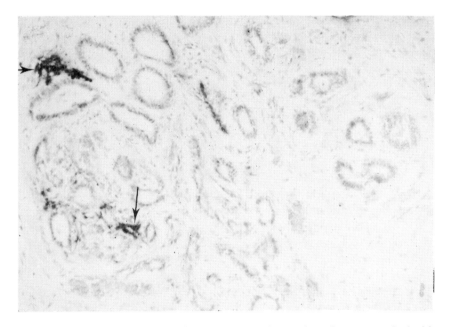

FIG. 24·10 Immunoperoxidase labelling of human breast tissue (cryostat section) with an antibody raised against human placental syncytiotrophoblast surface membrane (Sunderland *et al.*, 1981). The antibody reacts with two areas (arrowed) within the stroma around some of the glandular elements. This photomicrograph illustrates the way in which immunohistological staining may pick out small areas of labelling within an otherwise negative tissue section. Furthermore it serves as a reminder of the frequency with which monoclonal antibodies apparently specific for a single cell type may be shown on more extensive examination to react with unrelated tissue elements. Immunohistological labelling is particularly valuable in this context since it enables very large numbers of different tissue constituents to be rapidly tested for reactivity with a monoclonal antibody.

present which would escape detection by other methods. This point is illustrated by results obtained using the monoclonal antibody NDOG1 (Sunderland *et al.*, 1981) which initially appeared, on the basis of tissue homogenate absorption experiments, to be specific for human syncytiotrophoblast. However small areas of labelling (the precise cellular localization of which as yet remains uncertain) were subsequently found within the stroma of human breast tissue by immunoperoxidase staining (Fig. 24·10).

## 3. VISUALIZATION OF FIXED AND INTRACELLULAR TISSUE ELEMENTS

The preparation of a cell suspension from a tissue sample is a selective process which extracts only those cells or structures which are easily mobilized from the tissue, and which are not too fragile to survive the extraction procedure. In consequence analysis of a cell suspension using a monoclonal antibody provides a distorted view of the true antigenic content of the tissue.

An obvious practical example of this problem is encountered when studying thymic epithelial cells. A complex meshwork of these cells is found throughout the cortex of the thymus, where it can be revealed by staining for Ia (in the rat) or HLA-DR (in man) antigens (Fig. 24·11; see also Barclay, 1981; Bhan *et al.*, 1980, Janossy *et al.*, 1980). In thymic cell suspensions however, only a small minority of Ia or HLA-DR positive cells can be detected, clearly illustrating the difficulties of getting the thymic epithelial cells to enter suspension.

A further example of a fixed "framework" cell from lymphoid tissue which does not readily enter suspension is provided by the dendritic reticulum cell. A monoclonal antibody reactive with this important cellular constituent of follicular germinal centres has recently been raised in the authors' laboratories (Fig. 24·12; see also Naiem *et al.*. 1981a, Stein *et al.*, 1981 and section III C. 2 on *Immunohistological Analysis of Human Lymphoid Tissue Biopsies*).

Numerous other examples of antigenic fixed tissue constituents which do not readily enter suspension and are therefore best studied by immunohistological techniques must exist (Fig. 24·13). In screening primary hybridoma culture supernatants on lymphoid tissue sections we have frequently observed antibodies reactive with elements such as epithelium, vascular smooth muscle or unidentified fibre-like structures (Fig. 24·14). Immunohistological labelling using monoclonal antibodies is likely to throw considerable new light on these relatively neglected constituents of human tissue in the future.

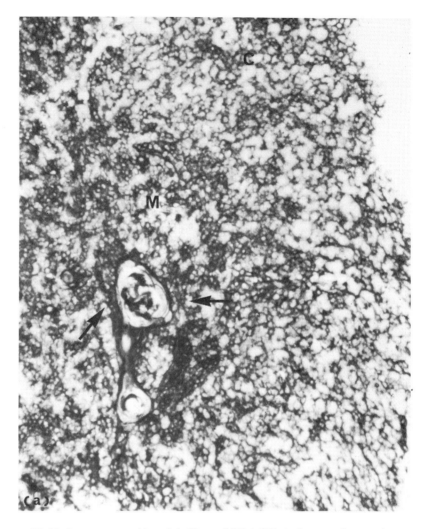

FIG. 24·11 Immunoperoxidase labelling of HLA-DR in human thymus (cryostat section). There is a strongly labelled meshwork of cells throughout the thymic cortex (C), representing thymic epithelium. The high power photomicrograph (b) shows unlabelled small thymocytes lying in between epithelial processes. In the thymic medulla (M), which can be recognized by the presence of Hassel's corpuscles

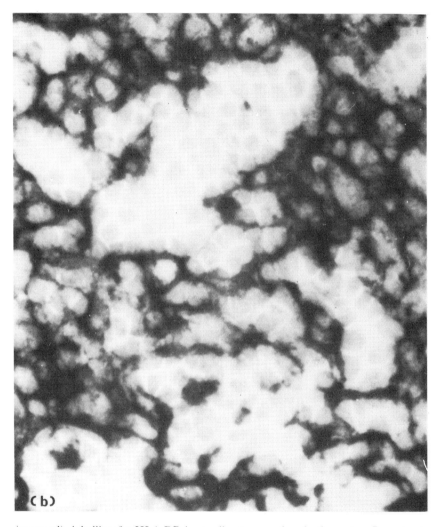

(b)

(arrowed), labelling for HLA-DR is usually stronger than in the cortex. Recent evidence from immunohistological studies of chimeric rats suggests that HLA-DR-positive cells in the medulla are bone-marrow-derived and unrelated in their development and turnover to HLA-DR-positive cortical cells (Barclay and Meyerhofer, 1981). Haematoxylin counterstain.

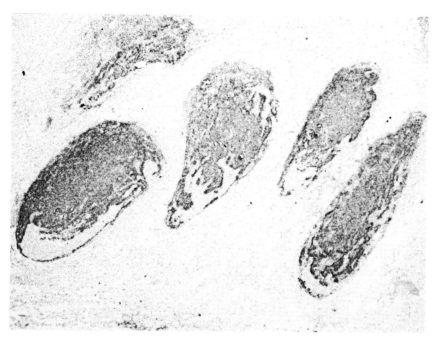

FIG. 24·12 Immunoperoxidase staining of human tonsil tissue (cryostat section) with an antibody which reacts with dendritic reticulum cells. These cells are confined to lymphoid follicles and their immunohistological detection is of value in the analysis of neoplastic lymphoid tissue (see text and figures Figs. 24·20 and 24·23). Haematoxylin counterstain. (Reproduced by permission from Naiem *et al.* (1982). *J. Immunol. Methods* (in press).

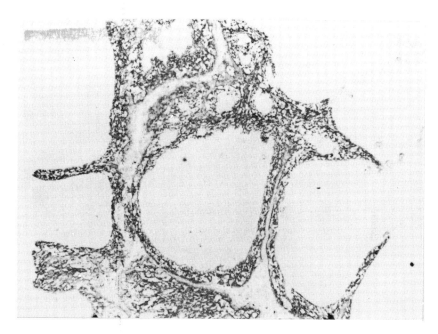

FIG. 24·13 Immunoperoxidase labelling of human tonsil (cryostat section) with an antibody (MHM8) which reacts primarily with epithelial cells. In this illustration the crypt epithelium is clearly delineated from the lymphoid elements of the tonsil, which are unreactive with this antibody. (Compare with Fig. 24·14a which shows tonsil tissue (at the same magnification) stained with a monoclonal antibody against a fibrillar component confined to lymphoid areas of the tonsil).

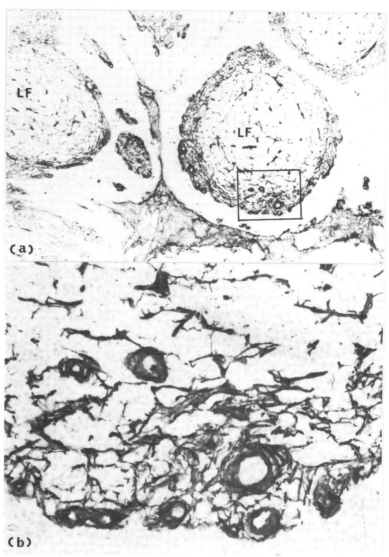

FIG. 24·14 Immunoperoxidase labelling pattern obtained when screening hybridoma culture supernatants (from a fusion aimed at producing anti-T cell antibodies) on cryostat sections of human tonsil (experiment in collaboration with J. Bastin and A. J. McMichael). The antibody (or antibodies) in this supernatant react strongly with an unidentified fibrillar element in the tissue which tends to be associated with lymphoid follicles (LF), although there is also some labelling of extrafollicular structures. The area marked in (a) at the margin of a follicle (where the reaction tends to be strongest) is shown in higher magnification in (b). Antibodies of this sort reacting with structural elements of human tissue are relatively frequently found when screening fusion experiments by immunohistological techniques. The specificity of this particular antibody has not been identified but the reaction pattern closely resembles that obtained using anti-fibronectin.

Immunohistological labelling may also be the most appropriate technique for detecting antibodies reactive with intracellular antigens (both cytoplasmic and nuclear—Fig. 24·15) since conventional binding assays based upon the use of whole cells will not detect antibodies reacting with antigens at these sites.

## B. Limitations of Immunohistological Labelling

### 1. limited sensitivity

The sensitivity of immunohistological techniques should not be overestimated. It is sometimes assumed that once a monoclonal antibody has been raised against a tissue constituent it will inevitably be possible to use the antibody for immunohistological analysis. However many tissue constituents are present at concentrations too low to be detectable by existing immunohistological techniques. This is particularly true of factors with high specific activity (e.g. growth factors, enzymes, modifiers of lymphoid cell function etc.) which are produced in small amounts and may have short half-lives. It would be more appropriate to analyse antibodies recognizing such constituents by a technique such as radioimmunoassay of tissue extracts than to use an immunohistological method. In this context it may also be noted that cell surface membrane constituents which are present at too low a concentration to be detectable on tissue sections may on occasion be demonstrable by immunofluorescent labelling of cells in suspension.

Realization of the limited sensitivity of immunohistological techniques leads to two practical conclusions. Firstly it should be appreciated that, whilst specific immunohistological labelling is always of significance, failure to obtain a labelling reaction cannot be interpreted as evidence that the tissue does not contain the relevant antigen. In this context it is important to realize that the preparation of tissue sections may itself denature an antigen. Even when cryostat sections are used in which antigenic reactivity tends to be particularly well preserved (see above) there is a risk of antigen loss. In most laboratories cryostat sections are fixed before staining and this step clearly introduces a risk of antigen destruction. In the authors' laboratory we have found acetone to be a good general purpose fixative but there may be occasions on which alternative fixatives are indicated.

A second point which follows from the preceding discussion is that immunohistological techniques are most efficient at detecting a small amount of antigen if it is present at a few sites in relatively high concen-

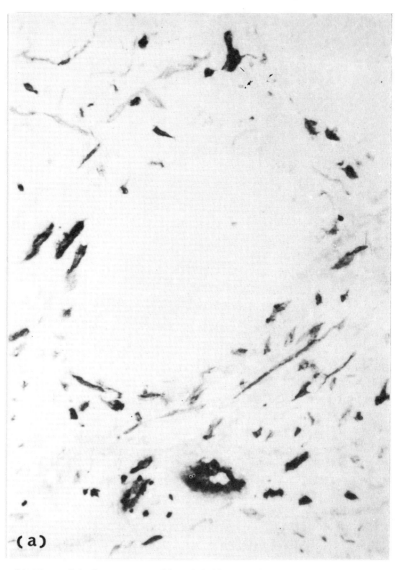

(a)

FIG. 24·15a and b Immunoperoxidase labelling of Factor VIII-related antigen in human tonsil (cryostat section). Vascular endothelium is strongly labelled. The higher power view (b) shows the characteristic granular pattern of intracytoplasmic labelling. (Reproduced by permission from Naiem *et al.*, (1982). *J. Immunol. Methods* (in press).

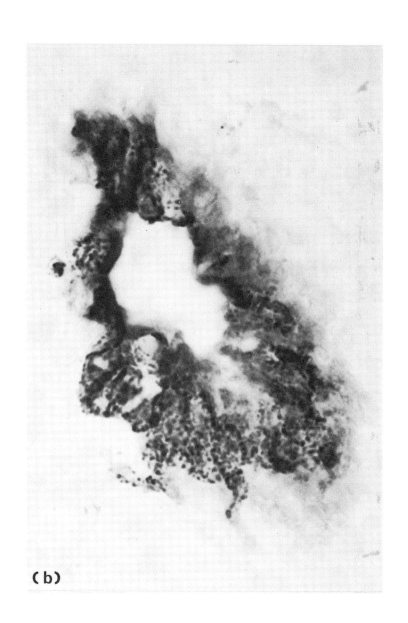

(b)

tration (e.g. on the membrane of a small minority of cells) rather than being diffusely distributed throughout the tissue.

## 2. BACKGROUND STAINING

This is a potential problem in all immunohistological studies but it should be eliminable by the use of an optimal technique (see Appendix). The advent of monoclonal antibodies has redefined the level of background staining which immunohistologists are prepared to accept. In the past, using polyclonal antisera, weak background staining was often considered inevitable; today, using monoclonal reagents, our expectations are higher.

It should be noted however that there is one type of background staining which, by its very nature, is not avoidable by improvement in technique. This arises when a cellular antigen is present at substantial concentration in the extracellular environment. A commonly encountered example in the field of human lymphoma immunohistology is provided by immunoglobulin. The demonstration that lymphoid cells carry Ig of a single light chain class provides strong evidence for their monoclonal (and hence neoplastic) nature. However light chains are ubiquitously present in human tissue (as part of normal immunoglobulin), particularly in association with collagen fibres and connective tissue (Fig. 24·16). In consequence it may be very difficult to label cell-surface light chains in some lymphoid tissue samples (e.g. when inflammation and fibrosis causes excessive background staining). This problem was well recognized in the past when polyclonal anti-Ig antisera were used, but it continues to represent a source of difficulty in the immunohistological analysis of human lymphoproliferative disorders with monoclonal antibodies.

Fortunately the majority of human lymphoid cell surface antigens detectable with currently available antibodies are not present at substantial concentration in the extracellular environment. Furthermore as the list of cell surface markers detectable with monoclonal antibodies lengthens it will become progressively less necessary to rely upon unsatisfactory antigens such as surface Ig light chains for analysing proliferating B cells.

## C. PRACTICAL APPLICATIONS OF MONOCLONAL ANTIBODY IMMUNOHISTOLOGY

In this concluding section details are given of two areas in which immunohistological labelling with monoclonal antibodies is already

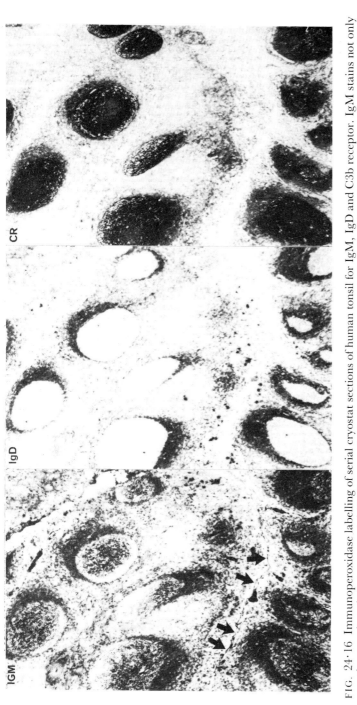

FIG. 24·16 Immunoperoxidase labelling of serial cryostat sections of human tonsil for IgM, IgD and C3b receptor. IgM stains not only mantle zone lymphocytes around follicular germinal centres but also a coarse meshwork within the germinal centres. This staining represents immune complexes bound by dendritic reticulum cells (see Fig. 24·12). IgD staining is localized to mantle zone lymphocytes, whilst complement receptor is present both on germinal centre and mantle zone cells. In the IgM stained preparation there is more background labelling than in the other two sections, and the position of an epithelial-lined crypt can be picked out because of its linear staining (arrowed). Background labelling for IgM (and also for IgG, kappa and lambda) is frequently seen in human tissues, particularly in association with collagen (see Figs. 24·21 and 24·23).

TABLE 24·4

Cell populations and other tissue elements detectable by immunohistological labelling in human tonsil

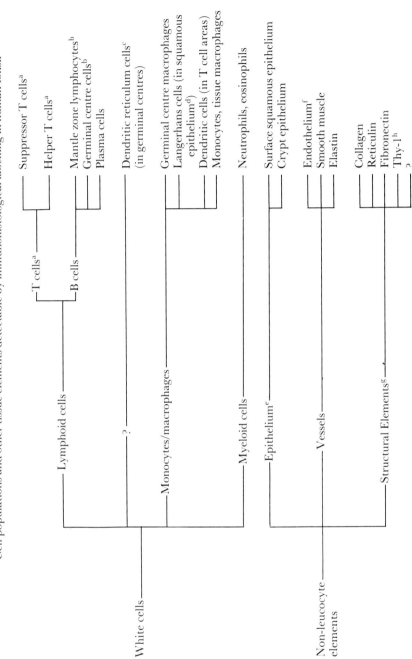

White cells

Lymphoid cells
— T cells[a]
— Suppressor T cells[a]
— Helper T cells[a]
— B cells
— Mantle zone lymphocytes[b]
— Germinal centre cells[b]
— Plasma cells
— ?
— Dendritic reticulum cells[c] (in germinal centres)
Monocytes/macrophages
— Germinal centre macrophages
— Langerhans cells (in squamous epithelium[d])
— Dendritic cells (in T cell areas)
— Monocytes, tissue macrophages
Myeloid cells
— Neutrophils, eosinophils

Non-leucocyte elements

Epithelium[e]
— Surface squamous epithelium
— Crypt epithelium
Vessels
— Endothelium[f]
— Smooth muscle
— Elastin
Structural Elements[g]
— Collagen
— Reticulin
— Fibronectin
— Thy-1[h]
— ?

a  Monoclonal antibodies reacting with all classes of T cells stain interfollicular areas, but also reveal scattered T cells within germinal centres (particularly at the boundary between germinal centres and the surrounding mantle zone of small lymphoid cells). Antibodies against helper T cells show a similar pattern, whilst anti-suppressor T cell antibodies stain small numbers of cells in the interfollicular regions and only very rare cells within lymphoid follicles (Poppema et al., 1981,. Stein et al., 1981).

b  Mantle zone lymphocytes may be distinguished from germinal centre B cells by the presence of surface IgD on the former cell type and by their more intense staining reaction with antibodies against the leucocyte-common antigen (Dalchau et al., 1980).

c  These cells, which are responsible for trapping immune complexes within germinal centres and thus enhancing the presentation of antigen to germinal centre lymphoid cells, can be detected by a dendritic reticulum cell-specific antibody (Fig. 24·12) and also by their reactivity with antibodies against IgM, IgG or C3b receptor (Gerdes et al., 1981).

d  These cells react strongly with anti-HLA-DR antibodies (Fig. 24·9) but also, unexpectedly, with monoclonal antibodies OKT6 and NA1/34, which were initially thought to be specific for cortical thymocytes (McMichael et al., 1979).

e  A number of monoclonal antibodies react with squamous epithelium and not infrequently the reaction intensity is related to maturation, either decreasing as these cells differentiate (Fig. 24·19) or showing the reverse pattern. Some monoclonal antibodies appear to distinguish between surface squamous epithelium and its reticular extensions into the tonsillar substance (crypt epithelium—Fig. 24·13).

f  Endothelium may be labelled using monoclonal antibody against human Factor VIII-related antigen (Fig. 24·15).

g  A number of antibodies reactive with unidentified fibrillar elements in lymphoid tissue have been detected by screening cell fusion supernatants on sections of human tonsil (Fig. 24·14).

h  See McKenzie and Fabre, 1981 for details of the monoclonal antibody F15-42-1 specific for human Thy-1.

proving to be of practical benefit. Firstly the value of monitoring monoclonal antibody production (at all stages from the initial primary screen to the evaluation of cloned antibodies) by immunohistological techniques will be described. Secondly details will be given of the use of monoclonal antibodies in the immunohistological analysis of human lymphoid tissue biopsies.

## 1. MONITORING OF MONOCLONAL ANTIBODY PRODUCTION

In order to appreciate the unique value of immunohistological techniques in the monitoring of monoclonal antibody production it is necessary to compare the procedure with the alternative assay methods currently used for the same purpose. In the majority of assays the target antigen (in the form of either whole cells or antigen immobilized on a solid surface) is incubated with hybridoma supernatant, followed by an enzyme- or radioisotope-conjugated antibody (with an intervening washing stage to remove unbound Ig). Less frequently used techniques include haemagglutination, cytotoxicity, indirect immunofluorescence on cells in suspension and inhibition of functional assays.

All of the assays provide, for each sample tested, a single numerical value, e.g. radioactive counts bound, percentage cytotoxicity, haemagglutination titre etc. In contrast when a culture supernatant is tested on a single tissue section by the immunohistological technique semi-quantitative information is obtained on the reactivity of antibody (or antibodies) in the supernatant against a wide variety of different antigenic constituents and cell populations in the tissue. It may be noted in this context that even the simplest tissue is histologically complex and contains numerous different cellular and noncellular elements. An example is provided by human tonsil, a tissue extensively used in the authors' laboratories for screening hybridoma supernatants. As can be seen from Table 24·4 this tissue contains not only a number of clearly distinguishable lymphoid cell compartments but also numerous other non-lymphoid elements, the immunohistological reactions of which are often highly informative (Figs. 24·16 and 24·17).

The value of immunohistologically screening hybridoma supernatants is often further enhanced when sections from more than one tissue are analysed. This is illustrated in Fig. 24·18 which demonstrates the way in which two antibodies (anti-HLA-DR and antibody to C3b receptor) which gave superficially similar staining patterns on tonsil sections could clearly be distinguished when tested on kidney sections. By selection of appropriate combinations of tissues in the initial immunohistological screening of culture supernatants it is possible to rapidly obtain a large amount of information about the probable specificity of new antibodies.

This discussion may be concluded by pointing out that immunohistological techniques are of value not only in the initial screening of hybridoma supernatants, but also during subsequent cloning and analysis of individual antibodies (see Table 24·5 for further details and Figs. 24·6 and 24·19).

## 2. IMMUNOHISTOLOGICAL ANALYSIS OF HUMAN LYMPHOID TISSUE BIOPSIES

Histopathological diagnosis plays a central role in clinical medicine. However the techniques on which it relies (tissue fixation in formalin, dehydration and embedding in paraffin, staining of sections with haematoxylin and eosin) were all introduced approximately 100 years ago. Specialized techniques such as enzyme cytochemistry or specific stains (e.g. silver stains for reticulin fibres, periodic acid-Schiff reaction for carbohydrate) have been added over the years to supplement conditional staining methods, but are only applied in a small minority of cases.

In the past 20 years immunohistological techniques have begun to be used in a limited way as an adjunct to routine histological examination. Initially these investigations were limited largely to immunofluorescent tracing of tissue immune complex deposits in diseases such as glomerulonephritis. In the early 1970's the field began to widen when immunoperoxidase techniques were applied for the first time to routine histopathological samples, and a variety of antigenic constituents in many different disease states have been analysed since that time. Examples include the demonstration of immunoglobulin, lysozyme, J chain and alpha-1-antitrypsin in lymphoproliferative diseases; carcinoembryonic antigen in gastrointestinal and other malignancies; milk proteins in breast carcinoma; and hormones such as chorionic gonadotrophin in teratomas. However although analysis of these markers is of some value from the point of view of fundamental research, it must be admitted that immunohistological labelling is still of relatively little diagnostic value in individual cases.

The advent of monoclonal antibodies has introduced an important new factor in this field and it appears likely that their use for the immunohistological staining of routine tissue sections will in the future transform the practice of diagnostic histopathology. Histopathological diagnosis is a highly subjective art and many year's training are required in order to achieve competence. The use of monoclonal anti-

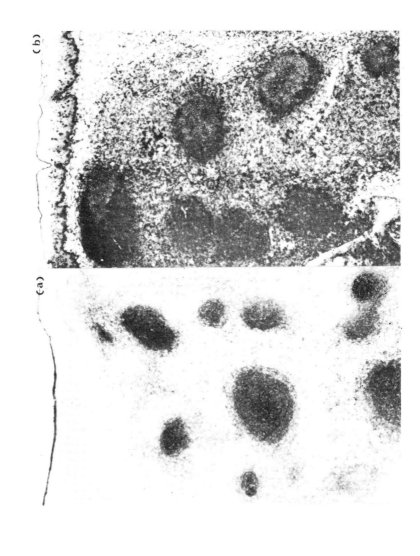

(a)

(b)

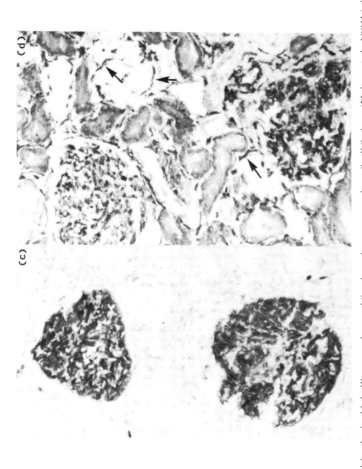

FIG. 24·18 Immunohistological labelling may be used for the primary screening of cell fusions (Naiem et al., 1981b). The aim of this fusion was to produce antibodies against human complement receptor (Gerdes et al., 1982). By screening on tonsil sections several supernatants were identified which labelled in the expected pattern, i.e. lymphoid follicles (a). Other supernatants also stained lymphoid follicles (b) but were reactive in addition with numerous cells in interfollicular regions and also with scattered cells in superficial squamous epithelium. This pattern is typical of anti-HLA-DR antibody. Further confirmation of these results came from screening these supernatants on human kidney sections. The antibody of presumed anti-C3 receptor specificity labelled only glomeruli (c) whereas the putative anti-HLA-DR antibody stained glomeruli, endothelium, probable dendritic cells (arrowed) and renal tubules (d)—see Hart et al., 1981. (Reproduced by permission, from Naiem et al., (1982). J. Immunol Methods (in press) ).

## TABLE 24·5

The use of immunohistological labelling for monitoring monoclonal antibody production

| Production stage | Practical application of immunohistological labelling |
|---|---|
| Primary screening of hybridoma supernatants for antibody activity | Positive supernatants can rapidly be identified. Their probable specificity can frequently be predicted from their reactivity against sections from one or more different tissues (Fig. 24·18). Unwanted antibodies, e.g. pan-reactive antibodies can be identified and eliminated at this stage. A permanent record of the primary screen is obtained which can be re-evaluated if necessary at a later date. |
| Cloning of primary cultures | Immunohistological screening of culture supernatants after cloning reveals whether the initial reactivity pattern · (identified in the primary screen) represented a single clone (in which case all positive daughter clones will give identical reactions) or multiple clones (in which case different patterns will separate on cloning). |
| Analysis of cloned antibodies | Immunohistological labelling allows minor differences in specificity between individual monoclonal antibodies to be detected. Such differences would be difficult to reveal by other techniques. Double immunohistological labelling may be of particular value when analysing the specificity of monoclonal antibodies. Fig. 24·16 illustrates the way in which evidence for the specificity of a monoclonal antibody against human lambda light chains was obtained by employing it in a double labelling system in conjunction with a well characterized rabbit antibody to human kappa chains. The demonstration of the expected ratio of kappa to lambda plasma cells (2:1) and the absence of double stained cells suggest that this antibody reacts with a determinant which is common to all lambda light chains but absent from kappa chains. |

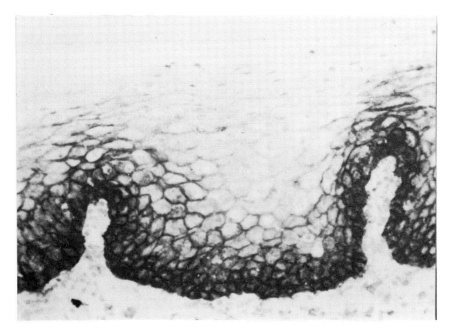

FIG. 24·19 Immunoperoxidase staining of human squamous epithelium with antibody BK19·9. This antibody (raised by Dr. G. Brown) was suspected (on the basis of binding assays against a range of human cell types) to be directed against a proliferation-associated glycoprotein (Omary *et al.*, 1980). Immunoperoxidase staining provided evidence for this supposition since labelling is strongest in the basal layers and becomes progressively weaker as the cells mature and cease to divide. Subsequent testing in Dr. Brown's laboratory confirmed the specificity of this antibody. (Reproduced by permission, from Naiem *et al.* (1982). *J. Immunol. Methods* (in press) ).

bodies should not only introduce a new objectivity to this field but will also allow new prognostically significant disease sub-groups (which cannot currently be recognized by conventional criteria) to be identified.

In the remaining section of this chapter examples will be given of the way in which monoclonal antibodies have been used in the author's laboratories for the analysis of human lymphoid tissue biopsies (Stein *et al.*, 1981). However it should be noted that these samples represent only a small proportion of the total workload of diagnostic biopsies analysed in histopathological laboratories and in consequence results reported below represent only a fraction of the potential field of application of immunohistological labelling techniques in diagnostic histopathology.

(a) *Non-Hodgkin's Lymphoma* (Table 24·6)

(b) *Follicular Lymphoma*

Approximately 25% of cases of non-Hodgkin's Lymphoma show a follicular growth pattern. Immunohistological labelling with mono-clonal antibodies demonstrates the close relationship which exists between these neoplastic follicles and normal lymphoid follicles. The proliferating cells are found initially within the germinal centres of the follicles leading to expansion and distortion of the peripheral corona of IgD/IgM positive small lymphocytes (Fig. 24·20). Furthermore the network of dendritic reticulum cells within the germinal centres (which are presumed to be innocent bystanders in the neoplastic process) is expanded and distorted, as revealed by staining with monoclonal anti-bodies against dendritic reticulum cells and C3b receptor (Fig. 24·20).

The neoplastic germinal centre cells in the majority of cases of follicular lymphoma express surface Ig (most frequently IgM, followed by IgG) of a single light chain type. It is of interest that although neoplastic germinal centres resemble normal germinal centres in con-taining dendritic reticulum cells (see above) these cells differ from those in normal tissue in that they do not carry surface immune complexes (staining for IgG, IgM, kappa and lambda). This may on occasion be of diagnostic importance when attempting to distinguish between neo-plastic and reactive germinal centres.

Other antigens associated with normal germinal centres (e.g. HLA-DR etc.) are also found on neoplastic follicles. Furthermore T cells are often plentiful within the neoplastic follicles and in the extrafollicular regions (Fig. 24·20), as is the case in normal reactive lymphoid tissue (Figs. 24·7 and 24·17).

(c) *Diffuse Lymphoma*

This is a very heterogeneous group of neoplasms. The majority of cases are revealed by immunohistological typing to be of B cell origin (Fig. 24·21). A minority however express little or no surface Ig. This is important for two reasons. Firstly, when such tumours are of anaplastic morphology, the absence of Ig staining may be taken as confirmatory evidence of their non-lymphoid origin. In such cases it is often of essential diagnostic importance to analyse their reactivity with anti-bodies reactive with leucocytes (e.g. antibodies F10-89-4, (Dalchau *et al.*, 1980) or 2DI (Pizzolo *et al.*, 1980) ), HLA-DR and B cells (e.g. antibody F8-11-13 (Dalchau and Fabre, 1981) ). Fig. 24·22 illustrates a case in which this type of analysis allowed the true diagnosis to be obtained in a

TABLE 24·6

Immunohistological reaction patterns of human non-Hodgkin's lymphoma
with monoclonal antibodies

| Histological category | Monoclonal antibody against: | | | |
|---|---|---|---|---|
| | Surface Ig | C3b receptor | HLA-DR | Dendritic reticulum cells |
| Chronic lymphatic leukaemia | + | + | + | ± |
| Hairy cell leukaemia | + | − | + | − |
| Centrocytic/ centroblastic lymphoma[a] | +(−) | + | + | +++ |
| Blastic B cell lymphoma[b] | +(−) | +(−) | +(−) | ± |

For further details see the text and Stein *et al.* (1981).
[a]  This category is approximately equivalent to "follicular cell lymphoma" in the Lukes and Collins classification of non-Hodgkin's lymphoma.
[b]  This category is approximately equivalent to "large non-cleaved follicle cell lymphoma" and "B immunoblastic lymphoma" in the Lukes and Collins classification.

lymphoma of primitive morphology which had initially been categorized as a metastatic carcinoma.

A second context in which the detection of Ig negative B cell lymphomas may be of importance comes from the work of Warnke and colleagues (1980) who have reported that diffuse large cell lymphomas appear to enjoy a better response to therapy and subsequent survival than do Ig positive cases. If these findings are confirmed in subsequent studies they will provide an obvious example of the way in which immunohistological typing with monoclonal antibodies can sub-divide an apparently homogeneous histological disease category into clinically distinct sub-groups.

(d) *Hodgkin's Disease*

Immunohistological studies of this disease in the past have been limited, because of the restricted range and availability of satisfactory polyclonal antisera (Poppema *et al.*, 1979, Curran and Jones, 1978). It is now possible, however, with the advent of monoclonal antibodies to obtain a much clearer idea of the immunohistological pattern in this disease. In many cases T cells are plentiful (both of helper and suppressor phenotype) whilst B cell areas are distorted and partially obliterated

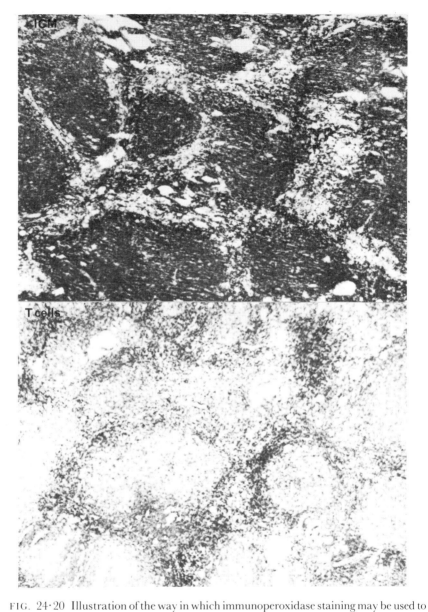

FIG. 24·20 Illustration of the way in which immunoperoxidase staining may be used to analyse human follicular lymphoma. Cryostat sections have been stained for IgM, IgD, C3b receptor and T cells. The neoplastic follicles are distorted and irregular in outline (compare with normal follicles in Figs. 24·4, 24·7, 24·16 and 24·17). However the basic structure is very similar to that of a normal follicle in that the IgD-positive mantle zone is still present, although thinned and partially destroyed by the neoplastic germinal centre cells. Dendritic reticulum cells are plentiful within neoplastic germinal centres as revealed by staining with the anti-C3b receptor, and also with the monoclonal antibody

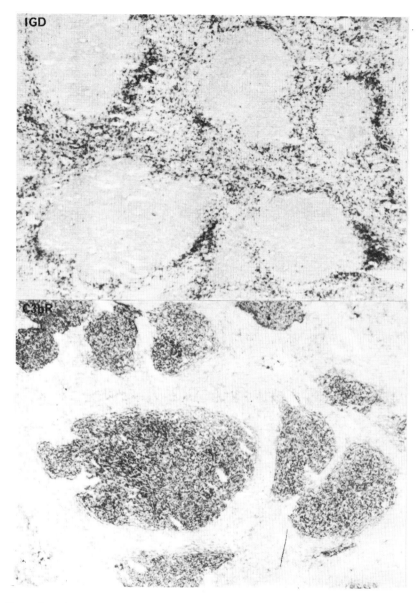

directed against this cell type (not shown—see Fig. 24·12). The neoplastic follicles in this case were also strongly stained for IgM, although this was accounted for by surface IgM on the neoplastic lymphoid cells rather than by polyclonal immune complexes bound to dendritic reticulum cells (which appear not to take up complexes when present in neoplastic follicles). Relatively large numbers of T cells are present around and within the neoplastic follicles. Immunohistological labelling with antibodies against kappa and lambda light chains (not shown) showed that this lymphoma expressed surface IgM of kappa type.

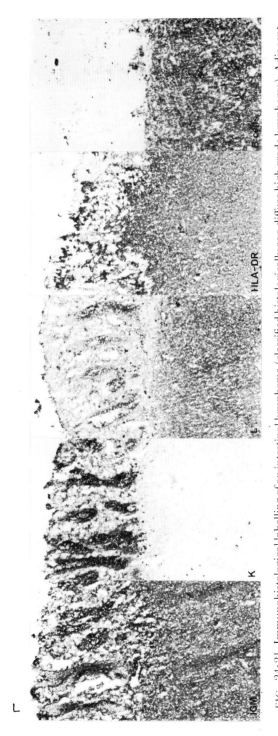

FIG. 24·21 Immunohistological labelling of an intestinal lymphoma (classified histologically as a diffuse high grade lymphoma). Adjacent sections have been stained for IgM, kappa chains, lambda chains, HLA-DR and a determinant found predominantly on B cells (antibody F8-11-13, Dalchau and Fabre, 1981). The neoplastic cells, which occupy the lower half of each figure, stain for IgM lambda, and also carry HLA-DR and the B cell antigen. Staining for kappa chains is negative. Staining for IgM, kappa and lambda, reflecting the presence of polyclonal immunoglobulin. In contrast staining for the B cell-related antigen is negative within the epithelium (in the upper part of each figure) stains for IgM, kappa and lambda, reflecting the presence of polyclonal immunoglobulin. In contrast staining for the B cell-related antigen is negative within the epithelium, demonstrating the value of using a marker which (unlike immunoglobulin) is not present in the serum at substantial concentration. Staining for HLA-DR reveals cells within the epithelium which are not (to judge from the B cell staining) part of the neoplastic population. They have the morphological appearance of normal resident mucosal macrophages, which are known to possess large amounts of this antigen.

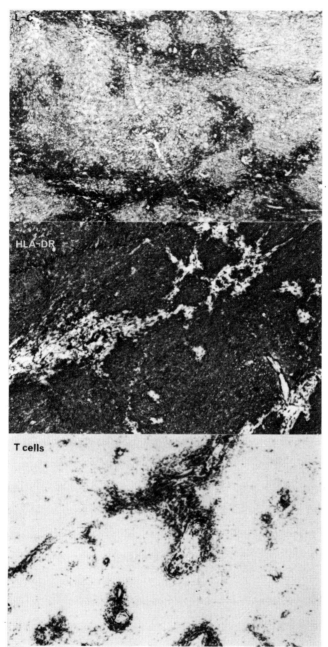

FIG. 24·22  Immunohistological labelling of an anaplastic tumour which was classified on conventional histological grounds as a metastatic carcinoma. However, labelling of cryostat sections for leucocytes (L-C), (Pizzolo *et al.*, 1980) HLA-DR, and T cells revealed that the section contains sheets of HLA-DR-positive white cells interspersed with islands of T cells. The latter population of host lymphocytes stains more strongly for leucocyte-common antigen than do the tumour cells, but is predominantly negative for HLA-DR antigen. These immunohistological staining reactions, together with results obtained (not shown) using other monoclonal antibodies, showed clearly that the tumour was a high grade B-cell lymphoma rather than an anaplastic carcinoma.

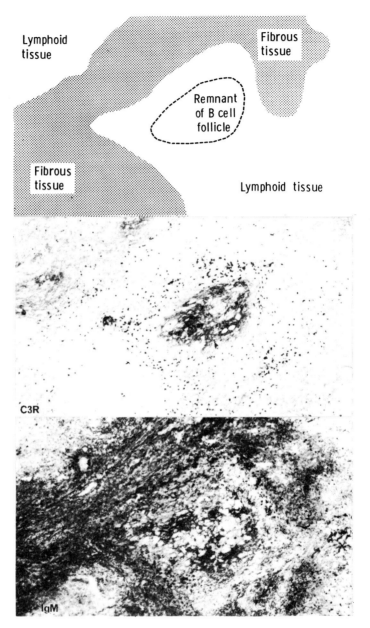

FIG. 24·23 Immunohistological labelling of a biopsy from a case of Hodgkin's disease (nodular sclerosing type). Each photomicrograph shows the same area stained for a different antigen. The line diagram indicates the relative positions of lymphoid tissue and of fibrous tissue. T cells are present in large numbers in the lymphoid regions. The distorted remnant of a lymphoid follicle is detectable by staining for C3b receptor and for dendritic reticulum cells (DRC). IgM staining also picks out the B cell area, although this reaction is partially obscured by the dense labelling for IgM on fibrous tissue. Staining for IgD and for a determinant found predominantly on B cells (F8-11-

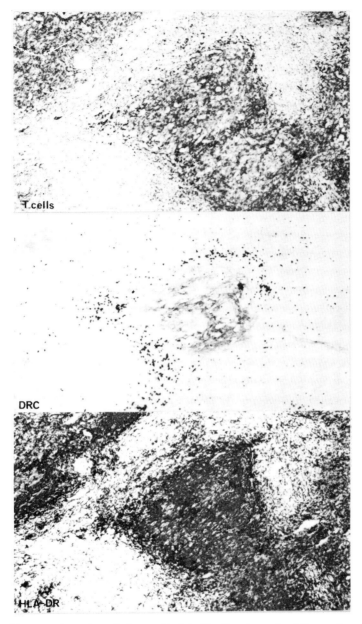

13) (neither reactions shown) also enabled the B cell region to be delineated, and these two antibodies gave cleaner reactions than anti-IgM in that they did not react with fibrous tissue. HLA-DR is strongly expressed throughout the lymphoid areas (presumably partially reflecting the presence of activated T cells) and also on scattered cells in the fibrous tissue.

N.B. Scattered myeloid cells (visualized because of their endogenous peroxidase activity) are present around the lymphoid areas (most clearly seen in the C3b receptor and DRC stained sections).

by the disease process (Fig. 24·23). However in a minority of cases (which appear to correspond to the lymphocyte predominant histological category) there is a clearly different pattern in that the areas of Hodgkin's tissue appear to be composed of enlarged primary lymphoid follicles. This is evident when monoclonal antibodies against IgM, IgD, B cells, dendritic reticulum cells and C3b receptor are used. These primary follicles are infiltrated with Reed Sternberg and Hodgkins cells, although the degree of this infiltration is less striking than in other types of Hodgkin's disease.

(e)  *Carcinomatous Metastasis*

As noted above metastatic carcinoma in lymph nodes may be difficult to distinguish from anaplastic lymphoma if the tumour is of primitive morphology and the node almost completely replaced by neoplasm. Fig. 24·24 illustrates the way in which such metastases may be clearly identified using monoclonal antibodies, since not only do they fail to react with antibodies against lymphoid antigens (e.g. the leucocyte-common antigen (Dalchau et al., 1980) ) but they are reactive with antibodies recognizing epithelial cells. This application of monoclonal antibody immunohistology is of obvious potential value not only in confirming the carcinomatous origin of lymph node metastasis, but also in searching for micrometastasis in regional lymph nodes removed during radical surgery for cancer (Sloane et al., 1980). Furthermore, as the range of monoclonal antibodies directed against epithelial cells enlarges, it should prove possible in the future to identify the probable primary site of origin of carcinomatous metastases.


# IV  CONCLUSIONS


This chapter has illustrated that recently developed immunohistological techniques make it possible to combine strong immunoenzymatic labelling of antigens recognized in a tissue section by a monoclonal antibody with good visualization of tissue morphological details. Of particular importance is the fact that non-specific background staining can be eliminated when using these methods. These techniques are likely to prove of increasing value in the future both in the monitoring and analysis of monoclonal antibodies during their production, and also in the histopathological diagnosis and assessment of a wide range of human diseases.

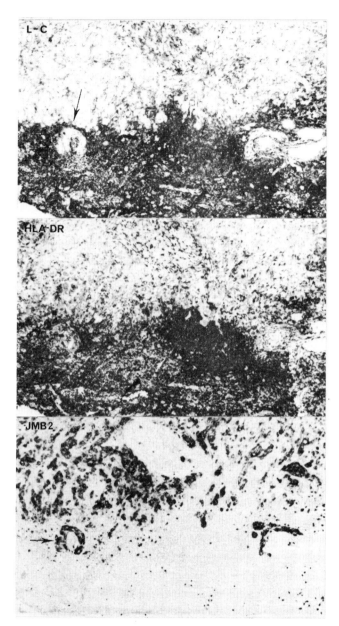

FIG. 24·24 Immunohistological identification of metastatic carcinoma in a lymph node. Staining for leucocytes (L-C) (Pizzolo *et al*., 1980) and for HLA-DR reveals normal lymphoid tissue (in the lower half of each figure) being infiltrated by carcinoma cells (upper half of each figure). In contrast antibody JMB2 (which reacts with human glandular epithelium) labels the carcinoma cells but gives no staining of uninvolved lymphoid tissue. A perivascular infiltrate of carcinoma cells (arrowed) can be identified both by negative staining for leucocyte-common antigen and by positive labelling with JMB2.

# APPENDIX

## Immunohistological Labelling of Cryostat Sections with Monoclonal Antibody

### 1. TISSUE PREPARATION

Tissue samples are frozen by direct immersion of small portions (usually not exceeding 1 cm in narrowest dimension) in liquid nitrogen. They are then wrapped in foil and stored in liquid nitrogen tanks until sectioning.

### 2. PREPARATION OF TISSUE SECTIONS

Tissue samples are sectioned in a conventional cryostat at 5–10 $\mu$ and picked up on gelatin coated slides. They are dessicated by leaving them in the vacuum chamber of a freeze dryer for a period of between 4 and 18 hours. The slides are then transferred to acetone at room temperature for ten minutes, and air dried. At this stage they may either be stained or wrapped in foil and frozen at $-20°C$ for future staining.

### 3. STAINING TECHNIQUE

Monoclonal antibodies are applied directly to dry sections and left at room temperature in a humid atmosphere for 30 minutes. In some cases (e.g. when staining surface kappa and lambda chains in lymphoid tissues, and when staining HLA-DR antigen) shorter incubation periods are optimal. In a few cases staining which is relatively weak after 30 minutes incubation can be improved by prolonging incubation to one hour. The slides are then washed in Tris buffered saline for one to two minutes and incubated with peroxidase-conjugated rabbit anti-mouse Ig (1/10 to 1/50). It is usually necessary to add human serum (at a final dilution of 1/3 to 1/25) to this conjugate to block cross-reactivity against human Ig which leads to excessive background staining, e.g. in germinal centres. After 30 minutes incubation with this reagent the slides are washed once more and incubated for ten minutes in diaminobenzidene ($0·3$ mg ml$^{-1}$) and hydrogen peroxide ($0·01\%$) diluted in Tris buffered saline. The slides are then washed in tap water or buffer, counterstained with haematoxylin, and mounted for microscopy.

DETAILS OF REAGENTS

*Tris buffered saline* consists of normal saline containing a tenth part of 0·5M Tris HCl buffer pH 7·6.

*Peroxidase conjugated anti-mouse Ig* is obtained from Dako Immunoglobulins (U.K. distributors: Mercia Brocades Limited).

*Diaminobenzidine Tetrahydrochloride* is obtained from Sigma Chemical Co. Ltd.

ACKNOWLEDGEMENTS

We are grateful to the following colleagues who kindly provided us with monoclonal antibodies for immunohistological use: Dr. P. C. L. Beverley (UCHT1 and 2D1); Dr. G. Brown (BK 19·9); Dr. J. W. Fabre (F8-11-13 F10-89-4 and F15-42-1); Mr. J. Hildreth (MHM 8); Dr. N. Ling (anti-$\kappa$ and anti-$\mu$) Dr. J. Morton (JMB 2) and Dr. C. A. Sunderland (NDOG1). The work described in this chapter was supported by the Leukaemia Research Fund, the Medical Research Council and the Deutsche Forschungsgemeinschaft.

REFERENCES

Arklie, J., Taylor-Papadimitriou, J., Bodmer, W. F., Egan, M. and Millis, R. (1981). *Int. J. Cancer* **28**, 23.
Avrameas, S. and Ternynck, T. (1971). *Immunochemistry* **8**, 1175.
Barclay, A. N. (1981). *Immunology* **42**, 593.
Barclay, A. N. and Meyerhofer, G. (1981). *J. exp. Med.* **153**, 1666.
Bhan, A. K., Reinherz, E. L., McClusky, R. T. and Schlossman, S. F. (1980). *J. exp. Med.* **152**, 771.
Boorsma, D. M. and Streefkerk, J. G. (1976). *J. Histochem. Cytochem.* **24**, 481.
Boorsma, D. M. and Streefkerk, J. G. (1979). *J. Immunol. Meth.* **30**, 245.
Brandtzaeg, P. (1974). *Immunology* **26**, 1101.
Carlsson, J., Drevin, H. and Axen, R. (1978). *Biochem. J.* **173**, 723.
Cuello, A. C., Milstein, C., Priestley, J. V. (1980). *Brain Res. Bull.* **5**, 575.
Curran, R. C. and Jones, E. L. (1978). *J. Path.* **125**, 39.
Dalchau, R. and Fabre, J. W. (1981). *J. exp. Med.* **153**, 753–765.
Dalchau, R., Kirkley, J. and Fabre, J. W. (1980). *Eur. J. Immunol.* **10**, 737–744.
Gerdes, J., Naiem, M., Mason, D. Y. and Stein, H. (1982). *Immunol.* **45**, 645
Gu, J., De Mey, J. and Polak, J. M. (1981). *Regulatory Peptides* (in press).
Guesdon, J. L., Ternynck, T., Avrameas, S. (1979). *J. Histochem. Cytochem.* **27**, 1131.

Hart, D. N. J., Fuggle, S. V., Williams, K. A., Fabre, J. W., Ting, A. and Moms, P. J. (1981). *Transplantation* **31**, 428–433.

Hoffman-Fezer, G., Thierfelder, S., Rodt, H., Kummer, U., Doxiadis, I., Stunkel, K., Evlitz, M. (1981). *In* "Leukaemia Markers" (W. Knapp Ed.), p. 405. Academic Press, London and New York.

Horisberger, M. (1979). *Biol. Cellulaire* **36**, 253.

Hsu, S-M., Raine, L., Fanger, H. (1981). *Amer. J. clin. Path.* **75**, 734.

Isaacson, P. and Judd, M. A. (1978). *Cancer* **42**, 1554.

Janossy, G., Thomas, J. A., Bollum, F. J., Granger, S., Pizzolo, G., Bradstock, K. F., Wong, L., McMichael, A., Ganeshaguru, K. and Hoffrand, A. V. (1980). *J. Immunol.* **125**, 202.

Kitagawa, T., Fujitake, T., Taniyama, H. and Aikawa (1978). *J. Biochem.* L2, 326.

McMichael, A. J., Pilch, J. R., Galfre, G., Mason, D. Y., Fabre, J. W. and Milstein, C. (1979). *Eur. J. Immunol.* **9**, 205.

Mason, D. Y. and Taylor, C. R. (1975). *J. clin. Path.* **28**, 124.

Mason, D. Y. and Sammons, R. E. (1978). *J. clin. Path.* **31**, 454.

Mason, D. Y. and Biberfeld, P. (1980). *J. Histochem. Cytochem.* **28**, 731.

Mason, D. Y., Bell, J. I., Christensson, B. and Biberfeld, P. (1980). *Clin. exp. Immunol.* **40**, 235.

Mason, D. Y., Stein, H., Naiem, M. and Abdulaziz, Z. (1981a). *J. Cancer Res. Clin. Oncol.* **101**, 13.

Mason, D. Y., Cordell, J. L., Abdulaziz, Z., Naiem, M. and Bordenave, G. (1982). *J. Histochem. Cytochem.* (in press).

McKenzie, J. L. and Fabre, J. W. (1981). *J. Immunol.* **126**, 843–850.

Morton, J. A., Bastin, J., Fleming, K. A., McMichael, A. J., Burns, J. and McGee, J. O'D. (1981). *Gut* **22**, 1.

Naiem, M., Gerdes, J., Abdulaziz, Z., Nash, J. R. G., Stein, H., Mason, D. Y. (1981a) *In* "Leukaemia Markers" (W. Knapp, Ed.), p. 117. Academic Press, London and New York.

Naiem, M., Gerdes, J., Abdulaziz, Z., Sunderland, C. A., Allington, M. J., Stein, H. and Mason, D. Y. (1982). *J. Immunol. Meth.* (in press).

Nygren, H. and Hansson, H. A. (1981). *J. Histochem. Cytochem.* **29**, 266.

Omary, M. B., Trowbridge, I. S. and Minowada, J. (1980). *Nature* **286**, 888.

Pearse, A. G. E., Polak, J. M., Adams, S. C. and Kendall, P. A. (1974). *Histochem. J.* **6**, 347.

Pizzolo, G., Sloane, J., Beverley, P., Thomas, J. A., Bradstock, K. F., Mattingly, S. and Janossy, G. (1980). *Cancer* **46**, 2640.

Ponder, B. A. and Wilkinson, M. M. (1981). *J. Histochem. Cytochem.* **29**, 981.

Poppema, S., Elema, J. D., Halie, M. D. (1979). *Int. J. Cancer* **24**, 532.

Poppema, S., Bhan, A. K., Reinherz, E. L., McClusky, R. T., Schlossman, S. F. (1981). *J. exp. Med.* **153**, 30.

Sloane, J. P., Ormerod, M. G., Imrie, S. and Coombes, R. C. (1980). *Brit. J. Cancer* **42**, 392.

Stein, H., Mason, D. Y., Gerdes, J., Ziegler, A., Naiem, M., Wernet, P. and Lennert, K. (1981). *In* "Leukaemia Markers" (W. Knapp, Ed.), p. 99. Academic Press, London and New York.

Stein, H., Bonk, A., Tolksdorf, G., Lennert, K., Rodt, H. and Gerdes, J. (1980). *J. Histochem. Cytochem.* **28**, 746.

Stenman, S. and Vaheri, A. (1981). *Int. J. Cancer* **27**, 427.

Sternberger, L. A. (1979). *J. Histochem. Cytochem.* **27**, 1657.

Sunderland, C. A., Redman, C. W. G., and Stirrat, G. M. (1981). *Immunology* **43**, 541.

Warnke, R. and Levy, R. (1980). *J. Histochem. Cytochem.* **28**, 771.

Warnke, R., Miller, R., Grogan, T., Pederson, M., Dilley, J. and Levy R. (1980). *New Engl. J. Med.* **303**, 293.

Wilson, M. B. and Nakane, P. K. (1978). *In* "Immunofluorescence and Related Staining Techniques" (W. Knapp, K. Holubar and G. Wick, Eds), pp. 215–224. Elsevier/North Holland, Amsterdam.

Wood, G. S., Warnke, R. (1981). *J. Histochem. Cytochem.* **29**, 1196.

# Appendix A: Monoclonal antibodies described

| Name of antibody | Specificity | Page reference |
|---|---|---|
| Unnamed | Blood group A | 246 |
| Unnamed | Blood group B | 246 |
| Unnamed | Alkaline phosphatase | 596 |
| Unnamed | Thy1.2 | 182, 185, 193, 195 |
| Unnamed | Immunoglobulin δ chain | 194, 195 |
| Unnamed | Thy1.1 | 180, 181, 187, 191, 193, 194 |
| 1C5 | Cardiac myosin | 488, 489 |
| 1E6 | Cardiac myosin | 487 |
| 1/6A | Erythrocyte | 132, 144 |
| 1.1 | HLA-DR | 352, 353 |
| 10G3 | Plasmodium gallinaceum | 325 |
| 10.2 | T lymphocyte (PAN) | 42, 84 |
| 11C7 | Plasmodium gallinaceum | 325 |
| 12E7 | X-Chromosome antigen | 42, 373–377 |
| 13CT1 | Plasmodium knowlesi | 323 |
| 16F8 | Plasmodium knowlesi | 323 |
| 17.5 | HLA-DR 4, 5, 7 | 352 |
| 110 | Influenza haemagglutinin | 266, 267 |
| 1083-17-1A | Colorectal carcinoma | 185 |
| 2D1 | Leucocytes | 622, 623 |
| 22 | Influenza haemagglutinin | 266 |
| 25.1 | Plasmodium yoelii | 321 |
| 25.23 | Plasmodium yoelii | 321 |
| 25.27 | Plasmodium yoelii | 321 |
| 25.54 | Plasmodium yoelii | 321 |
| 25.77 | Plasmodium yoelii | 321 |
| 289 | Cardiac myosin | 488, 489, 490 |
| 3A1 | T Lymphocyte | 42 |
| 4F10 | Cardiac myosin | 488, 489 |

| | | |
|---|---|---|
| 53B3 | Plasmodium knowlesi | 323 |
| 602–29 | MIC3 | 373 |
| 70 | Influenza haemagglutinin | 266 |
| 8w1247 | HLA-DR3, 5, 6 | 352 |
| 9.6 | T Lymphocyte (PAN) | 42, 84, 140 |
| A2B5 | Neuroblastoma | 188 |
| A50 | T Lymphocyte (PAN) | 84 |
| Ab89 | B-CLL, Non Hodgkin lymphoma | 159 |
| AN51 | Platelet (megakaryocyte) | 132, 144, 148, 149, 218–222, 224, 225, 230 |
| Anti-JMB1 | Mallory body | 434–438, 443, 447 |
| Anti-JMB2 | Mallory body, intermediate filaments | 434–441, 443–445, 631, 633 |
| Anti-JMB3 | Hepatic mesenchymal cells | 445 |
| Anti-$\kappa$ | Immunoglobulin $\kappa$ chain | 633 |
| Anti-$\mu$ | Immunoglobulin $\mu$ chain | 633 |
| ATM1 | T Lymphocyte (PAN) | 94 |
| ATM2 | T Lymphocyte (PAN) | 94 |
| B-1 | B Lymphocyte | 102 |
| B-2 | B Lymphocyte | 102 |
| B3/25 | Transferrin receptor | 153, 154 |
| BA-1 | B Lymphocyte | 50, 132 |
| BA-2 | Leukaemia (CALL) | 132, 142, 144, 145, 146 |
| BB5 | $\beta$2 Microglobulin | 132 |
| BB7.1 | HLA B7 | 346 |
| BB7.5 | HLA-ABC | 344 |
| BB7.7 | HLA-ABC | 132 |
| BBM1 | $\beta$2 Microglobulin | 344, 373 |
| BK19.9 | Proliferation antigen | 621, 633 |
| C13(L) | Influenza haemagglutinin | 260 |
| Ca1(N) | Influenza haemagglutinin | 260 |
| Ca10(T) | Influenza haemagglutinin | 260 |
| Ca4(D) | Influenza haemagglutinin | 260 |
| Cb5(R) | Influenza haemagglutinin | 260 |
| Ca6(S) | Influenza haemagglutinin | 260 |
| Cb14 | Influenza haemagglutinin | 260 |
| CR3-43 | HLA-DR | 461 |
| DA2 | HLA-DR | 132, 144, 145, 158, 352 |
| Dig25–54 | Digoxin | 482, 484, 486 |
| Dig26–10 | Digoxin | 482–484, 486 |
| Dig26–20 | Digoxin | 482, 484 |
| Dig26–30 | Digoxin | 482, 484 |

| Leu3 | T Lymphocyte, inducer | 83 |
|---|---|---|
| Leu3a | T Lymphocyte, inducer | 569, 572, 573 |
| | | 577, 578 |
| Leu4 | T Lymphocyte (PAN) | 83, 84 |
| Leu5 | T Lymphocyte (PAN) | 84 |
| M1/N1 | Granulocytes | 132, 157 |
| MA2.1 | HLA A2, B17 | 346 |
| MA28.1 | HLA A2, A28 | 346 |
| MB40.2 | HLA B7, B40 | 346 |
| MB40.3 | HLA B7, B40 | 346 |
| MBG6 | T Lymphocyte (PAN) | 83, 84, 88 |
| ME1 | HLA B27, B7, B22 | 346 |
| MHM.8 | Epithelium | 607, 633 |
| MRCOX3 | HLA-DR1, 2, 6 | 351–353 |
| MRCOX8 | T Lymphocyte, suppressor-cytotoxic rat | 188 |
| NA1/34 | Thymocytes | 42, 83, 85, 132, 140, 144, 156, 158, 179, 615 |
| NC1/34 | Substance P | 415, 416, 417, 419, 425 |
| NDOG1 | Syncytiotrophoblast | 459, 460, 462, 463, 469, 472, 603, 633 |
| NDOG2 | Syncytiotrophoblast | 459, 460, 462, 463, 469, 472 |
| NFK3 | HLA-DR2 | 352, 353 |
| OKI | HLA-DR | 42, 43, 48–50, 52, 132, 144, 145 |
| OKM1 | Monocyte-granulocyte | 42, 43, 132, 144, 155, 158 |
| OKT1 | T Lymphocyte (PAN) | 42, 43, 46, 64, 82–86, 93, 97, 132, 138, 140, 141, 144, 150, 151, 152, 156, 570, 571, 573 |
| OKT3 | T Lymphocyte (PAN) | 42, 43, 46, 47, 48, 53, 59, 60, 64, 78, 82–86, 88–92, 94, 95, 99, 100, 132, 136, 138, 141, 142, 144, 151, 156, 188, 570 |

| | | |
|---|---|---|
| OKT4 | T Lymphocyte, inducer | 42–64, 82, 83, 85, 86, 92, 94, 95, 132, 136, 138, 140, 141, 142, 144, 150, 151, 152, 156, 188, 573 |
| OKT5 | T Lymphocyte, suppressor-cytotoxic | 42, 43, 46, 56, 57, 82, 83, 85, 151, 156, 188 |
| OKT6 | Thymocyte | 42, 43, 47, 83, 85, 132, 136, 138, 140, 141, 142, 144, 156, 615 |
| OKT8 | T Lymphocyte, suppressor-cytotoxic | 42–64, 82, 83, 85, 86, 98, 132, 136, 138, 140, 141, 142, 144, 150, 151, 156, 570, 573, 579 |
| OKT9 | Transferrin receptor | 42, 43, 49, 50, 132, 138, 141, 144, 145, 146, 150–156, 373, 379, 380, 381 |
| OKT10 | Haemopoietic (PAN) | 42, 43, 46, 47, 49, 50, 53, 132, 136, 138, 141, 144, 151, 156 |
| OKT11 | T Lymphocyte (PAN) | 42, 46, 47, 50, 64, 82, 83, 85–88, 90, 94, 98, 132, 140, 142, 144, 151, 152, 156 |
| OKT11A | T Lymphocyte (PAN) | 43, 82, 84, 88, 90, 91, 99, 101, 132, 138, 140, 142, 144, 156 |
| P1153-3 | B Lymphocyte, neural | 132 |
| P17F12 | T Lymphocyte (PAN) | 140 |
| P6/38 | Peroxidase | 593, 594 |
| PA2.1 | HLA A2 | 346 |
| PA2.6 | HLA-ABC | 354, 448, 449, 451 |
| R1 | X-Linked antigen | 385, 387 |
| R1.3 | Erythrocyte | 240, 241, 245 |

| | | |
|---|---|---|
| R10 (LCR-LON) | Erythrocyte, glycophorin | 132, 144, 148, 149, 240, 241, 246 |
| R18 | Erythrocyte | 240, 241, 244, 246 |
| R2 | Erythrocyte | 240 |
| R20.16 | Erythrocyte | 240, 244, 245 |
| R23 | Erythrocyte | 240, 241 |
| R6A | Erythrocyte | 240, 244, 246 |
| R7 | Erythrocyte | 240, 246 |
| Sa4(P) | Influenza haemagglutinin | 260 |
| Sa6(K) | Influenza haemagglutinin | 260 |
| Sal(C) | Influenza haemagglutinin | 260 |
| Sb6(E) | Influenza haemagglutinin | 260 |
| Sb7(B) | Influenza haemagglutinin | 260 |
| SK1 | T Lymphocyte | 42 |
| SK2 | T Lymphocyte | 42 |
| SK3 | T Lymphocyte | 42 |
| SK4 | T Lymphocyte | 42 |
| SK5 | T Lymphocyte | 42 |
| T101 | T Lymphocyte (PAN) | 42, 83, 84, 132, 140 |
| Tab | Platelet | 231 |
| Tac | T Lymphocytes (activated) | 45 |
| TB23 | Mycobacterium tuberculosis | 304, 305, 306 |
| TB68 | Mycobacterium tuberculosis | 304, 306 |
| TB71 | Mycobacterium tuberculosis | 304, 306 |
| TB72 | Mycobacterium tuberculosis | 304, 306 |
| TB73 | Mycobacteria | 304, 306, 308 |
| TB77 | Mycobacterium bovis | 304 |
| TB78 | Mycobacterium bovis | 304, 306 |
| TG-1 | Granulocytes | 132, 575, 576 |
| Tu-1 | Lymphoma (BCLL, NHL) | 102 |
| UCHT1 | T Lymphocyte (PAN) | 42, 83, 84, 132, 156, 560, 561, 565, 570–573, 577 |
| UCHT2 | T Lymphocyte (PAN) | 132, 140, 572 |
| UCHT3 | T Lymphocyte (PAN) | 132, 140, 573 |
| VIL-A1 | Leukaemia (CALL) | 101 |
| W18 | Influenza haemagglutinin | 266 |
| W3/25 | T Lymphocyte inducer (RAT) | 188, 195 |
| W6/32 | HLA-ABC | 132, 144, 344, 373, 448, 449, 461 |

# Appendix B: Specificities of monoclonal antibodies described

| Name of antibody | Specificity | Page reference |
|---|---|---|
| Unnamed | Alkaline phosphatase | 596 |
| B-1 | B Lymphocyte | 102 |
| B-2 | B Lymphocyte | 102 |
| BA-1 | B Lymphocyte | 50, 132 |
| FMC1 | B Lymphocyte | 102, 132 |
| FMC7 | B Lymphocyte subset | 132, 159 |
| P1153-3 | B Lymphocyte, neural | 132 |
| Ab89 | B-CLL, Non Hodgkin lymphoma | 159 |
| BB5 | $\beta 2$ Microglobulin | 132 |
| BBM1 | $\beta 2$ Microglobulin | 344, 373 |
| EC3 | $\beta 2$ Microglobulin | 132 |
| Unnamed | Blood group A | 246 |
| Unnamed | Blood group B | 246 |
| F15-135-1 | Brain | 405, 407 |
| F3-87-8 | Brain | 400, 403, 404, 405, 407, 533 |
| 1C5 | Cardiac myosin | 488, 489 |
| 1E6 | Cardiac myosin | 487 |
| 2B9 | Cardiac myosin | 488, 489, 490 |
| IE6 | Cardiac myosin | 487 |
| 4F10 | Cardiac myosin | 488, 489 |
| W6/34 | Chromosome 11 marker | 373, 375, 388, 389 |
| 1083-17-1A | Colorectal carcinoma | 185 |
| WM1 | Complement C3 | 382, 384, 385 |
| Dig26-10 | Digoxin | 482–484, 486 |
| Dig26-20 | Digoxin | 482, 484 |
| Dig25-54 | Digoxin | 482, 484, 486 |
| Dig26-30 | Digoxin | 482, 484 |
| Dig35-20 | Digoxin | 482, 484 |

| | | |
|---|---|---|
| Dig26-40 | Digoxin | 482, 484 |
| EGFR1 | Epithelial growth factor receptor | 373, 379, 380, 386 |
| MHM.8 | Epithelium | 607, 633 |
| 1/6A | Erythrocyte | 132, 144 |
| R1.3 | Erythrocyte | 240, 241, 245 |
| R2 | Erythrocyte | 240 |
| R6A | Erythrocyte | 240, 244, 246 |
| R18 | Erythrocyte | 240, 241, 244, 246 |
| R23 | Erythrocyte | 240, 241 |
| R20.16 | Erythrocyte | 240, 244, 245 |
| R7 | Erythrocyte | 240, 246 |
| R10(LCR–LON) | Erythrocyte, glycophorin | 132, 144, 148, 149, 240, 241, 246 |
| M1/N1 | Granulocytes | 132, 157 |
| TG-1 | Granulocytes | 132, 575, 576 |
| HLe-1 | Haemopoietic (PAN) | 132, 575, 576 |
| OKT10 | Haemopoietic (PAN) | 42, 43, 46, 47, 49, 50, 53, 132, 136, 138, 141, 144, 151, 156 |
| Anti-JMB3 | Hepatic mesenchymal cells | 445 |
| FMC5 | HLA A2 | 346 |
| PA2.1 | HLA A2 | 346 |
| MA28.1 | HLA A2, A28 | 346 |
| MA2.1 | HLA A2, B17 | 346 |
| ME1 | HLA B27, B7, B22 | 346 |
| BB7.1 | HLA B7 | 346 |
| MB40.2 | HLA B7, B40 | 346 |
| MB40.3 | HLA B7, B40 | 346 |
| BB7.5 | HLA-ABC | 344 |
| BB7.7 | HLA-ABC | 132 |
| PA2.6 | HLA-ABC | 354, 448, 449, 451 |
| W6/32 | HLA-ABC | 132, 144, 344, 373, 448, 449, 461 |
| 1.1 | HLA-DR | 352, 353 |
| CR3-43 | HLA-DR | 461 |
| DA2 | HLA-DR | 132, 144, 145, 158, 352 |
| GENOX 3.32 | HLA-DR | 352, 353 |
| OKI | HLA-DR | 42, 43, 48–50, 52, 132, 144, 145 |
| 17.5 | HLA-DR 4, 5, 7 | 352 |

| | | |
|---|---|---|
| GENOX 3.53 | HLA-DR1, 2, 6 | 352 |
| MRCOX3 | HLA-DR1, 2, 6 | 351–353 |
| NFK3 | HLA-DR2 | 352, 353 |
| 8w1247 | HLA-DR3, 5, 6 | 352 |
| FMC2 | HLA-DR4 | 352 |
| Unnamed | Immunoglobulin $\delta$ | 194, 195 |
| Anti-$\kappa$ | Immunoglobulin $\kappa$ chain | 633 |
| Anti-$\mu$ | Immunoglobulin $\mu$ chain | 633 |
| 22 | Influenza haemagglutinin | 266 |
| 70 | Influenza haemagglutinin | 266 |
| 110 | Influenza haemagglutinin | 266, 267 |
| Ca1(N) | Influenza haemagglutinin | 260 |
| C13(L) | Influenza haemagglutinin | 260 |
| Ca4(D) | Influenza haemagglutinin | 260 |
| Ca6(S) | Influenza haemagglutinin | 260 |
| Ca10(T) | Influenza haemagglutinin | 260 |
| Cb5(R) | Influenza haemagglutinin | 260 |
| Cb14 | Influenza haemagglutinin | 260 |
| H2-4B3 | Influenza haemagglutinin | 257, 261, 263 |
| H2-4C2 | Influenza haemagglutinin | 261, 263 |
| H2-6C4 | Influenza haemagglutinin | 261, 263 |
| H9-D3 | Influenza haemagglutinin | 257 |
| H35-C7-2 | Influenza haemagglutinin | 272 |
| H35-C10-2 | Influenza haemagglutinin | 272 |
| H36-55-4 | Influenza haemagglutinin | 272 |
| H36-18-2 | Influenza haemagglutinin | 272 |
| Sa4(P) | Influenza haemagglutinin | 260 |
| Sa6(K) | Influenza haemagglutinin | 260 |
| Sa1(C) | Influenza haemagglutinin | 260 |
| Sb6(E) | Influenza haemagglutinin | 260 |
| Sb7(B) | Influenza haemagglutinin | 260 |
| W18 | Influenza haemagglutinin | 266 |
| 2D1 | Leucocytes | 622, 623 |
| F8-11-13 | Leucocyte | 622, 633 |
| F10-89-4 | Leucocyte common | 622, 633 |
| BA-2 | Leukaemia (CALL) | 132, 142, 144, 145, 146 |
| J-5 | Leukaemia (CALL) | 93, 101, 132, 133, 139, 141, 143, 144, 145, 158, 188 |
| VIL-A1 | Leukaemia (CALL) | 101 |
| F10-44-2 | Lymphocyte (MIC4) | 405, 407, 529 |
| Tu-1 | Lymphoma (BCLL, NHL) | 102 |
| Anti-JMB1 | Mallory body | 434–438, 443, 447 |

| | | |
|---|---|---|
| SK5 | T Lymphocyte | 42 |
| SK4 | T Lymphocyte | 42 |
| SK2 | T Lymphocyte | 42 |
| SK1 | T Lymphocyte | 42 |
| SK3 | T Lymphocyte | 42 |
| 9.6 | T Lymphocyte (PAN) | 42, 84, 140 |
| 10.2 | T Lymphocyte (PAN) | 42, 84 |
| A50 | T Lymphocyte (PAN) | 84 |
| ATM1 | T Lymphocyte (PAN) | 94 |
| ATM2 | T Lymphocyte (PAN) | 94 |
| Leu5 | T Lymphocyte (PAN) | 84 |
| HuLyt2 | T Lymphocyte (PAN) | 83 |
| HuLyt3 | T Lymphocyte (PAN) | 83 |
| L17 | T Lymphocyte (PAN) | 84 |
| Leu1 | T Lymphocyte (PAN) | 83, 84 |
| Leu4 | T Lymphocyte (PAN) | 83, 84 |
| L17F12 | T Lymphocyte (PAN) | 42, 83, 91, 93, 97, 132, 144, 156 |
| OKT1 | T Lymphocyte (PAN) | 42, 43, 46, 64, 82–86, 93, 97, 132, 138, 140, 141, 144, 150, 151, 152, 156, 570, 571, 573 |
| MBG6 | T Lymphocyte (PAN) | 83, 84, 88 |
| OKT3 | T Lymphocyte (PAN) | 42, 43, 46, 47, 48, 53, 59, 60, 64, 78, 82–86, 88–92, 94, 95, 99, 100, 132, 136, 138, 141, 142, 144, 151, 156, 188, 570 |
| OKT11 | T Lymphocyte (PAN) | 42, 46, 47, 50, 64, 82, 83, 85–88, 90, 94, 98, 132, 140, 142, 144, 151, 152, 156 |
| OKT11A | T Lymphocyte (PAN) | 43, 82, 84, 88, 90, 91, 99, 101, 132, 138, 140, 142, 144, 156 |
| P17F12 | T Lymphocyte (PAN) | 140 |
| T101 | T Lymphocyte (PAN) | 42, 83, 84, 132, 140 |

| UCHT1 | T Lymphocyte (PAN) | 42, 83, 84, 132, 156, 560, 561, 565, 570–573, 577 |
|---|---|---|
| UCHT3 | T Lymphocyte (PAN) | 132, 140, 573 |
| UCHT2 | T Lymphocyte (PAN) | 132, 140, 572 |
| LEU3A | T Lymphocyte, inducer | 569, 572, 573, 577, 578 |
| LEU3 | T Lymphocyte, inducer | 83 |
| OKT4 | T Lymphocyte, inducer | 42–64, 82, 83, 85, 86, 92, 94, 95, 132, 136, 138, 140, 141, 142, 144, 150, 151, 152, 156, 188, 573 |
| W3/25 | T Lymphocyte, inducer (RAT) | 188, 195 |
| MRCOX8 | T Lymphocyte, suppressor-cytotoxic | 188 |
| Leu2 | T Lymphocyte, suppressor-cytotoxic | 83, 85, 569, 572, 573, 578 |
| OKT5 | T Lymphocyte, suppressor-cytotoxic | 42, 43, 46, 56, 57, 82, 83, 85, 151, 156, 188 |
| OKT8 | T Lymphocyte, suppressor-cytotoxic | 42–64, 82, 83, 85, 86, 98, 132, 136, 138, 140, 141, 142, 144, 150, 151, 156, 570, 573, 579 |
| Tac | T Lymphocytes (activated) | 45 |
| F15-42-1 | THY-1 | 403, 404, 407, 615, 633 |
| Unnamed | THY1.1 | 180, 181, 187, 191, 193, 194 |
| Unnamed | THY1.2 | 182, 185, 193, 195 |
| OKT6 | Thymocyte | 42, 43, 47, 83, 85, 132, 136, 138, 140, 141, 142, 144, 156, 615 |
| NA1/34 | Thymocyte | 42, 83, 85, 132, 140, 144, 156, 158, 179, 615 |
| B3/25 | Transferrin receptor | 153, 154 |

| OKT9 | Transferrin receptor | 42, 43, 49, 50, 132, 138, 141, 144, 145, 146, 150–156, 373, 379, 380, 381 |
| 12E7 | X-Chromosome antigen | 42, 373–377 |
| R1 | X-Linked antigen | 385, 387 |

# Index